Clinical En Face OCT Atlas

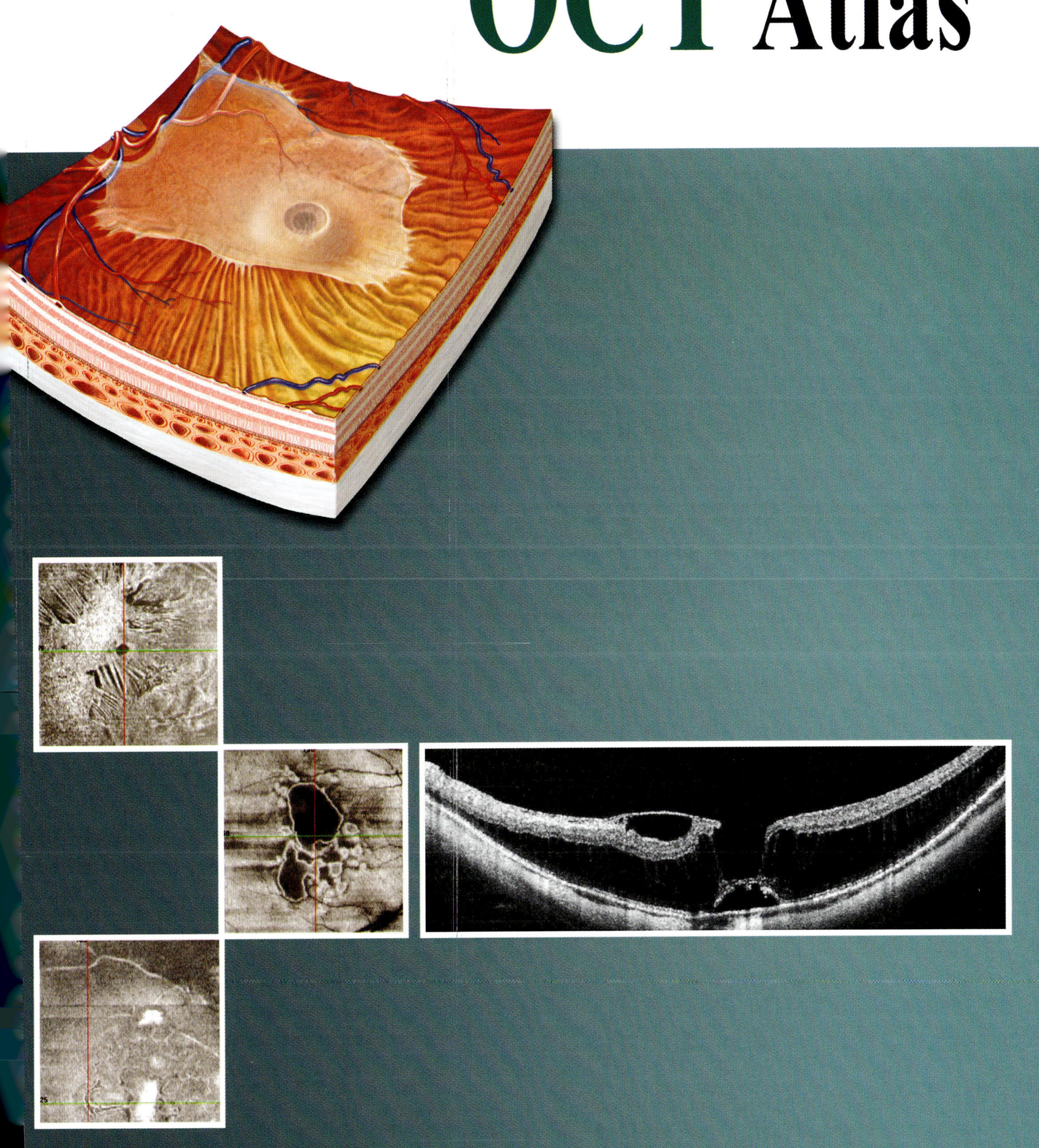

Clinical En Face OCT Atlas

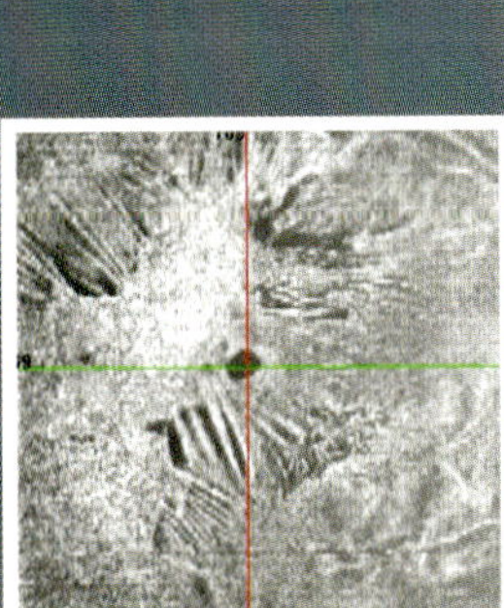

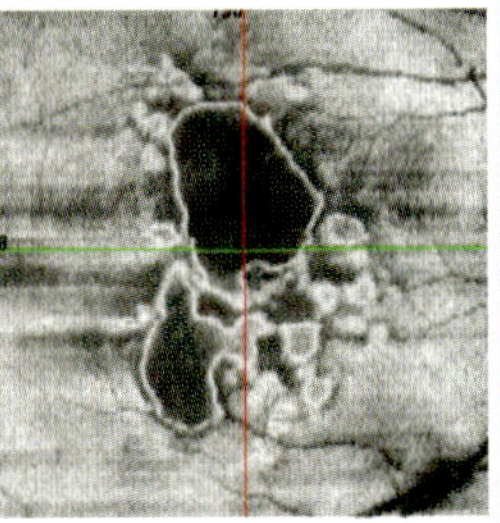

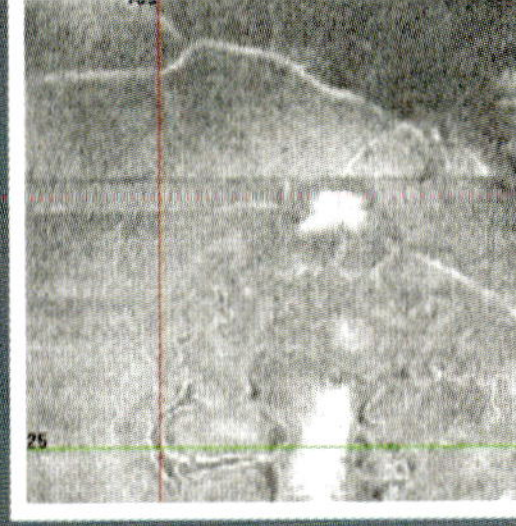

Editors

Bruno Lumbroso MD
Former Head of Department and Director
Rome Eye Hospital
Director, Centro Oftalmologico Mediterraneo
for Retinal Diseases, Rome, Italy

David Huang MD PhD
Professor of Ophthalmology
Casey Eye Institute
Oregon Health & Science University
Portland, USA

Andre Romano MD
Department of Ophthalmology
Federal University of Sao Paulo
Voluntary Adjunct Professor, University of Miami
Miller School of Medicine, and
Director, Neovista Eye Center
Americana, Brazil

Marco Rispoli MD
Ophthalmology Department
Ospedale Nuovo Regina Margherita, and
Centro Oftalmologico Mediterraneo for Retinal Diseases
Rome, Italy

Gabriel Coscas MD
Professor of Ophthalmology
Hôpital Intercommunal de Créteil
Service d'Ophtalmologie, France

Foreword

James G Fujimoto

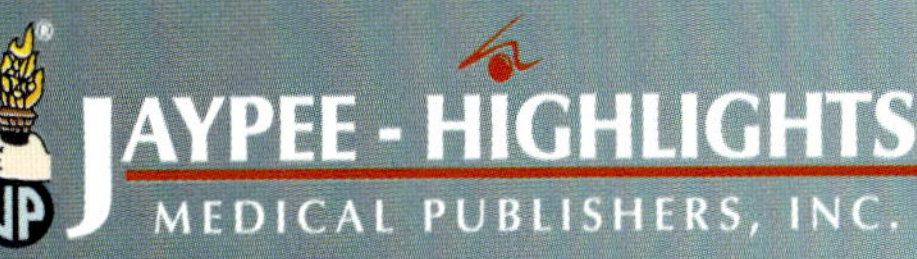

JAYPEE - HIGHLIGHTS
MEDICAL PUBLISHERS, INC.

New Delhi • London • Philadelphia • Panama

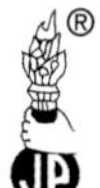

Jaypee Brothers Medical Publishers (P) Ltd

Headquarters

Jaypee Brothers Medical Publishers (P) Ltd
4838/24, Ansari Road, Daryaganj
New Delhi 110 002, India
Phone: +91-11-43574357
Fax: +91-11-43574314
Email: jaypee@jaypeebrothers.com

Overseas Offices

J.P. Medical Ltd.,
83 Victoria Street London
SW1H 0HW (UK)
Phone: +44-2031708910
Fax: +02-03-0086180
Email: info@jpmedpub.com

Jaypee-Highlights Medical Publishers Inc.
City of Knowledge, Bld. 237, Clayton
Panama City, Panama
Phone: +507-301-0496
Fax: +507-301-0499
Email: cservice@jphmedical.com

Jaypee Brothers Medical Publishers, Ltd
The Bourse
111 South Independence Mall East
Suite 835, Philadelphia, PA 19106, USA
Phone: + 267-519-9789
Email: joe.rusko@jaypeebrothers.com

Jaypee Brothers Medical Publishers (P) Ltd
17/1-B Babar Road, Block-B, Shaymali
Mohammadpur, Dhaka-1207
Bangladesh
Mobile: +08801912003485
Email: jaypeedhaka@gmail.com

Jaypee Brothers Medical Publishers (P) Ltd
Shorakhute, Kathmandu
Nepal
Phone: +00977-9841528578
Email: jaypee.nepal@gmail.com

Website: www.jaypeebrothers.com
Website: www.jaypeedigital.com

Clinical En Face OCT Atlas

First Edition : **2013**

ISBN: 978-93-5090-296-7

Printed at: Ajanta Offset & Packagings Ltd., New Delhi

Foreword

The *Clinical En Face OCT Atlas* is a bold and innovative step forward in the diagnosis and management of ocular disease. The pioneering efforts of the editors, Professors Bruno Lumbroso, David Huang, Andre Romano, Marco Rispoli and Gabriel Coscas, have made possible this publication, bringing together contributions from the world's leading clinicians and researchers in the field of ophthalmology and optical coherence tomography. En face OCT is an important new methodology which will play a key role in the clinical ophthalmological examination of ocular disease in the near future.

Recent advances in OCT technology have dramatically increased imaging speeds and now enable high density, three-dimensional volumetric OCT data sets to be acquired in clinical ophthalmic practice. Access to this three-dimensional OCT data provides comprehensive information on retinal pathology, but presents clinical challenges in order to rapidly and decisively interpret this large amount of data.

This clinical atlas is the first of its kind, presenting new examination and diagnostic protocols for interpreting OCT imaging based on en face visualization. Organized into three main parts, this text covers the technology and interpretation of en face OCT images; presents an atlas of retinal pathologies to guide clinical interpretation and diagnosis; and surveys future developments in en face OCT. The en face OCT paradigm presented in this atlas represents a powerful and elegant approach which connects three-dimensional volumetric OCT to classic methods of ophthalmic imaging built on en face views of the retinal fundus. It promises to be a landmark reference for clinical ophthalmology practice as well as research.

James G Fujimoto PhD
Elihu Thomson Professor of Electrical Engineering
and Computer Science
Massachusetts Institute of Technology
USA

Contributors

Massimo Accorinti MD PhD
Uveitis Department
La Sapienza University of Rome, Italy

Micol Alkabes MD
San Giuseppe Hospital
University Eye Clinic, Milan, Italy
IMO (Instituto de Microcirugia Ocular)
Barcelona, Spain

Camilla Alovisi MD
Department of Clinical Physiopathology
Eye Clinic, University of Torino, Italy

Chrysanthi Basdekidou MD
Professor Sahel Department
Rothschild Ophthalmologie Fondation
Paris, France

Rubens Belfort Jr. MD
Department of Ophthalmology
Hospital São Paulo
Federal University of São Paulo, Brazil
Member Academia Ophthalmologica Internationalis

Rubens N Belfort MD
Department of Ophthalmology
Hospital São Paulo
Federal University of São Paulo, Brazil

Bernardo Cavalcanti MD
Post-doctoral Research Fellow
Cornea and Refractive Surgery Service
Massachusetts Eye and Ear Infirmary
Harvard Medical School, Boston, USA

Gilda Cennamo MD PhD
Eye Department
Federico II University
Naples, Italy

Salomon Y Cohen MD PhD
Centre Ophtalmologique
d'Imagerie et de Laser
Paris, France

Florence Coscas MD
Hôpital Intercommunal de Créteil
Service d'Ophtalmologie
Créteil, France

Gabriel Coscas MD
Professor of Ophthalmology
Hôpital Intercommunal de Créteil
Service d'Ophtalmologie
Créteil, France

Umberto De Benedetto MD
Hôpital Intercommunal de Créteil
Service d'Ophtalmologie
Créteil, France

Giuseppe de Crecchio MD
Eye Department
Federico II University
Naples, Italy

Luca Di Antonio MD PhD
Ophthalmology Clinic
Department of Medicine and
Science of Ageing, University of "G. d'Annunzio"
of Chieti-Pescara, Italy

Ali R Djalilian MD
Associate Professor of Ophthalmology
Director, Limbal Stem Cell Biology &
Ocular Surface Transplantation
Department of Ophthalmology and Visual Sciences
University of Illinois at Chicago, Chicago, IL, USA

Lise Dubois
Orthoptist and OCT Specialist
Centre Ophtalmologique d'Imagerie et de Laser
Paris, France

Jay S Duker MD
Director, New England Eye Center
Professor and Chair of Ophthalmology
Tufts Medical Center
Tufts University School of Medicine
Boston, MA 02111, USA

Chiara M Eandi MD PhD
Department of Clinical Physiopathology
Eye Clinic, University of Torino, Italy

Adil El Maftouhi OD
Centre Explore Vision, Paris, France
Centre Hospitalier
National Ophtalmologique des XV XX
Service du Pr C Baudouin, Paris, France

Edgar M Espana MD
Assistant Professor of Ophthalmology
Cornea Service, University of South Florida
Tampa, USA

Michel E Farah MD
Department of Ophthalmology
Hospital São Paulo
Federal University of São Paulo
Brazil

Amani A Fawzi MD
Associate Professor of Ophthalmology
Northwestern University
Chicago, USA

Raimondo Forte MD PhD
Eye Department
Federico II University
Naples, Italy

James G Fujimoto PhD PhD
Professor of Electrical Engineering and Computer Science
Department of Electrical Engineering and Research
Laboratory of Electronics
Massachusetts Institute of Technology
Cambridge, USA

Marta Gilardi MD
Uveitis Department
La Sapienza University of Rome, Italy

Kyioko Gocho MD PhD
Clinical Investigation Center 503
Quinze-Vingts Hospital and University Pierre et Marie
Curie-Paris 6, Paris, France

Giovanni Gregori PhD
Bascom Palmer Eye Institute
Miami, Florida, USA

Federico M Grignolo MD
Professor and Chairman
Department of Clinical Physiopathology
Eye Clinic, University of Torino, Italy

Amod Gupta MD
Professor and Head
Advanced Eye Centre
Postgraduate Institute of Medical Education and
Research, Chandigarh, India

Vishali Gupta MD
Senior Vitreo-Retina Consultant
King Khaled Eye Specialist Hospital, Riyadh, KSA
Additional Professor, Advanced Eye Centre
Postgraduate Institute of Medical Education and
Research, Chandigarh, India

Pedram Hamrah MD
Director
Ocular Surface Imaging Center
Henry Allen Cornea Scholar, Cornea
and Refractive Surgery Service
Massachusetts Eye & Ear Infirmary
Visiting Scientist, Immune Disease Institute
Assistant Professor, Department of Ophthalmology
Harvard Medical School, USA

Mark Hathaway PhD
Senior Scientist
Optos, Inc, University of Kent
Canterbury, UK

Joachim Hornegger
Pattern Recognition Lab and
Erlangen Graduate School in Advanced Optical
Technologies (SAOT)
Friedrich-Alexander-University Erlangen
Erlangen, Germany

David Huang MD PhD
Professor of Ophthalmology
Casey Eye Institute
Oregon Health & Science University
Portland, USA

Yali Jia
Casey Eye Institute
Oregon Health & Science University
Portland, USA

Chunhui Jiang MD
Associated Professor
Ophthalmology Department
Eye & ENT Hospital of Fudan University
Shanghai, China

Martin F Kraus MD
Department of Electrical Engineering and
Computer Science, and Research Laboratory of
Electronics, Massachusetts Institute of Technology
Cambridge, MA, USA
Pattern Recognition Lab and Erlangen Graduate School
in Advanced Optical Technologies (SAOT)
Friedrich-Alexander-University Erlangen
Erlangen, Germany

Jean-Francois Le Rouic MD
Clinique Sourdille
Nantes, France

Mathieu Lehmann MD
Professor Sahel Department
Rothschild Ophtalmologie Fondation
Rothschild, Paris, France

Bruno Lumbroso MD
Former Head of Department and
Director, Rome Eye Hospital
Director, Centro Oftalmologico Mediterraneo
for Retinal Diseases
Rome, Italy

André Maia MD
Department of Ophthalmology
Hospital São Paulo
Federal University of São Paulo
Brazil

Nadine Manasseh MD
Professor Sahel Department
Rothschild Ophtalmologie Fondation, Rothschild
Paris, France

John Marshall PhD FRCPath FRCOphth (Hon)
Frost Professor of Ophthalmology and
Chairman of the Academic Department of
Ophthalmology at Kings College
St. Thomas' Hospital, London, UK

Virginie Martinet MD
Professor Sahel Department
Rothschild Ophtalmologie Fondation
Rothschild, Paris, France

Leonardo Mastropasqua MD
Professor and Chairman Ophthalmology Clinic
Department of Medicine and Science of Ageing
University of "G. d'Annunzio" of Chieti-Pescara, Italy

Carlos Mateo MD
IMO (Instituto de Microcirugia Ocular)
Barcelona, Spain

Alexandre Matet MD
Professor Sahel Department
Rothschild Ophtalmologie Fondation
Paris, France

Martine Mauget-Faÿsse MD
Professor Sahel Department
Rothschild Ophtalmologie Fondation, Rothschild
Paris, France

Cinzia Mazzini MD
Professor of Ophthalmology
Ophthalmic Ultrasound and Ocular Oncology Service
Eye Clinic of the University of Florence, Italy

Nalin J Mehta MD
The Colorado Retina Center
Lakewood, Colorado, USA

Ugo Menchini MD
Professor and Chairman
The Eye Clinic of the University of Florence, Italy

Paolo Nucci MD
Professor of Ophthalmology
University of Milan
Chairman, Eye Clinic, San Giuseppe Hospital, Italy

Vanessa Pala MD
Epidemiologist
Centro Oftalmologico Mediterraneo
Rome, Italy

Michel Paques MD PhD
Clinical Investigation Center 503
Quinze-Vingts Hospital and
University Pierre et Marie Curie-Paris
Paris, France

Swapnil Parchand MD
Advanced Eye Centre
Postgraduate Institute of Medical Education
and Research, Chandigarh, India

Lucia Pelosini MRCOphth
Ophthalmology Fellow
Western Eye Hospital
Imperial College, London

Fernando M Penha MD
Department of Ophthalmology
Hospital São Paulo
Federal University of São Paulo
Brazil

Adrian Gh Podoleanu FInstP FOSA FSPIE
Professor of Biomedical Optics
Head of the Applied Optics Group
School of Physical Sciences
University of Kent
Canterbury, Kent, UK

Michel Puech MD
Centre Explore Vision
Paris, France

Maddalena Quaranta-El Maftouhi MD
Centre Rabelais
Lyon, France

Marco Rispoli MD
Ophthalmology Department
Ospedale Nuovo Regina Margherita, and
Centro Oftalmologico Mediterraneo
for Retinal Diseases
Rome, Italy

Andre Romano MD
Vitreo-Retinal Surgeon
Department of Ophthalmology
Federal University of Sao Paulo
Voluntary Adjunct Professor, University of Miami
Miller School of Medicine, and
Director, Neovista Eye Center, Americana, Brazil

Richard Rosen MD FACS FASRS
Professor and Vice-Chairman
Surgeon Director, Chief of Retinal Services
Director of Research, Department of Ophthalmology
NY Eye & Ear Infirmary
New York Medical College, USA

Philip J Rosenfeld MD PhD
Professor of Ophthalmology
Bascom Palmer Eye Institute
Miami, Florida, USA

SriniVas R Sadda MD
Associate Professor of Ophthalmology
Director, Medical Retina Unit
Ophthalmic Imaging Unit
Doheny Image Reading Center
Doheny Eye Institute, Keck School of Medicine
University of Southern California, USA

José-Alain Sahel MD PhD
Rothschild Ophtalmologie Fondation
Paris, France

Maria Cristina Savastano MD PhD
Catholic University School of Medicine
Rome, Italy

Andrea Sodi MD
Department of Ophthalmology
Eye Clinic University of Florence, Florence, Italy

Mahsa Sohrab MD
Ophthalmology Department
Northwestern University
Feinberg School of Medicine
Chicago, USA

Eric Souied MD PhD
Head of the Department of Ophthalmology
Hopital Intercommunal de Creteil and
Ophthalmology Department, "Henri Mondor"
Hospital, Creteil, Paris, France

Anderson Teixeira MD
Assistant Professor
Universidade Catolica de Brasilia
Department of Ophthalmology
Hospital São Paulo
Federal University of São Paulo, Brazil

Federico Tridico MD
Department of Clinical Physiopathology
Eye Clinic, University of Torino, Italy

Vivien Vasseur
Professor Sahel Department
Rothschild Ophtalmologie Fondation
Paris, France

Roberta Velletri MD
Department of Ophthalmology
Hospital São Paulo
Federal University of São Paulo
Brazil

Min Wang MD PhD
Associate Professor
Department of Ophthalmology
Eye and ENT Hospital of Fudan University
Shanghai, China

Jay Wei PhD
President & CEO
Optovue, Inc., Fremont
California, USA

Rishard Weitz
Senior Technical Advisor for Retinal Imaging
New York Eye and Ear Infirmary
USA

Benjamin Wolff MD
Professor Sahel Department
Rothschild Ophtalmologie Fondation
Paris, France

Gezhi Xu MD
Professor
Vice-President of Eye and ENT Hospital of
Fudan University
Vice-President of Shanghai EENT Hospital
Director of Retinal Department
Shanghai, China

Zohar Yehoshua MD
Bascom Palmer Eye Institute
900 NW 17th St. Miami, FL 33136

Sonia H Yoo MD
Professor of Ophthalmology
Bascom Palmer Eye Institute
University of Miami
Miller School of Medicine, USA

Qienyuan Zhou PhD
Vice-President/Clinical Development
Optovue, Inc.,
Fremont, California, USA

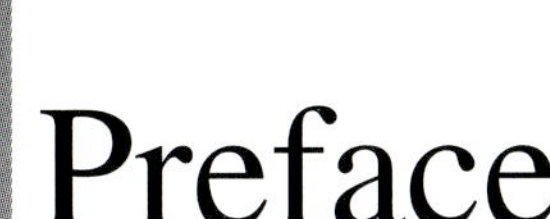

Preface

Current spectral domain optical coherence tomography (SD-OCT) devices already allow ophthalmologists to obtain good en face images of the retina and optic disk. En face OCT is no longer confined to a few retina specialists, but is widely available to all eye practitioners. As imaging speed and definition increases in the next generation of devices, the quality of en face views will further improve and their use will become even more important. All OCT users may get a different and new visualization of morphology, structure and topography of the eye. Everyday ophthalmologists will get an *in vivo* transverse layer-by-layer dissection of retina. This new way of seeing will help ophthalmologists localize and study lesions in individual layers of the retina.

The aim of the *Clinical En Face OCT Atlas* is to show everyday OCT users the utility of clinical en face imaging. The keyword is "clinical". We hope to develop interest in the use of en face OCT in everyday clinical work, and help users interpret en face OCT images. This Atlas should guide the general ophthalmologists to select the best en face views and read easily the typical and atypical aspects of en face images. Most OCT devices already have en face visualization capabilities. The use of these capabilities should be increased and applied to more types of pathologies.

This book is fortunate to have outstanding contributions from leaders in the field. The operating principles and the future of OCT are explained by some of the original developers of the technology. The retinal and macular diseases chapters are written by well-known authors from around the world.

We believe that en face imaging has practical clinical interest for everyday clinical ophthalmology. Our atlas addresses a vast audience and describes how to diagnose diseases and plan surgery for a variety of disorders. We hope that this atlas gives a timely answer to a widely felt clinical need.

Bruno Lumbroso
David Huang
Andre Romano
Marco Rispoli
Gabriel Coscas

Contents

PART III: Clinical *En Face* OCT Future Developments
Section 12: Future Developments in *En Face* Optical Coherence Tomography

PART I

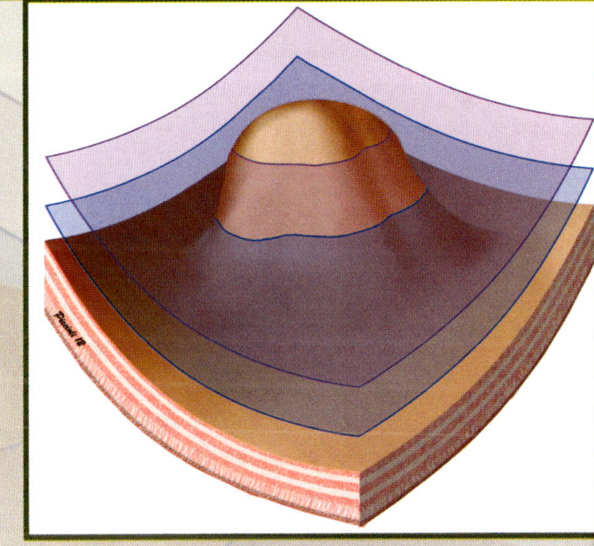

TECHNOLOGY
AND
INTERPRETATION

Section 1

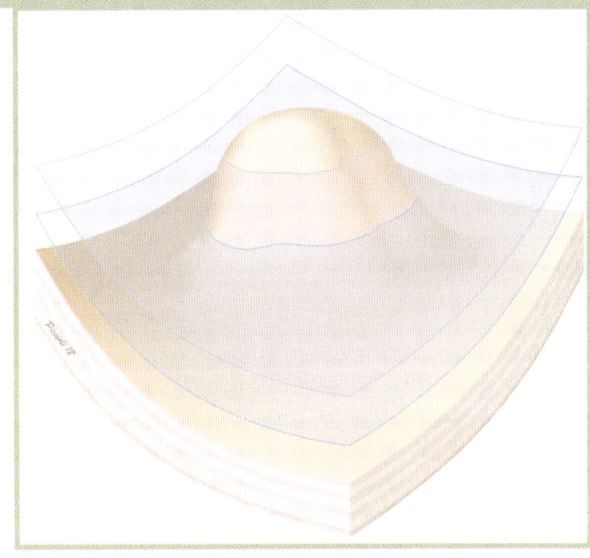

Methods and Techniques of *En Face* Optical Coherence Tomography Examination

Principles of *En Face* Optical Coherence Tomography: Real Time and Post-processing *En Face* Imaging in Ophthalmology

Adrian Gh Podoleanu

Introduction

The most natural view of inspecting the eye is the *en face*. Fundus cameras and scanning laser ophthalmoscopes present images of the retina oriented *en face*. The first optical coherence tomography (OCT) image of the retina was a cross section image obtained using time domain OCT (TD-OCT) and OCT technology progressed mainly along the direction of generating cross section images. The need to create an image of the fundus with *en face* orientation and axial resolution of OCT led to the development of *en face* OCT technology. Time domain OCT was initially used and this is still the only technology that can provide real time *en face* OCT images. Spectral OCT technology evolved along creating cross sections. In the last 5 years, the acquisition speed in spectral domain OCT (SD-OCT) reached line rates of MHz which reduced the time to acquire a significant three-dimensional (3D) volume to the time to produce a real time *en face* OCT image using the time domain technology. This has opened the avenue of generating *en face* images by post processing the volume of data captured, images which are now superior in density of pixels to the *en face* OCT images created by time domain OCT. The chapter presents succinctly the interplay of TD- and SD-OCT methods in shaping the *en face* OCT imaging employed today in ophthalmology.

Different Scanning Procedures

To obtain 3D information about the retina, any imaging system is equipped with three scanning means, one to scan the object in depth and two others to scan the object transversally.[1] Depending on the order these scanners are operated and on the scanning direction associated with the line displayed in the raster of the final image delivered, different possibilities exist. One-dimensional (1D) and two-dimensional (2D) scans are known. One-dimensional scans are labeled as A and T scans, while 2D scans are labeled as B and C scans and this terminology is explained below. Optical coherence tomography systems, using charge-coupled device (CCD) cameras, arrays of sensors or arrays of emitters eliminate the need of scanning the beam. However, the terminology below applies in such cases as well, where the ray scanning has been replaced by different forms of electronic scanning. The scanning terminology is illustrated in **Figure 1** and the utilization of the three scanners is described in **Figure 2**.

One Letter Terminology of Scanning (A, B, C and T)

A scan represents a reflectivity profile in depth. This scanning technology is used clinically for determining the eye length.

T scan represents the reflectivity profile obtained by scanning the beam transversally across the target.

B scan represents a cross section image, a (lateral X depth) map. This could be obtained by grouping T scans together from different depth values or A scans together for different lateral positions, both in use in the OCT practice. Historically, the first OCT image was a B scan image of the retina[2] made from A scans, using flying spot longitudinal OCT technology. B scan images, analogous to ultrasound B scan are generated by collecting many A scans **(Figure 1)** for different and adjacent transverse positions, as shown in **Figure 2(i)**. The lines in the raster generated correspond to A scans, i.e. the lines are oriented along the depth coordinate. The transverse scanner [operating along X or Y, or along the polar angle θ in polar coordinates in

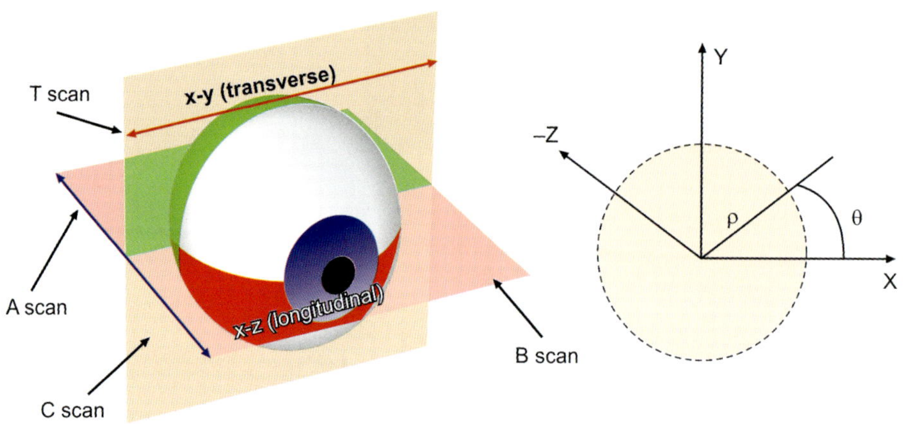

Figure 1: Relative orientation of the axial scan (A scan), transverse scan (T scan), longitudinal slice (B scan) and *en face* or transverse slice (C scan)

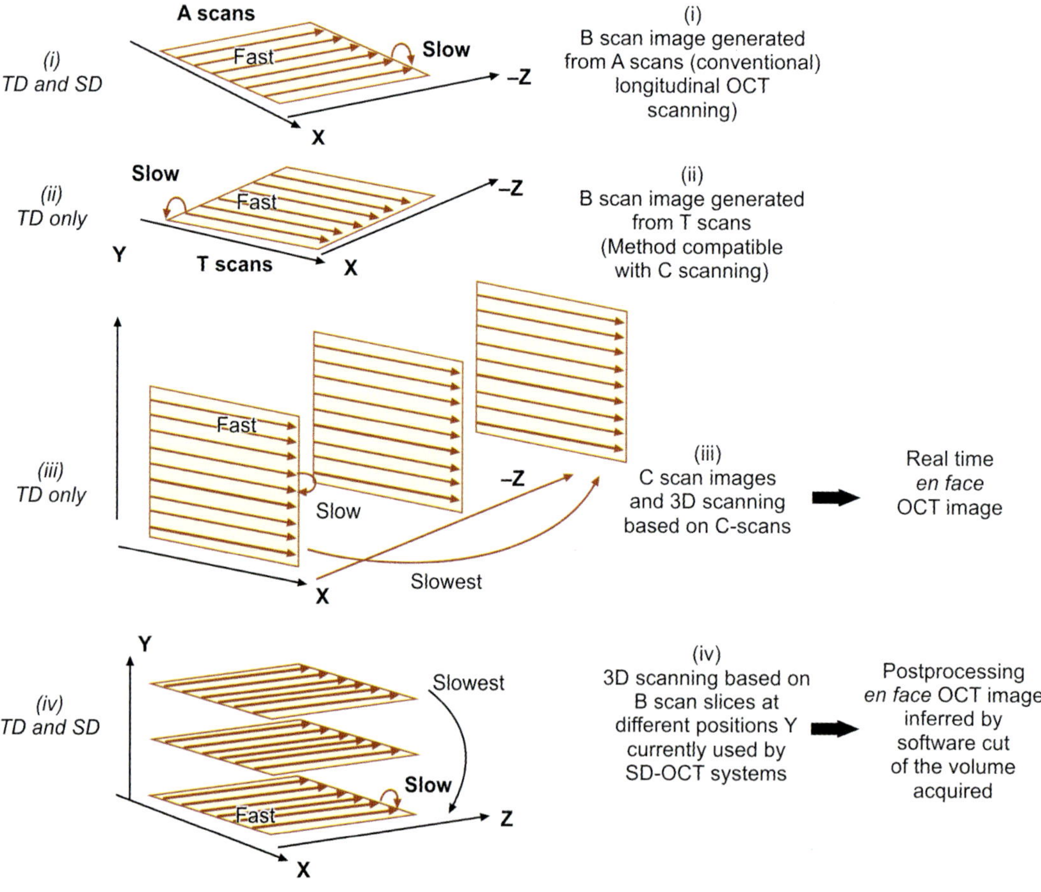

Figure 2: Different modes of operation of the three scanners in a three-dimensional (3D) imaging system and the two modalities of creating an *en face* image. Lateral scanning along the X and Y axes are implemented using an XY or two-dimensional (2D) transverse scanner. The 3D procedure in (iii) leads to a real time *en face* image. The 3D procedure in (iv) can lead to *en face* images by post processing only, after the whole volume was collected and software cuts are selected from such volumes
(*Abbreviations:* OCT: Optical coherence tomography; TD: Time domain; SD: Spectral domain)

Figure 1 (right), with X shown in **Figure 2(i)**] advances at a slower pace to build a B scan image. The majority of OCT reports in literature refer to this mode of operation.

C scan represents a raster image, with the same orientation as a TV image or image provided by microscopy, a (lateral × lateral) scanned map. Historically, the C scan has the native orientation for fundus cameras and scanning laser ophthalmoscopy (SLO) systems. C scans are provided by the flying spot *en face* OCT and the full field OCT. They can also be inferred post acquisition in longitudinal OCT, either time domain or spectral domain. C scans are made from many T scans along either of X, Y, ρ or θ coordinates, repeated for different values of the other transverse coordinate, Y, X, θ or ρ respectively in the transverse plane (with the most used case, oriented along the horizontal axis, X). The repetition of T scans along the other transverse coordinate is performed at a slower rate than that of the T scans **(Figure 2iii)**, which determines the frame rate. In this way, a complete raster is generated. For 3D imaging, several transversal slices are collected at different depths Z, either by advancing the optical path difference in the OCT in steps after each complete transverse (XY) or (ρ, θ) scan, or continuously at a much slower speed than the frame rate. The depth scanning is the slowest in this case.

Principles of Operation

There are two main OCT methods: TD-OCT and SD-OCT.[3] SD-OCT is attractive because it eliminates the need for depth scanning, which in case of TD-OCT is performed usually by mechanical means. Spectral domain methods can be implemented in two formats: (1) spectrometer based (SB) or (2) by using a tunable laser or a swept source (SS). Each method, SB-OCT or SS-OCT has its own merits and demerits. The depth resolution achieved depends on the bandwidth of the optical source in the TD-OCT and SB-OCT and on the tuning bandwidth in the SS-OCT.

Optical coherence tomography schematic diagrams implementing different OCT modalities are presented in **Figure 3(L and R)**. They consist of an optical source and a Michelson interferometer, where a *reference mirror* and an optical *splitter* are used to produce a reference beam.[4] *Interface optics* is employed to convey light from the *splitter* and from the *eye* to be examined to a *processing unit* that performs interference of light between the reference beam and the beam returned by the *object* (the eye), as well as processing of the interference signal and its analysis. The path traversed by the object wave from the splitter to the object and back represents the object path length (OPL). The path traversed by the reference wave from the *splitter* to the *reference mirror* and back represents the reference

path length (RPL). An optical path difference (OPD) in the interferometer is defined as, OPD = |OPL - RPL|.

Time Domain Optical Coherence Tomography

As shown in **Figure 3 (L and R)**, a TD-OCT setup uses a *broadband optical source* and the *processing unit* employs a *photodetector*. The principle of operation is based on partial coherence interferometry, where the *photodetector* senses variations in the interference result as long as the OPD is less than the coherence length of the *broadband source*, cl. Let us say that the *retina* is made from a structure of layers at different depths. Each layer returns a replica of the incoming wave train, delayed correspondingly. By scanning the RPL through moving the *reference mirror*, the layer satisfying the coherence gate condition, OPD < cl, can be selected. The layer selected is that wherein the back-scattered wave train is matched temporally by the reference wave train. Maxima of interference are obtained for each scattering point in depth that satisfies the condition OPD = 0. So far, such a configuration is that of a low coherence interferometer widely used in sensing. OCT was invented by adding a transversal scanner to the object arm of a low coherence interferometer to scan the beam laterally over the object.[2] By collecting adjacent A scans for successive pixels along a transversal coordinate, a B scan image is obtained. This imaging method has become what is now known as longitudinal (or axial) TD-OCT. Another version of TD-OCT is *en face* OCT[5] that can acquire a C scan image from 1D reflectivity profiles (T scans) collected by flying the spot transversally in two directions, while maintaining the axial coordinate fixed (*reference mirror* at rest). An *en face* OCT system presents the advantage that B scan images can also be constructed from many T scans repeated for successive pixels in depth, in other words, scanning fast laterally and slow axially using the *reference mirror*, as illustrated in **Figure 2(ii)**. Initially the method was applied to generate C scan OCT images of the retina *in vitro*,[6] of the retina *in vivo*[7] and then to provide both C scan and B scan OCT images of the retina *in vivo*.[8]

Spectral Domain Optical Coherence Tomography

Spectral domain OCT refers to spectral interrogation of the spectrum at the interferometer output. There are two possibilities. In **Figure 3(R)**, the *processing unit* employs a spectrometer, usually built using a prism or a diffraction grating and a linear photodetector array, using a CCD or a CMOS linear camera, method referred in what follows as spectrometer based (SB)-OCT. A second SD-OCT method consists in employing a *photodetector* in the *processing unit*, similar to the TD-OCT setup in **Figure 3(L)** and the OCT

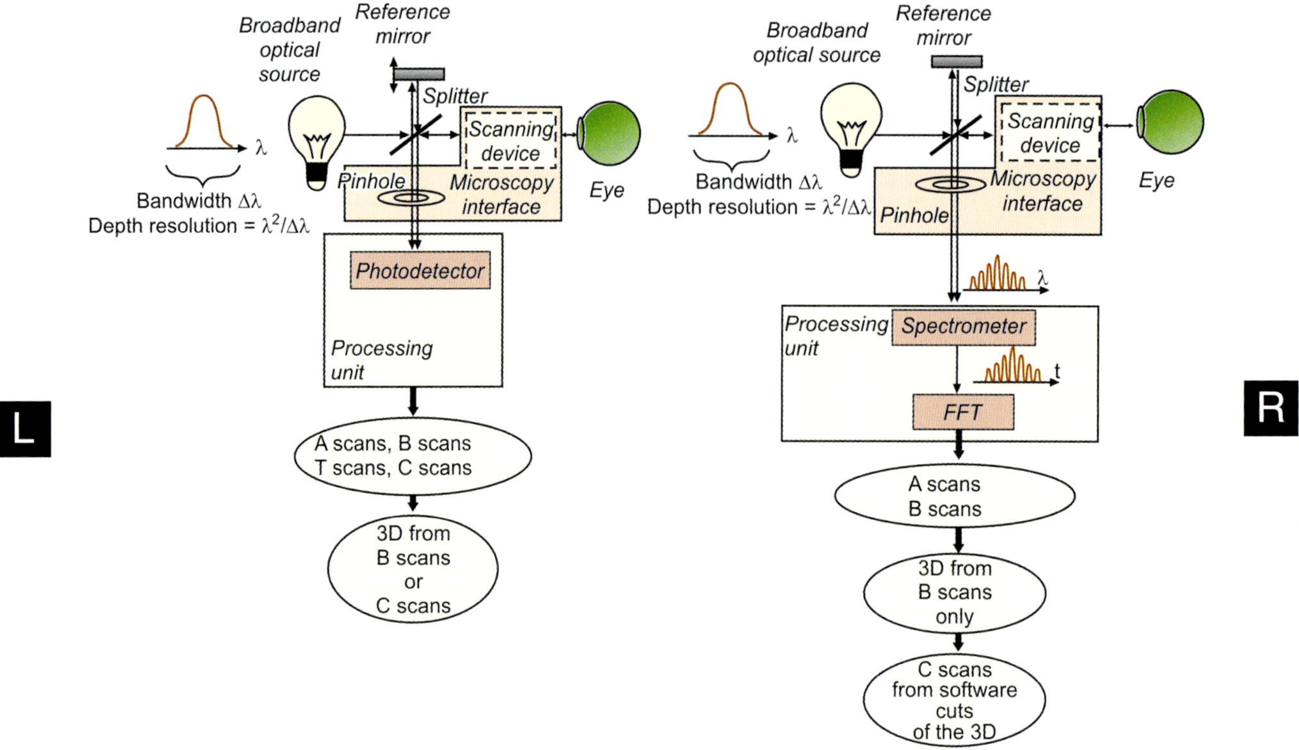

Figure 3: (L) Principle of time domain optical coherence tomography (OCT); (R) Principle of spectral domain OCT (spectrometer based)

setup being illuminated by a *swept source* (tunable laser), operating according to a method referred to as SS-OCT. Mechanical scanning of the OPD in TD-OCT in **Figure 3(L)** is replaced by reading the charges on the array in the spectrometer in SB-OCT in **Figure 3(R)** or by tuning the frequency of the laser source in SS-OCT (not shown).

Spectrometer Based Optical Coherence Tomography

The operation of the SB-OCT is based on the optical spectrum output demodulation of the low coherence interferometer. The spectrum exhibits peaks and troughs (channeled spectrum) and the period of such a modulation is proportional to the OPD in the interferometer.[9] Larger the OPD larger is the number of peaks in the spectrum. By downloading its charge content, the linear camera in the spectrometer transforms the optical spectrum into an electrical signal in time. If multilayered objects are imaged, such as retina, each layer imprints its own spectrum modulation periodicity, depending on its depth. A fast Fourier transform (FFT) of the spectrum of the linear camera signal translates the periodicity of the channeled spectrum into peaks of different frequency, related to the OPD. Such a profile is essentially the A scan profile of the square root of reflectivity in depth.

Due to its sensitivity advantage and availability of fast digital linear cameras, the SB-OCT became the method of choice in current OCT investigations of the retina with video-rate images from the retina demonstrated.[10] The majority of SB-OCT reports employ linear cameras at 20–70 kHz, which represents a line scan rate faster than maximum achievable by TD-OCT *en face* imaging using a resonant scanner at 16 kHz[11] and more than 20 times faster than line scan rates in *en face* OCT using galvanometer scanners. Progress in multi-tap cameras allowed 312.5 kHz line rate for OCT images collected from the retina.[12]

Swept Source Optical Coherence Tomography

The time required to tune the wavelength in the swept source determines the time to produce an A scan. Tuning speeds in excess of 3 MHz[13] makes the SS-OCT the fastest scanning OCT method that has proven sufficient quality of in vivo images of the retina.

Evolution of Optical Coherence Tomography *En Face* Imaging of the Retina

The evolution of OCT technology in imaging the retina *in vivo* based on data cumulated from a selection of reports is presented in **Table 1**. The first four columns show the acquisition rate and number of pixels in the image, depending on whether B scan or C scan, while the next two columns on the right display the time required to produce a C scan image, $T_{en\ face}$. The Table starts with the first report of OCT from retina at MIT[2] and ends with the highest OCT speed reported so far from the retina using SS-OCT.[13] Where the authors have not specified the numbers of pixels, such numbers were inferred from the data available in each report, as detailed in the footnotes. The size of the image varies across different reports therefore the number of Megavoxel/s in the last column represents a suitable performance to compare the different modalities involved. The number of pixels in **Table 1** are those specified in the images presented in the reports. A rigorous comparison would have required an evaluation of the techniques mentioned based on a similar size image, however this was not possible. Therefore, the order of magnitude of the Megavoxel/s and of the $T_{en\ face}$ should be considered and not their exact values.[1]

The graphs in **Figure 4** are assembled based on some of the exemplary reports in Table 1 only, for simplicity. In reality, a large spread of points could be placed in the graphs based on the articles mentioned in the reference list, however when completed, these would have displayed a similar trend to that shown that used only the few points representing the publications in **Table 1**. The graphs show the extraordinary progress in the number of Megavoxels acquired per second, due to the progress in SD-OCT and especially in the case of SS-OCT imaging using mode-locked swept source technology.[13]

For A scan based OCT systems, the time to collect the whole volume of voxels [as illustrated in **Figure 2(iv)**],

determines the minimum time required to produce a C scan image, $T_{en\ face}$, since such an image is only available once all data has been acquired. In addition to this time interval, the time required for the software cut of data should be added to (not incorporated in **Table 1**). Where data was not available, $T_{en\ face}$ in column 8 was inferred considering a number of 256 B scan frames.

The $T_{en\ face}$ graph in **Figure 4** illustrates the progress over the years in reducing the time to produce an *en face* cut. $T_{en\ face}$ for A scan based TD-OCT systems exceeds tens of seconds, too long for imaging a moving eye (although the majority of reports on OCT before 1998 required such large time intervals for acquiring multivoxel data). The progress in fast cameras and fast swept sources was so substantial in the last few years, that the time to acquire a decent volume of data required to produce a C scan image by software cut reached subsecond values, comparable or smaller than the time to produce a real time *en face* OCT image using time domain OCT with resonant scanners.[11]

Combining Optical Coherence Tomography with Scanning Laser Ophthalmoscopy

Three methods to achieve functionality similar to that of a dual channel OCT/SLO instrument have been developed, based on performing: (1) real time simultaneous C scan OCT with C scan SLO; (2) sequential real time B scan OCT with real time C scan SLO and (3) B scan OCT with post processing volumes of B scan OCT images to produce SLO images. The first two implementations, (1) and (2) require assembling dual channel instruments while the method (3)

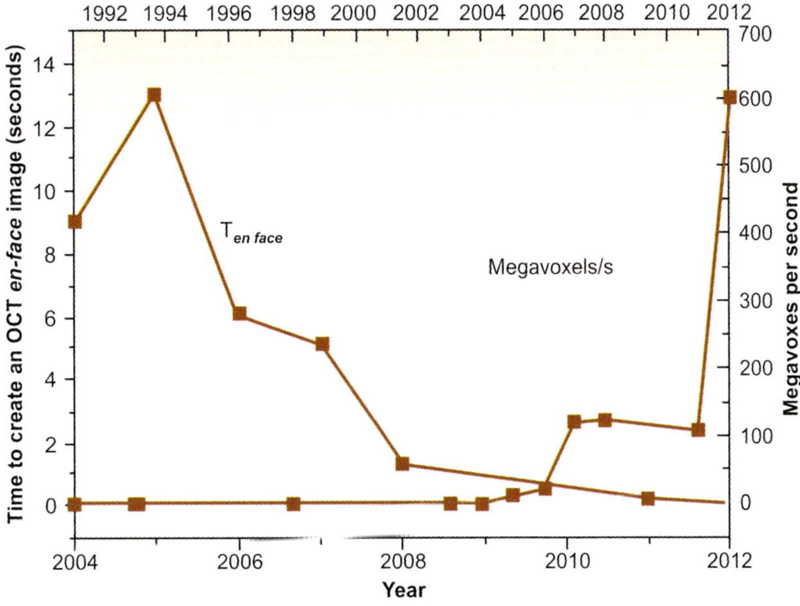

Figure 4: Evolution of the time interval to produce an *en face* optical coherence tomography image since 2004 and evolution of Megavoxels/second since 1991

Table 1: Evolution of the optical coherence tomography technology in imaging the retina in terms of the $T_{en\ face}$ and the number of Megavoxel/s

	Method employed	Line rate (kHz)	Frame rate (Hz)	Pixels in the B scan (N_x, N_z)	Pixels in the real time C scan (N_x, N_y)	$T_{en\ face}$ (s) (Time to produce an OCT C scan image, as reported)	Estimated $T_{en\ face}$ (s) to produce an OCT C scan image of 512 x 512 pixels[a]	Mvoxel/s $N_x N_y N_z$/Total time for 3D imaging
1	First report on OCT, longitudinal TD-OCT *in vitro* image of the retina[2]	0.0008	0.0053[b]	150 x 118[c]	n.a.	Not contemplated		0.000094
2	TD-OCT longitudinal OCT, in vivo[14]	0.042	0.42	100 x 285[d]	n.a.	6095[e]		0.012
3	[f]TD-OCT longitudinal OCT with fast axial scanning[15]	8	16 (32 possible)	250 x 250	n.a.	16 (8)[e]	32	1
4	*In vivo en face* TD-OCT image of the retina[8]	0.6	1.18	196 x 100	196 x 196	0.85	2.34	0.045
5	*En face* TD-OCT[16,18]	1	2(8)	512 x 250	512 x 512	0.5	0.5	0.52 (1.04 as OCT/SLO)
6	*En face* TD-OCT using a resonant galvoscanner[11]	4	53.3	Not contemplated, but possible	256 x 128	0.019	0.076	1.75
7	SB-OCT[10]	16	6.7 (or 31)	3000 x 1024 (or 512 x 1024)	n.a.	38.2[e](or 8.25)	16.4	21 (or 16.2)
8	SB-OCT[17]	29	29 (real time display 10)	1000 x 320	n.a.	8.83[e]	9	9.3
9	SB-OCT[19]	20	20	1000 x 292[g]	n.a	12.8[e]	13	5.84 (Considering two polarization channels gives: 11.7)
10	SB-OCT/Line-field SLO[20]	Not specified	15	1024 x 512	n.a.	17[e]	-	7.87 in the OCT 15.7 in the SLO
11	Line-field SB-OCT[21]	51.5 (single frame: 823.2)	201	128[h] x 108[i]	n.a.	1.27	5.1	2.8

Contd...

Table 1: *Contd...*

	Method employed	Line rate (kHz)	Frame rate (Hz)	Pixels in the B scan (N_x, N_z)	Pixels in the real time C scan (N_x, N_y)	$T_{en\ face}$ (s) (Time to produce an OCT C scan image, as reported)	Estimated $T_{en\ face}$ (s) to produce an OCT C scan image of 512 x 512 pixels[1]	Mvoxel/s $N_x N_y N_z$/Total time for 3D imaging
12	SS-OCT at 850 nm[22]	43.2	84	512 x 140[j]	n.a.	3[k]	6.07	6
13	SS-OCT at 1050 nm[23]	236	461	512 x 512	n.a	0.56[d]	1.1	122
14	SB-OCT, 2008[12]	312.15	610	512 x 167[l]	n.a.	1.3 (at 250 kHz with Nz = 400)	1.3 (at 250 kHz)	52125 (at 250 kHz)
15	SS-OCT at 1050 nm[24]	1,368.700 (1,190)	612	1900 x 90[m]	n.a.	3 (1900 x 1900)	0.22	107
16	Parallel SS-OCT [13] at 1050 nm	2 x 3,350	705	3168 x 90[n]	n.a.	0.33 (3168 x 708)	0.078	603

[a] Evaluated as $N_x N_y/F_z$

[b] Although potential to 5 Hz was also mentioned

[c] Evaluated using the values quoted in the paper of 2 mm depth range and 17 mm depth resolution in air

[d] Evaluated using the values quoted in the paper of 3 mm depth range and 10.5 mm depth resolution in air

[e] Not contemplated and evaluated for 256 frames using the frame rate for B scan imaging

[f] Although images from the anterior chamber of a murine eye are presented only and not from the retina, the fast scanning delay line method presents sufficient sensitivity to image the retina and was included here for comparison of technologies

[g] Evaluated from 1.75 mm depth range with 6 mm resolution quoted

[h] Dividing the line of 2.1 mm with the indicated value of transversal resolution, of 16.4 mm

[i] Evaluated from 0.8 mm depth range and 7.4 mm resolution quoted

[j] Evaluated from 1.4 mm depth range and 10 mm resolution in tissue

[k] Evaluated for 256 B scan frames

[l] Evaluated at max speed, where the axial range quoted is 1.5 mm with a 9 mm resolution

[m] Evaluated from 1.7 mm depth range and 19 mm resolution quoted

[n] Axial range not quoted, therefore the same N_z was used,[24] numerical values estimated could be better as here an improved depth resolution of 21 mm in air is quoted

(*Abbreviations:* OCT: Optical coherence tomography; SLO: Scanning laser ophthalmoscopy; n.a: Not applicable; TD-OCT: Time domain optical coherence tomography; SB-OCT: Spectrometer based optical coherence tomography; SS-OCT: Swept source optical coherence tomography)

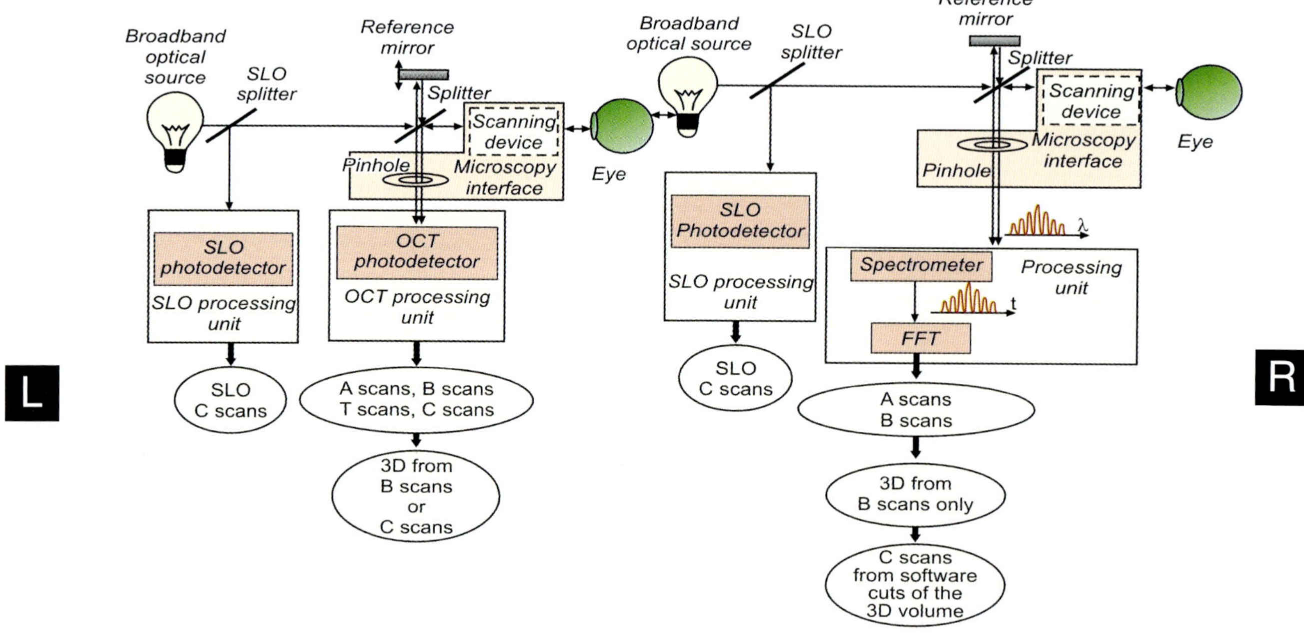

Figure 5: (L) Principle of a combined instrument time domain optical coherence tomography (OCT) and scanning laser ophthalmoscopy (SLO); (R) Principle of a combined instrument spectral domain OCT (spectrometer based) and SLO

operates on a single channel instrument, OCT, equipped with a post processing protocol.

Simultaneous Real Time Optical Coherence Tomography with Real Time Scanning Laser Ophthalmoscopy

Simultaneous acquisition of images in two channels, OCT and SLO requires configurations using splitters, as shown generically in **Figure 5(L)**. In this, a small fraction of the light returned is diverted towards the SLO channel using a separate splitter with an in-fiber OCT balanced interferometer.[25] There is an optimum splitting ratio which ensures sufficient and similar signal to noise ratio in both channels.[26] A bulk interferometer solution for simultaneous acquisition of an OCT and an SLO image was also reported.[27] The bulk configuration allows placing the optical splitter close to the optical source with the advantage of no signal loss towards the OCT channel (however requiring to compensate for loss of power by increasing the optical source power).

Recognizable Patterns

Several remarkable new aspects of clinical anatomy were revealed using the real time dual channel *en face* perspective.[28] After examining a diverse array of common clinic pathologies including macular degeneration, central serous retinopathy, macular hole, macular pucker, cystoid macular edema, diabetic maculopathy, hereditary maculopathies and macular trauma, a series of specific and recurring patterns for several pathologic entities became evident. Observation of uniquely specific and

recurring *en face* patterns for several pathologic entities has been reported for the first time.[1,29] The most notable examples were: the "*Chrysanthemum* flower" arrangement of cystic degeneration seen in macular holes, the "Swiss cheese wheel" cluster of cysts seen in cystoid macular edema, the "shining star" configuration of radiating epiretinal membrane folds, seen in macular pucker, the "bullseye target" pattern of concentric light and dark rings on the macula in central serous retinopathy, and the "ring of light" appearance of the slice through the bulge of a retinal pigment epithelium detachment). Other notable patterns which were recognizable but often variable enough to defy simple categorization include the "cluster of grapes" footprint of multiple retinal pigment epithelium bulges in polypoidal choroidopathy and the "islands in the stream" array of edema residues in diabetic macular edema.

Sequential Spectrometer Based Optical Coherence Tomography/ Scanning Laser Ophthalmoscopy (Sequential B Scan OCT with C Scan SLO)

This is implemented based on the generic configuration described in **Figure 5(R)** which operates in two sequential regimes. In the *en face* regime, both X and Y scanners are driven and the image displayed is provided by the SLO channel. In the cross-sectioning regime, the frame scanner is stopped and the image displayed is that of an SB-OCT channel. A B scan image is produced along a line placed above the SLO image displayed in the *en face* regime. Using the same pair of XY scanners, the pixel to pixel correspondence is ensured between the two images, i.e. the B scan OCT image is produced exactly along the contour drawn above the SLO image.[16] This can be a horizontal line, a vertical line, a line oriented at any arbitrary direction or a circle.

Historically, the first OCT/SLO instrument[25] employed the configuration in **Figure 5(L)**. It has taken almost a decade for the sequential version in **Figure 5(R)** to be implemented.[30]

Optical Coherence Tomography/Line-Scanning Laser Ophthalmoscopy (Sequential B Scan OCT with C Scan SLO)

A different sequential method is that where the linear camera is used for both a line-SLO (LSLO) channel and a SB-OCT channel.[20] The instrument can run in three modes: LSLO mode only, OCT mode only and frame/interleaved LSLO/ SB-OCT mode.

Image Generation from Optical Coherence Tomography Stacks

An equivalent SLO image can be generated from several OCT C scans or from several B scans. Using any OCT method, a 3D stack is first obtained. Then, by software means, an SLO image can be inferred without using a beam-splitter or a separate confocal receiver. Such an equivalent SLO image is obtained only after all the images in the stack have been acquired, determined by $T_{en\,face}$ (**Table 1**). Therefore, such a method can be implemented on a fast OCT system only. The transversal resolution along the synthesized axis of the SLO image is given by the spatial sampling, i.e. by the lateral interval from a B scan to the next B scan along a rectangular direction to that contained in the B scan image. Such SLO-like C scan images exhibit the normal transversal resolution (15–20 μm) along the B scan lateral coordinate (X) and the coarse sampling interval, along the lateral rectangular direction (Y).

Image Generation from Stacks of B Scan Spectrometer Based Optical Coherence Tomography Images

Several groups have reported inference of an SLO-like image from OCT B scans using SB-OCT systems.[31,32] A feature-based algorithm[33] was developed, which can register a high density OCT image of the fundus image from normal density scans. Both large and small blood vessels around the optic disk were imaged with good contrast.

Image Generation from Stacks of B Scan Swept Source Optical Coherence Tomography Images

Similar procedure was applied to generate an SLO-like image from a stack of SS-OCT images acquired with systems operating at 850 nm[22,34] and at 1 μm.[35] In the 3D measurement mode, a preview image of the fundus (fundus preview) was created immediately after acquisition. In the central 256 points were extracted from a single spectral interference signal and the signal power was obtained by squaring followed by its summation.

Synergies Provided by the Combination of Techniques

An OCT/SLO dual channel promotes synergy between the two images collected. This depends on the OCT technology employed and the procedure to provide the SLO signal. Irrespective of technology, depth location is provided by OCT B scans for patterns seen in the SLO images.

In the real time *en face* TD-OCT, the main motivation for OCT/SLO combination was to provide orientation to the OCT channel, which comes out fragmented. In addition, using the lateral shifts in the SLO image, lateral movement disturbances in the B scan OCT images can also be eliminated.

When using the sequential B scan SD-OCT/SLO, the SLO image is used to select the position of the subsequent B scan.

In the post processing instruments, the SLO inferred image is used to guide subsequent B scan sections.

Irrespective of the method used, the OCT/SLO has proved useful in allowing ophthalmologists and visions scientists to associate features seen in SLO systems to those highly fragmented in the OCT *en face* image, due to enhanced depth resolution of the OCT and curvature of the eye tissue.

As seen in this book, *en face* views derived from spectral domain OCT provide complementary information to the most traditional OCT cross sectioning, with a choice of: (1) high depth resolution, thin slicing of the volume investigated or (2) coarse depth resolution slicing, in which case averaged views over the scanning range provide images similar to those returned by a hardware SLO channel.

Acknowledgments

A Gh Podoleanu acknowledges support from the European Research Council-Advanced Fellowship Program, Engineering and Physical Sciences Research Council of the UK, Biotechnology and Biological Sciences Research Council of the UK, European Commission, New York Eye and Ear Infirmary and Ophthalmic Technology Inc., Toronto, Canada.

References

1. Podoleanu AG, Rosen RB. Combinations of techniques in imaging the retina with high resolution. Prog Retin Eye Res. 2008;27(4):464-99.
2. Huang D, Swanson EA, Lin CP, et al. Optical coherence tomography. Science. 1991;254:1178-81.
3. Rosen RB, Garcia P, Podoleanu AG, et al. In: Drexler W, Wolfgang W, Fujimoto J, James G (Eds). Optical Coherence Tomography Technology and Applications, in Series: Biological and Medical Physics, Biomedical Engineering, XXVIII. Berlin, Heidelberg: Springer; 2008.

4. Smith LM, Dobson CC. Absolute displacement measurements using modulation of the spectrum of white light in a Michelson interferometer. Appl Opt. 1989;28(16): 3339-42.

5. Podoleanu AG, Dobre GM, Webb DJ, et al. Coherence imaging by use of a Newton rings sampling function. Opt Lett. 1996;21:1789-91.

6. Podoleanu AG, Dobre GM, Webb DJ, et al. Simultaneous en-face imaging of two layers in the human retina by low-coherence reflectometry. Opt Lett. 1997;22:1039-41.

7. Podoleanu AG, Dobre GM, Jackson DA, et al. En-face coherence imaging using galvanometer scanner modulation. Opt Lett. 1998;23:147-9.

8. Podoleanu AG, Seeger M, Dobre GM, et al. Transversal and longitudinal images from the retina of the living eye using low coherence reflectometry. J Biomed Opt. 1998;3:12-20

9. Taplin S, Podoleanu A Gh, Webb DJ, et al. Displacement sensor using channeled spectrum dispersed on a linear CCD array. Electron Lett. 1993;29(10):896-7.

10. Wojtkowski M, Srinivasan V, Ko T, et al. Ultrahigh-resolution, high-speed, Fourier domain optical coherence tomography and methods for dispersion compensation. Opt Express. 2004;12(11):2404-22.

11. Hitzenberger C, Trost P, Lo PW, et al. Three-dimensional imaging of the human retina by high-speed optical coherence tomography. Opt Express. 2003;11:2753-61.

12. Potsaid B, Gorczynska I, Srinivasan VJ, et al. Ultrahigh speed spectral /Fourier domain OCT ophthalmic imaging at 70,000 to 312,500 axial scans per second. Opt Express. 2008;16(19):15149-69.

13. Klein T, Wieser W, André R, et al. Multi-MHz FDML OCT: Snapshot retinal imaging at 6.7 million axial-scans per second. Proc. SPIE. 2012;8427:84271D.

14. Swanson EA, Izatt JA, Hee MR, et al. In vivo retina imaging by optical coherence tomography. Opt Lett. 1993;18: 1864-6.

15. Rollins A, Yazdanfar S, Kulkarni M, et al. In vivo video rate optical coherence tomography. Opt Express. 1998;3:219-29.

16. Rosen RB, Podoleanu AG, Dunne S, et al. Optical coherence tomography ophthalmoscopy. In: Ciulla TA, Regillo CD, Harris A (Eds). Retina and Optic Nerve Imaging, 1st edition. Philadelphia: Lippincott Williams & Wilkins; 2003. pp. 119-36.

17. Nassif NA, Cense B, Park BH, et al. In vivo high-resolution video-rate spectral-domain optical coherence tomography of the human retina and optic nerve. Opt Express. 2004;12:367-76.

18. van Velthoven ME, Verbraak FD, Yannuzzi LA, et al. Imaging the retina by *en face* optical coherence tomography. Retina. 2006;26:129-36.

19. Götzinger E, Pircher M, Hitzenberger CK. High speed spectral domain polarization sensitive optical coherence tomography of the human retina. Opt Express. 2005;13: 10217-29.

20. Iftimia NV, Hammer DX, Bigelow CE, et al. Hybrid retinal imager using line-scanning laser ophthalmoscopy and spectral domain optical coherence tomography. Opt Express. 2006;4:12909-14.

21. Nakamura Y, Makita S, Yamanari M, et al. High-speed three-dimensional human retinal imaging by line-field spectral domain optical coherence tomography. Opt Express. 2007;15:7103-16.

22. Lim H, Mujat M, Kerbage C, et al. High-speed imaging of human retina in vivo with swept-source optical coherence tomography. Opt Express. 2006;14:12902-8.

23. Huber R, Adler DC, Srinivasan VJ, et al. Fourier domain mode locking at 1050 nm for ultra-high-speed optical coherence tomography of the human retina at 236,000 axial scans per second. Opt Lett. 2007;32:2049-51.

24. Klein T, Wieser W, Eigenwillig CM, et al. Megahertz OCT for ultrawide-field retinal imaging with a 1050 nm Fourier domain mode-locked laser. Opt Express. 2011;19:3044-62.

25. Podoleanu AG, Jackson DA. Combined optical coherence tomography and scanning laser ophthalmoscope. Electron Lett. 1998;34(11):1088-90.

26. Podoleanu AG, Jackson DA. Noise analysis of a combined optical coherence tomograph and a confocal scanning ophthalmoscope. Appl. Opt. 1999;38:2116-27.

27. Pircher M, Baumann B, Götzinger E, et al. Retinal cone mosaic imaged with transverse scanning optical coherence tomography. Opt Lett. 2006;31:1821-3.

28. Podoleanu AG, Dobre GM, Cucu RG, et al. Combined multiplanar optical coherence tomography and confocal scanning ophthalmoscopy. J Biomed Opt. 2004;9: 86-93.

29. Rosen RB, Podoleanu A Gh, Rogers JA, et al. Challenges and recognizable patterns in the en-face OCT of the retina. In: Tuchin VV, Izatt JA, Fujimoto JG (Eds). Coherence Domain Optical Methods and Optical Coherence Tomography, Conference in Biomedicine VIII. Proc. SPIE. 2004;5316:16-22.

30. Lumbroso B, Rosen R, Rispoli M. Spectral-domain OCT/ cSLO. In: Coscas G, Coscas F, Vismara S, Zourdani A, Calzi Cil (Eds). Optical Coherence Tomography in Age-Related Macular Degeneration, 2nd edition. New York: Springer; 2010. p. 233.

31. Hong Y, Makita S, Yamanari M, et al. Three-dimensional visualization of choroidal vessels by using standard and ultra-high resolution scattering optical coherence angiography. Opt Express. 2007;15:7538-50.

32. Wojtkowski M, Srinivasan V, Fujimoto JG, et al. Three dimensional retinal imaging with high-speed ultrahigh-resolution optical coherence tomography. Ophthalmology. 2005;112:1734-46.

33. Jiao S, Wu C, Knighton RW, et al. Registration of high-density cross sectional images to the fundus image in spectral-domain ophthalmic optical coherence tomography. Opt Express. 2006;14:3368-76.

34. Srinivasan VJ, Huber R, Gorczynska I, et al. High-speed, high-resolution optical coherence tomography retinal imaging with a frequency-swept laser at 850 nm. Opt Lett. 2007;32(4):361-3.

35. Yasuno Y, Hong Y, Makita S, et al. In vivo high-contrast imaging of deep posterior eye by 1-microm swept source optical coherence tomography and scattering optical coherence angiography. Opt Express. 2007;15:6121-39.

chapter 2

En Face Image Formation and Interpretation

Qienyuan Zhou, Jay Wei

Fourier domain optical coherence tomography (FD-OCT) refers to the technology to acquire entire A scan depth data in Fourier space and then through Fourier transform to realize the A scan distance profile in spatial space. It can be implemented with two different techniques: spectrometer based spectral domain OCT (SD-OCT) and tunable laser based swept source OCT (SS-OCT). While there is difference in technology, SD-OCT and SS-OCT are similar in the basic principle of operation. Regardless of the specific implementation, all FD-OCT devices share a common advantage over earlier time-domain OCT (TD-OCT) in that high data acquisition rate of the FD-OCT systems facilitates the acquisition of dense three-dimensional (3D) data set of ocular structures of the eye in a time frame tolerable to patients.

The 3D data set (**Figure 1A**) could be displayed in a series of two-dimensional (2D) cross-sectional images in any orientation desired. The most common cross-sectional images are referred to as B scan images (**Figure 1B**, B scans in X-Z plane and in Y-Z plane) in which the cross-sections are approximately perpendicular to the retinal surface and *en face* images (**Figure 1B**, *en face* image in X-Y plane) in which the cross-sections are approximately parallel to the retinal surface.

Intensity based *en face* images may serve as a condensed data set of the 3D data and facilitate assessment of retinal features or pathological changes with characteristics better represented in an *en face* view, for example, wedge defect of the retinal nerve fiber layer (RNFL) in glaucoma or area of geographic atrophy (GA) in dry age-related macular degeneration (AMD), etc.

There is a benefit to reducing the 3D data set to a few *en face* images at different depth without losing critical clinical information. While it is simple to generate *en face* images in flat cuts with varying Z-axis offset, much the same as the C scan images with TD-OCT in earlier days, the individual *en face* images generated this way could be difficult to interpret due to the fact that a C scan image is likely to cut through multiple tissue layers due to the natural curvature of the retina or pathology.

Instead of making a flat cut, the *en face* could be generated following a natural surface contour, with uniform thickness or varying thickness. As shown in **Figure 2**, the *en face* image of total intensity over the entire thickness range is similar to a scanning laser ophthalmoscope (SLO) fundus image; the advantage of OCT is the ability to generate depth resolved *en face* images with intensity integrated over a small depth range to visualize retinal structures layer-by-layer as shown in **Figure 2**. In the example, the 3D segmentation of retinal layers was used to set the range of intensity integration for the *en face* images. The inner limiting membrane (ILM) contour was followed to generate the *en face* image of RNFL; the RPE layer contour was followed to generate the outer plexiform layer (OPL) *en face* image, the RPE *en face* image, and the *en face* image from within the choroid.

The appearance of the *en face* image depends on surface contour it follows and the depth range of intensity integration for the *en face* image. For inner retinal layers such as the RNFL, the ILM could be a good contour surface to follow. For the outer retinal structures, the RPE or Bruch's membrane might be more appropriate surface contours to follow than the ILM. As illustrated in the case below of a 63-year-old male patient with polypoidal choroidal vasculopathy in the right eye. The *en face* image following Bruch's membrane surface contour (**Figure 3**, location of the *en face* slab indicated by red dotted contour line in the B scan) shows the features at fixed distance from the Bruch's membrane, while the *en face* image following the ILM contour (**Figure 3**, location of the *en face* slab indicated by yellow dotted line in the B scan) shows features at fixed distance from the ILM, cutting through RPE/Bruch's membrane into the

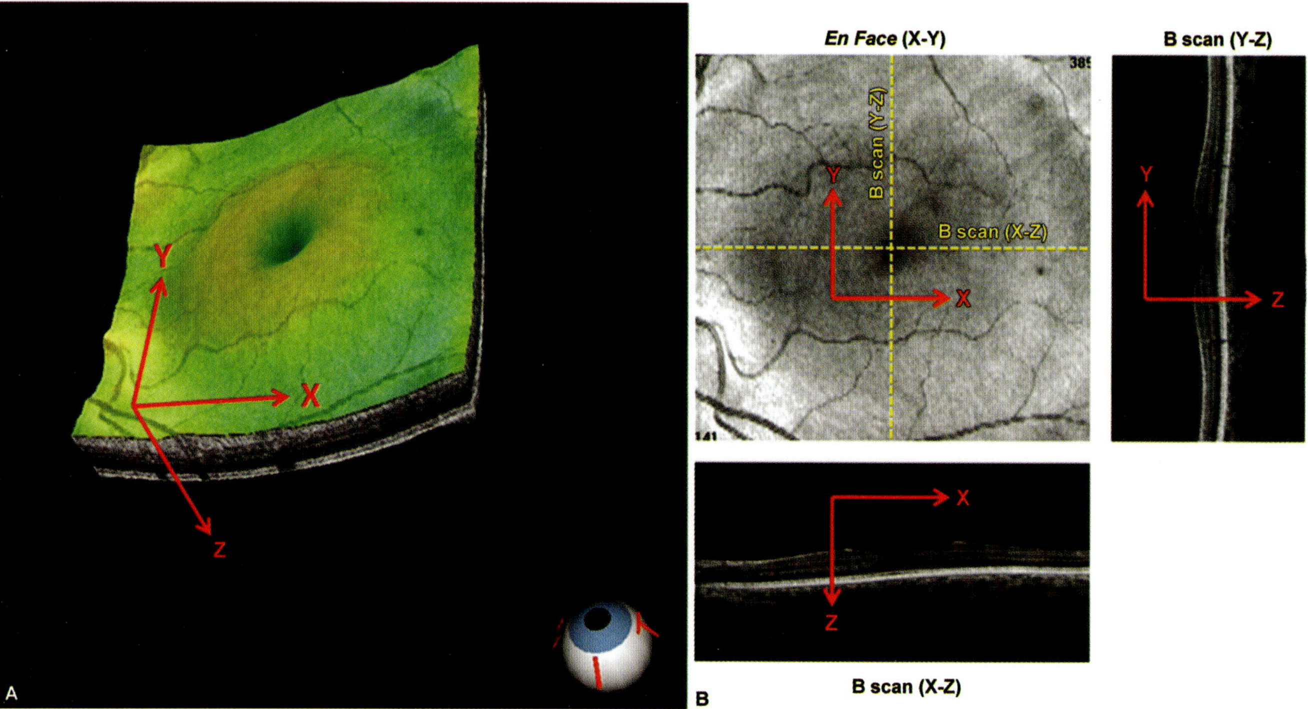

Figures 1A and B: (A) Three-dimensional volumetric data of the left eye of a healthy 55-year-old male volunteer subject; (B) Typical 2D display of the 3D data set, including *en face* images parallel to retinal surface in X-Y plane and B scan images in horizontal (X-Z plane) or vertical (Y-Z plane) directions
(*OCT Data Courtesy:* Dr Bruno Lumbroso, acquired with RTVue SD-OCT)

choroid. It often helps to understand the information in an *en face* image if the locations and the range of the *en face* image is indicated in a B scan image.

En face images may be generated to represent individual retinal layers, such as the RNFL, the inner and outer plexiform layers (IPL and OPL), the inner retina, the outer retina, the photoreceptor IS/OS junction, the RPE and the choroid. A benefit of the *en face* image representing a selected retinal tissue is to facilitate comparison of the same tissue across different eyes (subjects). To generate *en face* image of a specific retinal layer, segmentation should be performed based on the 3D data set to define layer boundaries which are then used to set the range of intensity integration for the *en face* image. As shown in **Figures 4A to D**, the choroidal *en face* images were generated by segmenting out the choroid anterior and posterior boundaries, and integrating the intensity between the two boundaries. The average choroidal thickness of the *en face* images ranged from 103 μm **(Figure 4C)** to 297 μm **(Figure 4D).**

Interpreting individual *en face* image in isolation could be difficult. Deeper layer intensity-based *en face* images may be affected by anterior structures. It is well understood that retinal blood vessels cast shadow on the deeper layers such as RPE. Pathological changes in the retina may also change the appearance of *en face* images posterior, as shown in

Figure 5. The highly scattering exudates adjacent to the OPL cast shadows in the RPE *en face* image, which could be mistakenly interpreted as change in the RPE, if the image is viewed in isolation, while the source of the change is actually in the space anterior to the RPE.

Another example of shadowing effect is illustrated in **Figure 6** of a 94-year-old patient with geographic atrophy in the left eye. The increased intensity in the choroid *en face* image is mostly due to the atrophy in the RPE layer resulting in greater penetration of light into the choroid. Note a few horizontal dark striations (red arrows) near the top of the *en face* images caused by eye motion in the Z-axis or RPE segmentation error.

Three-dimensional OCT intensity data set may be processed in different ways to generate a converted data set representing local tissue properties, such as attenuation coefficient, scattering coefficient, birefringence and depolarization, etc. *En face* images may be derived from the processed 3D data set based on a tissue property of interest. In such images, the shadowing effect would be minimized, making the *en face* images easier to interpret and analyze.

Eye motion during image acquisition could introduce artifacts in the *en face* image. Eye motion could cause distortion of retinal features, such as disruption of the blood

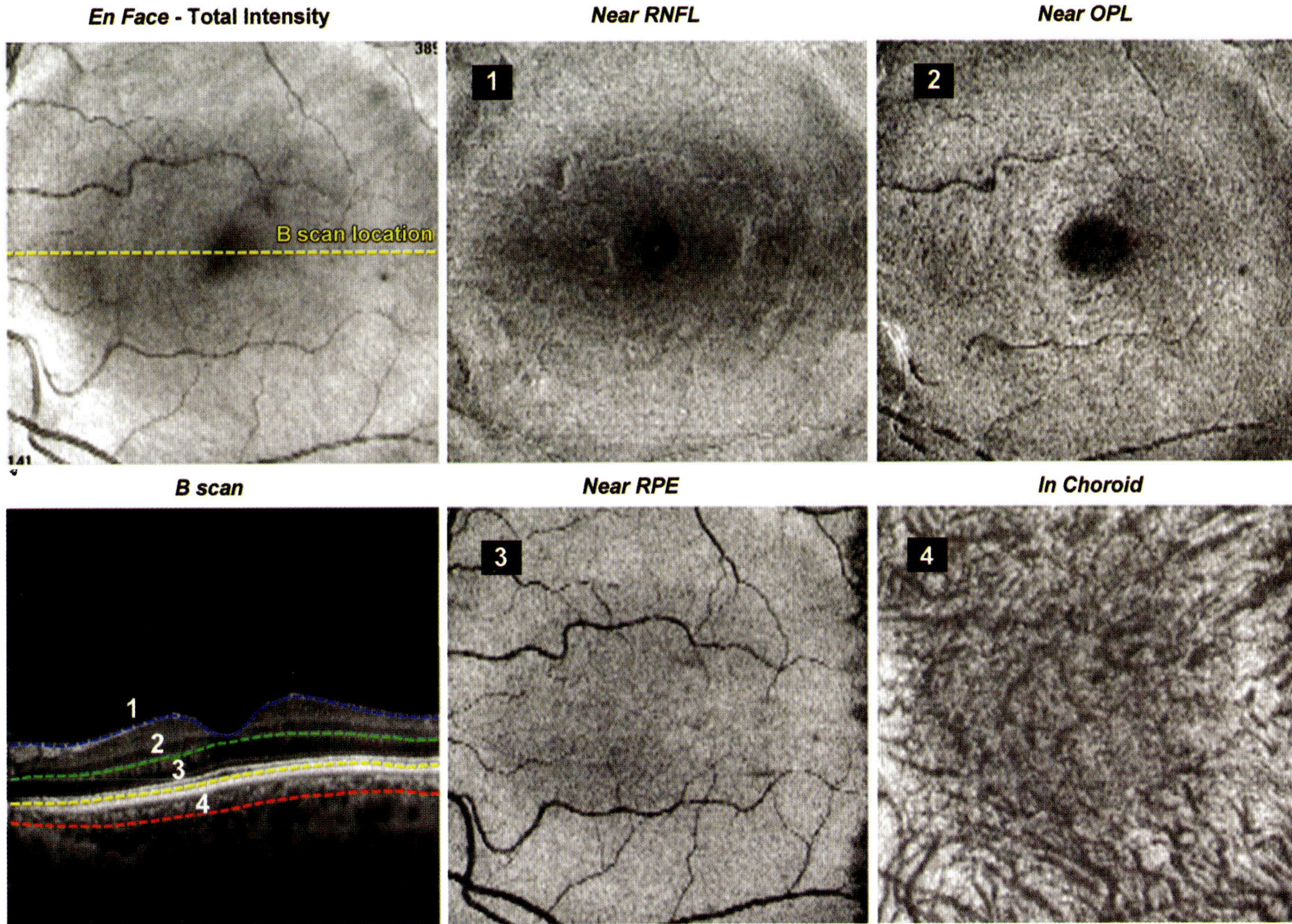

Figure 2: (Top-Left) *En face* image integrated over the full scan range, similar to SLO fundus image. (Bottom-Left) Horizontal B scan image through the center of the fovea with overlay of contour lines indicating the positions of four partial intensity *en face* images. (1) *En face* image of 30 μm thick slab immediately underneath the ILM; (2) *En face* image of 30 μm thick slab about the OPL; (3) *En face* image from 30 μm thick slab 40 μm above the RPE; (4) *En face* image of 30 μm thick slice in the choroid
(*OCT Data Courtesy:* Dr Bruno Lumbroso, acquired with RTVue SD-OCT)

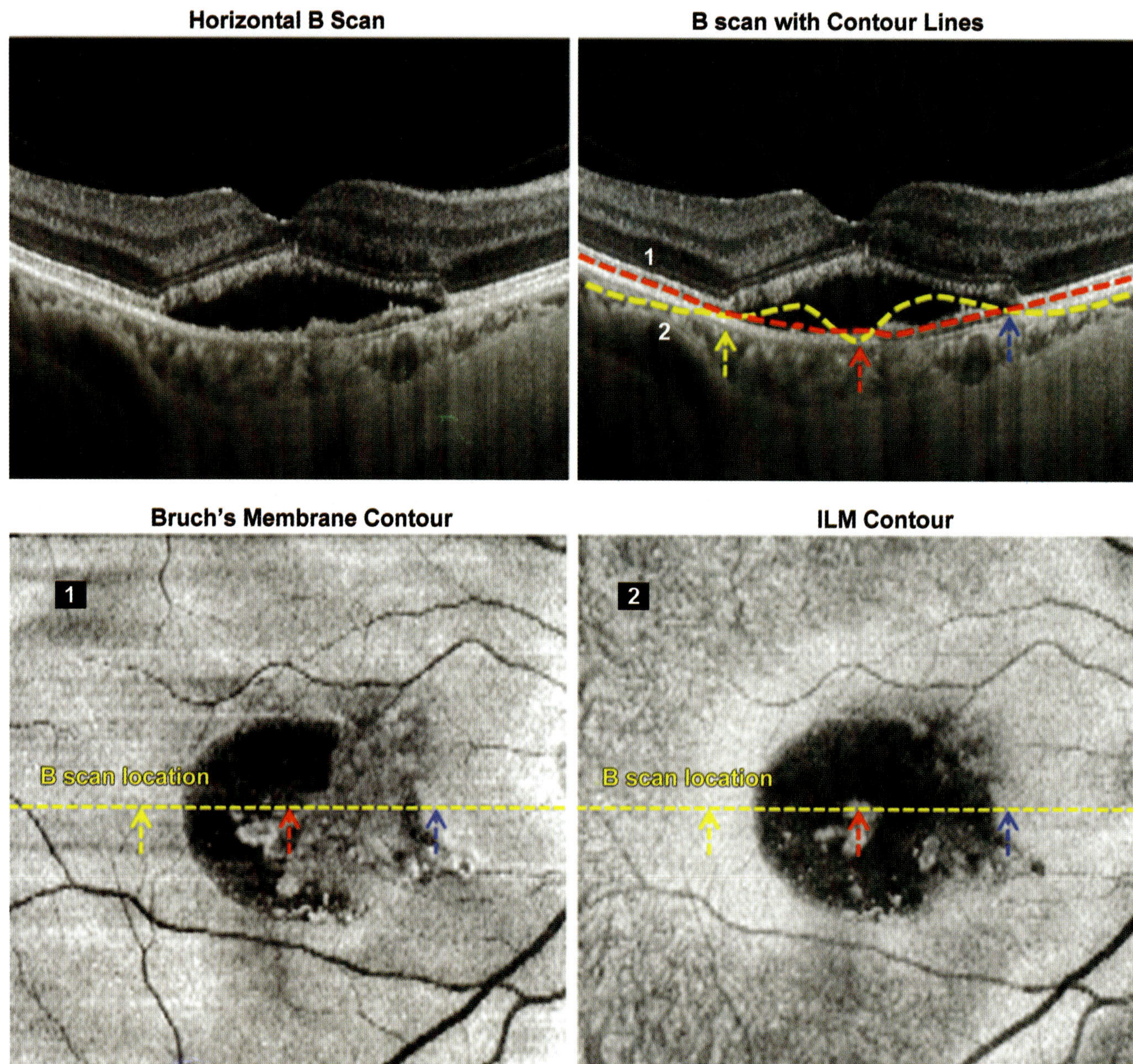

Figure 3: Illustration of the contour surface selection on the appearance of the *en face* image in a 63-year-old male patient with polypoidal choroidal vasculopathy in the right eye. (1) *En face* image of the RPE following the Bruch's membrane contour, showing the detached RPE from Bruch's membrane; (2) *En face* image of similar locations following the ILM surface contour missed the detached RPE and showing choroid in the periphery
(*OCT Data Courtesy:* Dr Bruno Lumbroso, acquired with RTVue SD-OCT)

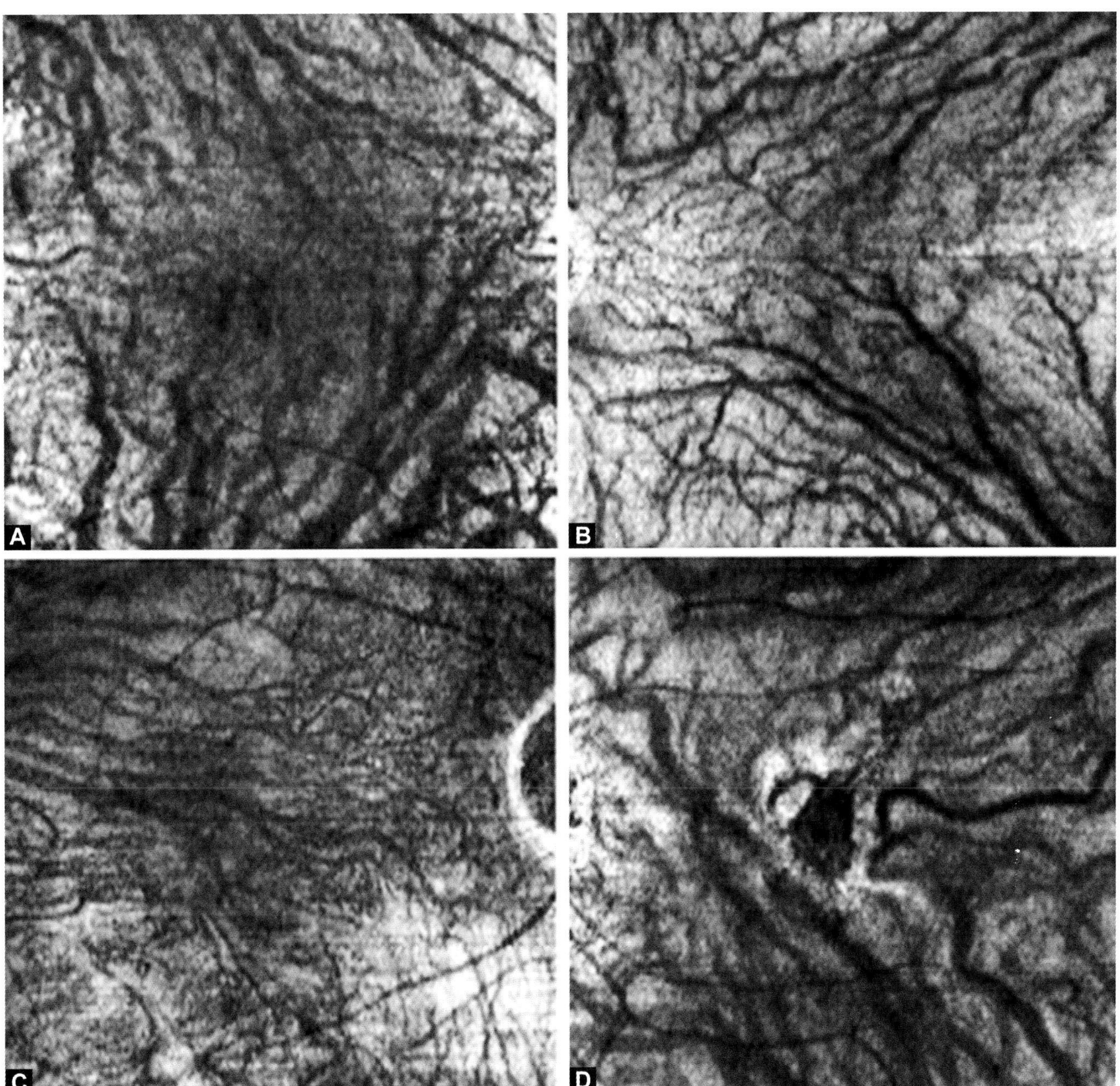

Figures 4A to D: Choroidal *en face* image based on intensity integration between the anterior and posterior boundaries of the choroid. (A) A normal emmetropic right eye of a 32-year-old subject with average choroid thickness of 295 μm; (B) A normal emmetropic left eye of a 55-year-old subject with average choroid thickness of 169 μm; (C) A normal myopic right eye of a 40-year-old female volunteer subject with average choroid thickness of 103 μm; (D) A myopic right eye with CNV of a 31-year-old patient with average choroid thickness of 297 μm
(Images adapted from a presentation given by Charles Guo from Optovue in Rome in 2010)

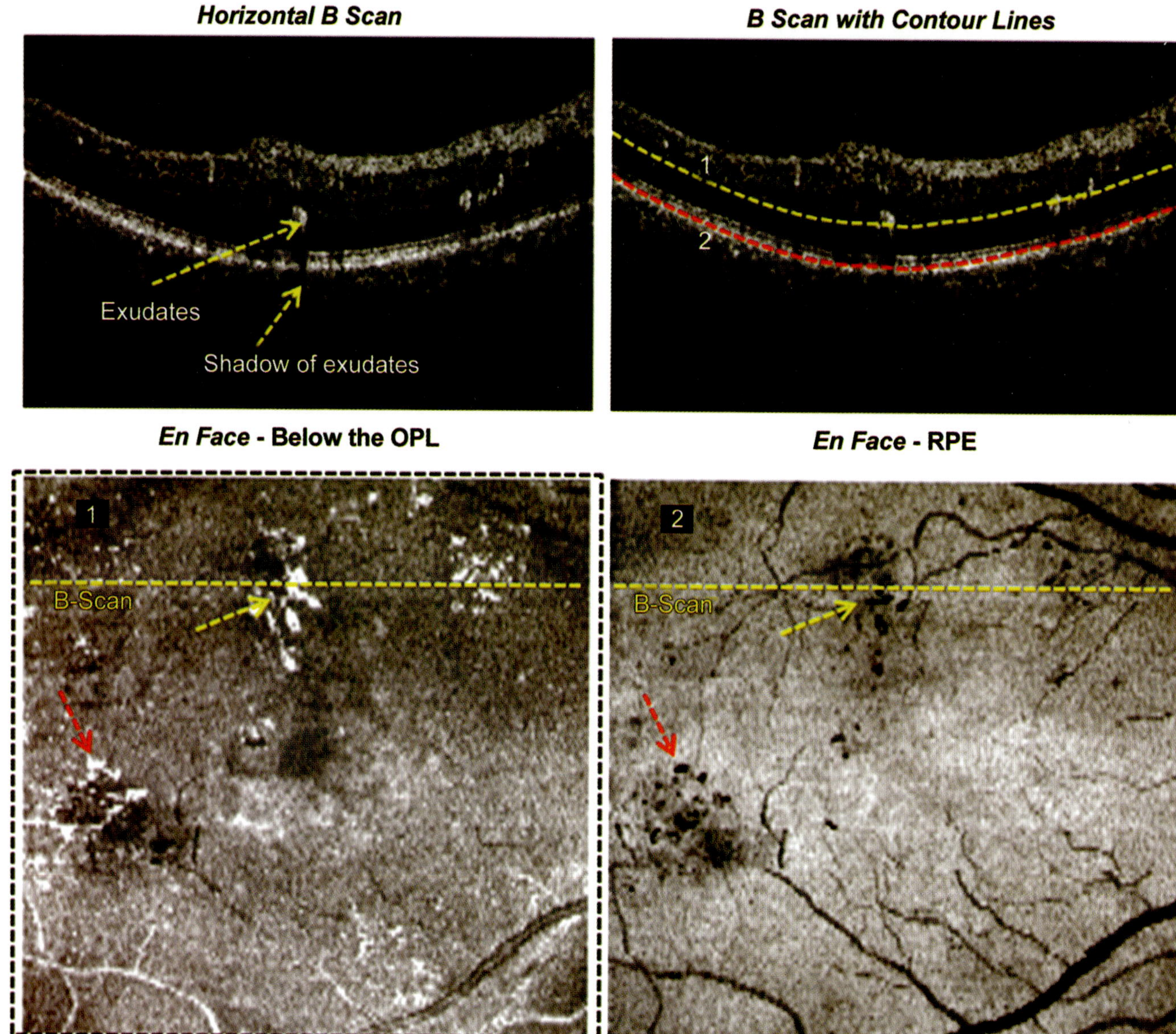

Figure 5: Shadowing effect of anterior structures on the deeper layer *en face* images of a 38-year-old male diabetic patient with clinically significant macular edema (CSME) in the right eye. (1) *En face* image immediately below the OPL showing the light scattering exudates due to CSME, marked with red and yellow arrows. (2) *En face* image of RPE layer with dark spots caused by the shadowing effect of the exudates rather than RPE defects, marked with red and yellow arrows (*OCT Data Courtesy:* Dr Nalin Mehta, acquired with RTVue SD-OCT)

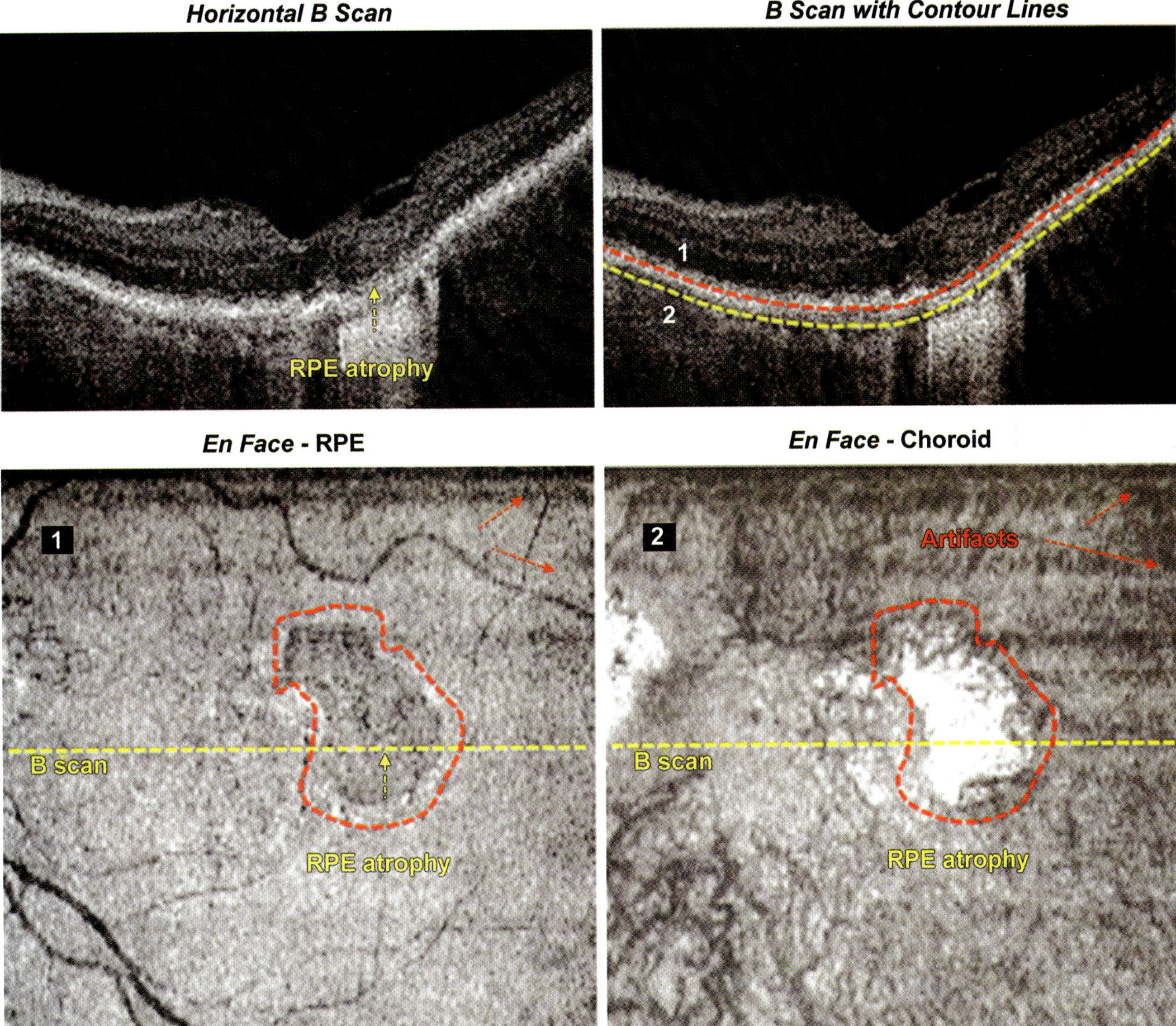

Figure 6: Effect of anterior structures on the deeper layer *en face* images of a 94-year-old female AMD patient with GA in the left eye. (1) *En face* image of the RPE showing an atrophic area (darker region outlined with red dotted line); (2) *En face* image of choroid with increased choroid reflection underneath the RPE atrophy (brighter region outlined with red dotted line).
(*OCT Data Courtesy*: Dr Nalin Mehta, acquired with RTVue SD-OCT)

vessel patterns, and intensity variation as illustrated in **Figure 6**. Motion corrected 3D data will have advantage over conventional 3D OCT data set in generating more accurate and reproducible *en face* images.

Finally, interpreting *en face* images needs to consider contour, thickness and location of the *en face* slab. Keeping in mind that the anterior retinal features could affect the appearance of the *en face* images of the posterior layers, B scan images can provide helpful complementing view when interpreting *en face* images.

Frontal Scans Clinical Applications: Plane Sections and Scans Generated to Follow a Retinal Surface Contour

Bruno Lumbroso, Andre Romano, Marco Rispoli

Introduction

Clinical retina specialist can today chose between different devices for *en face* study of ocular diseases; in *en face* images the sections are approximately parallel to the retinal surface or pigment epithelium. The images authors obtained differ from each other according to the technology used. The frontal scan clinical images can be plane sections, straightened images and scans adapted to pigment epithelium concavity (**Figure 1**). Authors will not try to explain the *en face* technology, which has been discussed in the first chapter by Adrian Podoleanu, and in chapter 2 by Qienyuan Zhou and Jay Wei. Authors will try to explain what is shown in the different sections obtained by each possibility. Each possibility has advantages and disadvantages.

The first clinically available retinal optical coherence tomography (OCT) scans show only cross-sectional images. Cross-section OCT imaging is very intuitive and apparently easy to understand. It is important to always remember that prudence is necessary when interpreting the OCT images and that it is difficult correlating them with histology data. Authors cannot be sure there is an immediate correlation. Cross-section OCT imaging gives a two-dimensional (2D) view of the retina.

A three-dimensional (3D) is given by frontal *en face* scans or C scans. *En face* technology constitutes a useful and necessary complement to the conventional cross-sectional B scan. It brings important new information to the clinician. Frontal scans highlight details of the retina that surgeons cannot see in B scans. Frontal *en face* scans provide a direct, front view of retinal layers.

Frontal *En Face* Plane C Scans

Frontal *en face* plane C scans are available since 2002 with some time domain OCT (TD-OCT) devices. They have a good clinical interest but image interpretation is difficult. Classical C scans are perfectly flat and present already a new vision of the ocular pathology. As the retina is cup shaped, the flat plane section cuts through all the retinal and choroidal layers giving complex planar C scans images difficult to understand.

Concavity of the posterior pole makes it impossible to study with flat scans more than a very small section of a retinal layer. At the immediate proximity of the area under study frontal flat scans cut through all the surrounding layers, going deeper as section goes progressively farther from the zone under study (**Figure 2**). In the OCT scans obtained sugeons see on the same image different layers, some located at distance from the one they want to study (**Figures 3 and 4**).

It is not always easy to get a section parallel to the posterior pole.

Difficulties in Flat C Scan Interpretation

C scan is flat and posterior pole is concave. Retinal surface at the posterior pole shows two depressions that are well evident on the flat sections: the macular depression and the depression between fovea and optic nerve. The flat section will show the macula as a round depression and the inter papillomacular concavity as a bean-shaped depression (**Figures 5A to C**). The nerve fiber layer has not a constant thickness and will show on the C scan.

A problem more important is that rarely the planar section is perfectly parallel to the posterior pole. Very frequently the section plane is vertically or laterally tilted (**Figures 6 and 7**).

If the ocular concavity is marked, due to high myopia, it is even more difficult to get a section parallel to the posterior

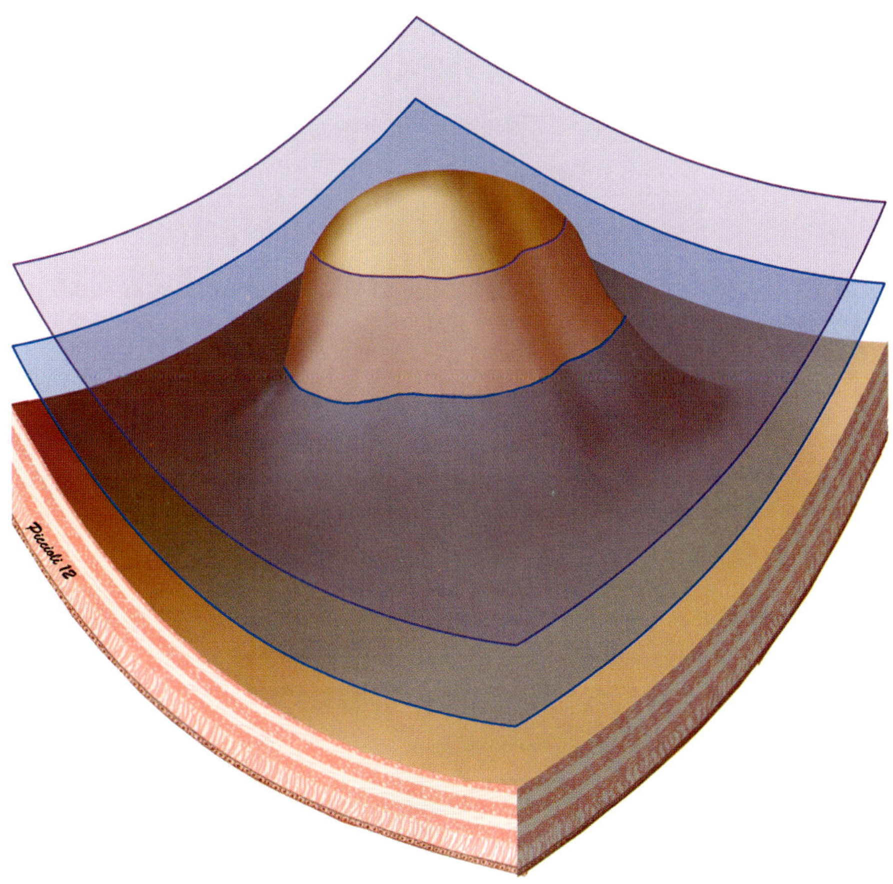

Figure 1: Detachment of the pigment epithelium. Frontal scans adapted to pigment epithelium shape may be at will placed at any constant depth in the retina or choroid and are always parallel to RPE. In this figure two *en face* scans cut frontally a detachment of the pigment epithelium

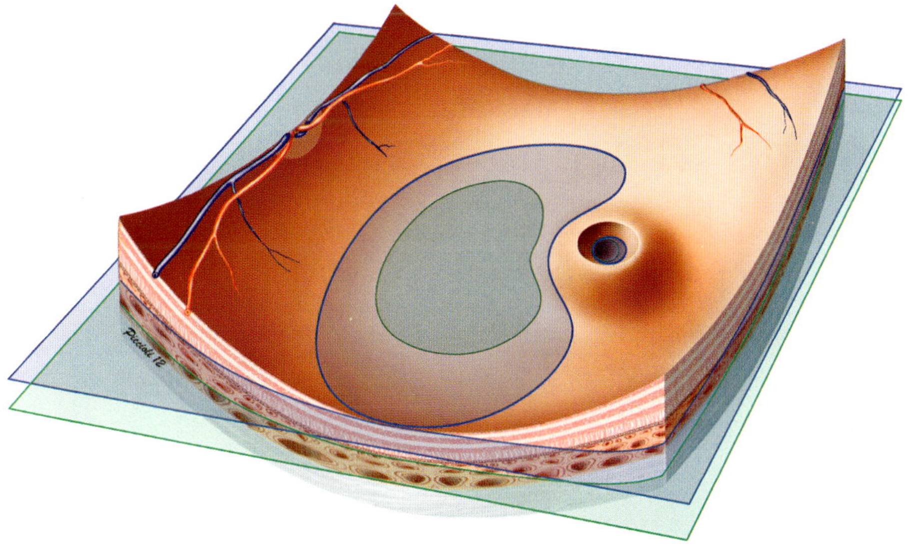

Figure 2: Flat C scan sections are flat and posterior pole is concave. Retinal surface at the posterior pole shows two depressions that are well evident on the flat sections: the macular depression and the depression between fovea and optic nerve. Concavity of the posterior pole makes it impossible to study with flat scans more than a very small section of a retinal layer. At the immediate proximity of the area under study frontal flat scans cut through all the surrounding layers, going deeper as authors go progressively farther from the zone under study

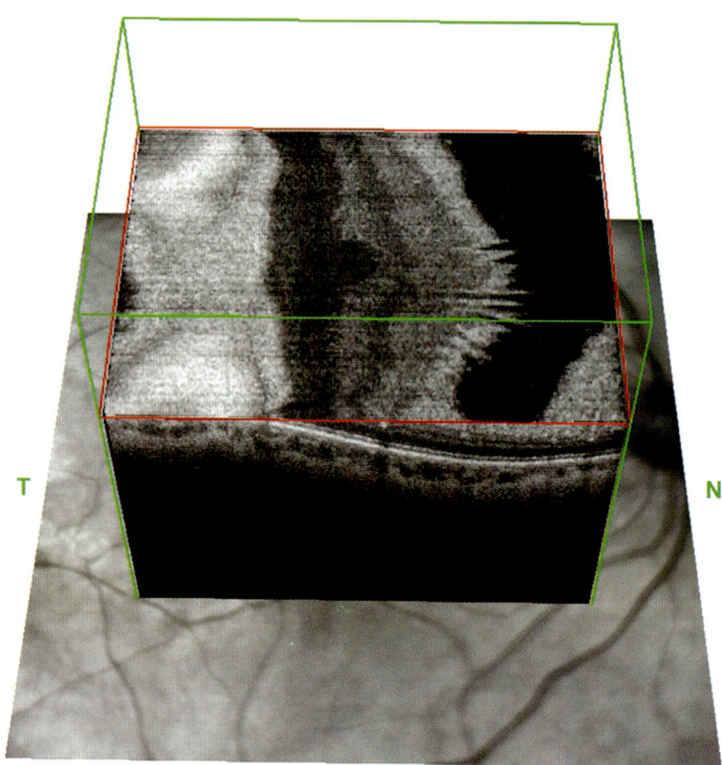

Figure 3: Flat C scan section only a small central part of the scan centers exactly the layer under study; at the immediate proximity of the area under study frontal flat scans cut through all the surrounding layers, going deeper as authors go progressively farther from the zone under study. In the flat OCT scans authors see on the same image different layers, some located at distance from the one authors want to study

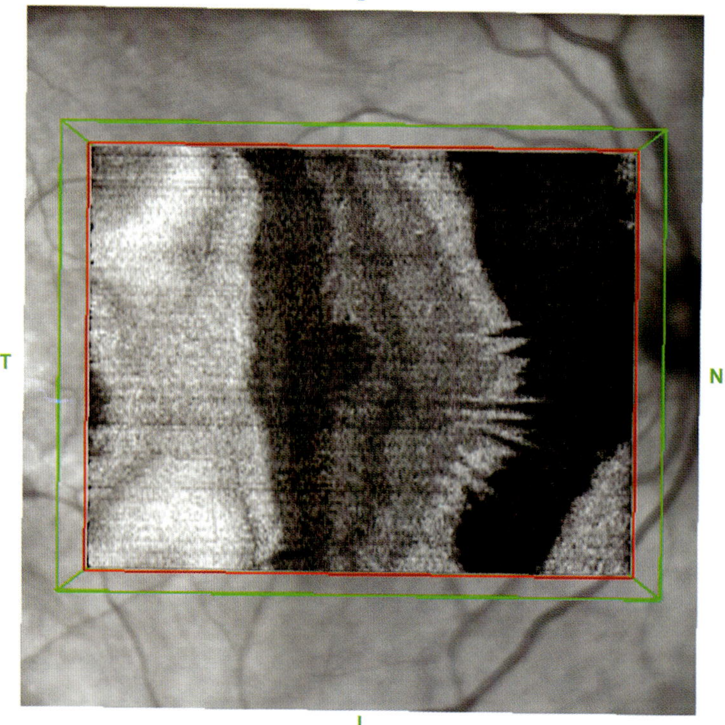

Figure 4: Flat section HRA Heidelberg Spectralis; in the planar scans, the section cannot follow a retinal layer that is normally cup shaped as the posterior pole of the eye. The section is flat and cuts through different layers, some located at distance from the one authors want to study, going from ILM (at right hand side) to RPE to choroid (left hand side)

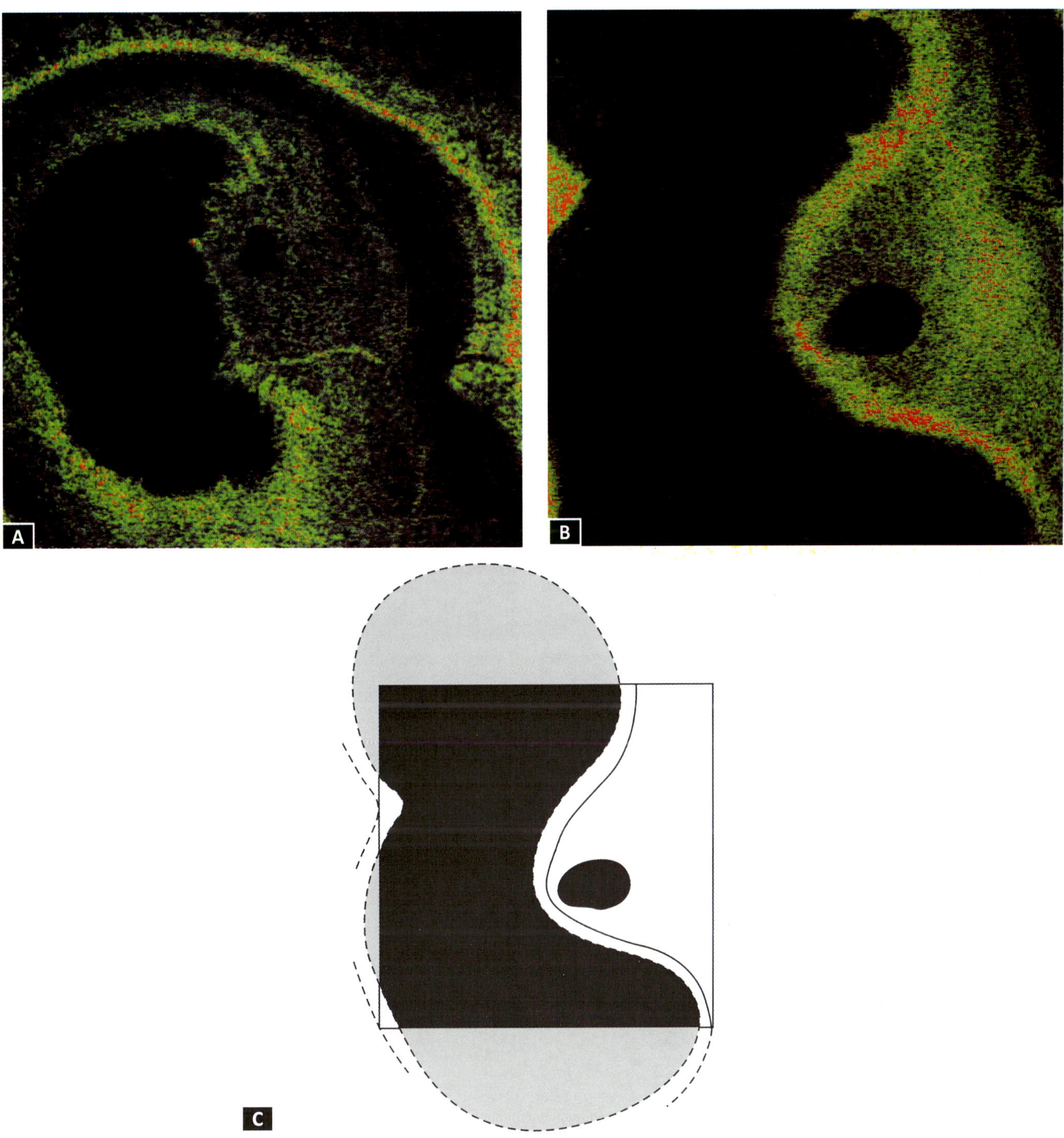

Figures 5A to C: Flat scans; The flat section at the posterior pole of the retina shows the macula as a round depression and the interpapillomacular concavity as a bean-shaped depression (OTI)

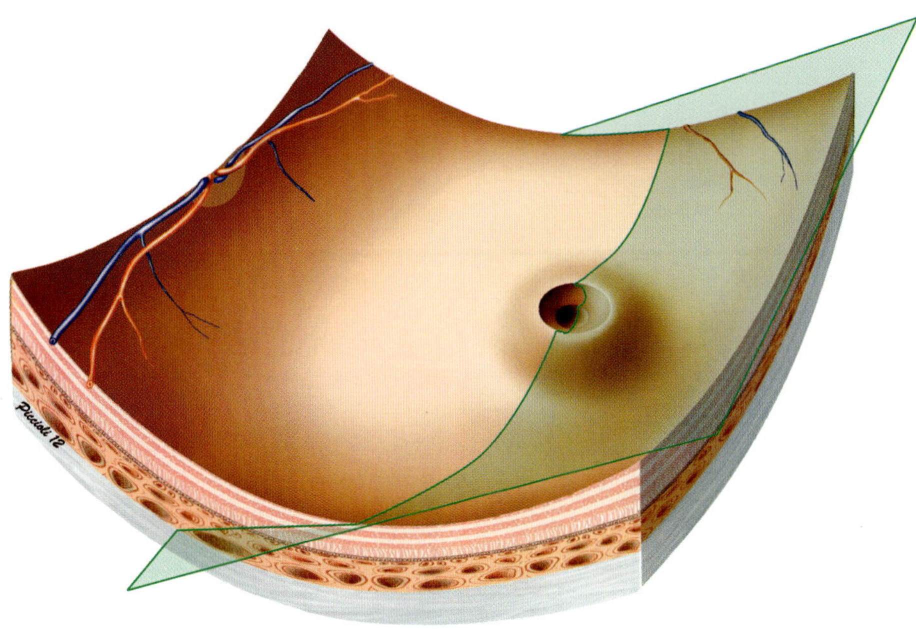

Figure 6: Tilted planar frontal scans. The planar section is rarely perfectly parallel to the posterior pole and perpendicular to visual axis. Here the section plane is laterally tilted. Tilted plane sections are difficult to analyze and understand

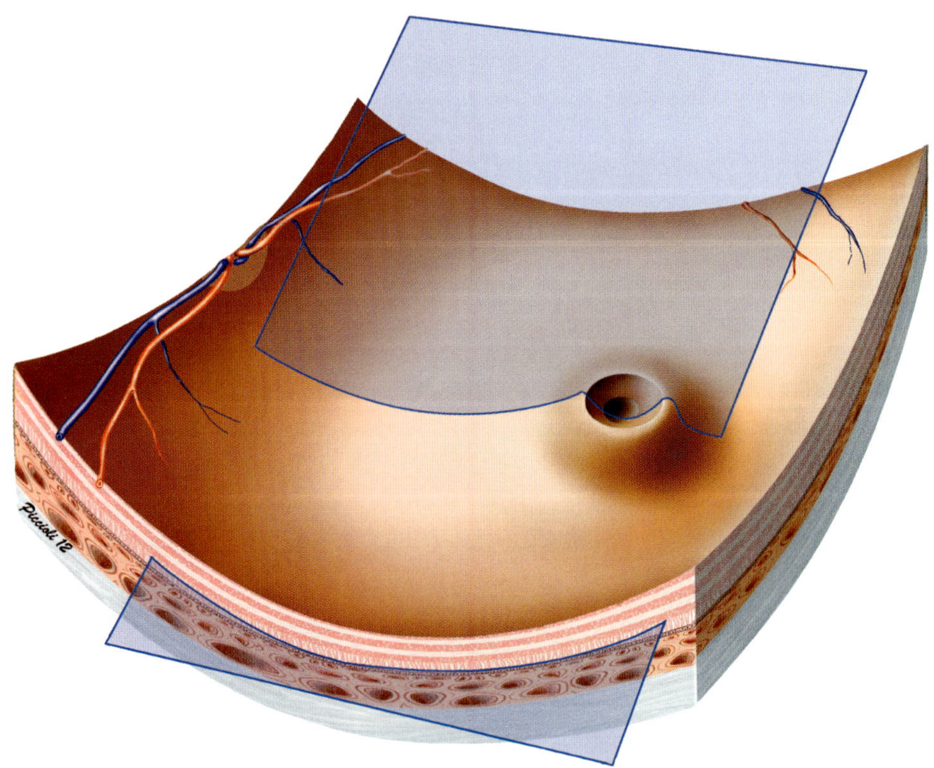

Figure 7: Tilted planar scan. The planar section is not parallel to the posterior pole: here the scan is vertically tilted. If the ocular concavity is marked, due to high myopia, it is even more difficult to get a section parallel to the posterior pole. Images from myopic, emmetropic and hypermetropic eyes are very different

pole. Tilted plane sections are difficult to analyze and understand. Images from myopic, emmetropic and hypermetropic eyes are very different.

Artifacts are frequent and sometimes difficult to distinguish from pathological retinal anomalies. For these reasons flat C scans are not very much used anymore. They are considered obsolete.

En Face Frontal Scans Generated to Follow the Cup-shaped Pigment Epithelium Contour

Instead of making a section, the *en face* scan may be generated following a natural surface contour. Its thickness is generally uniform. Most *en face* scans (Optovue RTVue, Zeiss Cirrus) adapt the retinal section authors want to study the actual shape of the pigment epithelium surgeons decided to use as basis of our scans. OCT scans adapted to the normal concavity of the retinal pigment epithelium (RPE) or of the inner limiting membrane (ILM) enable imaging the finer details of epiretinal membranes, macular edema, pigmented epithelial detachment (PED) and drusen.

En face images, adapted to the cup-shaped retina are an improvement on plane scans for clinical and research purposes. They bring to frontal scan the possibility to obtain a retinal or choroidal section that follows the RPE curve and is parallel to it. Frontal scans adapted to pigment epithelium shape, may be at will placed at any constant depth in the retina or choroid and are always parallel to RPE. Surgeons obtain thus an optical *in vivo* dissection of the layer of the retina or choroid they want to study, the possibility to isolate a layer from the other layers and look it from any direction, rotating it **(Figures 8 to 10)**.

Frontal scans generated to follow a retinal surface contour or adapted to pigment epithelium shape are placed at constant depth in the retina or choroid and parallel to RPE.

Frontal scans adapted to pigment epithelium shape bring new elements for the diagnosis and follow-up of retinal diseases and provide a good overview of the retina under study, allowing the assessment of all the scanned area within the retinal cube. They give us unusual points of view of the ocular pathologies and highlight details surgeons could not have seen without this technology **(Figures 11A and C)**.

En face scan procedures are easy to perform and images easy to understand after a short learning period. The first time authors see *en face* images they could seem strange. They are not as intuitive to understand as classical cross-section scans. In fact the only difficulty is in interpretation of the scans because the global aspects of the retina were

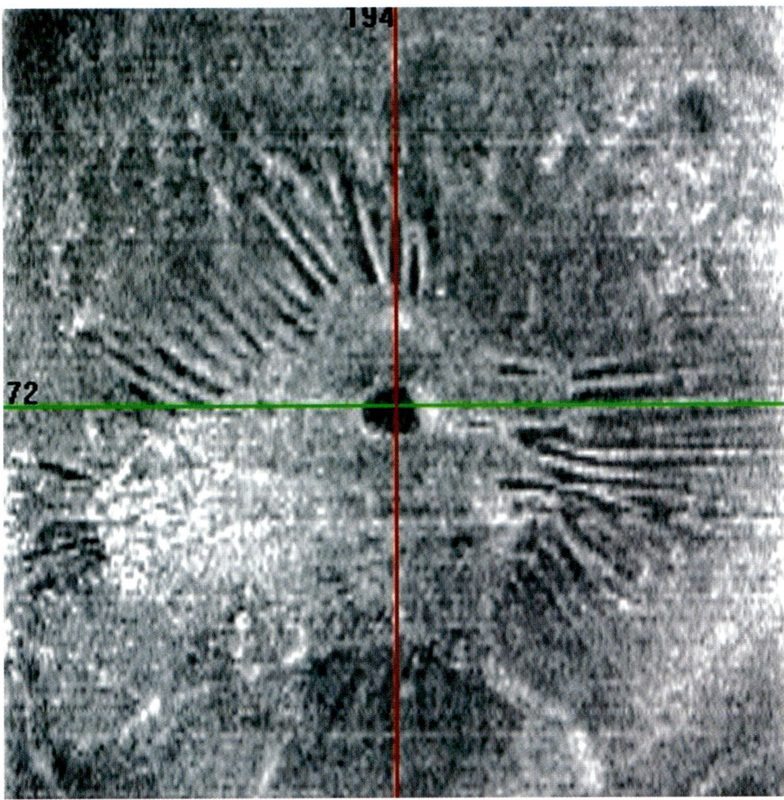

Figure 8: Frontal ILM scan; *en face* technology (Optovue RTVue) can follow the irregularities of a pathologic vitreoretinal boundary obtaining a delineation of the epiretinal membranes and vitreoretinal tractions

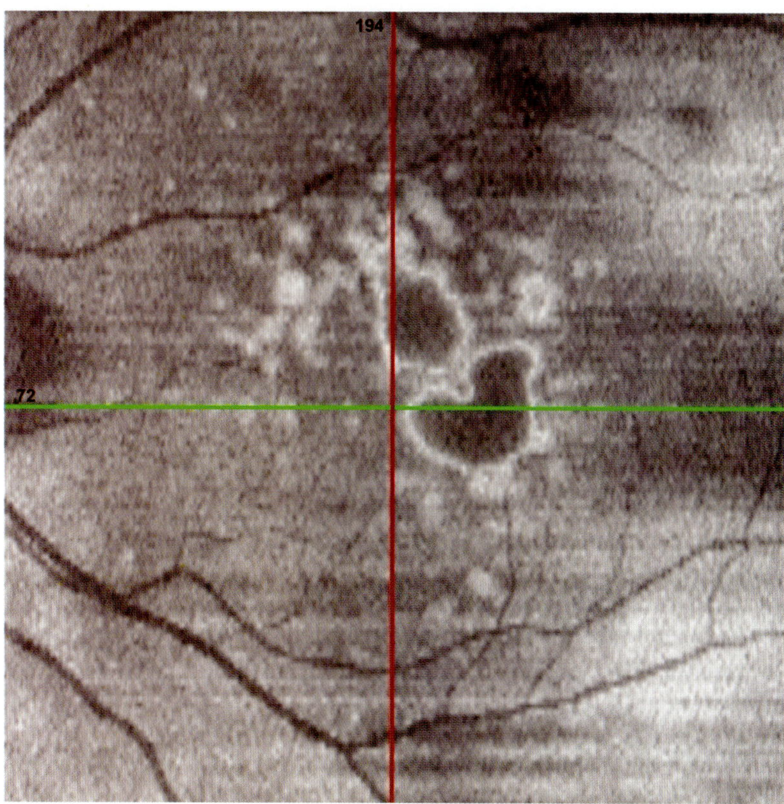

Figure 9: Frontal RPE scan (Optovue RTVue) *en face* scan follow the irregularities of a pathologic RPE obtaining a delineation of the pigment epithelium irregularities, drusen detachments. The bigger pigment epithelium detachments are cut through by the scan section

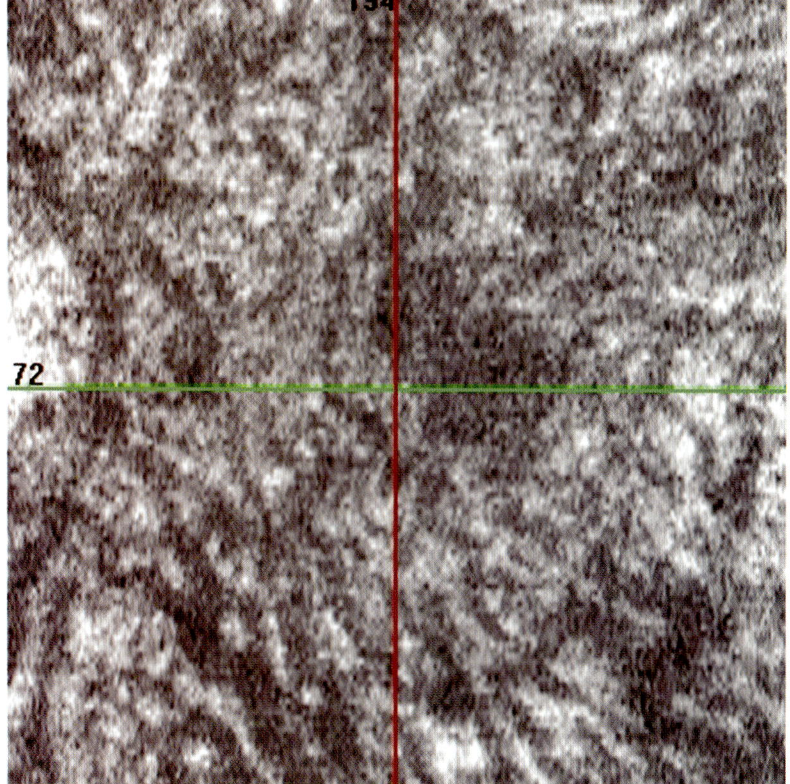

Figure 10: Frontal choroid scan (Optovue RTVue) frontal scan of the choroid at the large vessels level (Haller layer)

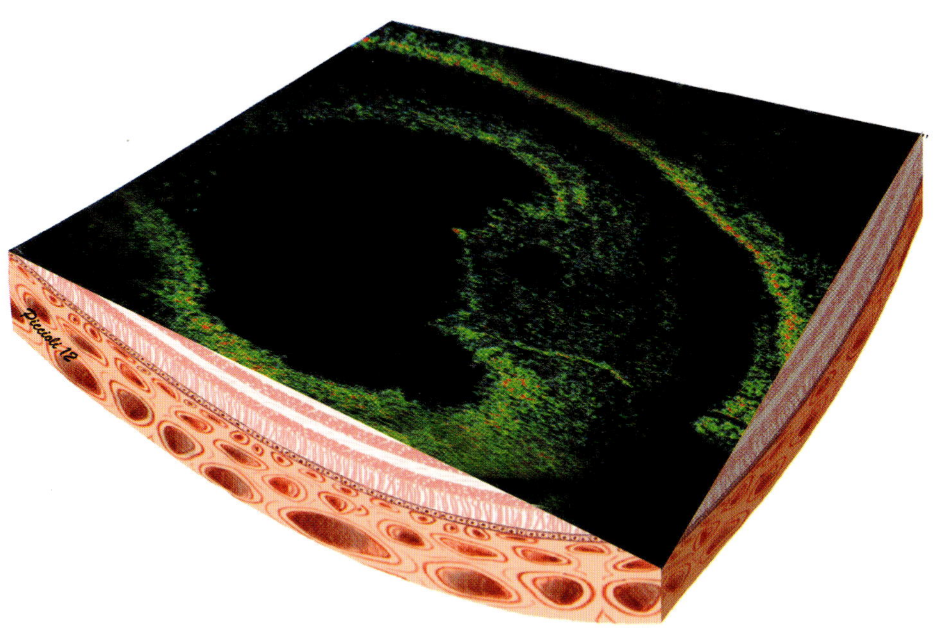

Figure 11A: Flat C scan; the drawing shows a flat section of the retina. The frontal flat scans cut through all surrounding layers, going deeper in the retina and in choroid as authors go progressively farther from the fovea

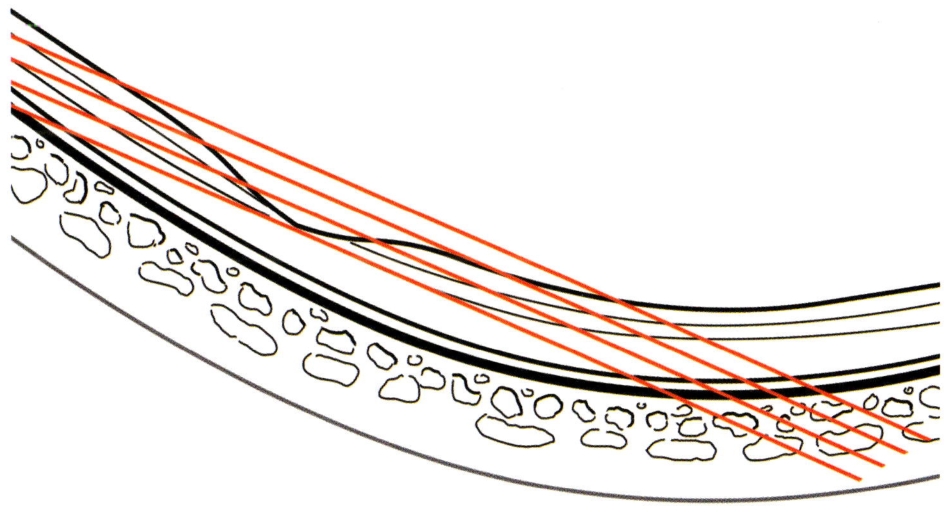

Figure 11B: Posterior pole cross section; flat C scan sections and concave posterior pole

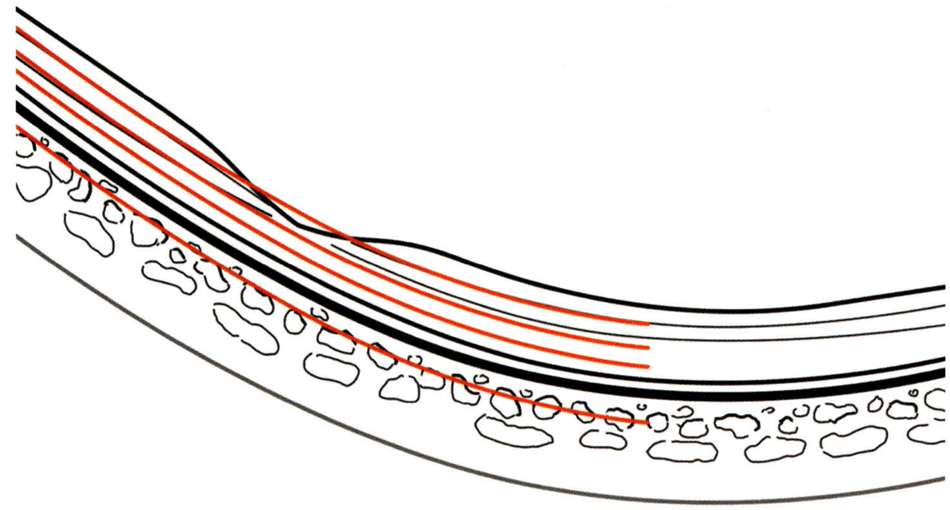

Figure 11C: Posterior pole cross section; OCT sections adapted to RPE ideal concavity and concave posterior pole. The OCT concave scan can be placed at any level in retina or choroid to study any layer

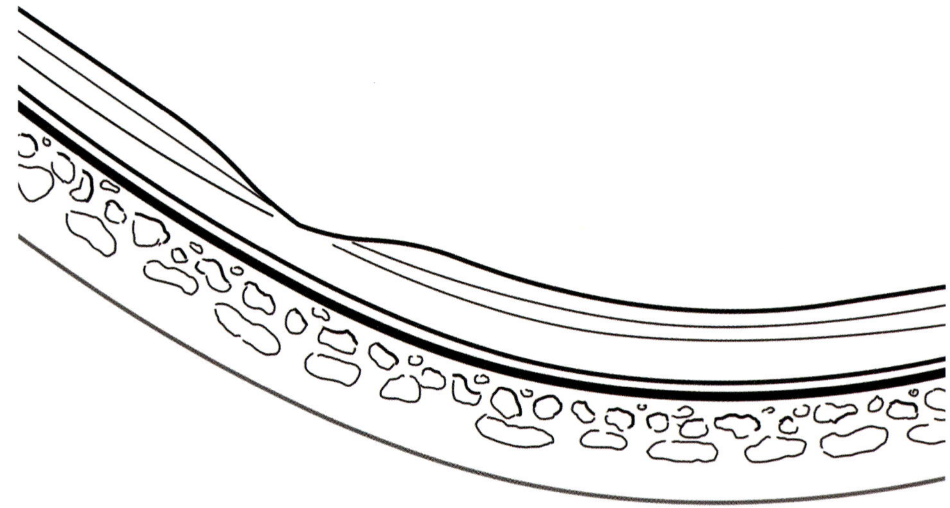

Figure 11D: Posterior pole cross section; concave posterior pole

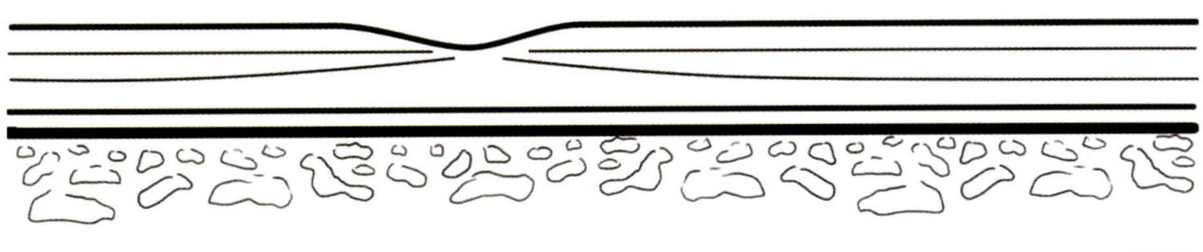

Figure 11E: Posterior pole cross section; the drawing gives an artist interpretation of how the software straightens the retinal cube and align it parallel to horizontal structures such as the RPE. Retina is ideally flattened to RPE. The drawing is an artist interpretation that does not represent the actual software action. The artist tries to show frontal scans aligned or flattened to pigment epithelium

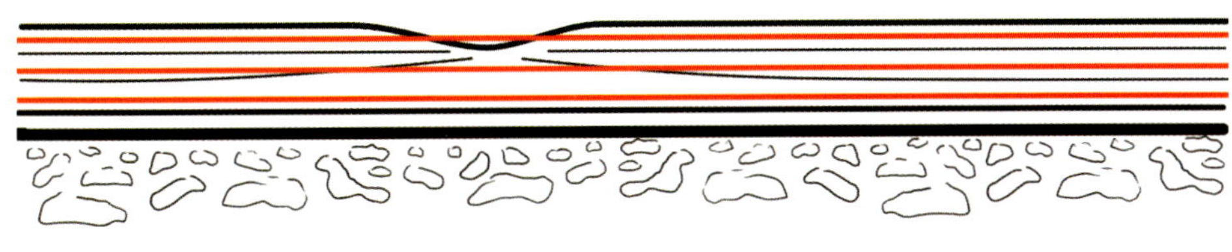

Figure 11F: Posterior pole cross section; flat frontal scans aligned to pigment epithelium, may be placed at any constant depth in the retina or choroid. The artist tries to show frontal scans aligned or flattened to pigment epithelium

until recently unknown to the clinicians, but the learning curve is fast.

Frontal *en face* scans give clinical information on retinal disturbances and are very important for research. Moreover, the 3D cube allows retinal segmentation, delineating the individual retinal layers. *En face* scans (frontal scans adapted to pigment epithelium paraboloid shape) help diagnose retinal and choroidal diseases.

En face technology can follow the irregularities of a pathologic RPE: obtaining a delineation of the drusen or of the PED. *En face* scans are clinically important because they can give quantitative information.

But, it is even more important to have an *en face* frontal scan following the ideal RPE concavity and cutting through pathologic alterations. The frontal scans are parallel to RPE, at a constant depth in the retina.

En face technology can follow the irregularities of a pathologic vitreoretinal boundary obtaining a delineation of the epiretinal membranes and vitreoretinal tractions. *En face* OCT of the retinal surface allows visualization of the retinal surface following the concavity of the posterior pole of the eye with high quality imaging that would not be obtained from longitudinal scans alone. *En face* scans are clinically important because they can give quantitative information.

For the moment only Optovue and Zeiss OCT devices give frontal scans adapted to retinal concavity, scans generated to follow a retinal surface contour. All the other clinically available devices produce classical planar C scans.

The frontal scans are parallel to ideal pigment epithelium, at a constant depth in the retina or choroid and thus study each retinal and choroidal layer separately. *En face* scan procedures are easy to perform and images easy to analyze. *En face* frontal scans that follow the ideal pigment epithelium concavity and cut through pathologic alterations are easy to understand.

After the macular cube acquisition the *en face* images are reconstructed from the cube data.

En face scan may follow the inner limiting membrane (ILM) curvature or the pigment epithelium concavity. The profile should be selected according to the retinal or choroidal layers under study.

Inner limiting membrane scan will be used in case of vitreal or vitreoretinal anomalies; inner plexiform layer (IPL) in case of edema or exudates, pigment epithelium scan will be used in outer retina or choroid diseases.

En face technology can follow the irregularities of a pathologic RPE or the ILM. It will give three-dimensional (3D) images useful to understand the lesion shape and dimensions and perfect as teaching tool.

Authors normally choose as reference the pigment epithelium ideal concavity for the section they want to obtain. It cancels the abnormalities of the pigment epithelium in the eye under study and gives a theoretical ideal 3D reference.

Scan Thickness

Reducing the scan thickness surgeons obtain a thin retinal slice. The image may be noisy but the sensitivity will be very high. If surgeons increase the scan thickness the image will be smoother but little details may be lost as they will not have a thin slice to study but a thick retinal slab.

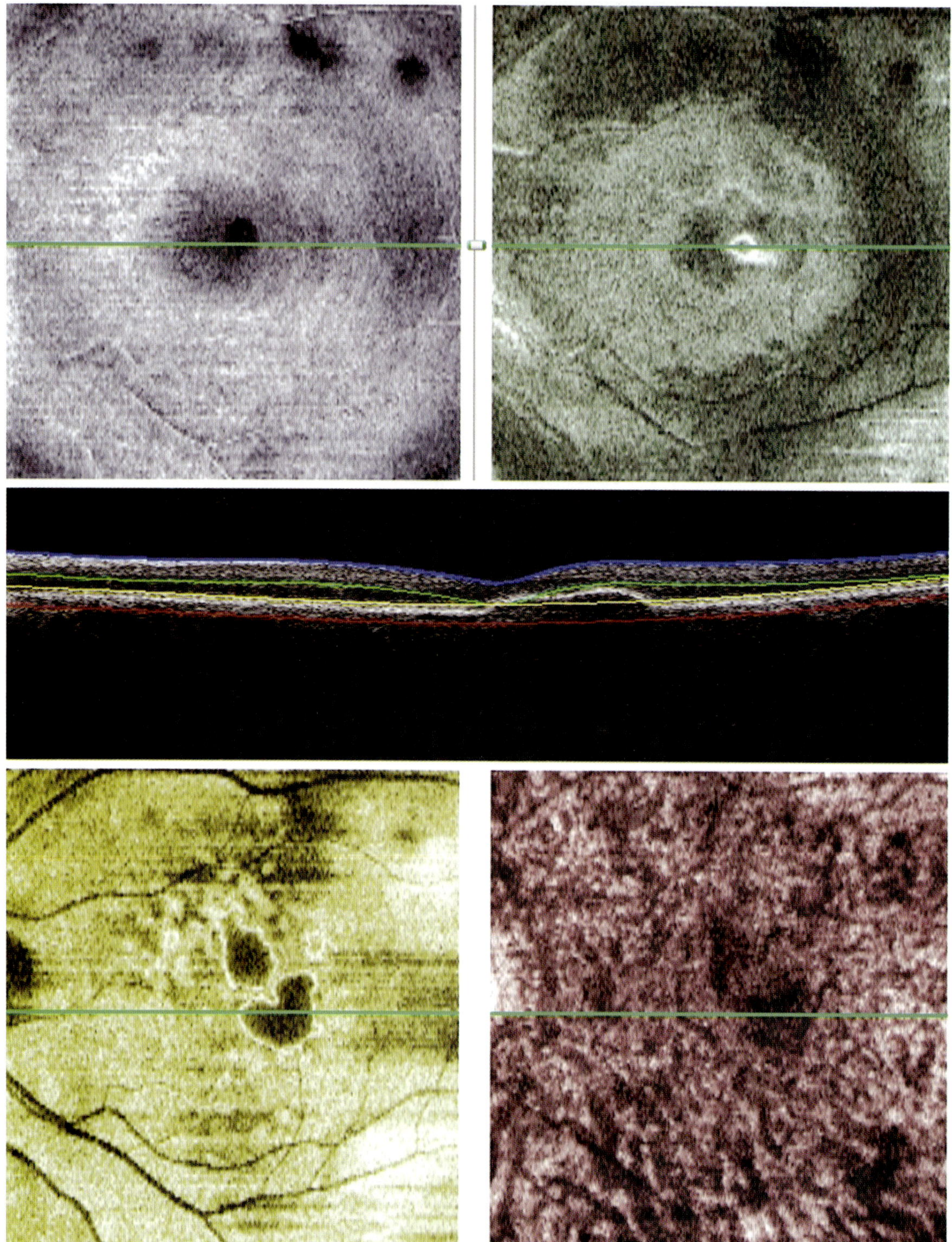

Figure 12: *En face* one click mode (Optovue RTVue): Pigment epithelium detachment in AMD

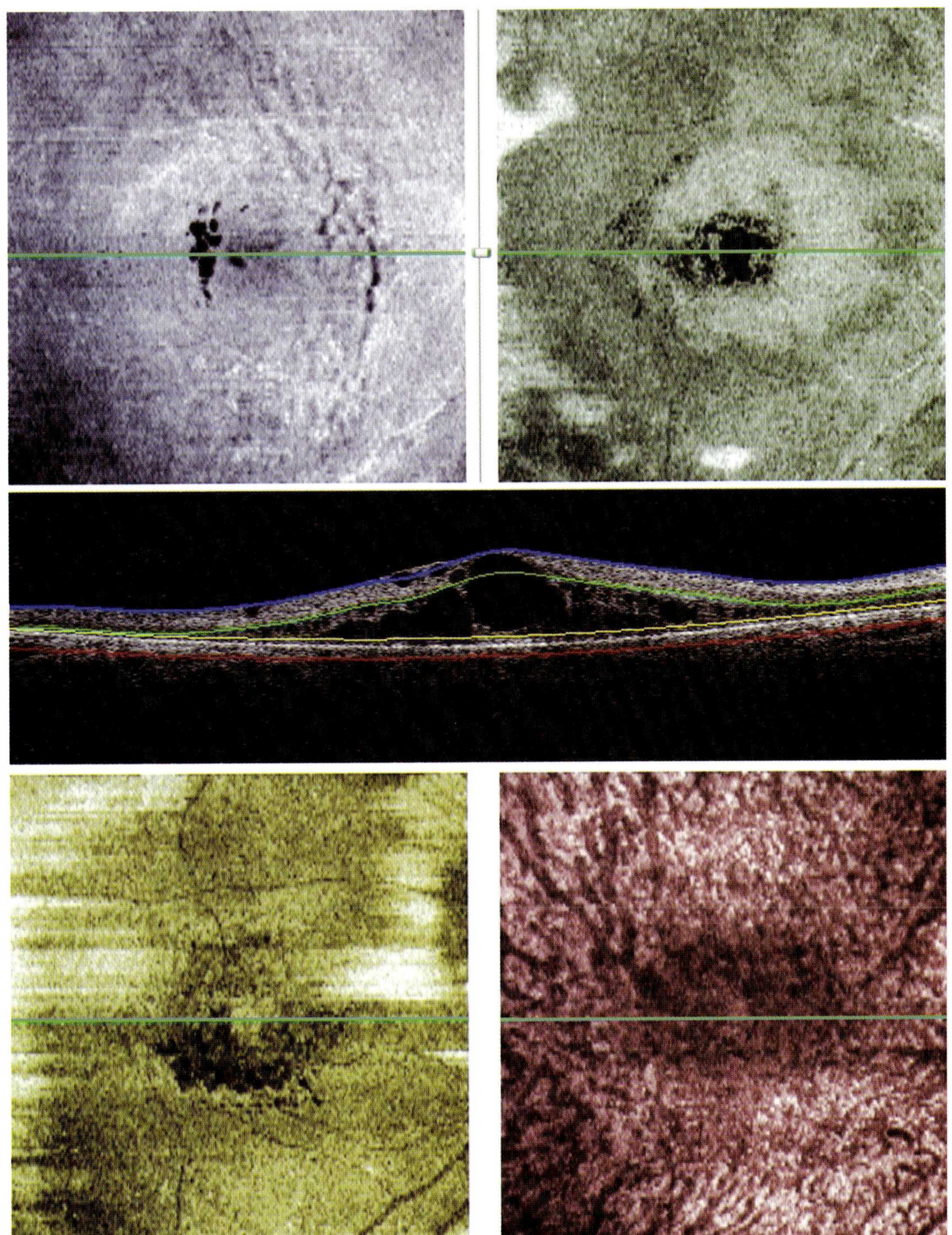

Figure 13: *En face* one click mode (Optovue RTVue): Cystoid edema

Figures 12 and 13: Lumbroso vue *en face* one click mode (Optovue RTVue).

The *en face* one click mode gives in a single move five scans: four *en face* scans illustrating to the most clinically important frontal sections, and a cross line scan.

The first *en face* scan is taken at retinal surface level and shows retina vitreous interface alterations, retinal folds, parallel or stellate. The second is placed deeper in retina shows eventually diffuse edema, cystoid edema and exudates. The third *en face* scan is parallel to retinal pigment. It cuts through drusen and RPEDs. It is useful in AMD, choroidal polypoidal vasculopathy, central serous retinopathy, diffuse chronic epitheliopathy. The fourth scan is in the choroid, parallel to RPE at level of Haller vascular layer. It shows choroid condition: choroid vessels are dilated in central serous retinopathy, diffuse chronic epitheliopathy. Choroid vessels are thinner in retinal atrophies and dystrophies. One cross section scan helps understand the frontal sections

Scan Depth

It is possible to shif forward or backward the *en face* cup-shaped lamina to the retinal layer surgeons want to study or to the different layers of the choroid. The device shows automatically on the screen the exact depth location inside the retina or the choroid and the slice thickness.

En face **One Click Mode**

RTVue-100 new software makes simpler and faster acquisition and use of *en face* images. It created the *en face* one click mode (Lumbroso-vue) that gives in a single move five scans: four *en face* scans illustrating to the most clinically important frontal sections, and a cross line scan (**Figures 12 and 13**).

The first *en face* scan is taken at retinal surface level, the second is placed deeper in retina. The third *en face* scan is parallel to retinal pigment. The fourth scan is in the choroid, parallel to RPE at level of Haller vascular layer.

The OCT cross line scan shows the exact level in the retina of the four frontal scans.

Thus in an immediate and easy way the normal OCT user will get immediately the *en face* images clinically useful for diagnosis, and will know their exact position in relation to retina and choroid layers. Expert OCT users will be able to fine-tune diagnosis modifying scan thickness and depth of acquisition.

En Face Frontal Scans Aligned (Straightened) Parallel to Pigment Epithelium

Heidelberg Engineering introduced recently another technique of frontal imaging. They released a new software module that allows to view transverse sections of OCT volume scans acquired with Spectralis. The special settings allow to view volume scan data in a variety of different ways. The transverse sections that are aligned parallel to structures such as the RPE. The transverse section module takes full advantage of the Spectralis ability to acquire OCT volume scans with a B scan distance as small as 11 µm. With this acquisition it is possible to get an isotropic transverse section image of 11 µm lateral resolution. Frontal scans aligned or flattened to pigment epithelium shape, can be at will placed at any distance within the retina or choroid and are always parallel to RPE (**Figures 14 to 17**).

En face technology allows to obtain frontal scans adapted to the concavity of the eye posterior pole. Standard retina and macula analysis should always include en face analysis.

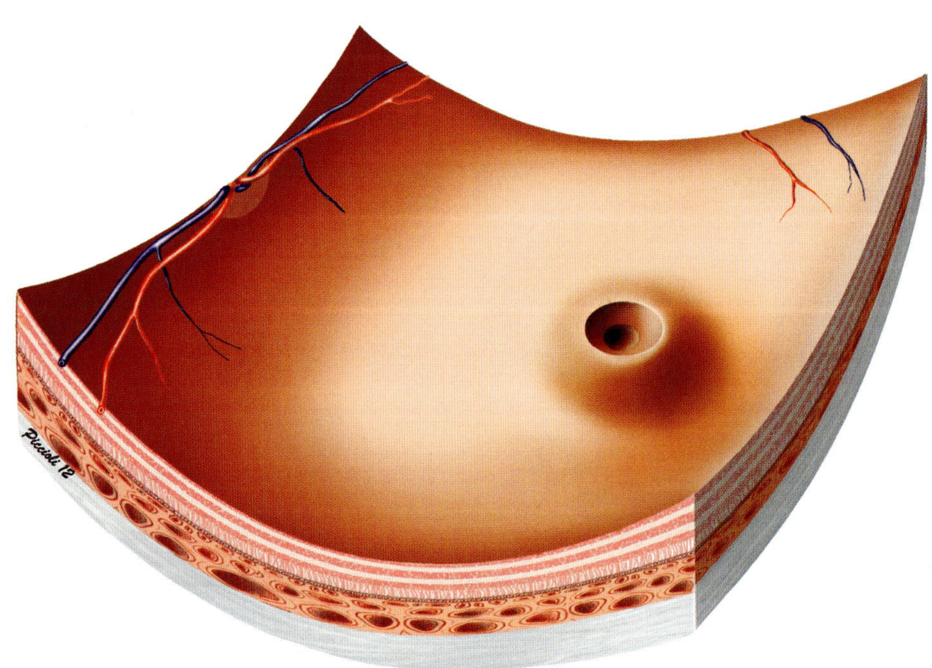

Figure 14: Spectralis software normal retinal concavity

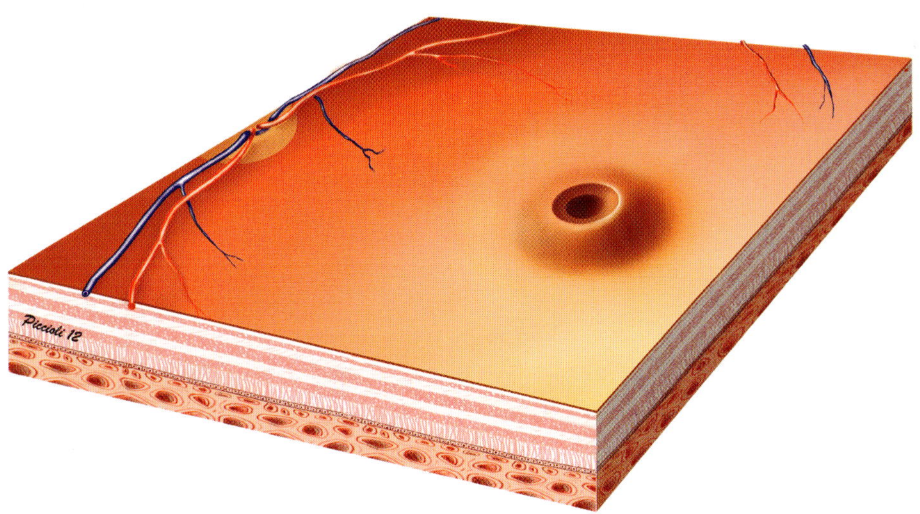

Figure 15: Spectralis aligned (straightened) cube. The drawing gives an artist interpretation of how the software straightens the retinal cube and align it parallel to horizontal structures such as the RPE. Retina is ideally flattened to RPE. The drawing does not represent the actual software action

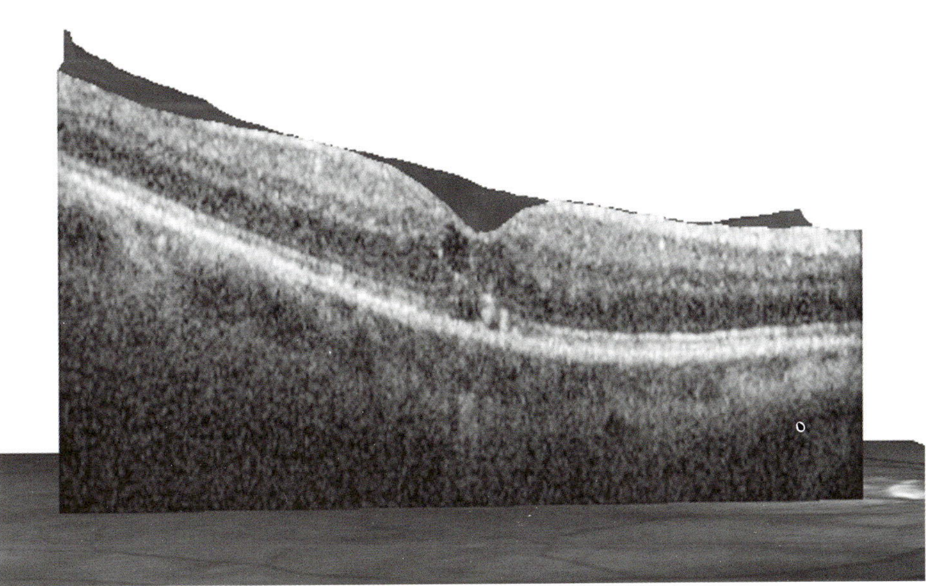

Figure 16: Spectralis cross-section showing pigment epithelium and IS/OS segment normal concavity

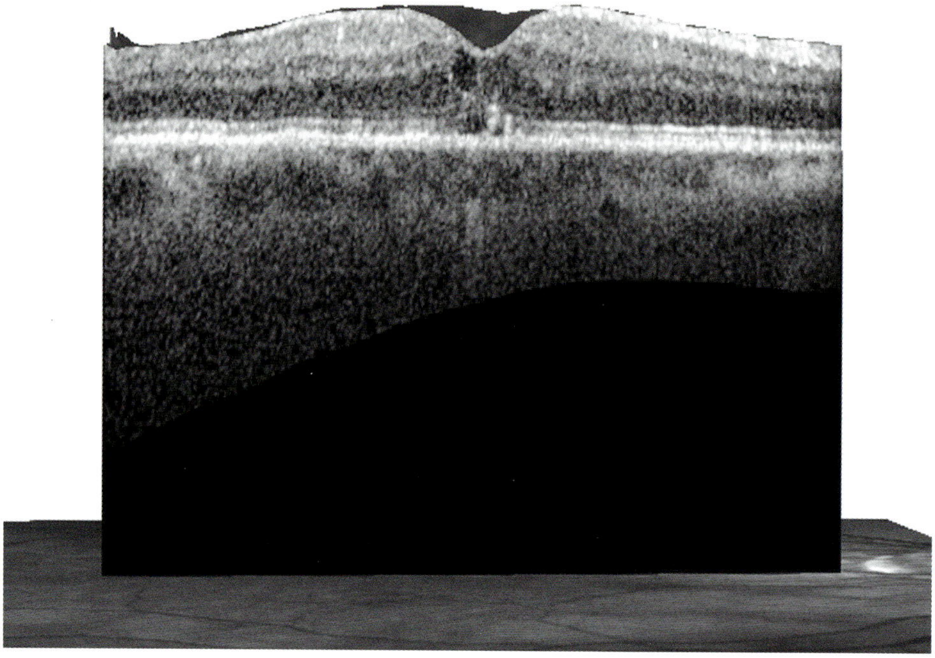

Figure 17: Spectralis cross-section showing pigment epithelium and IS/OS segment after straightening (aligning) by software

Section 2

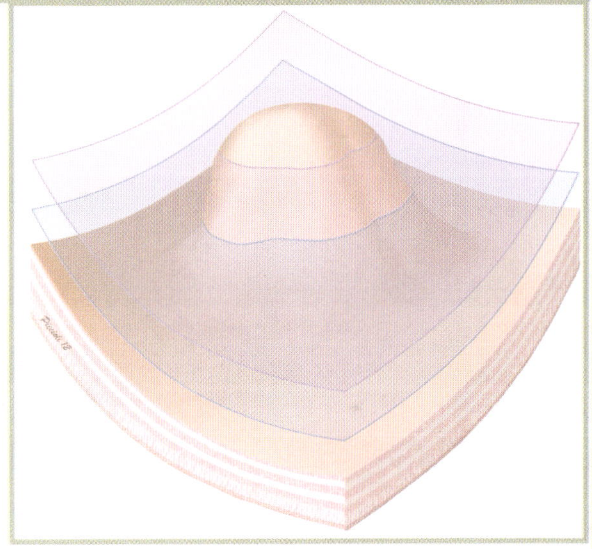

En Face Optical Coherence Tomography Structure and Histology

chapter 4

Retinal Structures and *En Face* Optical Coherence Tomography Features

Bruno Lumbroso, Marco Rispoli

Introduction

In order to understand *en face* optical coherence tomography (OCT) morphology it is indispensable to know frontal retinal anatomy and histology. In this chapter authors illustrate the frontal structures that need to be known to allow a correct interpretation and understanding of *en face* images. The transition from cross section OCT imaging to *en face* imaging involves a qualitative intellectual shift. Modern OCTs can reliably image not only ocular surfaces, but also the transversal (frontal) intraretinal structures with the quality of histological sections. The *en face* OCT is designed to virtually dissect retina. The development of sophisticated software capable of processing large data loads makes it possible to virtually dissect the vitreous, retina and retinal pigment epithelium (RPE), choroid and sclera.

There is not an immediate correlation between virtual OCT dissection and histology. Prudence is necessary when interpreting the OCT images and correlating them with histology data. Authors cannot be sure there is always a correlation.

Segmentation of the tissue makes it easier to visually understand the repercussions that pathological structures have on surrounding retinal layers.

En Face Optical Coherence Tomography Representation of the Retina

Optical tomography of the posterior pole of a normal retina seems to reveal a correlation between the anatomy of the eye and the structures that are observed via OCT retinal scanning. The study of retinal anatomy in relation to *en face* OCT involves subdivisions consisting of the macula, the area inside the vascular arcades and the retinal periphery outside of these structures.

Retinal Structures and their *En Face* Optical Coherence Tomography Features from Sclera to Vitreous

Choroid Arteries

The macula is supplied by the temporal peripapillary arteries. Ducournau (1980)[1,2] demonstrated that the short posterior ciliary arteries, on both the nasal and temporal sides, can be divided into two groups, one arranged around the papilla and one around the macula. One group perforates the sclera close to the optic nerve. The second group enters into the choroid beneath the macula. After entering the choroid most of the arteries describe a bend or knee before running to the retinal periphery (**Figure 1**).

Choroid Veins

There are four to eight vortex veins and a drainage area allocated to approximately four quadrants. At the posterior pole veins run diagonally across the macular area (**Figure 2**).

Watersheds

According to Hayreh,[3] watersheds exist between these venous outflow system. Indocyanine green (ICG) angiographs show them running horizontally through the macula and disk at the level of the lateral long posterior ciliary artery and also vertically through the papillomacular region. Thus the papillomacular region lies at a watershed of the arterial as the venous vessel supply (**Figure 3**).

Choriocapillaris

It consists of polygonal vascular lobules which independently receive blood from the short posterior ciliary arteries. The

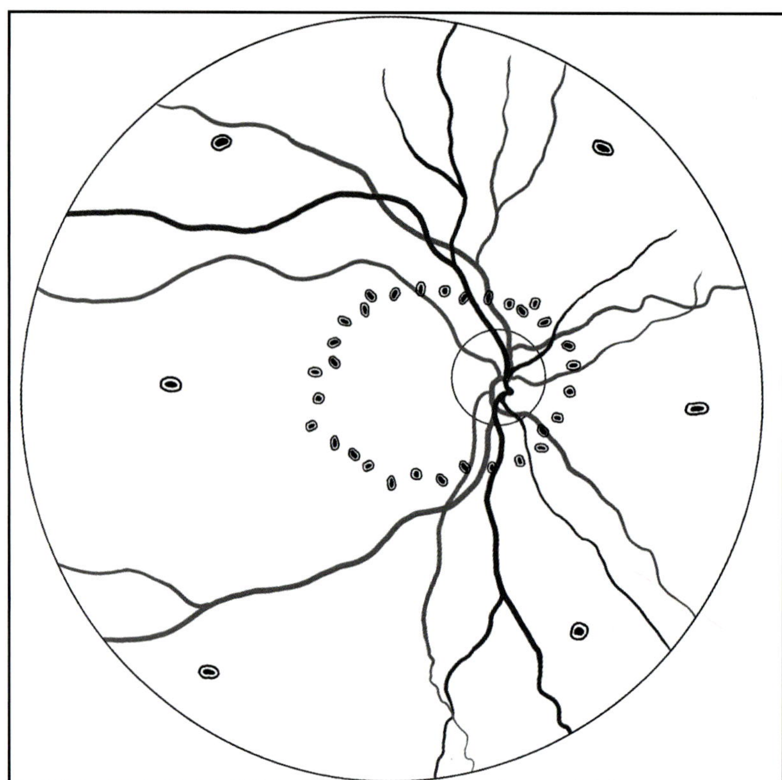

Figure 1: Choroid arteries; the macula is supplied by the temporal peripapillary arteries. The short posterior ciliary arteries, on both the nasal and temporal sides, can be divided into two groups, one arranged around the papilla and one around the macula. One group perforates the sclera close to the optic nerve. The second group enters into the choroid beneath the macula. After entering the choroid most of the arteries describe a bend or knee before running to the retinal periphery

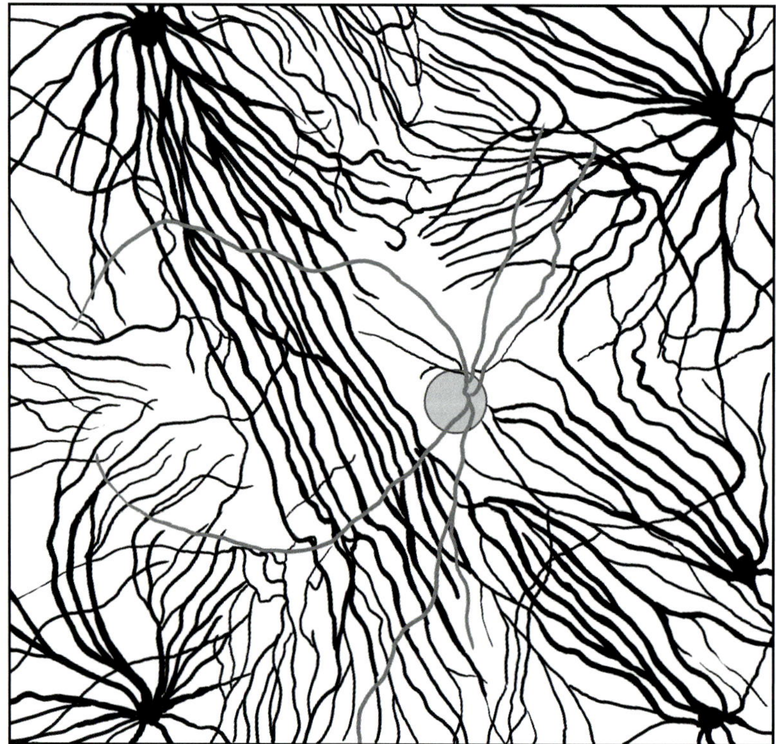

Figure 2: Choroid veins; at the posterior pole veins run diagonally across the macular area. There are four to eight vortex veins and a drainage area allocated to approximately four quadrants

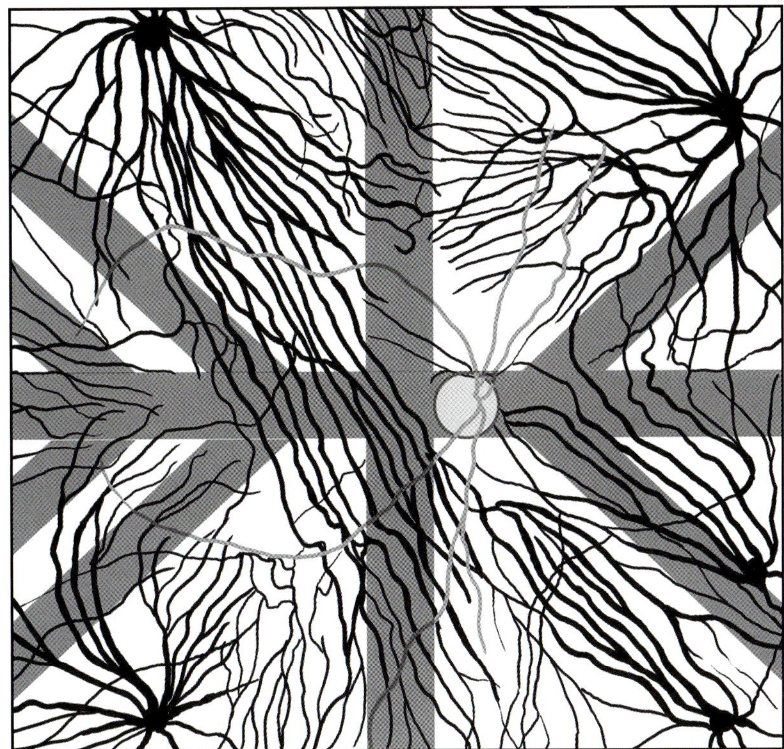

Figure 3: Watersheds exist between venous outflow systems. They run horizontally through the macula and disk at the level of the lateral long posterior ciliary artery and also vertically through the papillomacular region. Thus the papillomacular region lies at a watershed of the arterial as the venous vessel supply

venous blood is drained from the smaller veins into the vortex veins, of which there are one or two per quadrant. The choriocapillaris not always identified.

Retinal Pigment Epithelium

The retinal pigment epithelium (RPE) consists of a single layer of polygonal cells, some 15 microns wide with the nucleus being in the basal side. The inner side of the cell is deeply cupped and consists of villi tightly surrounding the tips of the rods and cones. At the fovea, each cell of the RPE surrounds a single cone whereas toward the periphery each cell accommodates more than one cone and rod thus forming small nests at each end. The outer surface of the pigment epithelium is flat and rests upon Bruch's membrane. Along the lateral walls of the RPE cells are tight junctions that block the free exchange of ions and macromolecules between the choriocapillaris and the photoreceptors. As a layer, the pigment epithelium forms the outer blood-retinal barrier.

Outer Retinal Layers

Photoreceptors—junction between inner and outer segment of the photoreceptors: En face OCT scans adapted to the concavity of the posterior pole and passing exactly through the level of the junction between inner and outer segment of the photoreceptors normally show only a gray uniform sheet. In case of lesions localized to the junction they allow to exactly localize and map the lesions of the photoreceptors as dark areas. They show the lesion shape, extension, surface and localization. *The study and mapping of photoreceptor lesions constitute one of the major achievements of En face OCT.* Authors recently renamed the photoreceptors junction: "Ellipsoid zone".

Ganglion Cells Layer

These rather bulky cells are multilayered in the macula but toward the ora serrata they are sparse and spread out. Their axons constitute the retinal nerve fiber layer (RNFL).

Retinal Veins, Arteries and Capillaries

The sensory retina is supplied by two distinctly different systems. The external third of the retina, receives its nutrients from the choroidal vascular system. The deeper outer retinal layers are avascular and are nourished by transudation from the choroid.

The inner layers, apart from the avascular zone around the fovea are supplied by the retinal arterial capillaries that penetrate to the inner nuclear layer. The largest branches

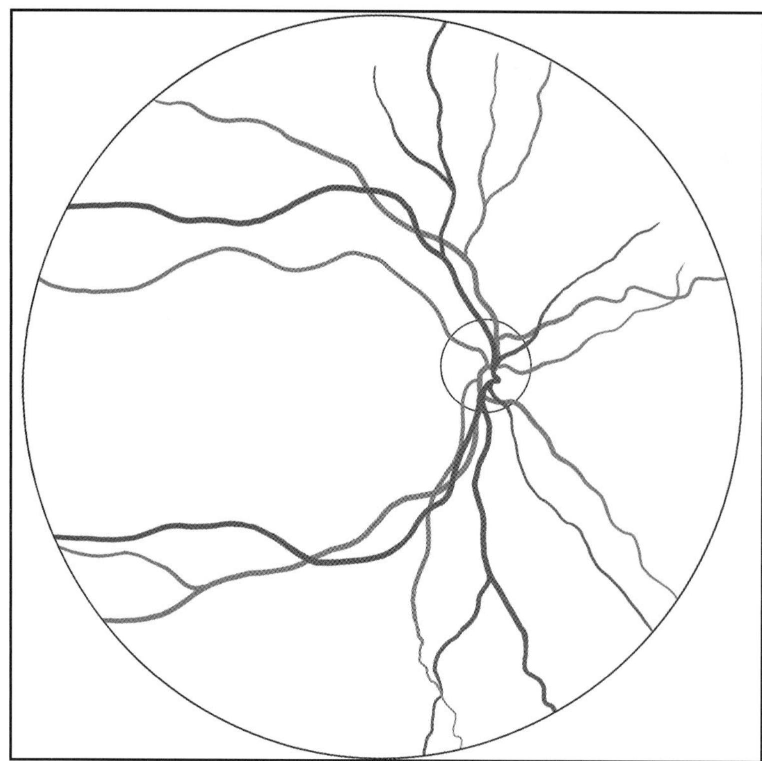

Figure 4: Retinal veins, arteries and capillaries; the inner retinal layers, apart from the avascular zone around the fovea are supplied by the retinal arterial capillaries that penetrate to the inner nuclear layer. The largest branches are located in the nerve-fiber layer and form a network with large links, while the capillaries form a more closely-knit network

are located in the nerve-fiber layer, and form a loosely-knit network with large links, while the capillaries are observed in the inner half of the retina, extending to the nuclear layer, and form a more closely-knit network. The retinal capillaries are from 5–10 microns in diameter (**Figure 4**).

The retina is interrupted at the limits of the papilla. The pigmented epithelium and the choriocapillaris are truncated, while the superficial nerve fibers display continuity with the fibers of the optic nerve. The scleral ring can be seen.

The posterior pole, cup-shaped, with the long axis oriented horizontally, is approximately 8–10 millimeters in size. It is now possible to study by *en face* OCT the entire posterior pole.

Macular Area

The macula, which is 150–190 microns thick, is located at the center of the posterior pole, where it forms a slight depression centered on the fovea and the foveola. It is 1,200 microns in diameter. Inside the macular area is located the avascular area which is 450–500 microns in diameter. This avascular area limits are defined by a continuous ring of very fine anastomoses of the perifoveal vascular network, consisting of a single layer of capillaries.

The fovea itself is 350 microns in diameter and located inside the avascular area while the foveola, which corresponds to the macular center, measures approximately 120–150 microns. Inside the macular area are retinal capillaries 5–10 microns in diameter.

The **avascular area** inside macular area is 450–500 microns in diameter (**Figure 5**).

Outside the macular area, the thickness of the retina is 270–280 microns. The interpapillomacular region is slightly thicker.

Retinal Nerve Fiber Layer

This layer consists of nerve axons that run from the ganglion cell bodies to the optic nerve. This is a very hyper-reflective layer consisting of horizontal structures and its thickness increases as it approaches the papilla. Nerve fibers run radially from the nerve fiber layer to the optic disc. This pattern is evident in the nasal half of the retina, but disturbed in the temporal half in reason of the high number of fibers that originate from the macular area. Fibers originating from the macula form the papillomacular bundle running directly from the fovea to the optic disc. Above and below the papillomacular bundle the fibers from the temporal periphery make an arcuate pattern toward the disc. There is an horizontal

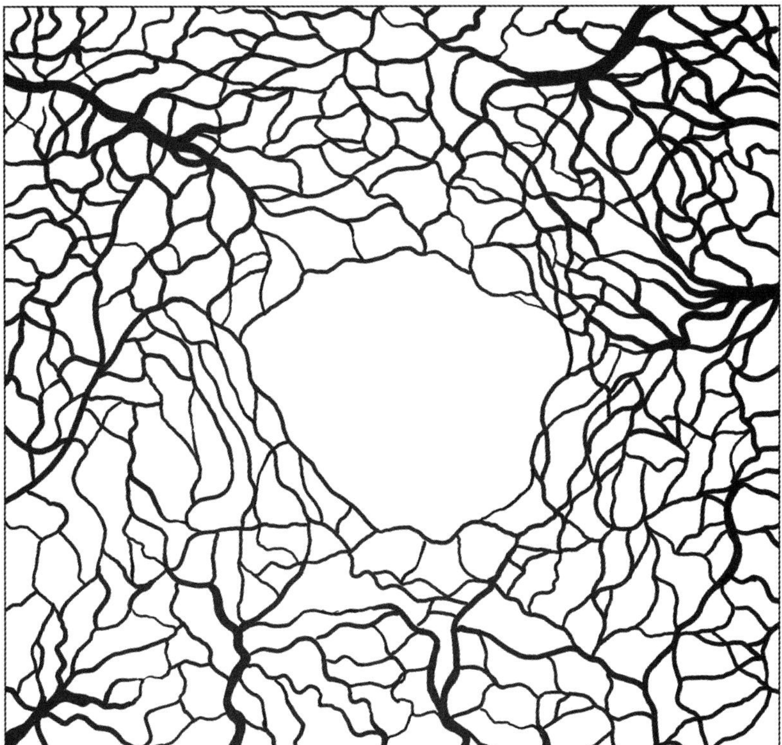

Figure 5: Avascular macular area; inside the macular area is located the avascular area which is 450–500 microns in diameter. This avascular area limits are defined by a continuous ring of very fine anastomoses of the perifoveal vascular network, consisting of a single layer of capillaries

line running from the fovea to the retinal temporal periphery that separate fibers bundles going to the optic disc, passing above or below the fovea (**Figure 6**).

Müller Cells

The Müller cells are fibrous elongated vertical cells that unite the inner and outer limiting membranes. Their nuclei are located in the bipolar cell layer. Their fibers fan out frontally increasing in width up to the outer limiting membrane.

On the vitreal side of the retina Müller's fiber terminate in large conical or bulbous expansions which are continued as a dense network of glial ridges forming a mosaic-like pattern lying upon the external surface of the internal limiting membrane (ILM). Müller cells constitute an important element in the support structure of the retina. They are vertical fibers that span the inner and outer limiting membranes. In case of cystoid edema they form the wall of the pseudocysts.

The Henle fibers and Müller cells frontal radial structure at the macula: The Henle fibers structure, seen frontally, is radial, star-shaped, centering on the foveola. On the edge of the fovea the Müller cells are radially disposed, following Henle fibers radial pattern. Müller cells and Henle fibers form a radial framework that is important in shaping the cystoid spaces patterns (**Figures 7A to I**).

At the center of the macula the Müller cells form a truncated inverted cone, described by Gass,[5,6] shaped as a plug that binds together the receptor cells in the foveola. According to Gass *"the Müller cell cone is the primary structural support for the fovea. The Müller cell cone serves as a plug to bind together the receptor cells in the foveola. Without this plug of glial cells, the retinal receptor cell layer with its thin layer of horizontally radiating nerve fibers would be highly susceptible to disruption at the umbo and hole formation under a variety of circumstances, including sensory retinal detachment, minor trauma, cystoid macular edema, and macular degeneration."* Gass hypothesized that fluid into the capillary free zone in the macula may disrupt the photoreceptor external limiting membrane (ELM) complex and lead to cystoid macular edema. Congenital abnormalities affecting the Müller cell cone and are also responsible for the pathognomonic biomicroscopic and OCT picture of foveo-macular schisis.

In the fovea, Henle's fibers disposition leads to the characteristic star-like appearance of cystoid macular edema, degenerative processes of the macula and juvenile or adult retinoschisis and the appearance of some lamellar holes, cystoid edema patterns and macular and retinal infrastructure framework. The shape, dimensions and extension of the cystoid edema cavities depend directly on the framework of retinal structures and layers.[6-10]

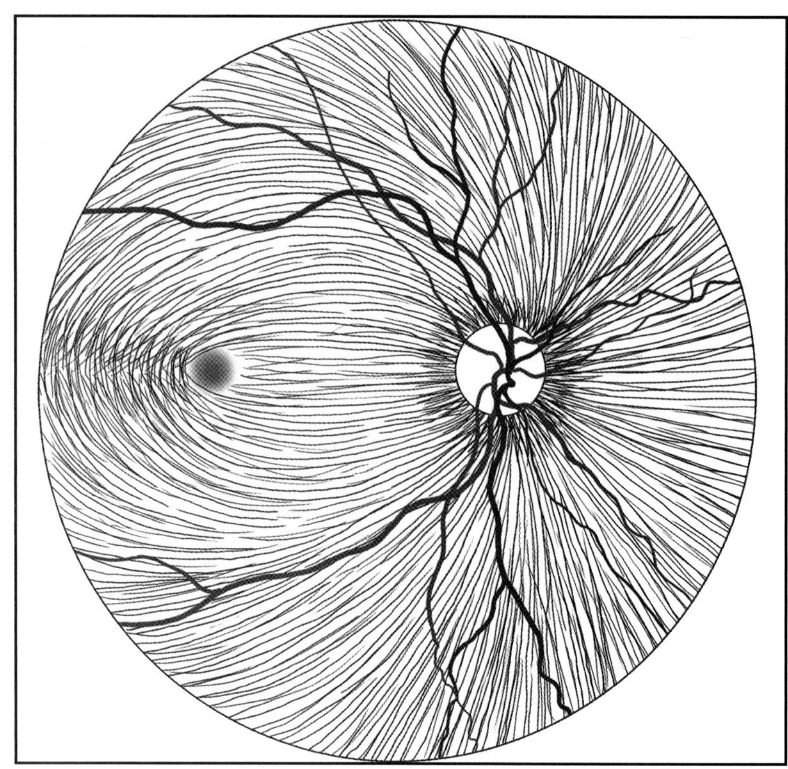

Figure 6: Retinal nerve fiber layer; nerve fibers run radially from the nerve fiber layer to the optic disc. Nerve axons run from the ganglion cell bodies to the papilla. This pattern is evident in the nasal half of the retina but it is not evident in the temporal half in reason of the high number of fibers that originate from the macular area. Fibers originating from the macula form the papillomacular bundle running directly from the fovea to the optic disc. Above and below the papillomacular bundle the fibers from the temporal periphery make an arcuate pattern toward the disc. There is an horizontal line running from the fovea to the retinal temporal periphery that separate fibers bundles going to the optic disc, passing above or below the fovea

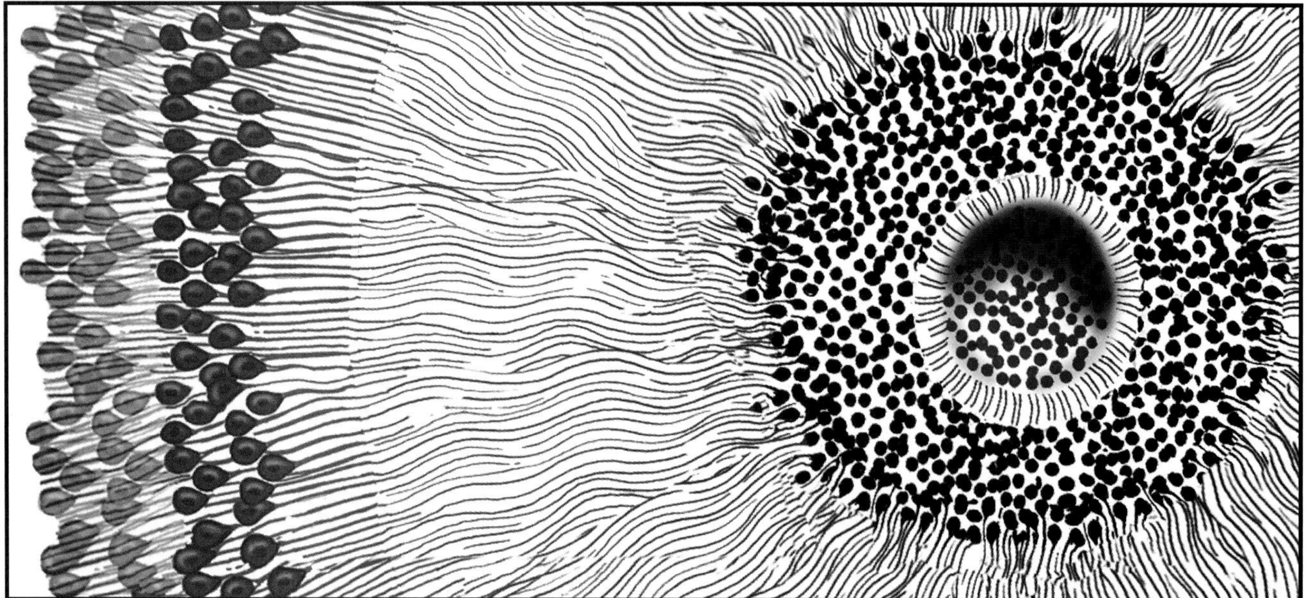

Figure 7A: The Henle fibers and Müller cells radial structure at the macula; the Henle fibers structure, seen frontally, is radial, star-shaped, centering on the foveola. On the edge of the fovea the Müller cells are radially disposed, following Henle fibers radial pattern

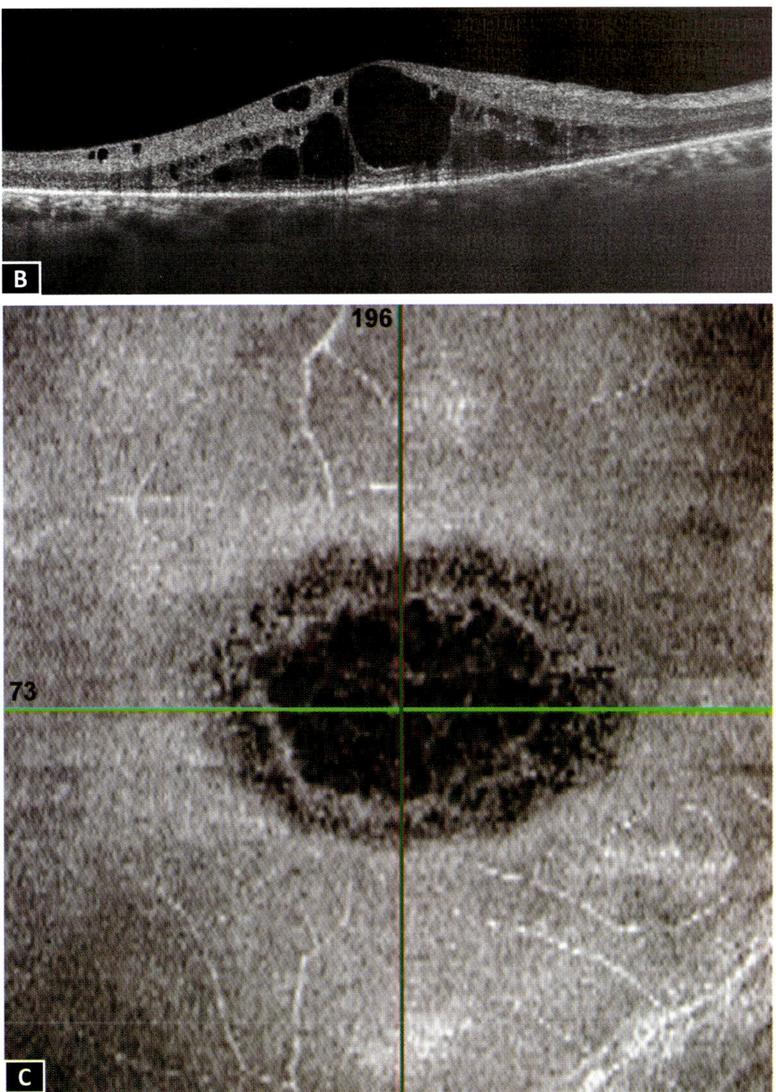

Figures 7B and C: The Henle fibers and Müller cells radial structure and macular edema; OCT *en face* scans show that the radial structure of Henle fibers and Müller cells is basic in shaping the layout of pseudocystic cavities. The frontal scan parallel shows inner nuclear layer cystoid cells. These cells are petal-shaped grossly ovoid with tips converging toward the fovea or flower-shaped. Around it are placed numerous smaller rounded cavities (Optovue RTVue)

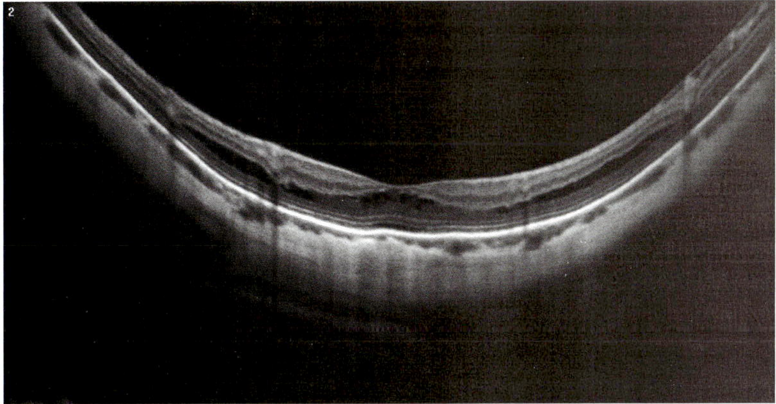

Figure 7D: The Henle fibers and Müller cells radial and macular retinoschisis; on *en face* scans typical retinoschisis OCT images show star-shaped or wheel-shaped, elongated cavities following the radial structure of Henle fibers and Müller cells (Optovue RTVue)

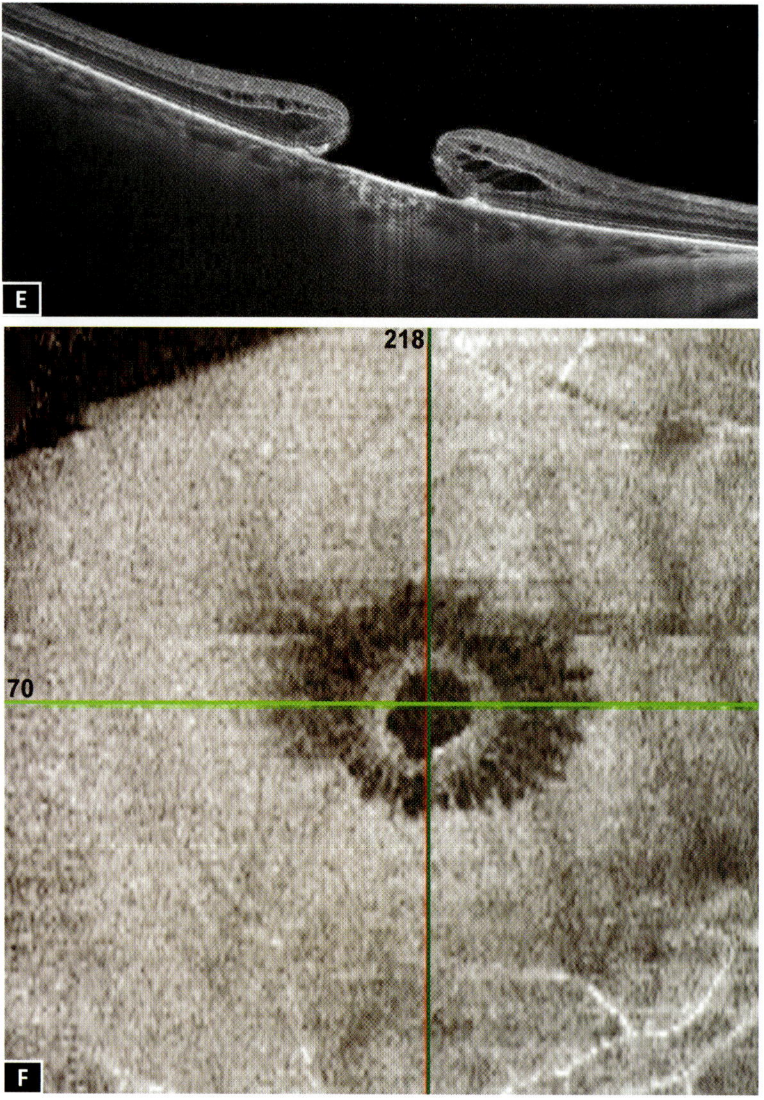

Figures 7E and F: The Henle fibers and Müller cells radial structure and macular hole; on *en face* scan retinal macular hole OCT image with section parallel to RPE about 30 micron above pigment epithelium. It shows a central rounded hole surrounded by wheel-shaped, elongated cavities following the radial structure of Henle fibers and Müller cells (Optovue RTVue)

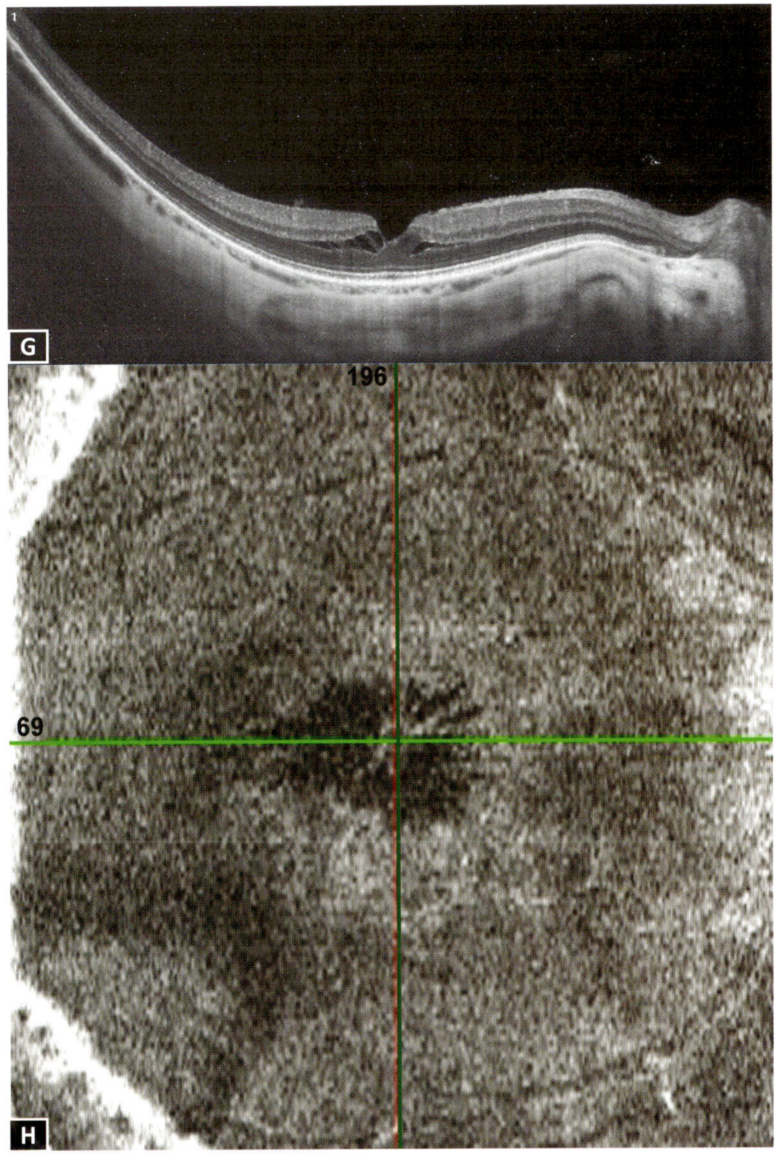

Figures 7G and H: The Henle fibers and Müller cells radial structure and lamellar macular hole; In this case of lamellar macular hole *en face* scans fissures enlarge laterally the lamellar hole, penetrating under the inner layers, simulating the retinoschisis wheel-shaped appearance. Lamellar holes can appear wheel-shaped, following the radial structure of Henle fibers and Müller cells (Optovue RTVue)

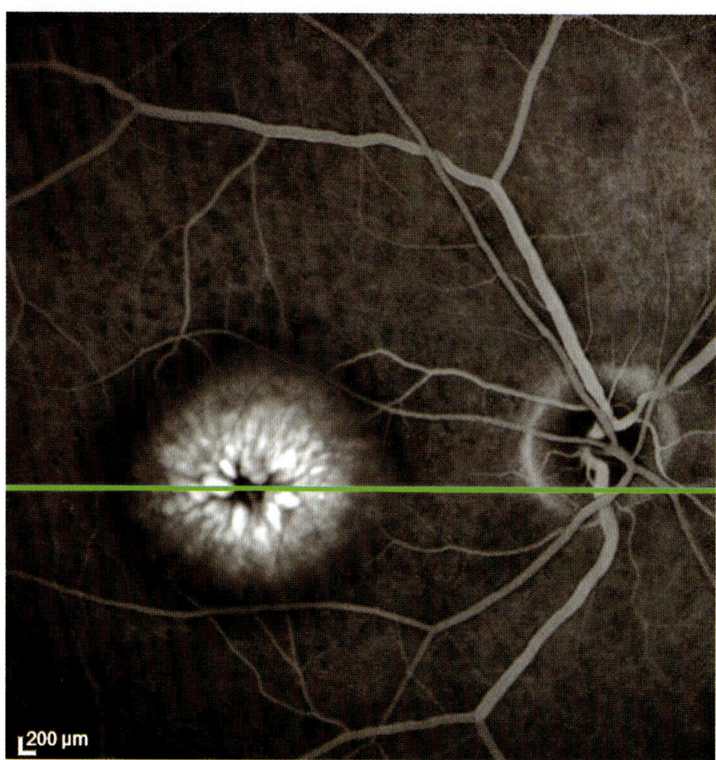

Figure 7I: The Henle fibers and Müller cells radial structure and cystoid macular edema in fluorescein angiography; Fluorescein angiography shows that the radial structure of Henle fibers and Müller cells is basic in shaping the layout of pseudo-cystic cavities. The dye shows petal-shaped cells with tips converging toward the fovea, flower-shaped

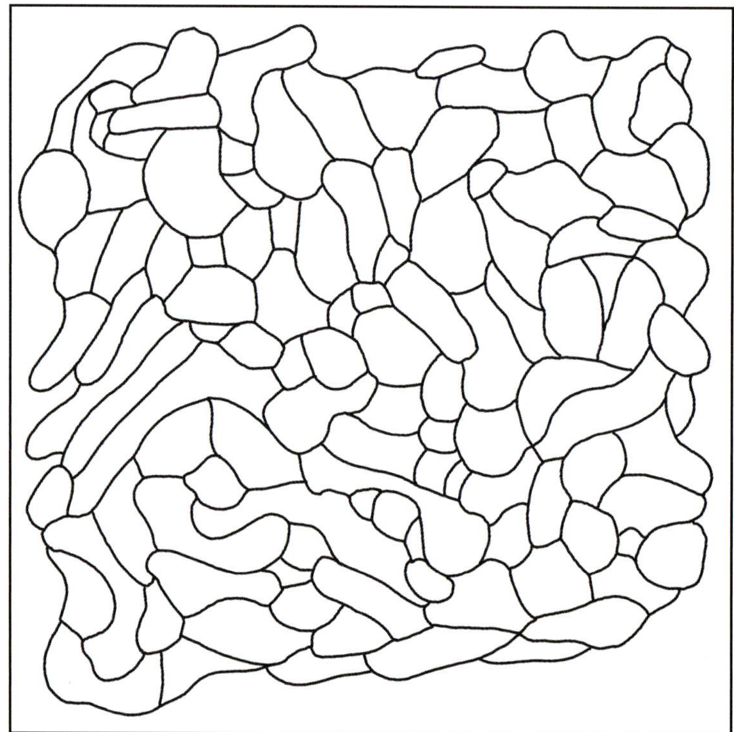

Figure 8A: Internal limiting membrane is a very thin acellular membrane which is connected at its outer surface to the polygonal inner ends of Müller's fibers. The polygonal inner ends of Müller's fibers take shape of a characteristic mosaic formation

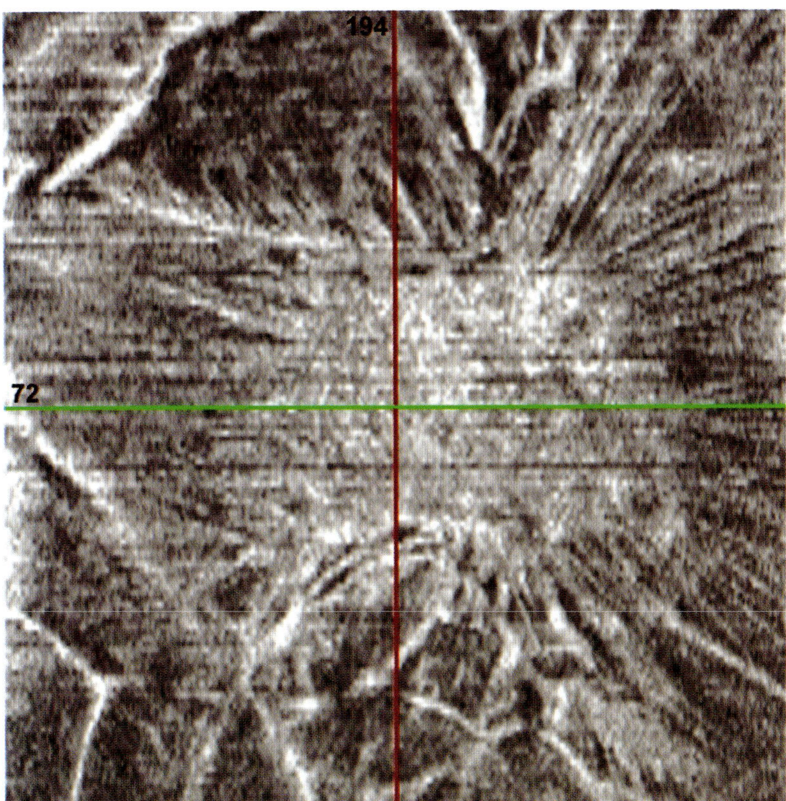

Figure 8B: Internal limiting membrane; vitreoretinal interface as seen with frontal scan in a case of pucker with retinal folds (Optovue RTVue)

Internal Limiting Membrane

Internal limiting membrane (ILM) is a very thin acellular membrane which is difficult to distinguish from the layer of nerve fibers. It is connected at its outer surface to the polygonal inner ends of Müller's fibers. In flat sections shows a curious and quite characteristic mosaic formation in the form of an irregular network of darkly staining lines with an average mesh size varying approximately between 4 and 12 micron. This pattern is found in all regions of the retina and is continuous over nerve fibers blood vessels and glial tissue. The shape and size of the reticulation varies over the large vessels and in the central area (**Figures 8A and B**).

References

1. Ducournau D. Short para-optic posterior ciliary arteries. An anatomo-clinical entity. Bull Soc Ophtalmol Fr. 1982;82(12):1527.
2. Hayreh SS. Posterior ciliary artery circulation in health and disease: the Weisenfeld lecture. Invest Ophthalmol Vis Sci. 2004; 45(3):749-57;748.
3. Hayreh SS. In vivo choroidal circulation and its watershed zones. Eye. 1990;4:273-89.
4. Gass JD. Müller cell cone, an overlooked part of the anatomy of the fovea centralis: hypotheses concerning its role in the pathogenesis of macular hole and foveomacualr retinoschisis. Arch Ophthalmol. 1999; 117(6):821-3.
5. Yamada E. Some structural features of the fovea centralis in the human retina. Arch Ophthalmol. 1969;82(2):151-9.
6. Pelosini L, Hull CC, Boyce JF, et al. Optical coherence tomography may be used to predict visual acuity in patients with macular edema. Invest Ophthalmol Vis Sci. 2011;52(5);2741-8.
7. Koleva-Georgieva D, Sivkova N. Assessment of serous macular detachment in eyes with diabetic macular edema by use of spectral-domain optical coherence tomography. Graefes Arch Clin Exp Ophthalmol. 2009;247(11); 1461-9.
8. Yeung L, Lima VC, Garcia P, et al. Correlation between spectral domain optical coherence tomography findings and fluorescein angiography patterns in diabetic macular edema. Ophthalmol. 2009;116(6):1158-67.
9. Bringmann A, Reichenbach A, Wiedemann P. Pathomechanisms of cystoid macular edema. Ophthalmic Res. 2004;36(5):241-9.
10. Reichenbach A, Wurm A, Pannicke T, et al. Müller cells as players in retinal degeneration and edema. Graefes Arch Clin Exp Ophthalmol. 2007;245 (5):627-36.

chapter 5

En Face SD-OCT and Green Angiography

Maria Cristina Savastano, Bruno Lumbroso

Vasculature aspect of the choroid has attracted significant interest since several years due to its potential involvement in single diseases.

Some investigators have pointed out that circulatory choroid abnormalities might play an essential role in the origin and development of the neuroretinal pathologies.[1,2]

The choroid circulation is well appreciable by the means of indocyanine green angiography (ICG), first described in 1972.[3] Moreover, digital ICG videoangiography is able to detect step-by-step all the circulation phases in filling recirculation, staining and clearing.[4]

The ICG, commonly performed in clinical practice, has improved our understanding of disorders as wet age related macular degeneration (AMD) (especially RAP and polypoidal choroidal vasculopathy), CSC and other chorioretinal disorders.[5]

The introduction of OCT tools, allowed the clinicians to investigate the retinal stroma in cross-sectional non-invasive approach by the means of B scan (**Figure 1**); moreover the introduction of C scan (coronal and C scan) investigation, opened new frontiers of interpretation and analysis.[6]

According to the study of Rosen et al. simultaneous visualization of *en face* OCT images and ICG angiogram, displayed more precise correlations between fluorescence anomalies and OCT changes.[7] In this paper the alteration of choroid vasculature was not studied by the means of OCT *en face*.

Several other studies considered the alteration of choroid by the means of OCT although their attention was centered on B scan.[8-12] The new OCT tools, by the means of *en face* scan analysis, allow *in vivo* reconstruction of the human choroid microvasculature exclusively on vessel reflectivity and without the use of contrast agents. This analysis revealed three interconnected capillary meshworks simultaneously in the choroid: the structure of the ***choriocapillaris*** differentiated

into ***Sattler's*** and ***Haller's*** layers and ***choroidal-scleral interface*** clearly delineated.

As reported by Považay et al. only advanced and noncommercial tools, may provide superior clinical feasibility to available 800 nm devices due to wavelength increasing at 1060 nm. The result of the increasing was the combination of better penetration, high speed and high resolution.[13] In authors experience some OCT devices are able to show the *under retinal structures* without changes in wavelength.

In this chapter authors would describe the images resulting by both ICG and C scan OCT analysis in normal and different eye diseases. Authors tried to study if there was precise overlapping of Sattler, Haller and choroidal-scleral interface layers between ICG and SD-OCT *en face* images or if only similarities could be found. The OCT-SD authors used was Optovue RTVue (Optovue Inc., Fremont, CA).

The ICG most significative images to study the Sattler morphology are appreciable at real early recirculation phase: 1–5 sec; while Haller structure at 5–20 sec.

Authors observation showed the importance to establish a correct reference plane on *en face* analysis to study the retroretinal structures (**Figure 2**).

In order to *en face* OCT images the better visualization images of the Sattler and Haller layers are appreciable between 10–80 μm and between 80–115 μm under the RPE boundary respectively. The described range are related to age of patient eye analysis and probably to the pulsation of choroid.[14,15] Not always and easily is to distinguish the choroidal-scleral interface; it results achievable especially in myopic eyes or in choroid thinner eyes (**Figures 3A to D**).

The **Figures 3A to D** showed the network of metarterioles in Sattler layer weakly hyporeflective tiny capillary; the Haller layer with bigger arterioles pronounced hyporeflective vessels exactly corresponding to ICG early phase. Moreover, the choroidal-scleral interface, not always visible due to the

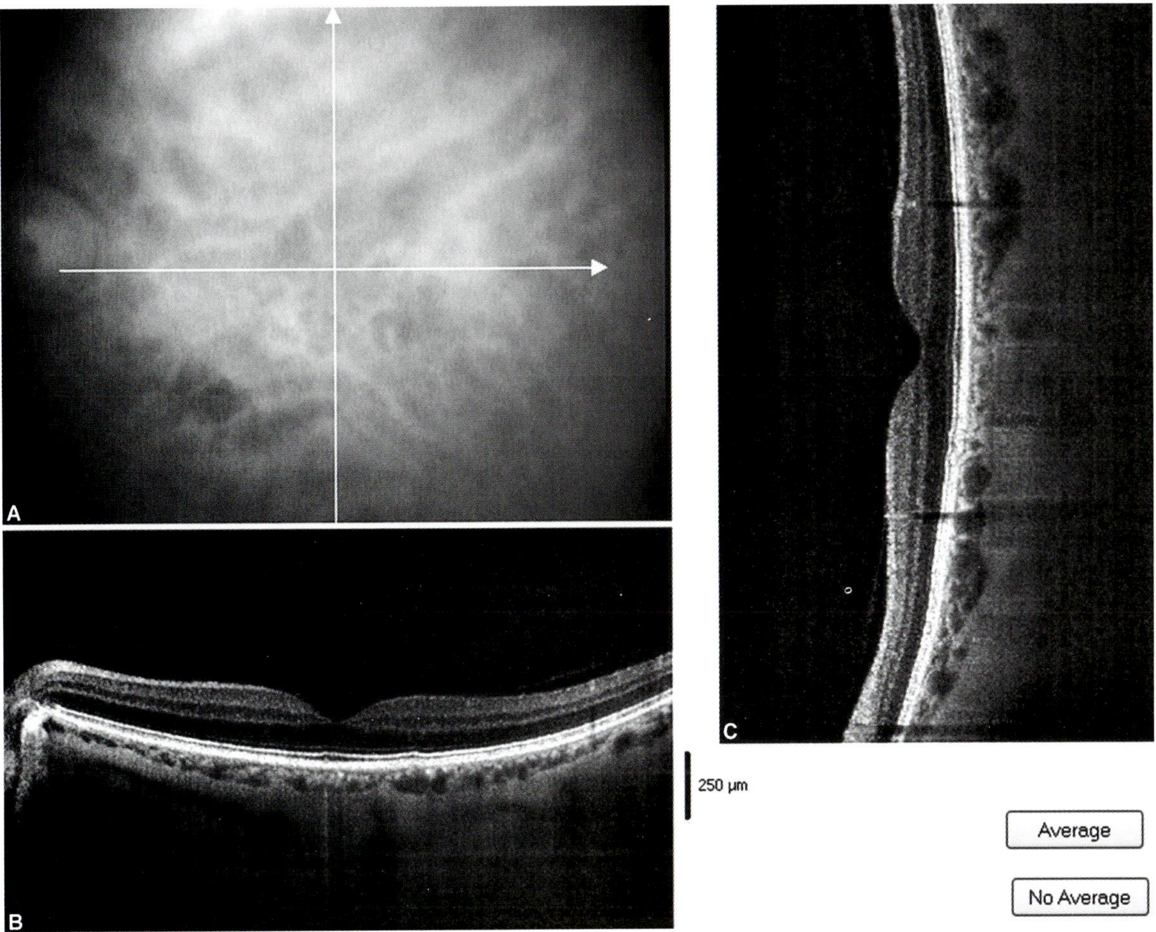

Figure 1: Cross-sectional scan of healthy left eye through the central fovea. Both horizontal and vertical tomograms showing the retinal stroma details, the choriocapillaris and choroidal visualization and sclera boundary

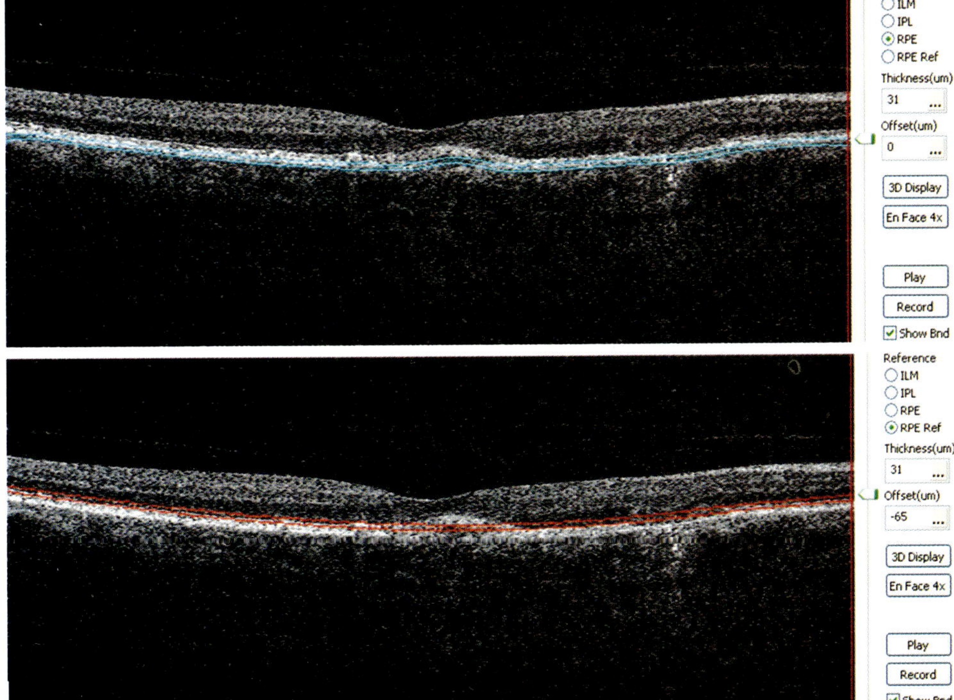

Figure 2: The reference plane RPE (top) and RPE-fit (bottom) of eye with subfoveal retinal pigment epithelium profile alteration (drusen). The RPE plane (blue lines) following the retinal pigment epithelium while RPE-ref the scleral profile

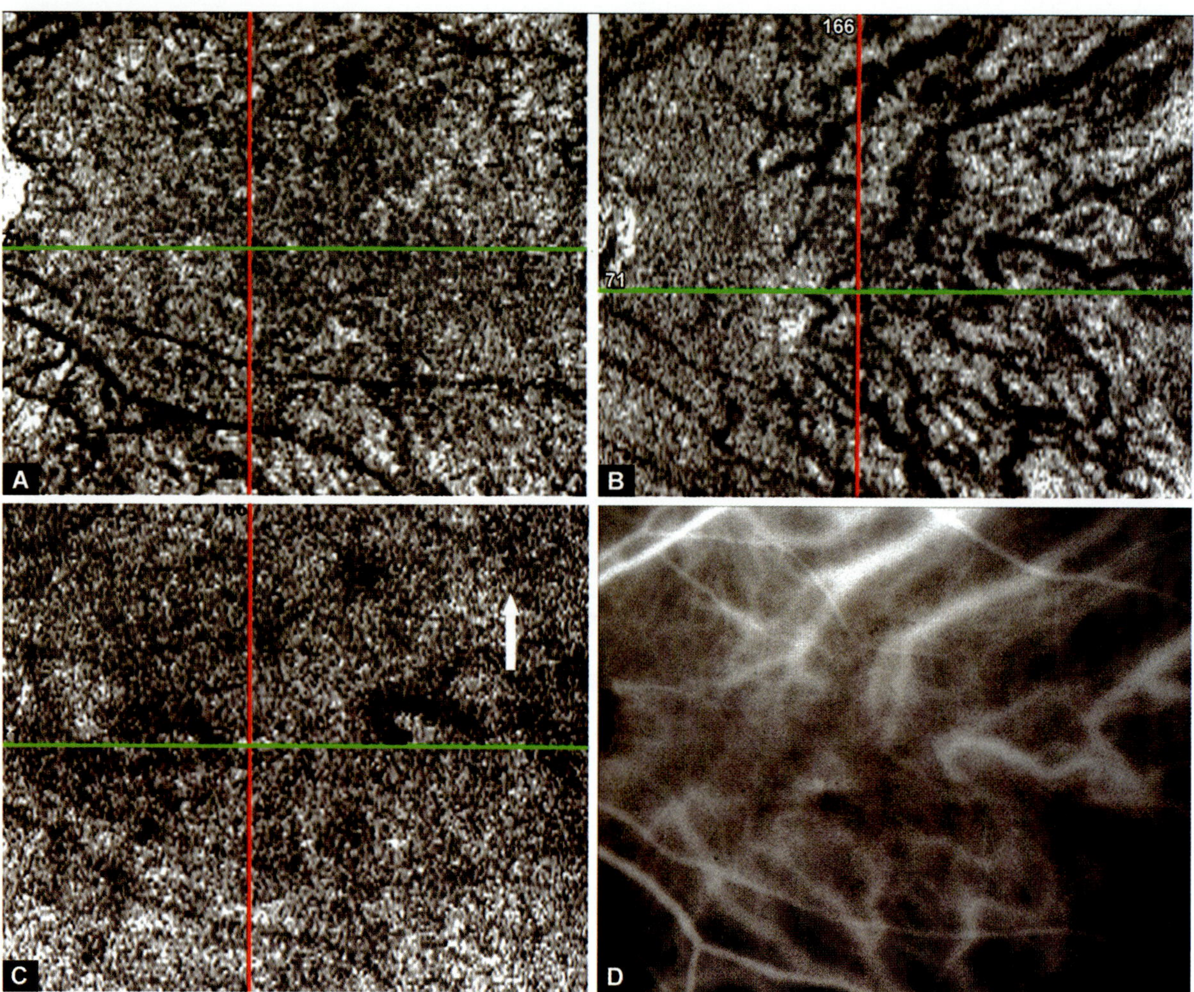

Figures 3A to D: The OCT *en face* and early ICG phase of healthy left eye. (A) The coronal scan was delineated at 25 μm under the retinal pigment epithelium (RPE) corresponding to the metarterioles of Sattler layer. At this plane are evident the retinal vessel (shadow effect) and the fine capillary network of inner choriocapillary. (B) The *en face* scan through the Haller layer showing the bigger arterioles corresponding at 80 μm reference plane under the RPE. (C) The *en face* scan at 194 μm under the RPE corresponding to choroidal-scleral interface where only the posterior ciliary arteries perforating the sclera at the lamina suprachoroidea were visualized (white arrow). (D) ICG early recirculation phase ("5") showing overlapping between the 3 *en face* scans (A-B-C) and vessels observable after the ICG vein injection

stronger absorption in the previous layers, could be observed especially when the posterior ciliary arteries perforating the sclera, run horizontally. **Figures 4, 5 and 6** showed normal eye, vessel dilatation and CNV details respectively evaluated by ICG, OCT B scan and C scan.

The **Figures 7A to C** showed the visualization capability of C scan in case of RPE tears. The precise location of tears is not observable in B scan although could be suspected. In C scan the dimension, the position and shape of tear are accurately approachable according to ICG evaluation.

Conclusion

The clinical evaluation of choroid vasculature details by using combined ICG and OCT coronal plane (*en face* view),

allowed to capture images able to provide overlapping informations about the "under retinal structures" specifically the Haller layer and in many cases the Sattler and choroidal-scleral interface. **Figures 8, 9 and 10** showed posterior pole laser treatment, occult CNV and polipoidal choroidal vasculopathy respectively by ICG, OCT B scan and C scan analysis.

In future possible combinations with optional Doppler flow measurements, opens the possibility to reduce the risk of invasive fluorescein angiography and/or ICG angiography by a completely noninvasive technique. The ability to visualize the blood vessels has great potential in order to improve diagnostic abilities such as AMD diabetes and several other diseases.

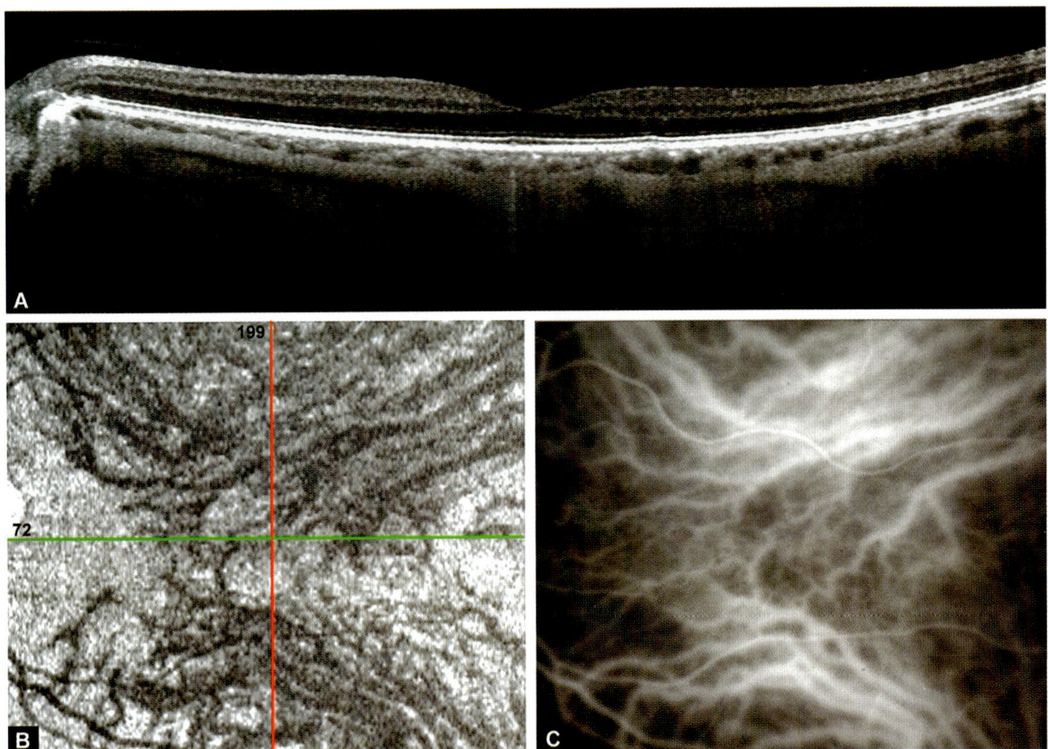

Figures 4A to C: Left normal eye by B scan (A) and *en face* (B) OCT and ICG (C) choroid early recirculation phase. The choroid circulation observable to ICG invasive analysis is overlapping to *en face* analysis scan at 98 µm under EPR

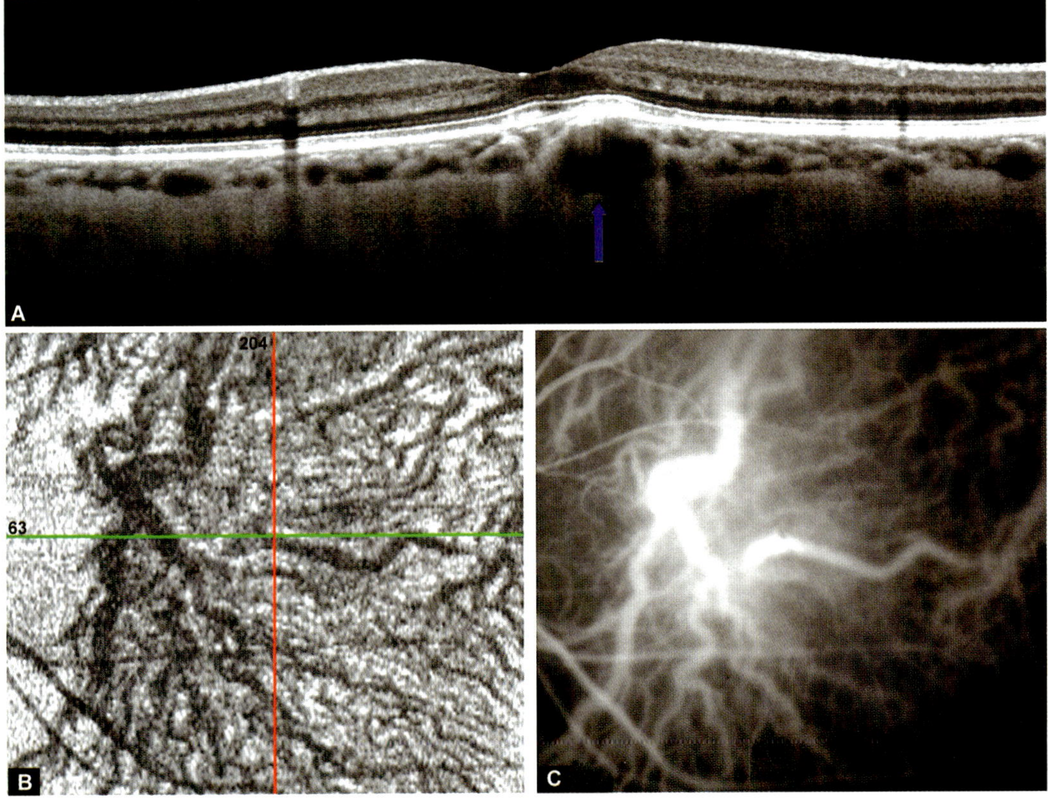

Figures 5A to C: (A) Left eye of choroidal localized vessel dilatation by B scan (B) *en face* OCT and (C) ICG. Horizontal B scan showing the deformation of chorioretinal profile due to a dilatation of choroidal vessel (Blue arrow). The reference plane (RPE-fit) on *en face* scan at 92 µm under RPE displayed a point-by-point overlapping with ICG image

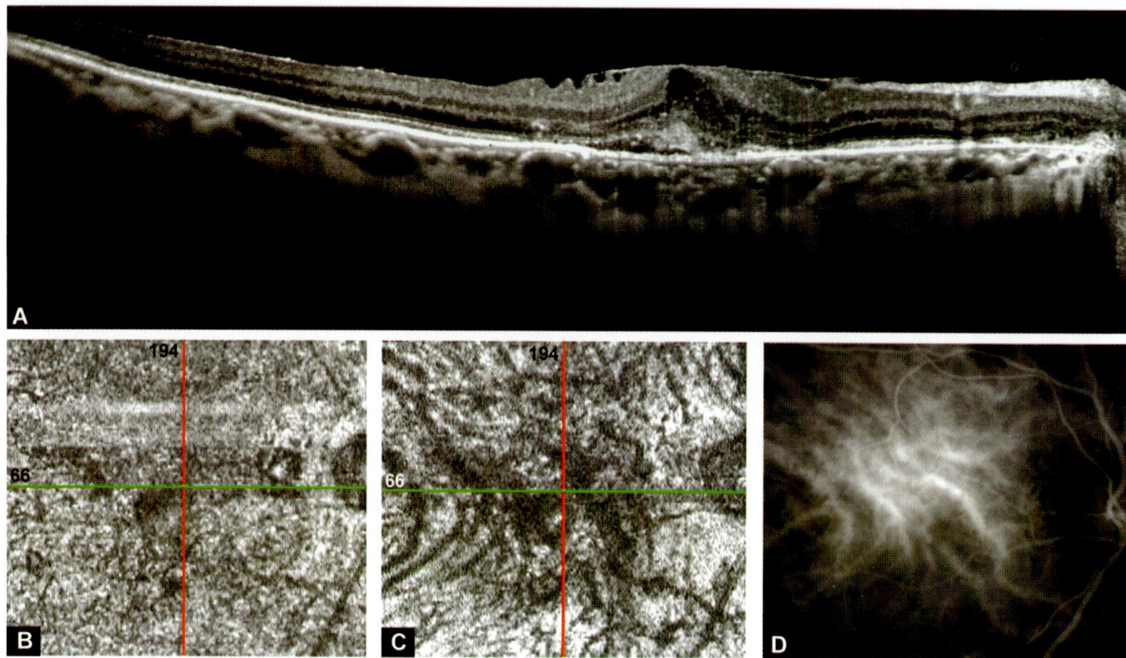

Figures 6A to D: (A) Choroidal neovascularization by B scan. The B scan showing the changes in profile and intraretinal structure related to neovascular activity. C scan (B) showing the Sattler layer revealed focal vascularization anomalies which corresponding to Haller layer (C) and ICG evaluation (D)

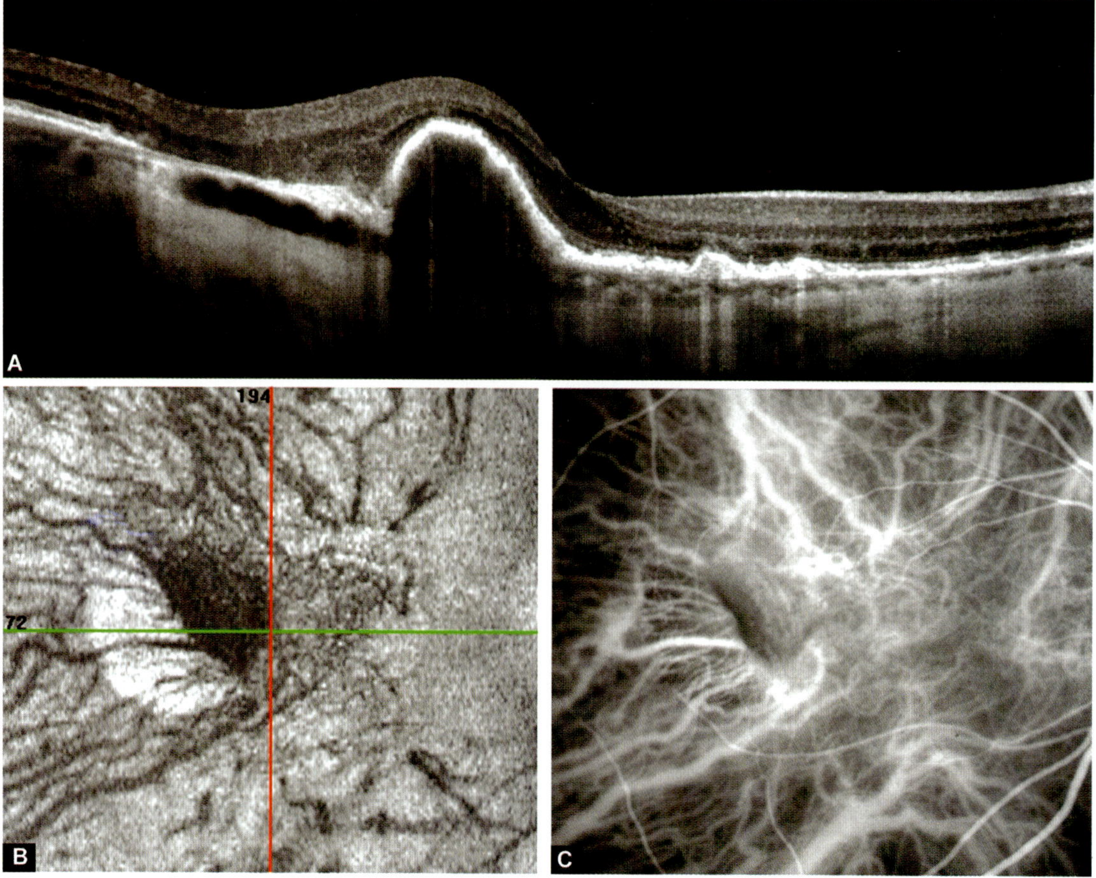

Figures 7A to C: Pigment epithelium tear. (A) B scan showing pigment epithelium detachment and several backscattering effect in correspondence of tears. (B) The *en face* scan reporting the precise location of RPE tear. (C) ICG early phase showing the choroid bed under the RPE tear

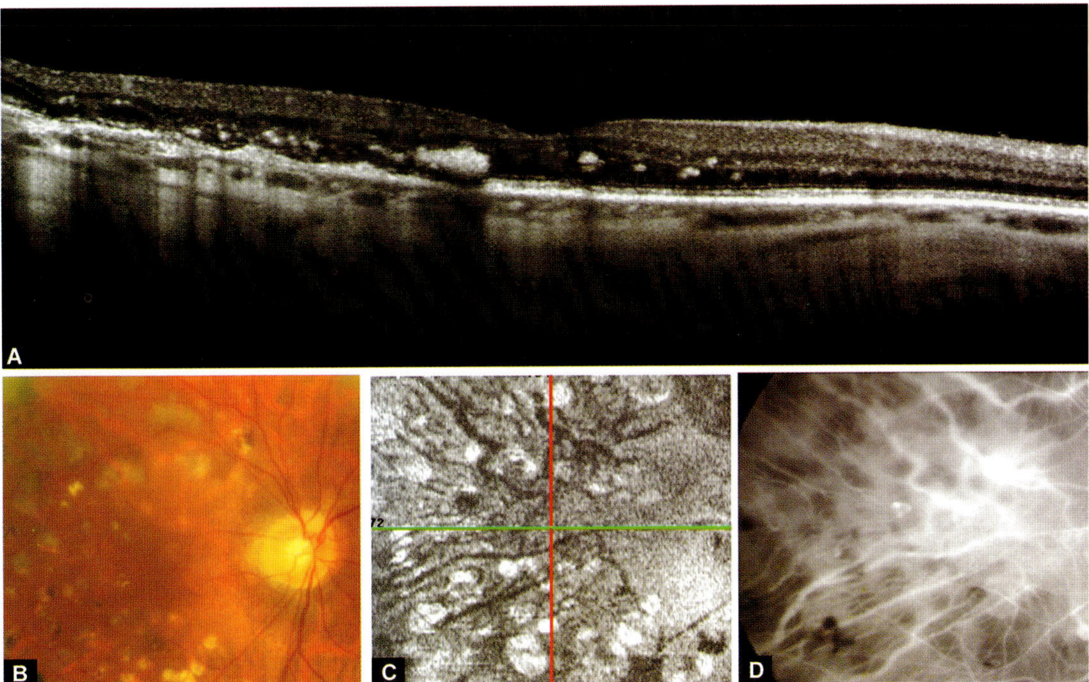

Figures 8A to D: (A) Right eye of laser treatment central vein occlusion. (B) The B scan showing the hard exudate and the backscattering effect spots secondary to focal laser treatment moreover detectable at retinography. (C) The C scan image at 82 µm displaying the exact localization of laser scars. (D) The ICG early phase demonstrating the retinal pigment epithelium laser defects

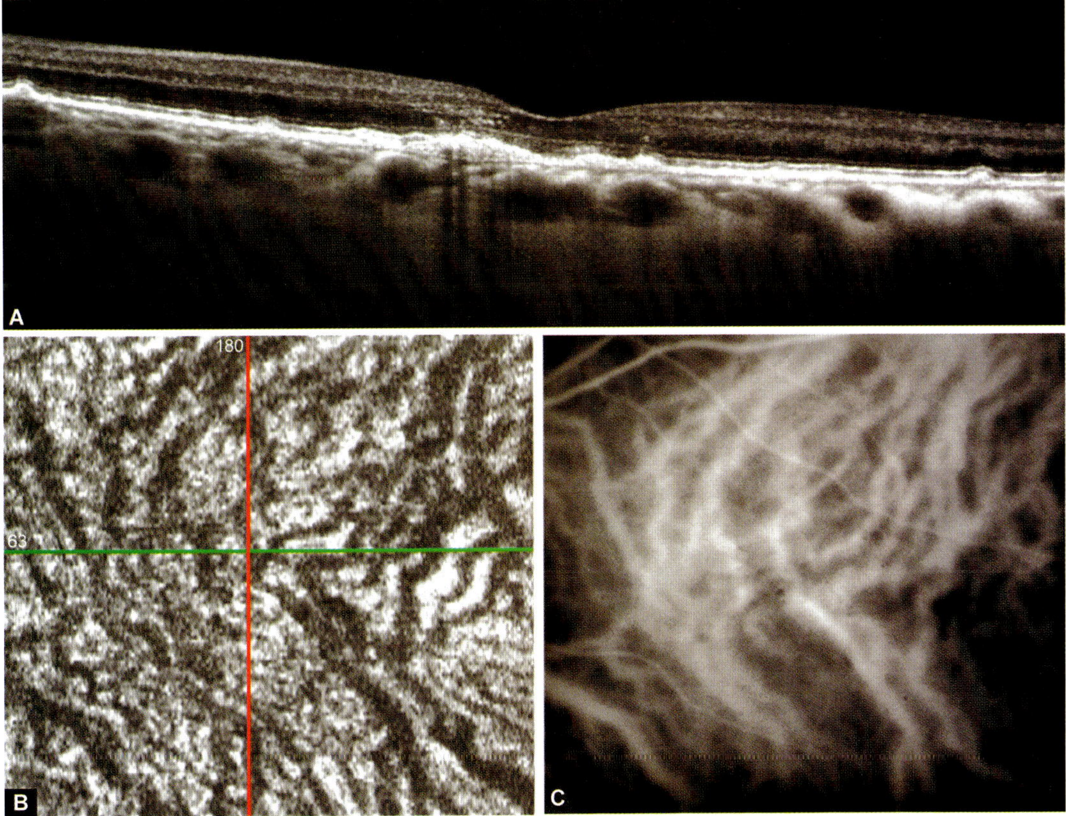

Figures 9A to C: Occult choroidal neovascularization. (A) The B scan revealed the irregular profile of preparticularly under the fovea are appreciable small dots around the hyper-reflectivity area due to the CNV activity. (B and C) The C scan and ICG showing the blood choroidal vessel dilatation

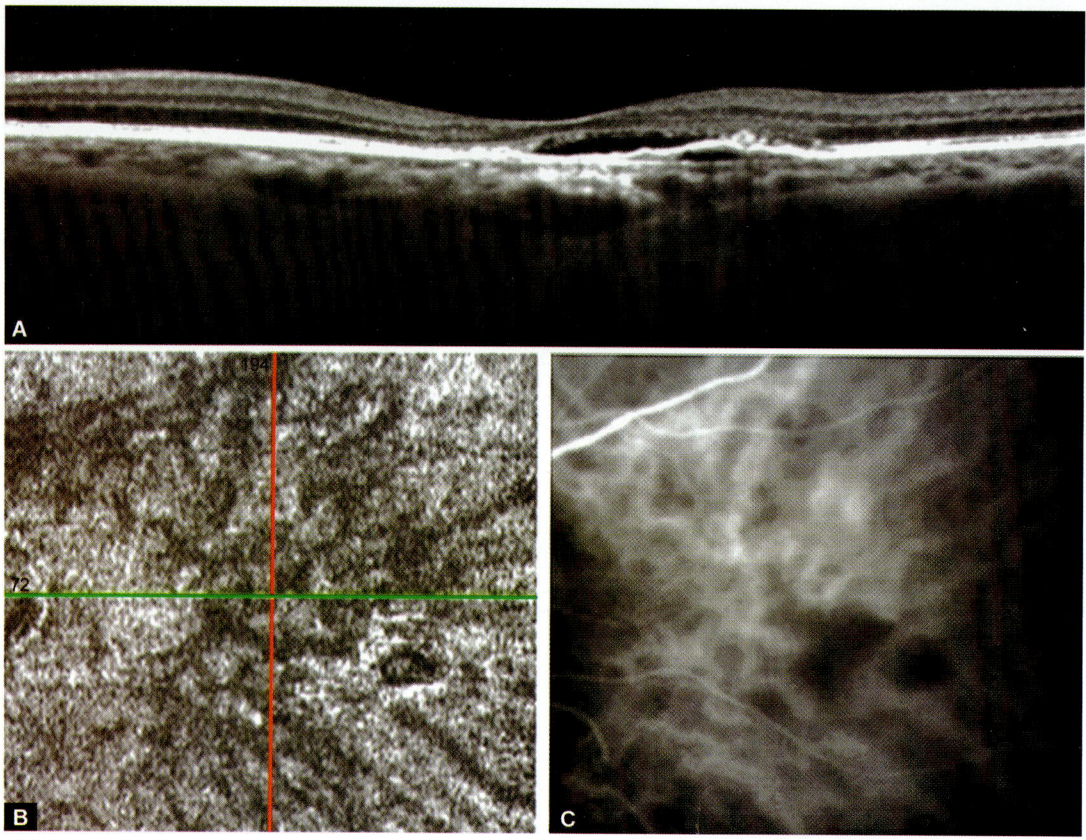

Figures 10A to C: Polypoidal choroidal vasculopathy. (A) The B scan showing the RPE tear with vascular notching upon the apex around the polypoidal lesion is appreciable the subretinal fluid. (B and C) The C scan and ICG revealed the exact topographic localization of polypoidal choroidal vasculopathy with detail about the dimension, shape, allocation and distribution

References

1. Mullins RF, Johnson MN, Faidley EA, et al. Choriocapillaris vascular dropout related to density of drusen in human eyes with early age-related macular degeneration. Invest Ophthalmol Vis Sci. 2011;52(3):1606-12.

2. Keane PA, Sadda SR. Imaging chorioretinal vascular disease. Eye. 2010;24(3):422-7.

3. Flower RW, Hochheimer BF. Clinical infrared absorption angiography of the choroid. Am J Ophthalmol. 1972;73: 458-9.

4. Yannuzzi LA, Slakter JS, Sorenson JA, et al. Digital indocyanine green videoangiography and choroidal neovascularization. Retina. 1992;12(3):191-223.

5. Stanga PE, Lim JI, Hamilton P. Indocyanine green angiography in chorioretinal diseases: indications and interpretation: an evidence-based update. Ophthalmology. 2003;110:15-21.

6. Rosen RB, Hathaway M, Rogers J, et al. Multidimensional en-face OCT imaging of the retina.Opt Express. 2009; 17:4112-33.

7. Rosen RB, Hathaway M, Rogers J, et al. Simultaneous OCT/SLO/ICG imaging. Invest Ophthalmol Vis Sci. 2009;50:851-60.

8. Margolis R, Spaide RF. A pilot study of enhanced depth imaging optical coherence tomography of the choroid in normal eyes. Am J Ophthalmol. 2009;147:811-5.

9. Fujiwara T, Imamura Y, Margolis R, et al. Enhanced depth imaging optical coherence tomography of the choroid in highly myopic eyes. Am J Ophthalmol. 2009;148:445-50.

10. Spaide RF. Age-related choroidal atrophy. Am J Ophthalmol. 2009;147:801-10.

11. Imamura Y, Fujiwara T, Margolis R, et al. Enhanced depth imaging optical coherence tomography of the choroid in central serous chorioretinopathy. Retina. 2009;29:149-73.

12. Ikuno Y, Kawaguchi K, Yasuno Y, et al. Choroidal thickness in healthy Japanese subjects. Invest Ophthalmol Vis Sci. 2010;51:2173-6.

13. Povazay B, Hermann B, Hofer B, et al. Wide-field optical coherence tomography of the choroid in vivo. Invest Ophthalmol Vis Sci. 2009;50:1856-63.

14. Kim SW, Oh J, Kwon SS, et al. Comparison of choroidal thickness among patients with healthy eyes, early age-related maculopathy, neovascular age-related macular degeneration, central serous chorioretinopathy, and polypoidal choroidal vasculopathy. Retina. 2011;31:1904-11.

15. Shahbazi S, Mokhtari-Dizaji M, Mansori MR. Noninvasive estimation of the ocular elastic modulus for age-related macular degeneration in the human eye using sequential ultrasound imaging. Ultrasonics. 2012;52:208-14.

Part **II**

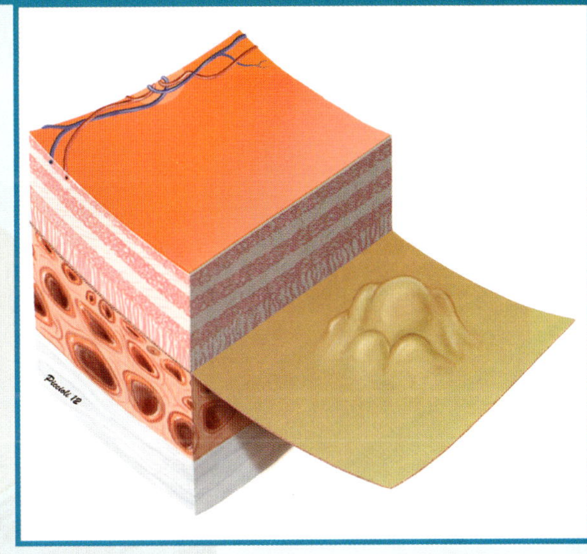

En Face Optical Coherence Tomography Study of Diseases and Disorders

Section 3

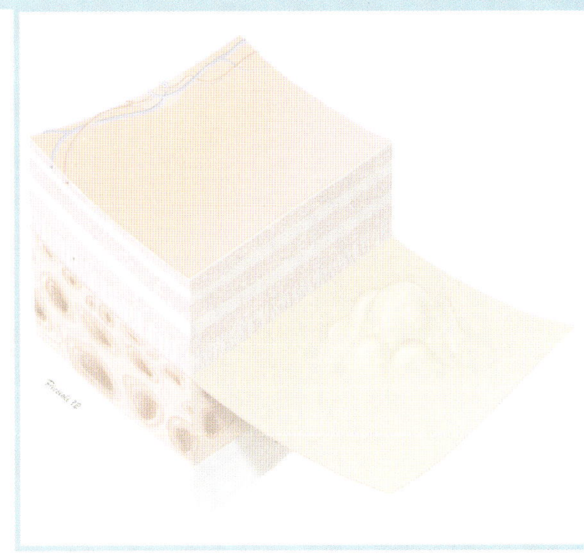

Anterior Segment *En Face* Optical Coherence Tomography Examination

chapter 6

Corneal and Anterior Segment *En Face* Optical Coherence Tomography

Bernardo Cavalcanti, Andre Romano, Pedram Hamrah

Anterior Segment Optical Coherence Tomography

The first report of optical coherence tomography (OCT) imaging of the cornea and anterior segment was published in 1994 using the Time domain OCT (TD-OCT) technology.[1] Since then, this technology has evolved rapidly with the development of the Fourier domain OCT (FD-OCT) that allows a higher resolution (5 μm FD-OCT vs. 18 μm TD-OCT) and faster speed of A scans (26,000 scan/sec FD-OCT vs. 2,000 scan/sec TD-OCT), resulting in less motion artifacts and the capability to obtain three-dimensional (3D) images of ocular tissues. However, TD-OCT still has the advantage over FD-OCT in that it allows deeper tissue penetration and in its use in anterior chamber biometry.

Anterior segment OCT (AS-OCT) is a new *in vivo* non-contact imaging system that provides detailed, high-resolution, cross-sectional anatomical images of the cornea and anterior segment, using an interference pattern of reflected light. AS-OCT usually uses a longer wavelength (1310 nm) as compared to posterior segment models, thus allowing better light absorption of the corneal stroma, resulting in reduced light penetration to the retina. However, lower wavelength (830 nm) AS-OCT systems are available (RTVue; Optovue Inc., Fremont, CA), which use a corneal adaptor module (CAM). The CAM consists of two adaptor lenses: a wider angle and a high magnification lens that provide scan width of up to 6 mm and 4 mm respectively, and a transverse resolution of 15 μm and 10 μm, respectively. The lenses provide telocentric scanning, allowing the OCT beam to be parallel to the central axis across the transverse scan. Currently commercially available AS-OCT devices are summarized in **Table 1**.

Anterior segment OCT has rapidly been adapted in clinical practice for diagnosis of cornea and anterior segment pathologies, as well as for surgical planning, by providing spatial arrangement of ocular tissues. Most commonly, AS-OCT has been used clinically for measuring corneal and

Table 1: Currently commercially available anterior-segment optical coherence tomographs (AS-OCT)

Device	Type	Wave-length (nm)	Range: Horizontal x Vertical (mm)	Transverse x Axial resolution (μm)	Scan speed (A scan/sec)	3D/*En face* technology
SL-OCT (Heidelberg Engineering)	TD	1,310	15 x 7	100 x 25	200	No
Visante OCT (Carl Zeiss Meditec)	TD	1,310	16 x 6 (10 x 3 for high resolution)	60 x 18	2,000	No
CASIA SS-1000 (Tomey)	FD	1,310	16 x 8	30 x 10	30,000	No
Cirrus HD-OCT (Carl Zeiss Meditec)	FD	840	3 x 2	15 x 5	27,000	Yes
RTVue (Optovue)	FD	830	6 x 2	8 x 5	26,000	Yes
iVue (Optovue)	FD	840	6 x 2	15 x 5	26,000	Yes
3D OCT-2000 (Topcon)	FD	840	6 x 3	20 x 5	27,000	Yes

Abbreviations: TD: Time domain; FD: Fourier domain; OCT: Optical coherence tomography; SL: Slit-lamp

sub-layer thickness to define the depth and composition of corneal lesions, to assess pre- and post-surgical anatomical changes for refractive surgery, and to define the configuration of the iris root and the angle.[2-10] Recently popularized lamellar surgical techniques, such as deep anterior lamellar keratoplasty (DALK) and endothelial keratoplasties, have used AS-OCT as a tool to assess tissue apposition,[11] resulting in improved patient outcome. Furthermore, few recent reports have demonstrated the advantages of using 3D reconstruction for the cornea and anterior segment.[12-14]

En Face Technique

Currently, the AS-OCT technology relies on images reconstructed from cross-sectional scans (A scans). However, the *en face* technique uses a reference path from multiple axial scanning depths, derived from a sequence of A and B scans. Normally, more time is required to acquire the necessary A scans needed to create 3D images. Further, acquisition of high-quality images requires a steady patient gaze. Once the volume-rendering procedure of the images is completed, cross-sectional images, 3D images, or movie clips of the *en face* images can be demonstrated from reconstructed data. The *en face* technique provides a layer-by-layer horizontal sectioning of the tissue. These sections allow identification of microstructural information throughout the scanned area that is not available with standard AS-OCT scans. Thus, *en face* AS-OCT images provide clinicians with a better understanding of a specific area of interest in the cornea, similar to *in vivo* confocal microscopy.

Vertex flare, the reflection from the anterior vertex of the cornea, may induce errors in the recognition of the tissue surface, appearing as artifacts on *en face* images. In a well-centered cross-sectional scan, this reflection from the corneal vertex may saturate the imaging system and produce the vertical flare **(Figures 1A to C)**. The precisely defined corneal vertex is an important centration point. However, for corneal thickness measurements, the pupil may be used as an alternate primary centration reference. Hence the primary centration reference can be modified for refractive [Laser assisted *in situ* keratomileusis (LASIK), photorefractive keratectomy (PRK) and phototherapeutic keratectomy (PTK)] and corneal (keratoplasty) surgeries, or diseases such as keratoconus or corneal scarring.

Clinical Applications of *En Face* Anterior Segment Optical Coherence Tomography

The ability to carry out non-invasive serial examinations makes AS-OCT a unique, and valuable modality for studying the cornea and anterior segment. The novel *en face* AS-OCT technique can thus be used in several ocular surface and anterior segment diseases.

Dry Eye Disease

Dry eye disease is a multifactorial condition of the tear film and ocular surface, with the tear film playing an important role in ocular surface maintenance. Assessment of the tear film meniscus has previously been performed by cross-sectional scans with AS-OCT.[15-18] Further, conjunctival conditions, such as conjunctivochalasis, have been shown to benefit from objective assessment of the tear meniscus area in the cross-sectional mode.[19] However, *en face* imaging in a patient with conjunctivochalasis in 3D provides a more detailed and extensive reconstruction of conjunctival folds as compared to cross-sectional imaging **(Figures 2A to C)** and is able to detect a larger tear meniscus.

Conjunctival Lesions

A wide variety of benign and malignant lesions can affect the conjunctiva. The most common lesions in order of frequency are: pterygium, nevus, dysplasia, nonspecific nongranulomatous inflammation and epithelial inclusion cysts. Anterior segment OCT is able to differentiate solid (hyper-reflective) from cystic (hyporeflective) lesions, and recent reports show the importance of this technology for the anterior segment tumors.[20,21] In addition, *en face* imaging is able to detect cystic formation and presence of vascularization **(Figures 3A and B)** in a suspicious conjunctival lesion. Intrinsic cystic formation is important, as it generally suggests

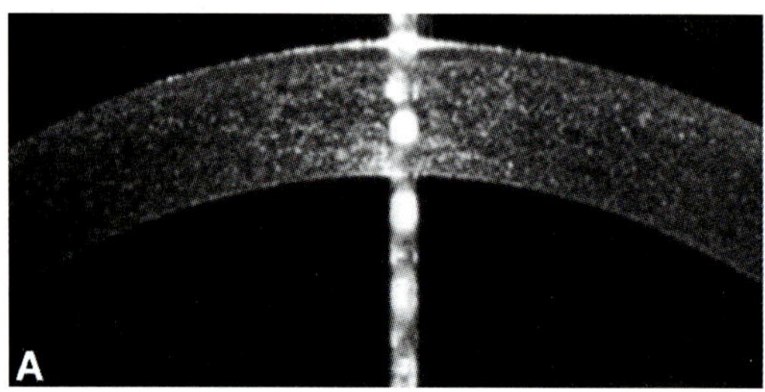
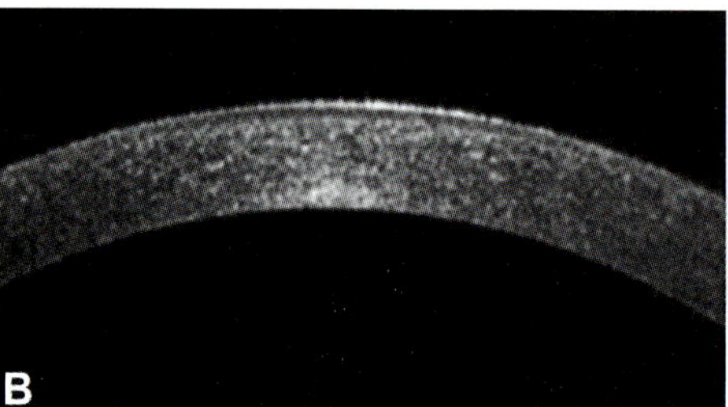
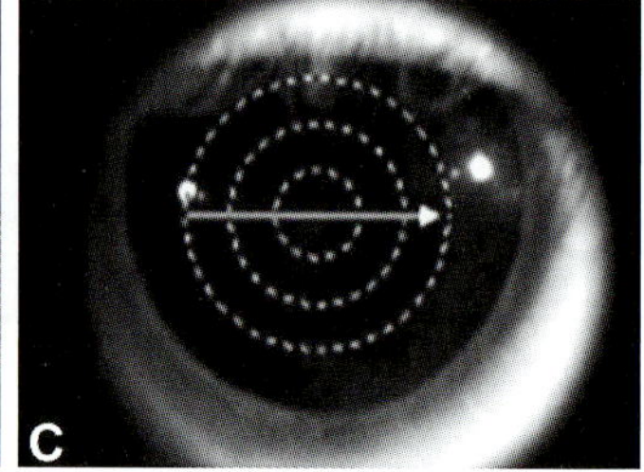

Figures 1A to C: Optical coherence tomography images showing the vertical flare from an apex centration (A) and no flare with the pupil centration (B and C)

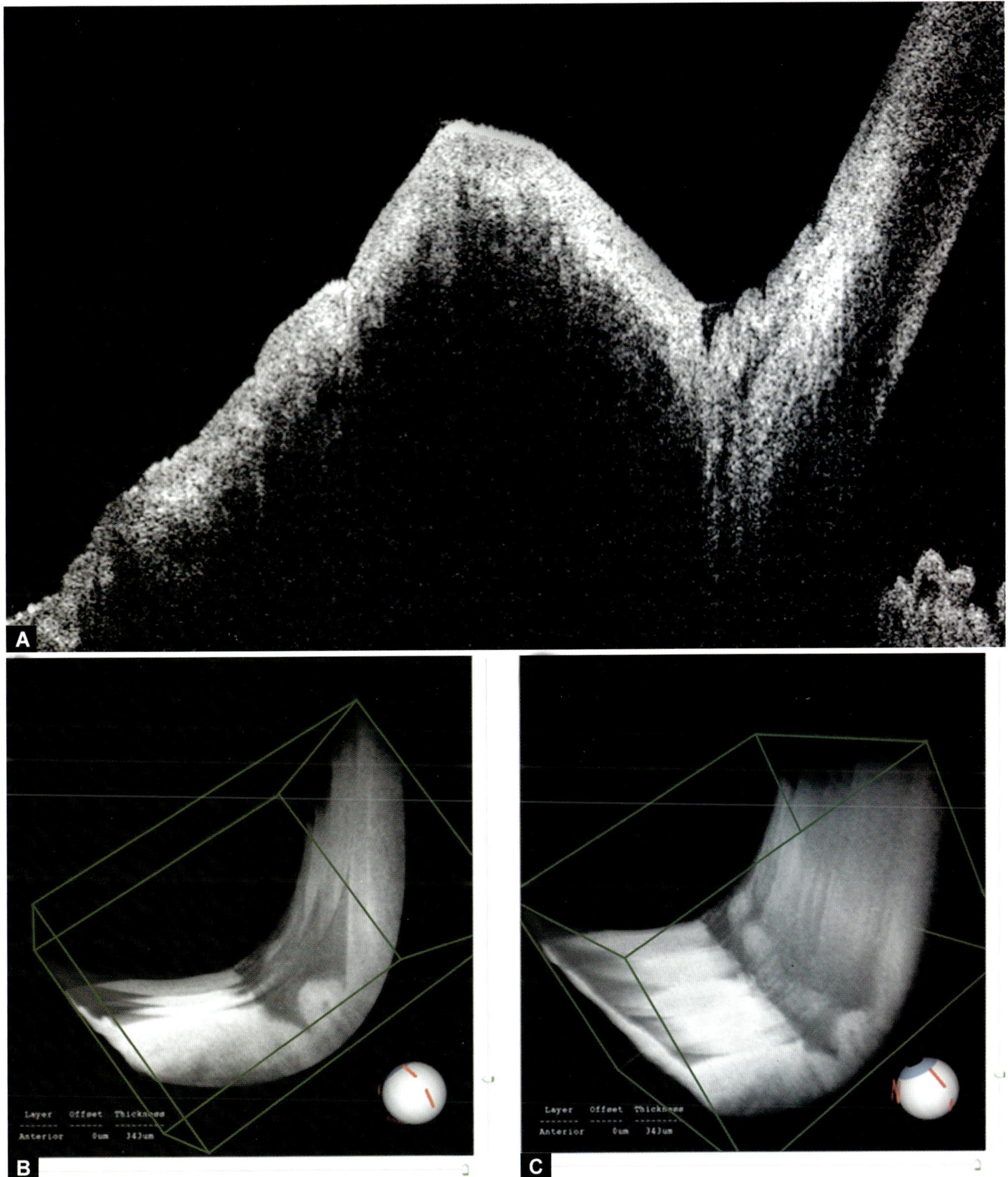

Figures 2A to C: Conjunctivochalasis. (A) Reduced inferior tear film meniscus and conjunctival folds are shown in a cross-section scan; (B and C) *En face* image with 3D imaging provides a more detailed reconstruction as compared to cross-sectional imaging. In addition, 3D imaging is able to detect a larger tear meniscus in comparison to cross-section (0.087 vs 0.047 mm^2)

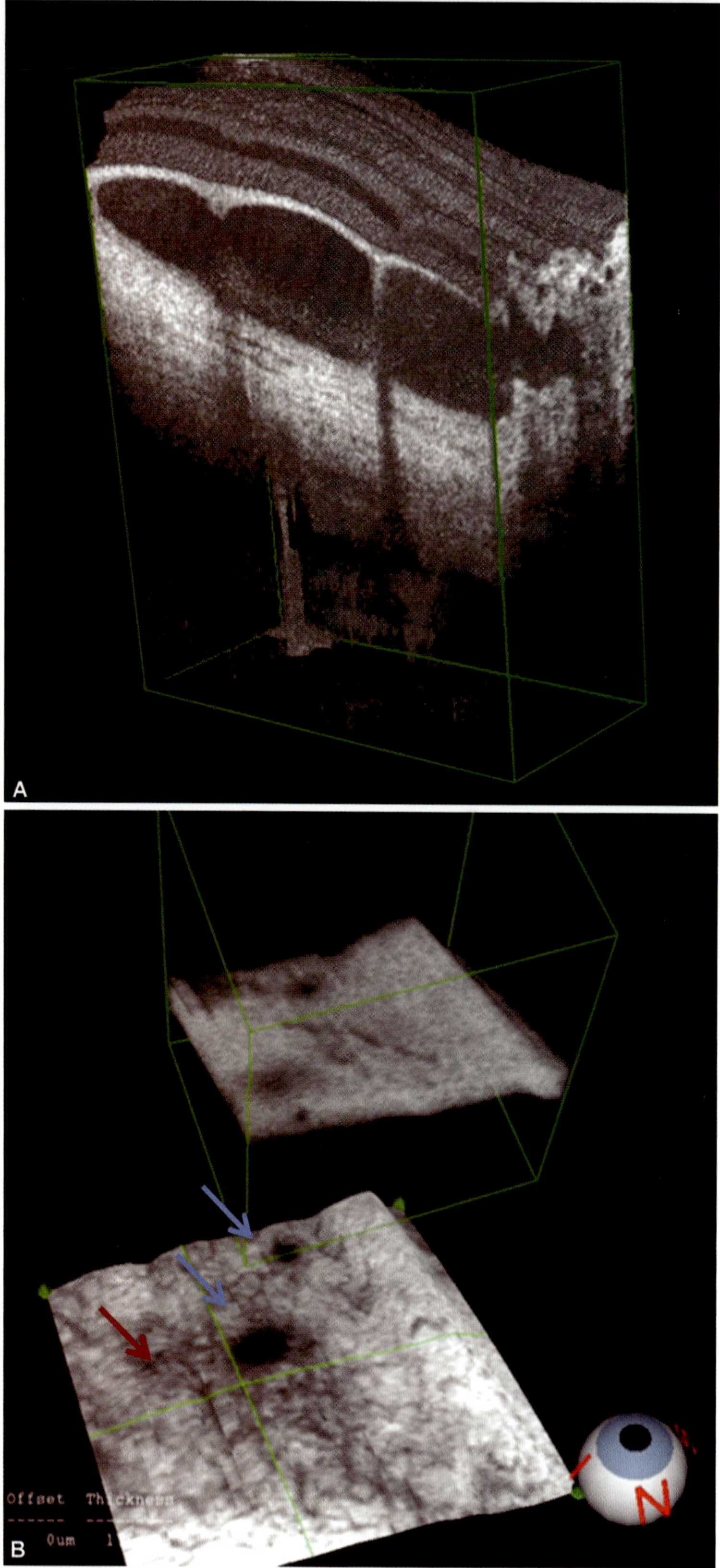

Figures 3A and B: Conjunctival cyst and pigmented conjunctival lesion. (A) Three cystic formations with visualization of cystic walls are shown by 3D imaging. (B, blue arrows) Optical shadowing of pigmented lesions and (B, red arrow) vascularization (red arrow) are visualized with the *en face* technique

a rather benign lesion.[22] Moreover, useful information can be derived with regards to tumor size, shape, internal features and extension if possible.

Infectious Keratitis

Infectious diseases of the cornea are a potentially blinding condition. As such, the outcome is correlated to rapid diagnosis, and to prompt and effective treatment.[23-27] Although AS-OCT is not able to detect the causative agent, images may reveal the extent of ulceration and corneal infiltrate size and depth.[28,29] Coronal sections can be obtained with the *en face* technique, improving visualization of epithelial irregularity or the absence of the epithelium in corneal ulcers, aiding in the evaluation of the extent and patter of epithelium defects in corneal ulcers (**Figures 4A and B**). In addition, the tissue around infiltrates reveals a granular pattern, demonstrating active disease and likely the presence of inflammatory cells. This technique may allow differentiation between corneal scars and active inflammation, as scar tissue presents a more homogenous pattern with a well-defined border, while inflammation is seen with a granular pattern (**Figures 5A and B**).

Corneal Neovascularization

Corneal neovascularization is a pathological response to a variety of insults, such as trauma, chemical burns, inflammation and infection. It may lead to corneal scarring and vision loss, and plays a significant role in corneal graft rejection. In fact around 20% of host corneal specimens obtained during corneal transplantation showed histopathologic evidence of some degree of corneal neovascularization.[30] Currently, visualization of corneal vessels is possible by slit-lamp biomicroscopy, and more detailed by fluorescein angiography (FA) and indocyanine green (ICG) angiography. Nevertheless, slit-lamp biomicroscopy only visualizes some of the vessels, while FA and ICG angiography are invasive techniques, requiring the use of intravenous dyes.[31] *En face* imaging, however, provides coronal sections with excellent visualization of vessels, not possible with standard cross-sectional AS-OCT imaging (**Figures 6A to E**). With the advent of anti-angiogenic treatments of the cornea, new techniques are needed to measure drug efficacy through quantification of vascular parameters, such as vessel caliper and assessment of blood flow. Current advances in *en face* imaging and the merging of AS-OCT with Doppler technology will enhance image quality and provide quantitative tools for evaluation of corneal neovascularization.

Corneal Edema

Corneal thickness reflects the corneal metabolic function, since corneal deturgescence is tightly controlled. With loss of metabolic and endothelial cell function, the hydration state changes, leading to increased corneal thickness and edema.[32] Anterior segment OCT can be used to detect the overall pachymetric changes.[33-35] Hutchings et al,[36] for example, reported acute changes in corneal thickness. Layer-by-layer measurements demonstrated that the corneal epithelial layer thickness increased approximately 3.5% in contact lens related hypoxia. Further, chronic corneal edema leads to changes in the epithelial and stromal reflectivity that can be visualized in cross-sectional AS-OCT images. Coronal sections by AS-OCT with *en face* imaging are able to show layer-by-layer changes, similar to *in vivo* confocal microscopy. The presence of areas suggestive of microcystic edema in a patient with a recent corneal abrasion indicates that epithelial recovery is not complete and further treatment is required (**Figures 7A and B**).

Uveitis

Anterior segment OCT is able to detect cellular anterior chamber reaction and the presence of keratic precipitates in the cornea. Recently, Agarwal et al[37] demonstrated the use of AS-OCT for visualization of corneal and anterior chamber inflammatory reaction using cross-sectional imaging. Although, currently it is not possible to differentiate pigments from keratic precipitates, there is evidence that AS-OCT can be used as a diagnostic tool to evaluate anterior uveitis in opaque corneas such as in patients with corneal edema. The presence and extent of keratic precipitates in a patient with herpetic anterior uveitis can be demonstrated by *en face* imaging and is superior to cross-sectional imaging (**Figures 8A and B**).

Corneal Transplantation

Anterior segment OCT imaging allows evaluation of corneal grafts. Historically, pachymetry has been used to assess the increase in corneal thickness in patients after corneal transplantation. Further, recent advances in corneal surgery have led to the emergence of deep anterior and endothelial lamellar keratoplasty. These procedures are technically difficult and AS-OCT has been applied as a tool in the diagnosis and management of possible complications. In lamellar procedures, especially in endothelial keratoplasty, the apposition and adhesion between donor endothelial layer and the recipient corneal stroma is accepted as a necessity to achieve corneal clearance, resulting in visual improvement. AS-OCT images are able to detect fluid in interface of posterior and anterior lamellar procedures.[11,38] Furthermore, 3D reconstruction can be used to evaluate graft apposition after endothelial keratoplasty (**Figure 9A**). Moreover, after penetrating keratoplasty, the graft-host junction remains vulnerable and is a potential area for wound dehiscence.[39-41]

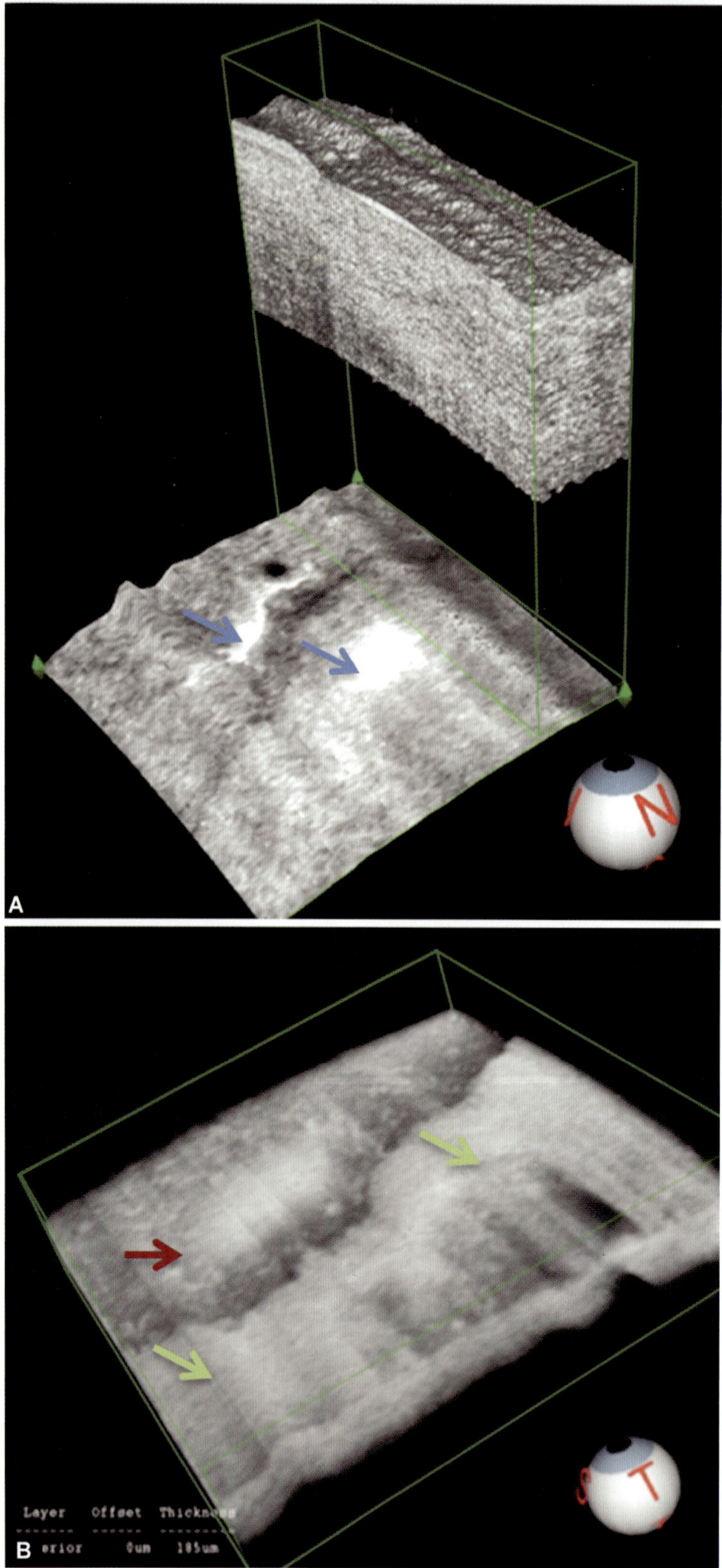

Figures 4A and B: Epithelial defect and corneal infiltrate in a patient with infectious keratitis. (A) 3D reconstruction with shadowing is demonstrated, allowing visualization of the irregular epithelial layer and two hyper-reflective infiltrates (blue arrows). A thin layer of epithelium covering the ulcer base is seen. (B) *En face* image of the infiltrate and irregular epithelium shows granularity around an infiltrate with a more heterogeneous hyper-reflective center (red arrow), and demonstrates the border and extent of the epithelial defect (green arrows)

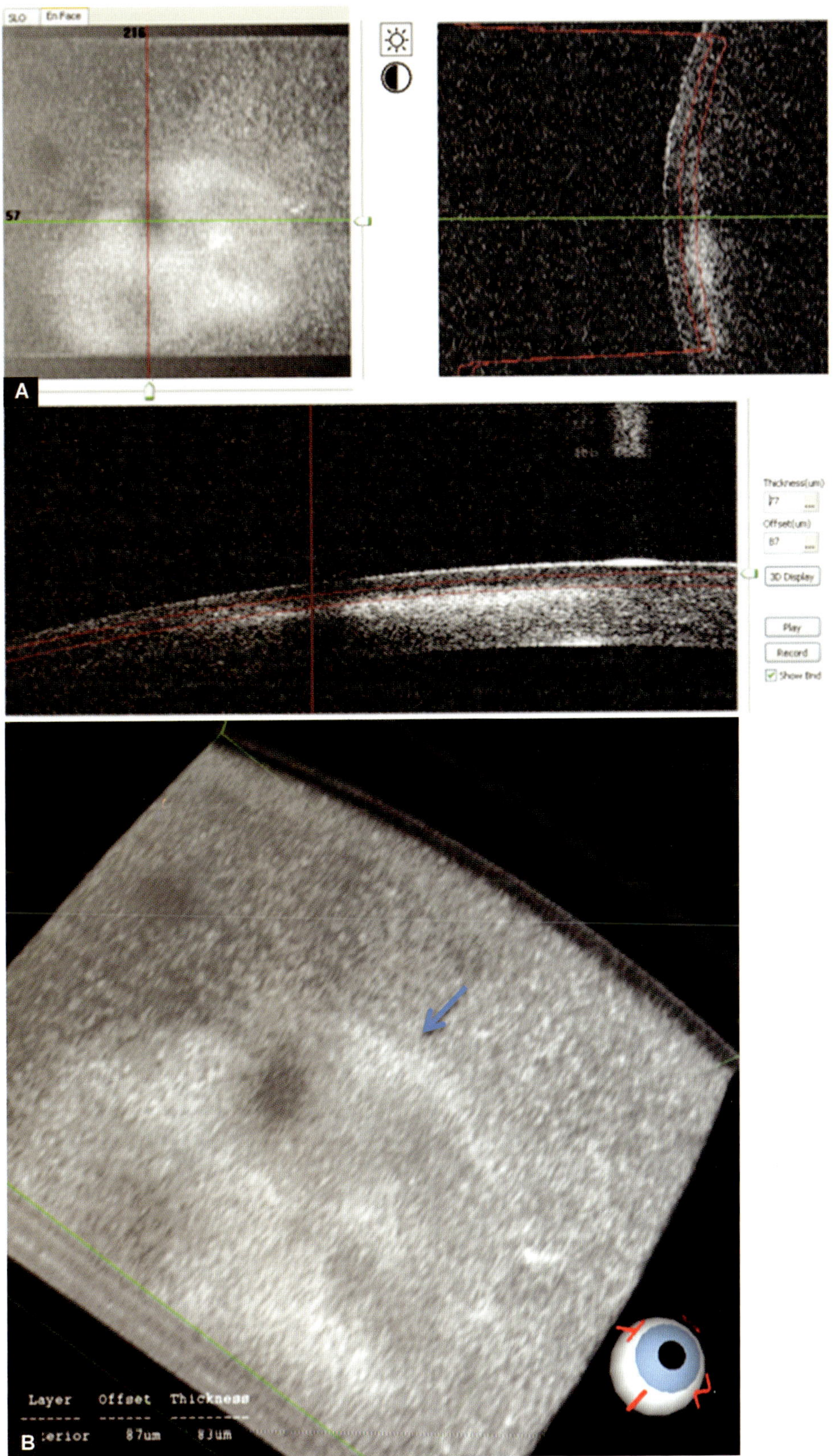

Figures 5A and B: Corneal scar. (A) Location, depth and width of the corneal scar is seen here. (B) *En face* image of the corneal scar reveals a homogenous hyper-reflective circular area with a well-defined border (blue arrow); no granular pattern is seen in surrounding the tissue

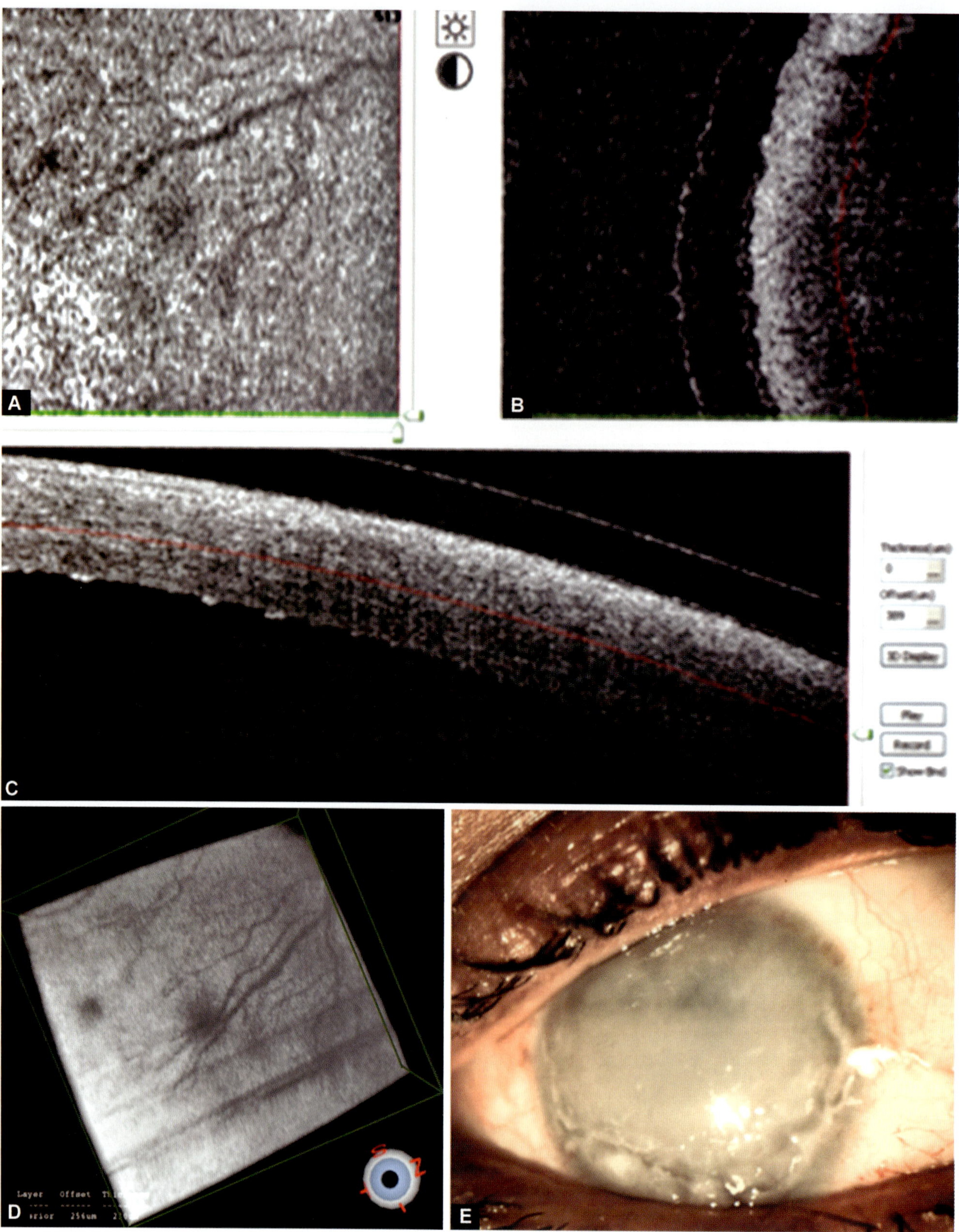

Figures 6A to E: Corneal neovascularization. (A to C) The location of the scan (389 μm), a preview of the coronal section and two cross-sectional images are shown. (D) *En face* image of deep stromal vessels is shown, demonstrating vessel length and caliper. (E) Slit-lamp photograph showing a dense scar in a neurotrophic ulcer did not allow identifying the deep corneal vessels shown by *en face* imaging

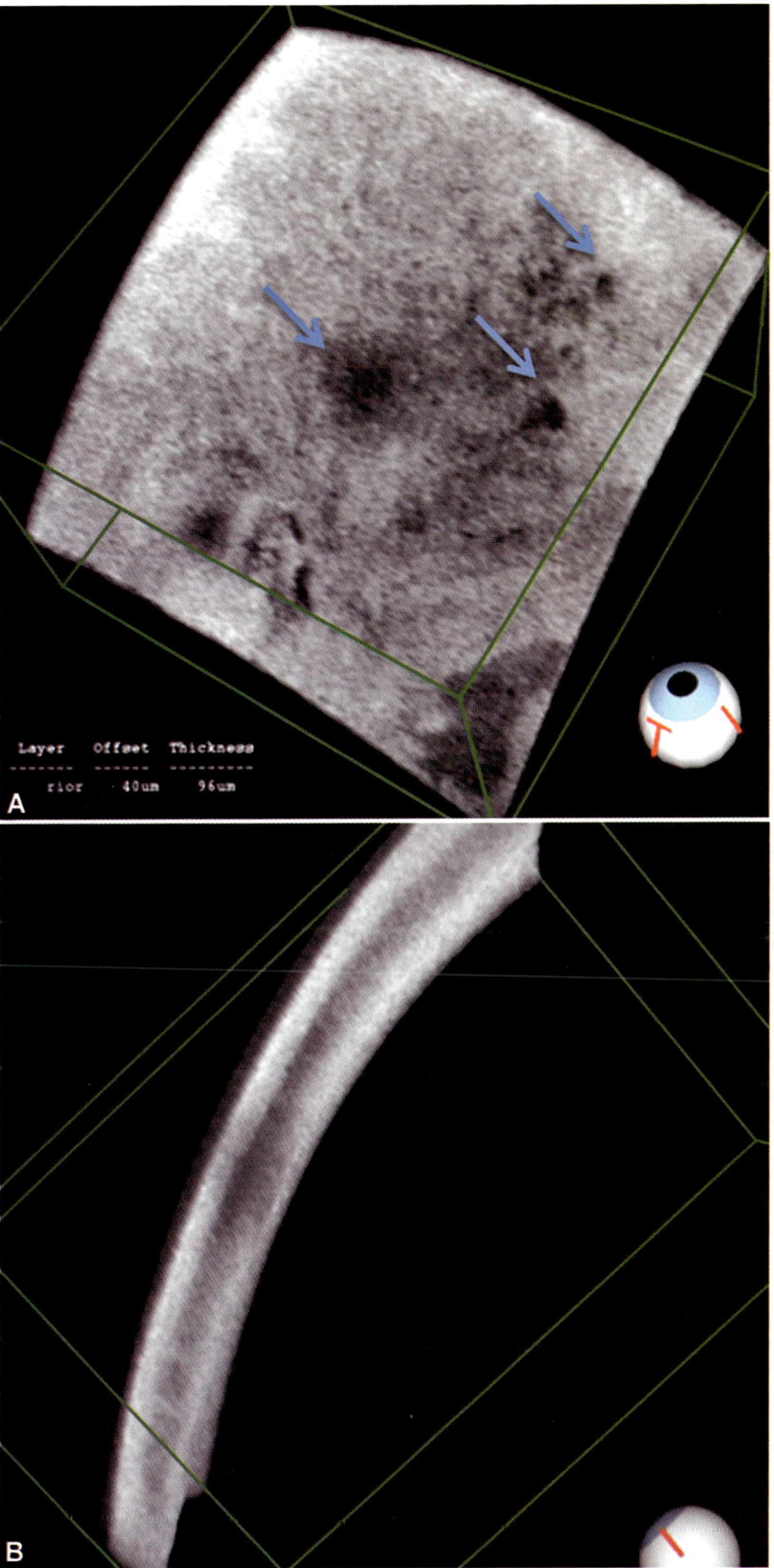

Figures 7A and B: Microcystic corneal edema in a patient with corneal abrasion. (A) Hyporeflective areas (blue arrows) in coronal sections are suggestive of microcystic corneal edema at 40 μm depth. (B) Cross-sectional imaging reveals a thin hyper-reflective epithelium and a hyporeflective stroma, but is not able to detect the microcystic epithelial edema

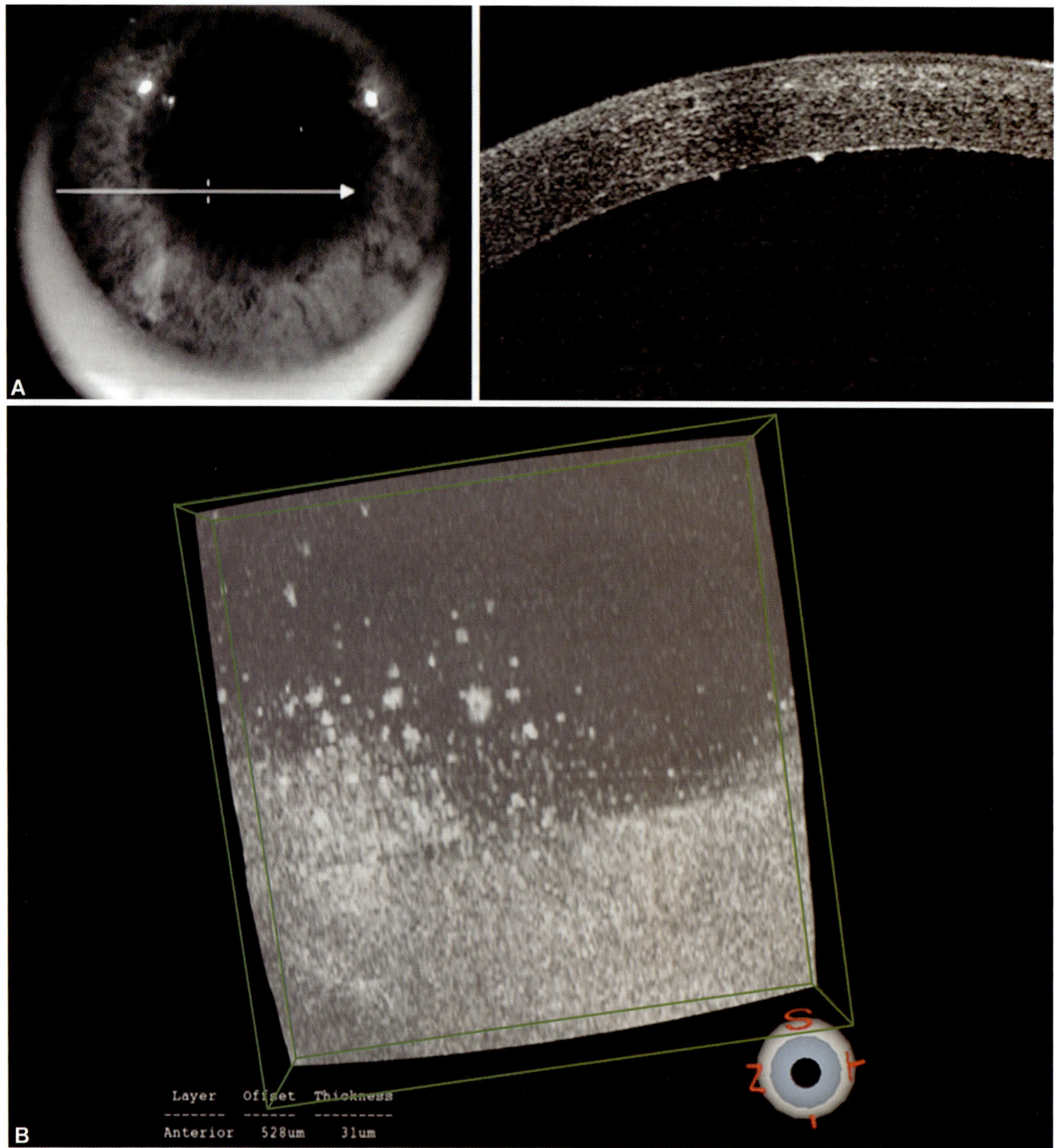

Figures 8A and B: Keratic precipitates in a patient with herpetic anterior uveitis. Presence of hyper-reflective areas adjacent to the corneal endothelium in (A) cross-sectional and (B) *en face* at 528 µm depth are shown

Several factors, such as poor wound apposition, suture failure, infection and melting may affect corneal wound construction after penetrating keratoplasty. A thick hyper-reflective line can be seen with *en face* AS-OCT as evidence of a good graft-host apposition at the graft host junction (**Figures 9B and C**). In addition, an irregular line with a surrounded hyporeflective area (gap) can be seen in a patient with minor graft dehiscence (**Figures 10A to C**).

Keratoprosthesis

Patients with multiples graft failures and moderate to severe ocular surface disease may not be good candidates for corneal transplantation. The Boston type 1 keratoprosthesis (Kpro I) is an "artificial cornea" used to replace the cornea in such cases. Cornea melting is one of the complications with this procedure, although the frequency has declined with the use of the bandage contact lens.[42,43] Clinical examination of the area behind the front plate is difficult, and early stages of melting may not be detected by slit-lamp biomicroscopy alone. AS-OCT imaging may be able to provide sufficient and superior detail of the KPRO and the surrounding donor corneal tissue, allowing clinicians to detect early melting before it is clinically apparent (**Figures 11A to D**).[44] *En face* imaging can further provide details regarding the extent and the dimensions of melting, and may allow determination of progression.

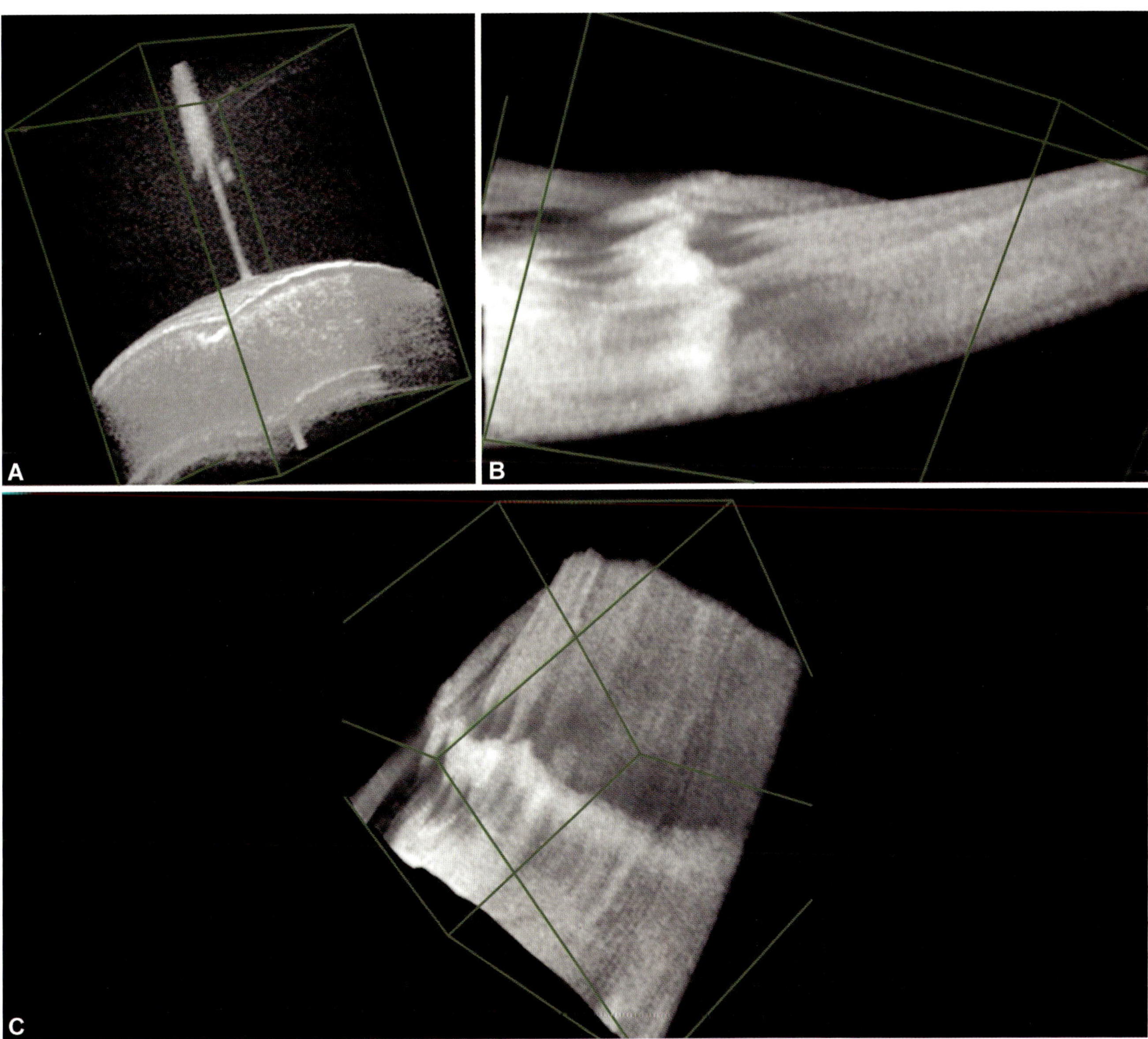

Figures 9A to C: Graft-host junction in penetrating and endothelial keratoplasty. (A) Three-dimensional reconstruction after endothelial keratoplasty shows good apposition of donor with no interface fluid. (B and C) A hyper-reflective line demonstrates the graft junction in a patient after penetrating keratoplasty

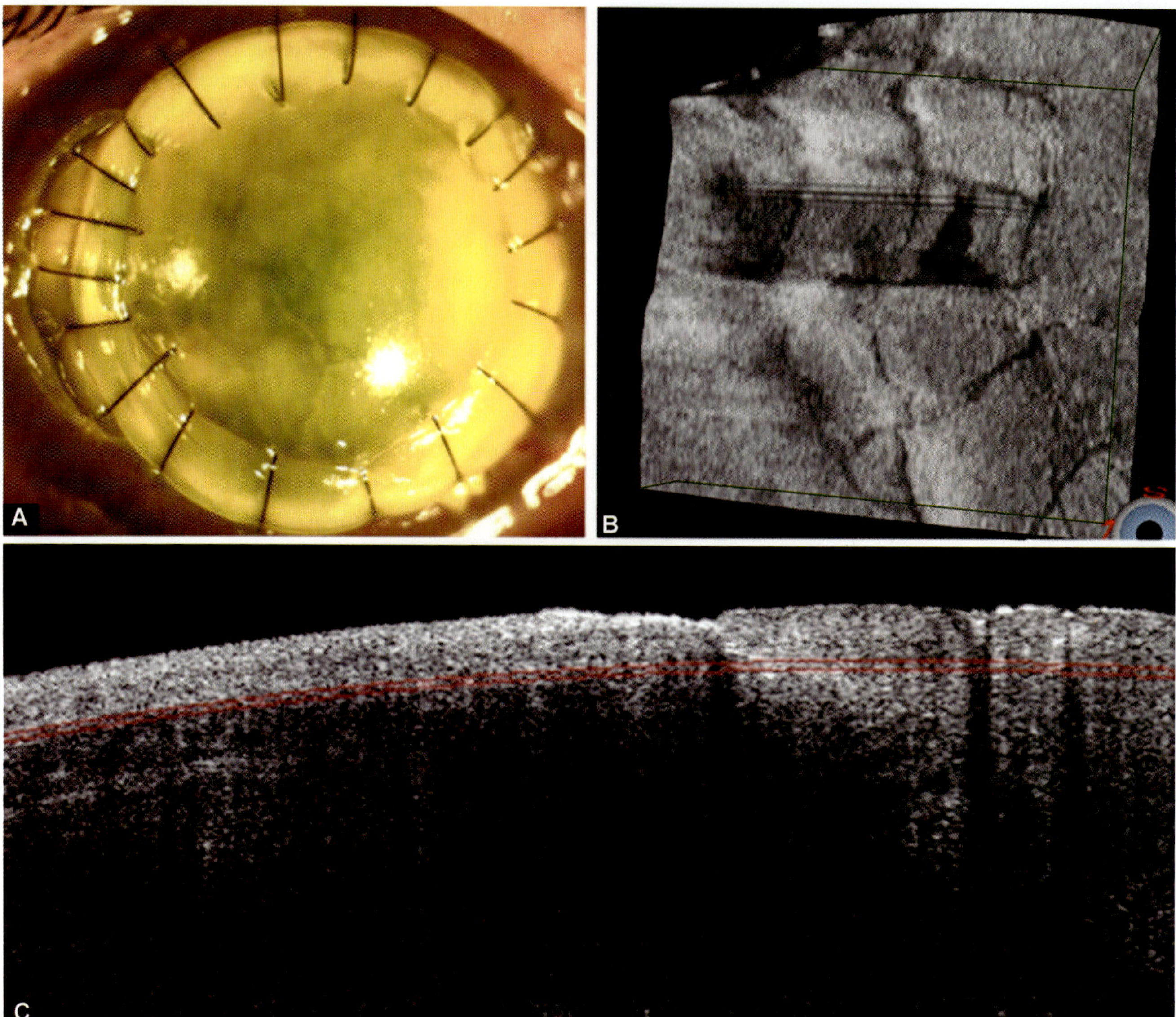

Figures 10A to C: Graft-host junction in a patient after penetrating keratoplasty. (A) Slit-lamp photo showing an epithelium defect in the nasal area of the graft. (B) *En face* image demonstrates improved visualization as compared to (C) cross-sectional imaging of the graft-host junction, showing a thin irregular line with a small gap between the donor and host cornea

Corneal Trauma

Corneal perforation is a cause of ocular morbidity and profound visual loss, thus requiring prompt management and in many cases necessitates urgent surgical intervention.[45-47] Currently slit-lamp evaluation is used to diagnose globe perforation. However, as it is important to minimize pressure on the eye, non-invasive AS-OCT would allow a more detailed measurement of wounds. This is particularly important when decision on surgical vs. medical treatment needs to be rendered. **Figures 12A to D** show a case of corneal perforation. Detailed analysis of the 3D imaging demonstrates self-sealing with iris plugging the site of corneal perforation.

Future

Anterior segment OCT is a new non-invasive technology that utilizes propagated infrared light waves onto a scattering medium, such as corneal tissue. The emergence of *en face* imaging will aid clinicians in medical and surgical management of corneal and anterior segment diseases beyond cross-sectional AS-OCT imaging, as detailed in this chapter. However, increased light reflectance and the requirement for a steady gaze for at least 2 seconds are some of the limitations for this technique. New swept source technology is currently being developed for the cornea and anterior segment. Swept source OCT uses a wavelength swept laser, single or dual

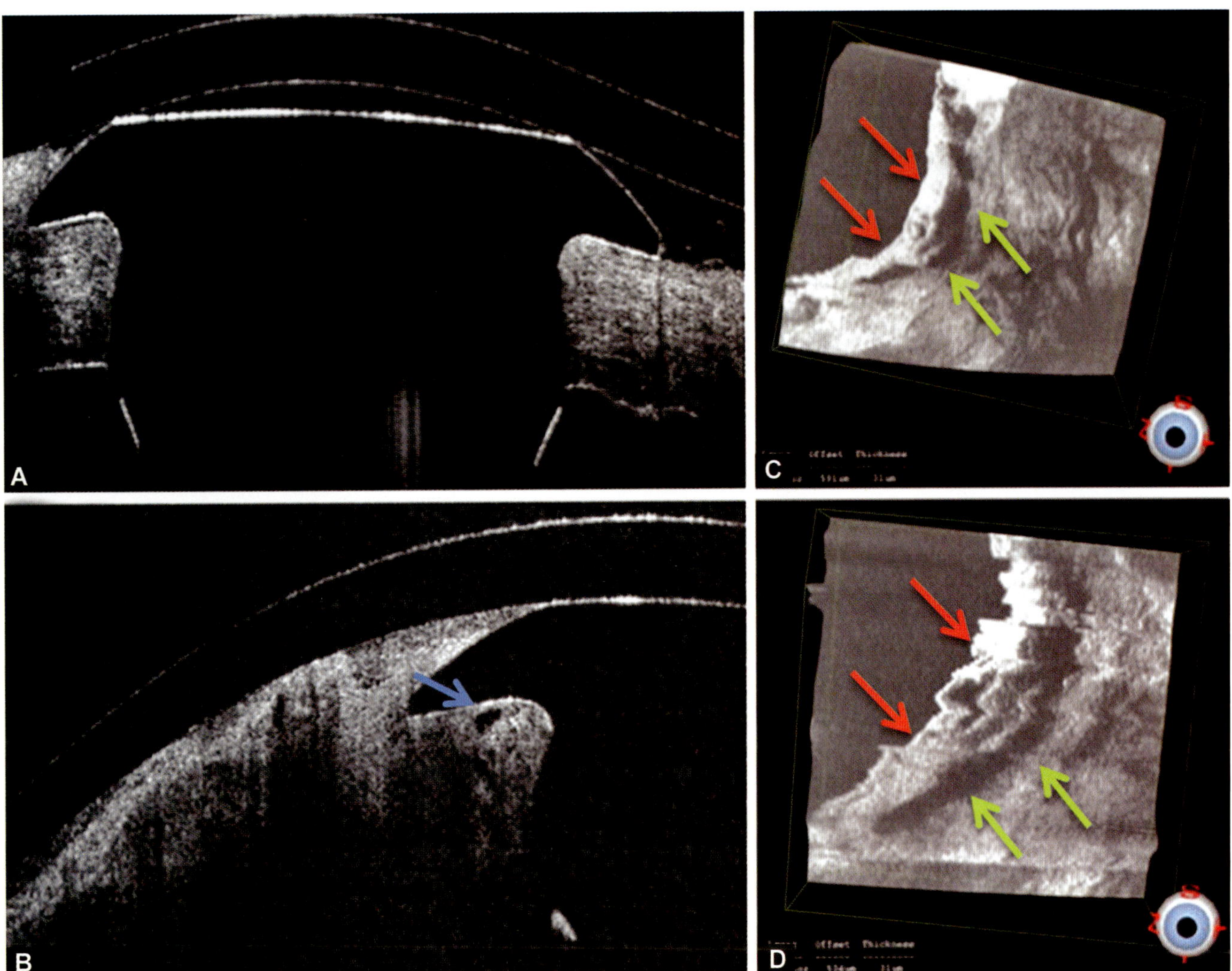

Figures 11A to D: Boston type 1 keratoprosthesis (Kpro I). (A) Normal cross-sectional imaging of Kpro type 1 showing good apposition of graft and poly(methyl methacrylate) (PMMA) front plate. (C) Early corneal melting can be detected as a hyporeflective area under the Kpro front plate (blue arrow). (B and D) *En face* imaging of the Kpro-graft junction shows evidence and the extent of corneal melting as an irregular hyporeflective area (green arrows), the appearance of adjacent hyper-reflectivity (red arrows) that could demonstrate scarring or inflammation

balanced detector and high speed A/D,[48] leading to improvement in *en face* imaging. Thus, promising future applications will be possible in the near future with the increased speed of scans (200,000 lines per second) and will enable high-sampling density in 3D imaging of the entire cornea.[49,50] The resulting superior quality of coronal sections will likely revolutionize anterior segment imaging and its impact on daily clinical decision-making.

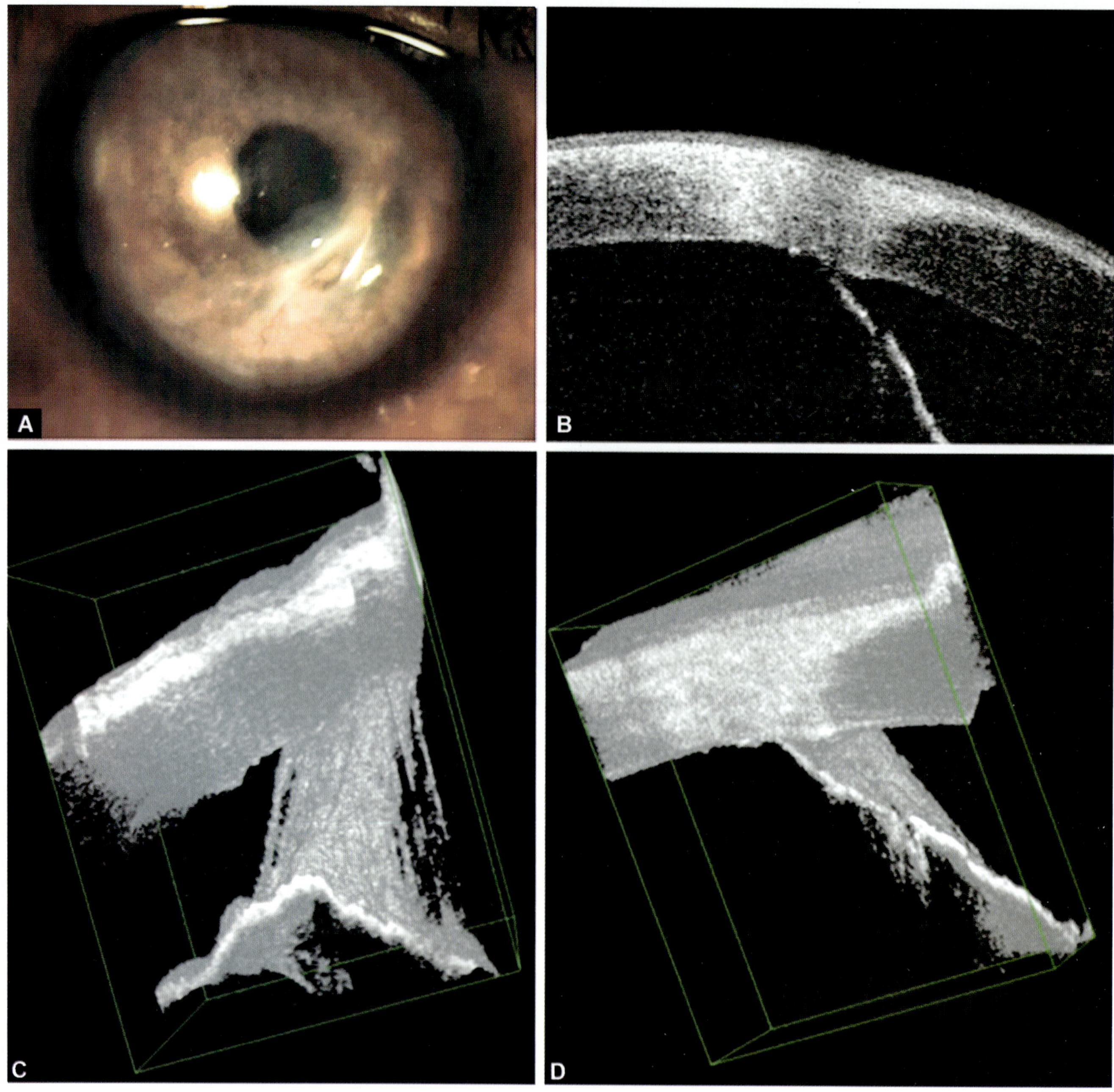

Figures 12A to D: Corneal perforation. (A) Slit-lamp photo of cornea perforation with deep anterior chamber. (B) Anterior segment optical coherence tomography imaging reveals anterior synechiae and iris plugging the site of corneal perforation in cross-sectional and 3D reconstruction (C and D)

References

1. Izatt JA, Hee MR, Swanson EA, et al. Micrometer-scale resolution imaging of the anterior eye *in vivo* with optical coherence tomography. Arch Ophthalmol. 1994;112:1584-9.

2. Wang J, Thomas J, Cox I, et al. Noncontact measurements of central corneal epithelial and flap thickness after laser *in situ* keratomileusis. Invest Ophthalmol Vis Sci. 2004;45:1812-6.

3. Chen HJ, Xia YJ, Zhong YY, et al. Anterior segment optical coherence tomography measurement of flap thickness after myopic LASIK using the Moria one use-plus microkeratome. J Refract Surg. 2010;26:403-10.

4. Li Y, Netto MV, Shekhar R, et al. A longitudinal study of LASIK flap and stromal thickness with high-speed optical coherence tomography. Ophthalmology. 2007;114:1124-32.

5. Li Y, Meisler DM, Tang M, et al. Keratoconus diagnosis with optical coherence tomography pachymetry mapping. Ophthalmology. 2008;115:2159-66.

6. Wirbelauer C, Pham DT. Imaging and quantification of calcified corneal lesions with optical coherence tomography. Cornea. 2004;23:439-42.

7. Khurana RN, Li Y, Tang M, et al. High-speed optical coherence tomography of corneal opacities. Ophthalmology. 2007;114:1278-85.

8. Reddy HS, Li Y, Yiu SC, et al. Optical coherence tomography of corneal and scleral melts. Ophthalmic Surg Lasers Imaging. 2007;38:514-7.

9. Wong HT, Lim MC, Sakata LM, et al. High-definition optical coherence tomography imaging of the iridocorneal angle of the eye. Arch Ophthalmol. 2009;127:256-60.

10. Radhakrishnan S, See J, Smith SD, et al. Reproducibility of anterior chamber angle measurements obtained with anterior segment optical coherence tomography. Invest Ophthalmol Vis Sci. 2007;48:3683-8.

11. Lim LS, Aung HT, Aung T, et al. Corneal imaging with anterior segment optical coherence tomography for lamellar keratoplasty procedures. Am J Ophthalmol. 2008;145:81-90.

12. Yasuno Y, Madjarova VD, Makita S, et al. Three-dimensional and high-speed swept-source optical coherence tomography for *in vivo* investigation of human anterior eye segments. Opt Express. 2005;13:10652-64.

13. Kawana K, Kiuchi T, Yasuno Y, et al. Evaluation of trabeculectomy blebs using 3-dimensional cornea and anterior segment optical coherence tomography. Ophthalmology. 2009;116:848-55.

14. Fukuda S, Kawana K, Yasuno Y, et al. Anterior ocular biometry using 3-dimensional optical coherence tomography. Ophthalmology. 2009;116:882-9.

15. Wang J, Aquavella J, Palakuru J, et al. Repeated measurements of dynamic tear distribution on the ocular surface after instillation of artificial tears. Invest Ophthalmol Vis Sci. 2006;47:3325-9.

16. Chen Q, Wang J, Shen M, et al. Lower volumes of tear menisci in contact lens wearers with dry eye symptoms. Invest Ophthalmol Vis Sci. 2009;50:3159-63.

17. Wang J, Cox I, Reindel WT. Upper and lower tear menisci on contact lenses. Invest Ophthalmol Vis Sci. 2009;50:1106-11.

18. Wang J, Palakuru JR, Aquavella JV. Correlations among upper and lower tear menisci, noninvasive tear break-up time, and the Schirmer test. Am J Ophthalmol. 2008;145:795-800.

19. Gumus K, Crockett CH, Pflugfelder SC. Anterior segment optical coherence tomography: a diagnostic instrument for conjunctivochalasis. Am J Ophthalmol. 2010;150:798-806.

20. Siahmed K, Berges O, Desjardins L, et al. Anterior segment tumor imaging: advantages of ultrasound (10, 20 and 50 MHz) and optical coherence tomography. J Fr Ophtalmol. 2004;27:169-73.

21. Bianciotto C, Shields CL, Guzman JM, et al. Assessment of anterior segment tumors with ultrasound biomicroscopy versus anterior segment optical coherence tomography in 200 cases. Ophthalmology. 2011;118:1297-302.

22. Shields CL, Belinsky I, Romanelli-Gobbi M, et al. Anterior segment optical coherence tomography of conjunctival nevus. Ophthalmology. 2011;118:915-9.

23. Whitcher JP, Srinivasan M. Corneal ulceration in the developing world—a silent epidemic. Br J Ophthalmol. 1997;81:622-3.

24. Thomas PA, Geraldine P. Infectious keratitis. Curr Opin Infect Dis. 2007;20:129-41.

25. Radford CF, Minassian DC, Dart JK. Acanthamoeba keratitis in England and Wales: incidence, outcome, and risk factors. Br J Ophthalmol. 2002;86:536-42.

26. Garg P. Diagnosis of microbial keratitis. Br J Ophthalmol. 2010;94:961-2.

27. Whitcher JP, Srinivasan M, Upadhyay MP. Corneal blindness: a global perspective. Bull World Health Org. 2001;79:214-21.

28. Konstantopoulos A, Yadegarfar G, Fievez M, et al. *In vivo* quantification of bacterial keratitis with optical coherence tomography. Invest Ophthalmol Vis Sci. 2011;52:1093-7.

29. Konstantopoulos A, Kuo J, Anderson D, et al. Assessment of the use of anterior segment optical coherence tomography in microbial keratitis. Am J Ophthalmol. 2008;146:534-42.

30. Cursiefen C, Küchle M, Naumann GO. Angiogenesis in corneal diseases: histopathologic evaluation of 254 human corneal buttons with neovascularization. Cornea. 1998;17:611-3.

31. Anijeet DR, Zheng Y, Tey A, et al. Imaging and evaluation of corneal vascularization using fluorescein and indocyanine green angiography. Invest Ophthalmol Vis Sci. 2012;53:650-8.

32. Huff JW. Contact lens-induced edema *in vitro*. Pharmacology and metabolic considerations. Invest Ophthalmol Vis Sci. 1991;32:346-53.

33. Li YJ, Kim HJ, Joo CK. Early changes in corneal edema following torsional phacoemulsification using anterior segment optical coherence tomography and Scheimpflug photography. Jpn J Ophthalmol. 2011;55:196-204.

34. Huang JY, Pekmezci M, Yaplee S, et al. Intra-examiner repeatability and agreement of corneal pachymetry map measurement by time-domain and Fourier-domain optical coherence tomography. Graefes Arch Clin Exp Ophthalmol. 2010; 248:1647-56.

35. Bechmann M, Thiel MJ, Neubauer AS, et al. Central corneal thickness measurement with a retinal optical coherence tomography device versus standard ultrasonic pachymetry. Cornea. 2001;20:50-4.

36. Hutchings N, Simpson TL, Hyun C, et al. Swelling of the human cornea revealed by high-speed, ultrahigh-resolution optical coherence tomography. Invest Ophthalmol Vis Sci. 2010;51:4579-84.

37. Agarwal A, Ashokkumar D, Jacob S, et al. High-speed optical coherence tomography for imaging anterior chamber inflammatory reaction in uveitis: clinical correlation and grading. Am J Ophthalmol. 2009;147:413-6.

38. Hurmeric V, Wang J, Kymionis GD, et al. Persistent lamellar interface fluid with clear cornea after Descemet stripping automated endothelial keratoplasty. Cornea. 2011;30: 1485-7.

39. Renucci AM, Marangon FB, Culbertson WW. Wound dehiscence after penetrating keratoplasty: clinical characteristics of 51 cases treated at Bascom Palmer Eye Institute. Cornea. 2006;25:524-9.

40. Rehany U, Rumelt S. Ocular trauma following penetrating keratoplasty: incidence, outcome, and postoperative recommendations. Arch Ophthalmol. 1998;116:1282-6.

41. Tseng SH, Lin SC, Chen FK. Traumatic wound dehiscence after penetrating keratoplasty: clinical features and outcome in 21 cases. Cornea. 1999;18:553-8.

42. Doane MG, Dohlman CH, Bearse G. Fabrication of a keratoprosthesis. Cornea. 1996;15:179-84.

43. Dohlman CH, Dudenhoefer EJ, Khan BF, et al. Protection of the ocular surface after keratoprosthesis surgery: the role of soft contact lenses. CLAO J. 2002;28:72-4.

44. Garcia JP, de la Cruz J, Rosen RB, et al. Imaging implanted keratoprostheses with anterior-segment optical coherence tomography and ultrasound biomicroscopy. Cornea. 2008;27:180-8.

45. Panda A, Khokhar S, Rao V, et al. Therapeutic penetrating keratoplasty in nonhealing corneal ulcer. Ophthalmic Surg. 1995;26:325-9.

46. Portnoy SL, Insler MS, Kaufman HE. Surgical management of corneal ulceration and perforation. Surv Ophthalmol. 1989;34:47-58.

47. Sall K, Stevenson OD, Mundorf TK, et al. Two multicenter, randomized studies of the efficacy and safety of cyclosporine ophthalmic emulsion in moderate to severe dry eye disease. CsA Phase 3 Study Group. Ophthalmology. 2000;107:631-9.

48. Chinn SR, Swanson EA, Fujimoto JG. Optical coherence tomography using a frequency-tunable optical source. Opt Lett. 1997;22:340-2.

49. Huber R, Wojtkowski M, Fujimoto JG. Fourier Domain Mode Locking (FDML): A new laser operating regime and applications for optical coherence tomography. Opt Express. 2006;14:3225-37.

50. Gora M, Karnowski K, Szkulmowski M, et al. Ultra high-speed swept source OCT imaging of the anterior segment of human eye at 200 kHz with adjustable imaging range. Opt Express. 2009;17:14880-94.

En Face Optical Coherence Tomography Imaging of Corneal Limbal Stem Cell Niche

Edgar M Espana, Ali R Djalilian, Sonia H Yoo, Andre Romano

Introduction

The corneal epithelium, like many other epithelial surfaces, undergoes constant renewal by a population of local adult stem cells. The corneal epithelial stem cells are located primarily at the limbus, the junction between the cornea and the conjunctiva, hence they are known as the limbal stem cells. Under various pathologic conditions, such as severe immunologic disorders or chemical injuries, the limbal stem cells may be damaged or destroyed. In such situations, the corneal epithelium is gradually replaced by conjunctival epithelium which has significant visual consequences. In particular, patients with limbal stem cell deficiency (LSCD), develop nonhealing epithelial defects, neovascularization and scarring of the cornea resulting in profound loss of vision.[1] Currently, most treatments for LSCD involve surgical replacement of the limbal stem cells from a healthy donor eye.[2] There are very few nonsurgical treatment options available especially for patients who have subtotal LSCD or those with localized dysfunction of the limbus. Most nonsurgical treatments, such as anti-inflammatory therapy, autologous serum tears, or scleral contact lenses, are aimed at restoring a healthy ocular surface and environment for the limbal stem cells.

There has been an increasing awareness of the role of the limbal stem cell microenvironment (aka limbal stem cell niche) in the maintenance and homeostasis of the corneal and limbal epithelial stem cells. This limbal niche consists of both cellular (e.g. limbal fibroblasts) as well as noncellular (e.g. extracellular matrix) components.[3] Major insults to the ocular surface, such as chemical injuries or severe autoimmune reactions, typically destroy the limbal epithelial stem cells along with their niche. In mild or localized LSCD, however, the limbal epithelial stem cells may be partially or completely preserved, yet their function compromised because of presumed disturbances to the limbal niche.

An important landmark that includes the limbal stem cell niche is the limbal palisades of Vogt. These are visible at the slit lamp as radial lines in the limbal regions with different degrees of pigmentation, characteristically more pigmented cells are noted in individuals with more skin pigmentation. Histologically, this corresponds to undulations in the underlying stroma. Another important histologic feature that has been recently proposed for a more specific location of limbal stem cells niche is the limbal crypt.[4]

A number of studies have described the use of confocal scanning microscopy to image the limbus and limbal epithelium *in vivo* and *ex vivo*.[5,6] One recent study has used OCT *ex vivo* to image the limbal palisades of Vogt.[7] However, there are no studies describing the use of OCT for *en face* imaging of the limbus in humans *in vivo*.[8] In this chapter we present *in vivo en face* imaging of the limbal palisades of Vogt for the first time. We describe the findings and the potential clinical application of this technology for diagnosis and management of patients with limbal dysfunction.[9-13]

In Vivo En Face Imaging of the Limbus in Healthy Eyes

Using the cornea anterior module (CAM) on an RTVue OCT system (Optovue), the corneal limbus was scanned in several healthy volunteers (**Figure 1A**). The *en face* images were typically reconstructed for a 2×2 mm^2 area, however the dimensions can range from X to Y. The most important anatomical features that were visualized in the *en face* images included the limbal palisades of Vogt, the limbal vasculature and the sub-basal nerve plexus (**Figures 1B and C**). The palisades were visible as regions of alternating high and low intensity signal corresponding to the topographic appearance of the palisades. Reconstructed *en face* images from deeper layers in the limbal region revealed islands of small epithelial-

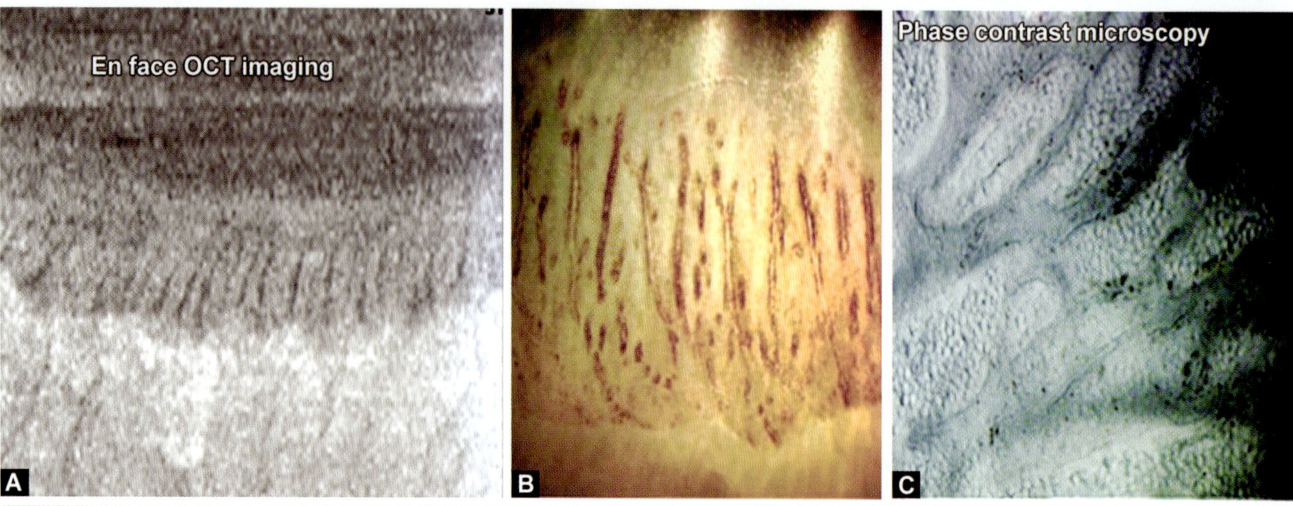

Figures 1A to C: Illustrative image of normal palisades of Vogt in a 37-year-old male with a healthy limbus. (A) Upper left image shows undulated radial lines at the junction of the cornea and conjunctiva. (B and C) Phase contrast microscopy depicts the undulating configuration of the palisades with cells within limbal crypts which one could speculate as containing the limbal stem cells

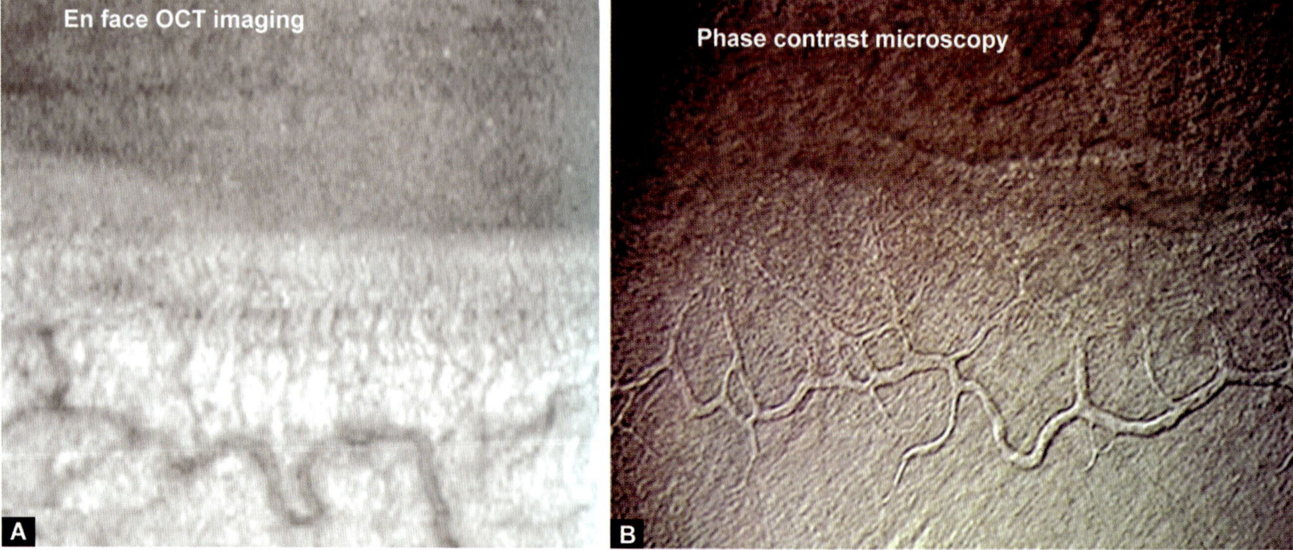

Figures 2A and B: (A) The limbal vascular arcades can be clearly visualized looping around and within the limbus with *en face* reference place located underneath the epithelium layer; (B) The same configuration can be appreciated with phase contrast microscopy

like structures which could represent inferior limbal basal cells or cells within limbal crypts which one could speculate as containing the limbal stem cells. However, the quality of images obtained from the deeper structures within the cornea were not high enough to completely resolve the nature of these structures. The limbal vascular arcades could be clearly visualized looping around and within the limbus. Likewise, the sub-basal nerve plexus in the limbal region were seen as areas of higher intensity signal at the level of the basement membrane **(Figures 2A and B).**

Potential Clinical Applications of *In Vivo En Face* Optical Coherence Tomography Imaging

Diagnosis of LSCD: Evaluating the normal anatomy of the limbus is one of the most important clues for the diagnosis of either partial or total limbal insufficiency. The presence of a normal conjunctival to corneal transition in the limbal area and the normal anatomy of limbal blood vessels can be easily appreciated with this novel, no touch *en face* imaging technique.

Assessment of medical therapies aimed at restoring the limbal niche: This imaging technique may be useful to assess the success of different treatments aimed to restore the limbal stem cells environment and ocular surface health. The effect of anti-inflammatory therapy, autologous serum tears, or scleral contact lenses on the anatomy of the limbal niche could easily be assessed with this technique.

Evaluation and quantification of limbal structures for transplantation: The presence of limbal structures associated with the presence of stem cells like the limbal crypts can be better evaluated and selected for limbal transplantation.

Evaluation of keratolimbal and limbal grafts vitality and survival: This method can potentially become an accurate method to evaluate the survival of stem cell grafts into the ocular surface. The presence of vascularization into the grafts can also be assessed and quantified.

Objective measurement of ocular surface inflammation: Patients with limbitis, measurement of limbal blood vessels diameter and tortuosity may correlate with the degree of inflammation.

References

1. Hatch KM, Dana R. The structure and function of the limbal stem cell and the disease states associated with limbal stem cell deficiency. Int Ophthalmol Clin. 2009;49:43-52.
2. Holland EJ. Epithelial transplantation for the management of severe ocular surface disease. Trans Am Ophthalmol Soc. 1996;94:677-743.
3. Li W, Hayashida Y, Chen YT, et al. Niche regulation of corneal epithelial stem cells at the limbus. Cell Res. 2007;17:26-36.
4. Dua HS, Shanmuganathan VA, Powell-Richards AO, et al. Limbal epithelial crypts: a novel anatomical structure and a putative limbal stem cell niche. Br J Ophthalmol. 2005;89:529-32.
5. Romano AC, Espana EM, Yoo SH, et al. Different cell sizes in human limbal and central corneal basal epithelia measured by confocal microscopy and flow cytometry. Invest Ophthalmol Vis Sci. 2003;44(12):5125-9.
6. Miri A, Alomar T, Nubile M, et al. In vivo confocal microscopic findings in patients with limbal stem cell deficiency. Br J Ophthalmol. 2012;96(4):523-9.
7. Lathrop KL, Gupta D, Kagemann L, et al. Optical coherence tomography as a rapid, accurate, noncontact method of visualizing the palisades of Vogt. Invest Ophthalmol Vis Sci. 2012;53(3):1381-7.
8. Notara M, Shortt AJ, O'Callaghan AR, et al. The impact of age on the physical and cellular properties of the human limbal stem cell niche. Age (Dordr). 2012.
9. Deng SX, Sejpal KD, Tang Q, et al. Characterization of limbal stem cell deficiency by in vivo laser scanning confocal microscopy: a microstructural approach. Arch Ophthalmol. 2012;130(4):440-5.
10. Zarei-Ghanavati S, Ramirez-Miranda A, Deng SX. Limbal lacuna: a novel limbal structure detected by in vivo laser scanning confocal microscopy. Ophthalmic Surg Lasers Imaging. 2011;42 Online:e129-31. doi: 10.3928/15428877-20111201-07.
11. Hong J, Zheng T, Xu J, et al. Assessment of limbus and central cornea in patients with keratolimbal allograft transplantation using in vivo laser scanning confocal microscopy: an observational study. Graefes Arch Clin Exp Ophthalmol. 2011;249(5):701-8.
12. Huang HW, Hu FR, Wang IJ, et al. Migration of limbal melanocytes onto the central cornea after ocular surface reconstruction: an in vivo confocal microscopic case report. Cornea. 2010;29(2):204-6.
13. Takahashi N, Chikama T, Yanai R, et al. Structures of the corneal limbus detected by laser-scanning confocal biomicroscopy as related to the palisades of Vogt detected by slit-lamp microscopy. Jpn J Ophthalmol. 2009;53(3): 199-203.

Section 4

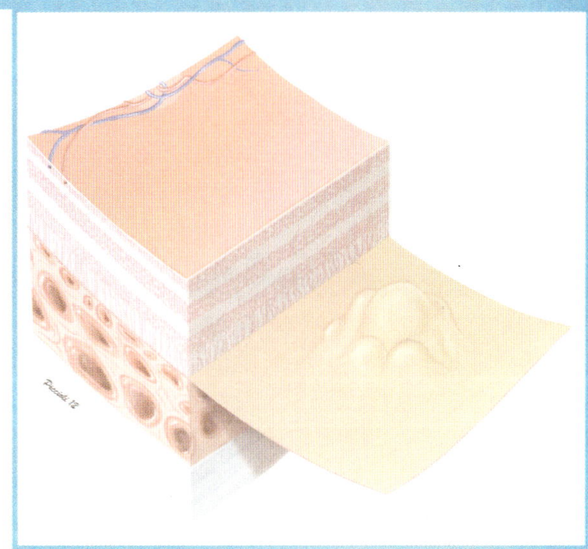

Retinal *En Face* Optical Coherence Tomography: General Syndromes

Pigment Epithelium Detachments *En Face* Optical Coherence Tomography Analysis

Bruno Lumbroso, Marco Rispoli, Maria Cristina Savastano

Introduction

Pigment epithelium detachments (PEDs) vary according to the retinal disease in which they are observed and the age of the patient, but PED having the same etiology may show different shapes. Their shape ranges from a simple rounded elevation to complex polylobular and cluster patterns. *En face* scans help delineate diagnosis in PED. They provide important information on the retinal PED structure and morphology.

Retinal PED is seen when retinal pigment epithelium (RPE) basement membrane separates from inner Bruch's membrane.[1,2] Pigment epithelium detachment is considered to be an important clinical condition of retinal-choriocapillaris suffering as outcome of disorders in fluid flow from retina to Bruch's membrane.[3]

We find in literature few reports about retinal PED analysis with *en face*. Van Velthoven et al. described advantages to detect tiny protrusions of RPE, by sequences of multiple scans in macular area with *en face* optical coherence tomography (OCT). High recurrences of retinal PED in central serous chorioretinopathy (CSC) eyes, 52% in active CSC and 100% in inactive CSC, were reported.[1-7]

Mitrai and colleagues described retinal PED irregularity (96%) and retinal PED (63%) related to fluorescein angiography (FA) leakage point in acute CSC.[4] Characteristic pinpoint FA leakage on RPE (69%) correlated to retinal PED (25%) and a bulge of RPE (45%), as seen with *en face* analysis, were reported by Hirami et al. in CSC patients.[5] Montero et al reported a small bulge of RPE on stratus OCT images related by leaking point seen on FA in acute CSC patients.[6] Probably the details observable, only with *en face* OCT, reveal more recurrent retinal PED in CSC than previously observed. The authors, Lumbroso and colleagues, reported in 2011[8] the morphologic differences, according to etiology, in pigment epithelial detachment by means of *en face* optical coherence tomography.

En Face Scans in Pigment Epithelium Detachments

En face scans adapted to cup-shaped pigment epithelium are easy to perform and to read. They bring important new insights and may help in the study of morphological and structural alterations in PED in CSC, diffuse retinal pigment epitheliopathy (DRPE), polypoidal chorioretinopathy and age-related macular degeneration (AMD). Thus, a series of cross-sectional scans and *en face* scans are necessary.

En face sections should be made at different levels; one scan parallel to the pigment epithelium and a few micron in front of it to cut through the detachment basis, another scan parallel to the pigment epithelium but placed 50 micron in front of it to cut through the detachment walls while other scans at different detachment levels and at the cupola level. These scans show different aspects of detachment and its contents in relation to the section level.

Normally choroidal neovascularization (CNV) is adherent to the superior part (dome) of the detachment; below its contents are generally clear allowing a good perception of the Bruch's membrane. The different scans must be confronted against one another.

Central Serous Chorioretinopathy

In CSC, frontal scans show the structure and dimensions of pigment epithelium detachments. Shape is predominantly perfectly circular or circular (90%) and never acquires multilobular or cluster aspects. Few cases have irregular oval shape (10%). Retinal PED dimensions are smaller than in DRPE and AMD. These measurements are based on maximum dimensions selected at the detachment's base.

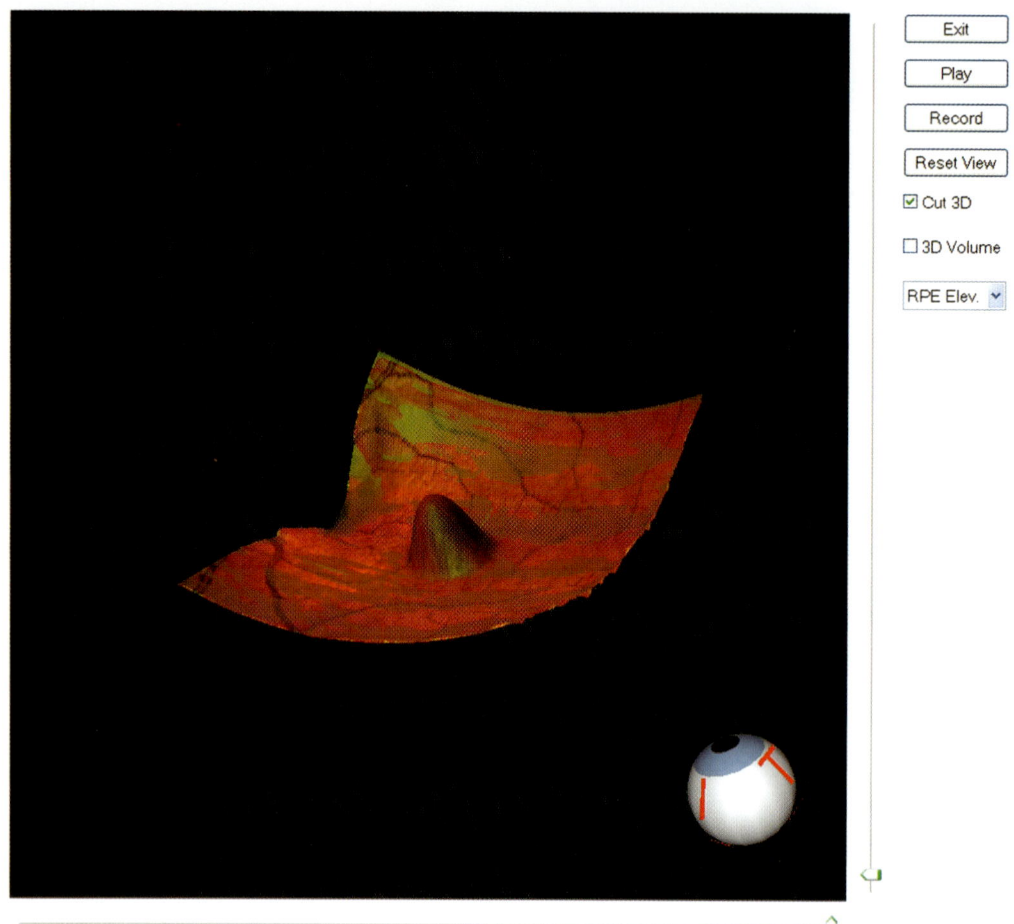

Figure 1A

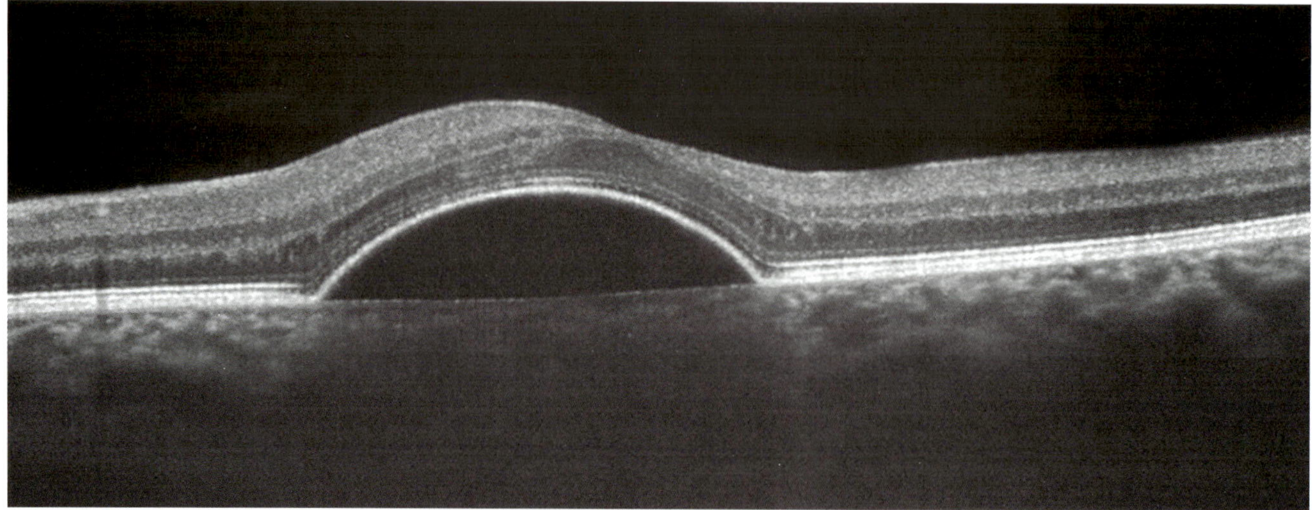

Figure 1B

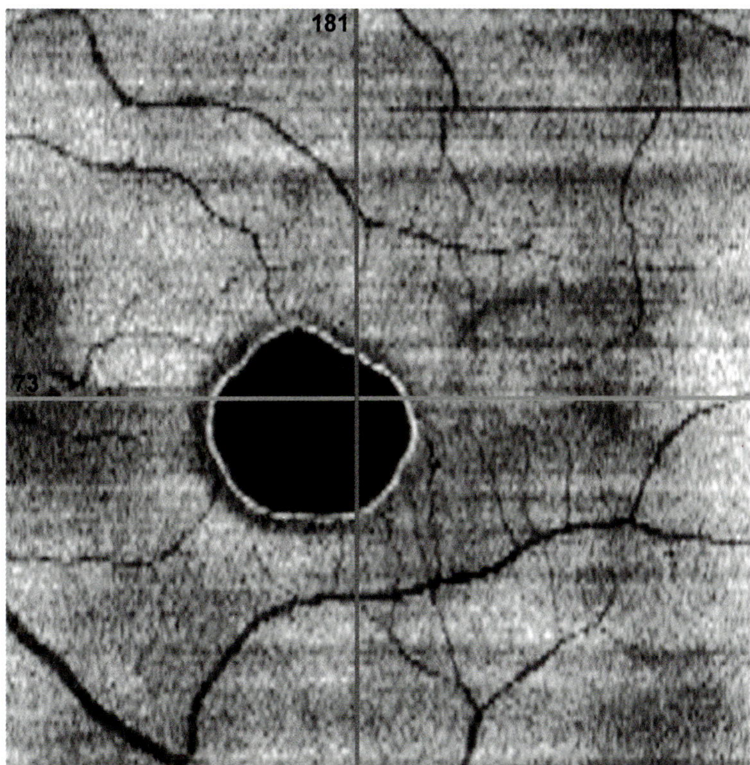

Figure 1C

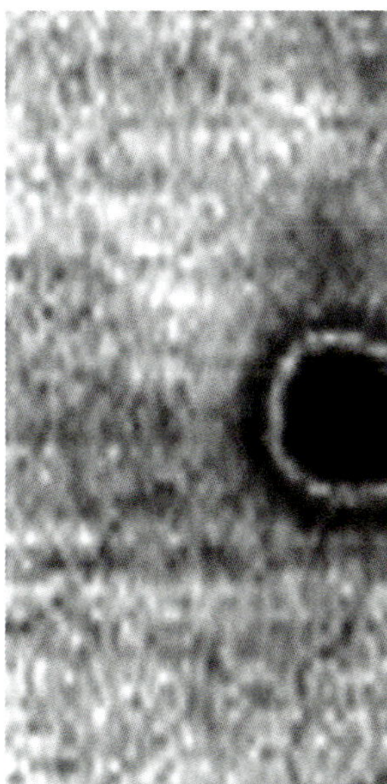

Figure 1D1

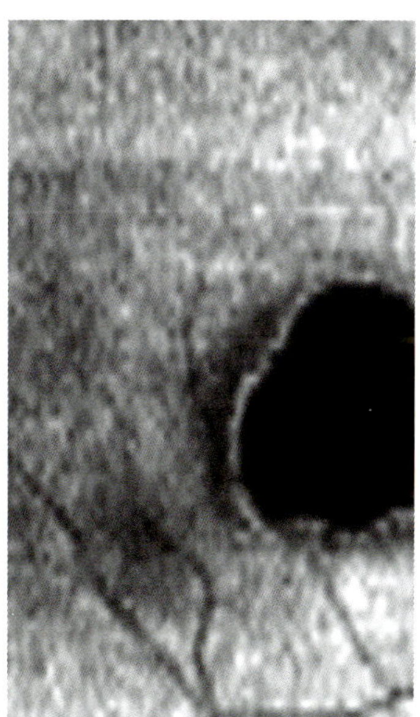

Figure 1D2

Figures 1A to D: Pigment epithelium detachments (PEDs) as seen in central serous chorioretinopathy. (A) Three-dimensional PED scan showing regular and smooth structure, and dimensions of PEDs (Optovue RTVue); (B) Cross-section scan showing the regular shape and smooth structure, and dimensions of walls of the PEDs (Optovue RTVue); (C) *En face* scan showing the shape: circular, very regular and smooth; it never acquires multilobular or cluster aspects. PED walls are thin smooth and regular. Retinal PED dimensions are smaller than in diffuse retinal pigment epitheliopathy and age-related macular degeneration (Optovue RTVue); (D) *En face* scan showing the wall features. Inner silhouette has smooth features, walls are regular, PED wall thickness is thinner than in the other considered diseases and the contents are clear (Optovue RTVue)

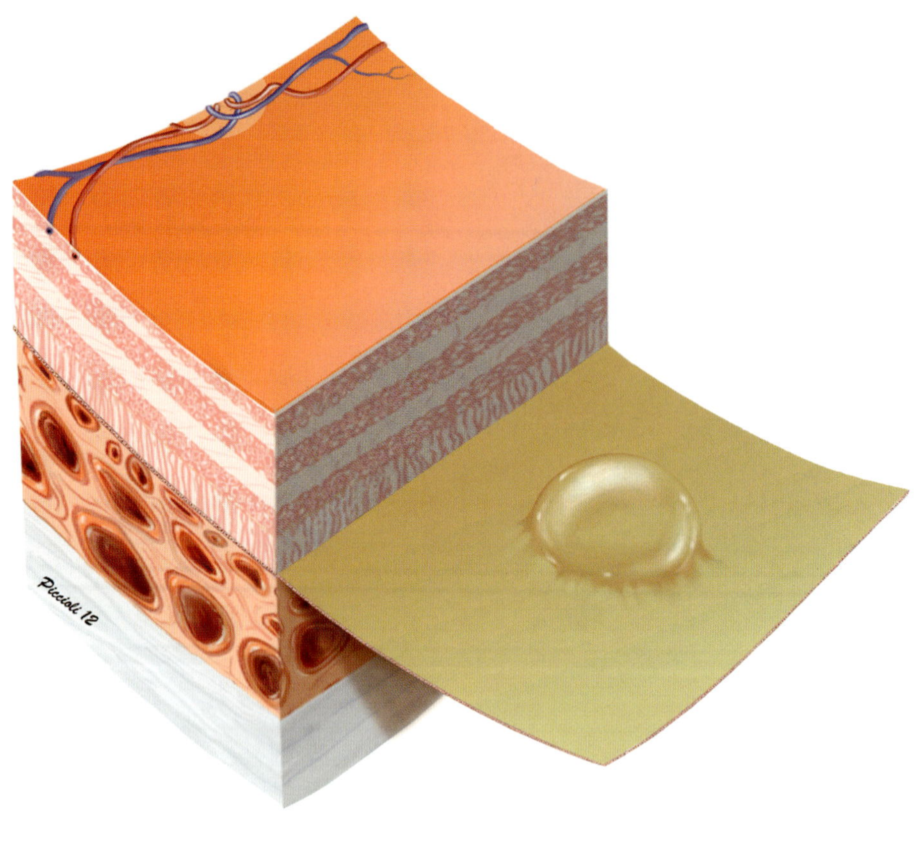

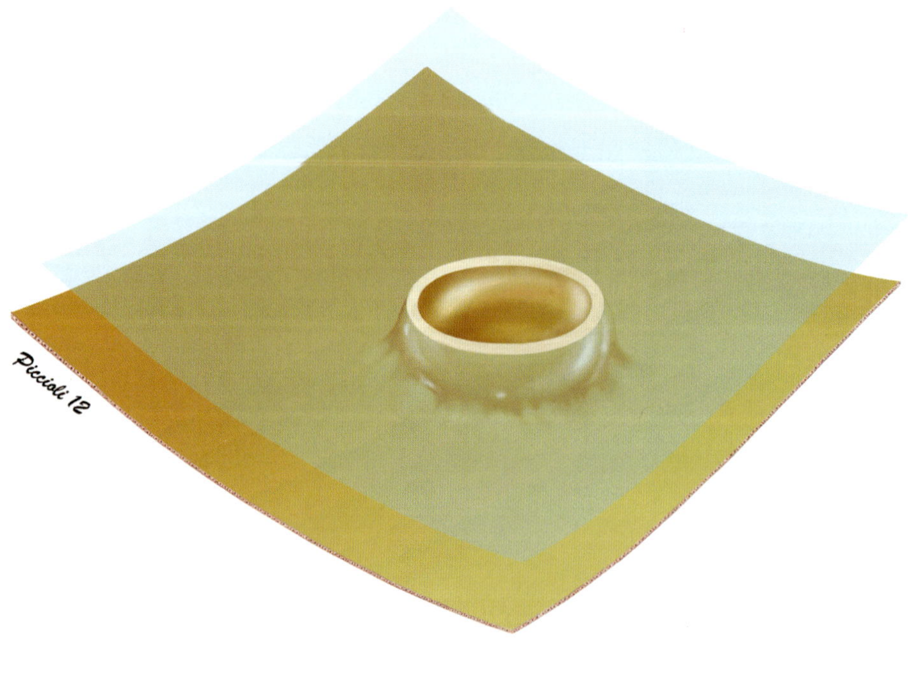

Figures 2A and B: In central serous chorioretinopathy, three-dimensional view shows the regular and smooth structure and dimensions of pigment epithelium detachments. The fundus examination shows a globular transparent detachment

PED's walls are thin smooth and regular. Inner silhouette has smooth aspect (89%), is rarely lightly granular (11%) and never takes rough or granular characteristics. Walls are regular or lightly irregular (95%) and acquire exceptionally irregular features. PED wall is thinner than in the other considered diseases and contents are clear (89%) (**Figures 1 and 2**).

Chronic Diffuse Epitheliopathy

Retinal PED shape in chronic diffuse epitheliopathy can be circular (33%), irregular oval (33%) or multilobular (34%). Dimensions are bigger and more irregular than in CSC. Wall inner silhouette shows a distribution midway lightly granular (67%) and granular (33%). Lightly irregular (67%) or irregular (33%) wall aspects are evident. PED wall is thinner in chronic diffuse epitheliopathy than in AMD and other considered diseases. Contents are generally clear (67%) or may contain flare 33% (**Figures 3 and 4**).

Polypoidal Choroidal Vasculopathy

Pigment epithelium detachments in polypoidal choroidal vasculopathy are generally ovoid with smooth and thin walls, more similar to CSC than to AMD. Shape never acquires multilobular or cluster aspects. Few cases have irregular oval shape (10%). PED dimensions in polypoidal choroidal vasculopathy are smaller than in AMD. PED walls in polypoidal choroidal vasculopathy are thin, smooth and lightly irregular. Inner silhouette has mostly a smooth aspect, in rare cases light granular features and never reveal granular features. Lightly irregular (67%) aspects are evident. Thickness at PED base is larger than in the other considered diseases except AMD. Contents are generally clear at basis level with presence of dense hyper-reflective vascular tissue towards cupola. **Vascular tissue (angioma) is found close or against the detachment dome.** Sometimes a vascular stalk can be seen connecting choroid and Bruch's membrane to the choroidal angioma in the cupola of the detachment (**Figures 5 and 6**).

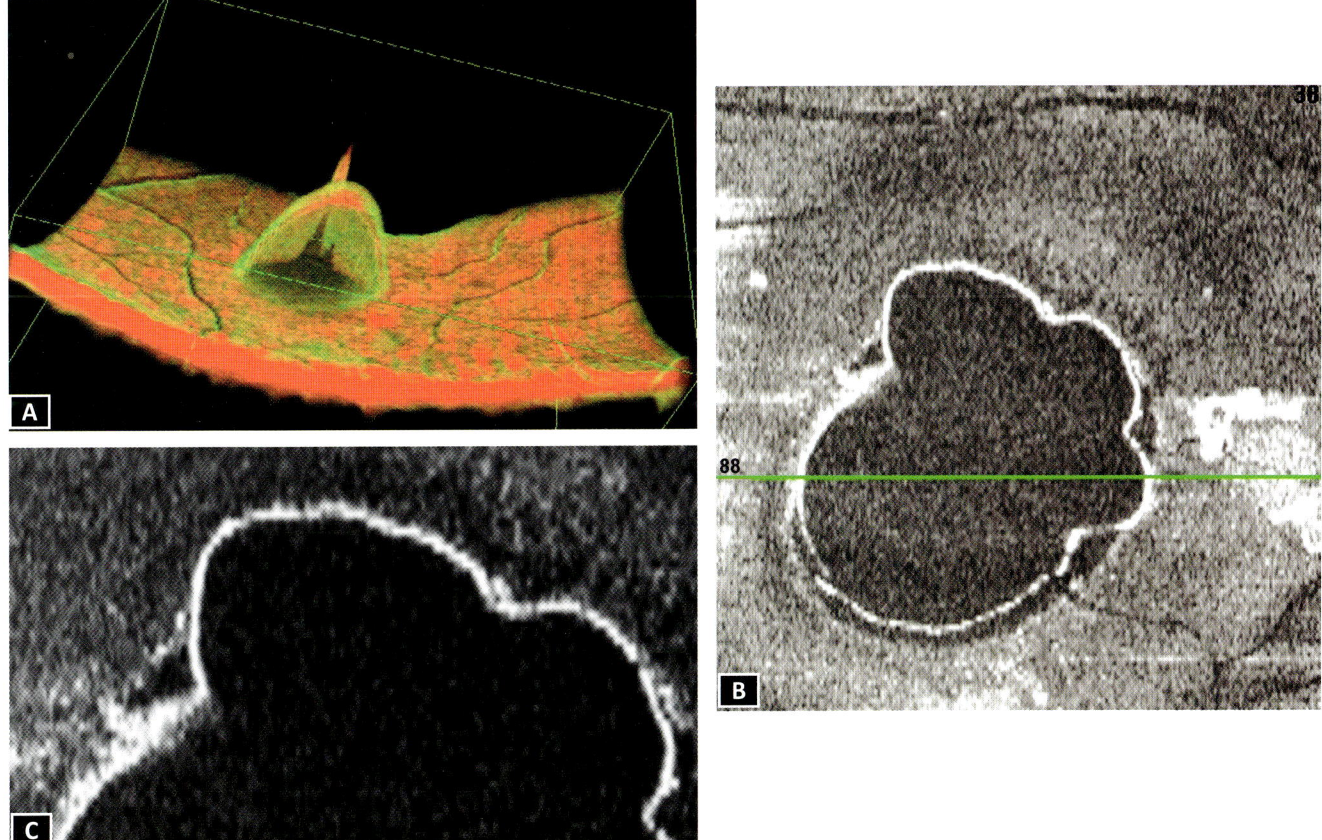

Figures 3A to C: Pigment epithelium detachments (PEDs) as seen in chronic diffuse epitheliopathy. (A) Three-dimensional PED scan showing slightly irregular structure and dimensions of PEDs (Optovue RTVue); (B) *En face* scan showing slightly irregular ovoid shape. Dimensions are bigger and more irregular than in central serous chorioretinopathy (Optovue RTVue); (C) *En face* scan showing wall features. Inner silhouette: an appearance midway between smooth and lightly granular may be seen, aspects lightly irregular, thickness walls are thinner than in age-related macular degeneration. Contents shown here are clear and they may contain flare (Optovue RTVue)

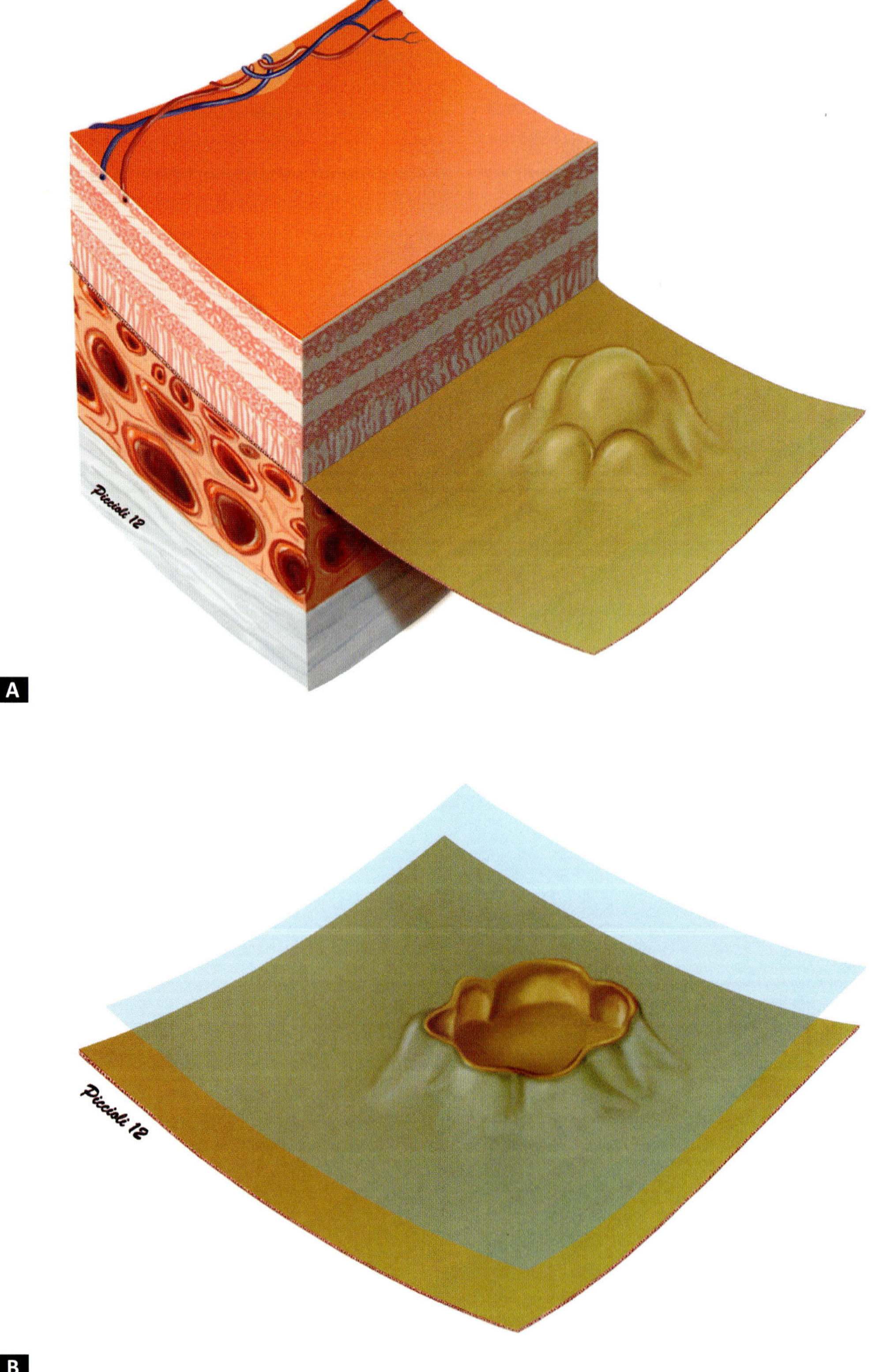

Figures 4A and B: In chronic diffuse epitheliopathy, a slightly irregular structure is seen. Dimensions of pigment epithelium detachments are bigger than central serous chorioretinopathy, smaller than age-related macular detachments

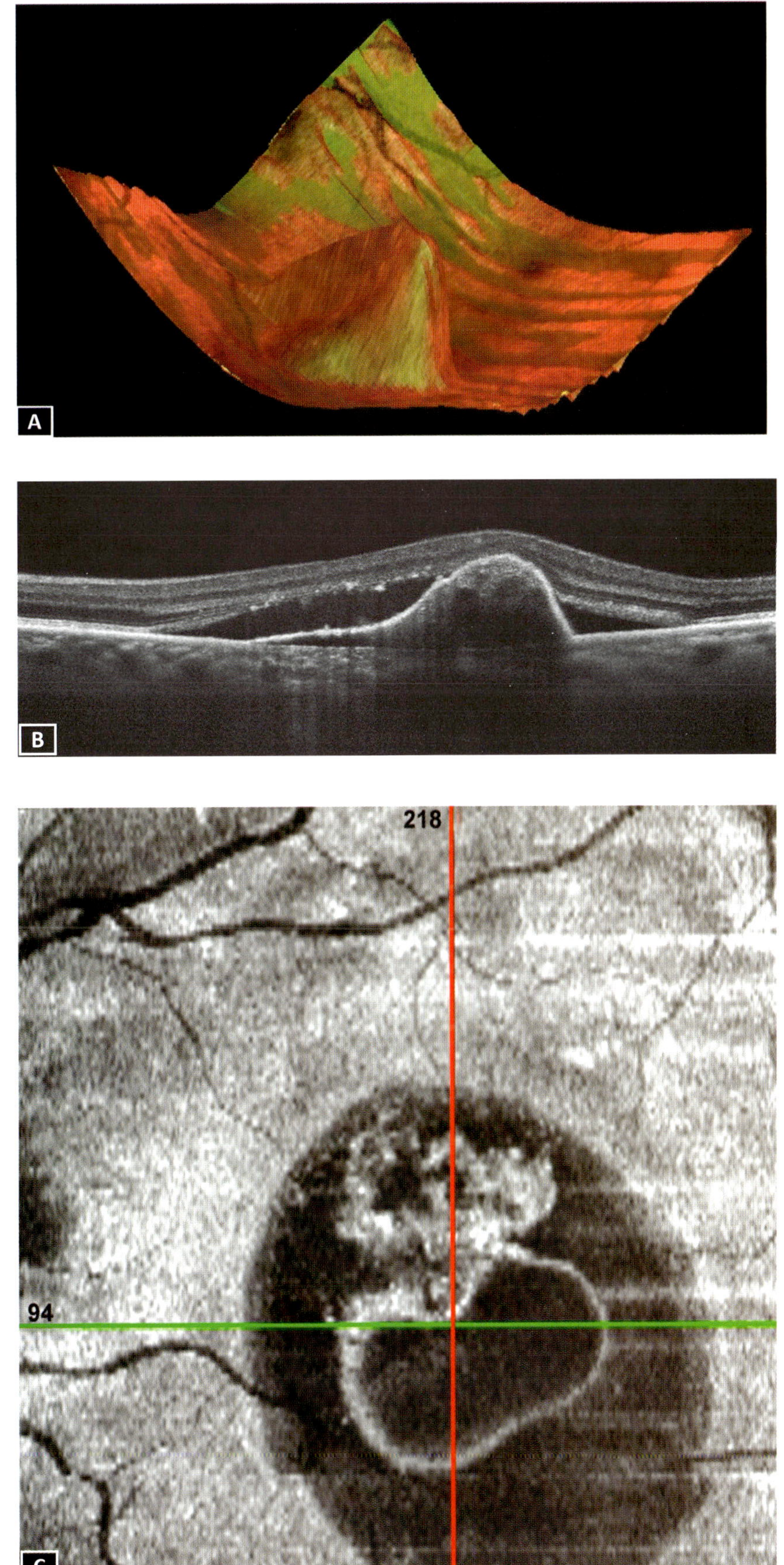

Figures 5A to C: PED in polypoidal choroidal vasculopathy

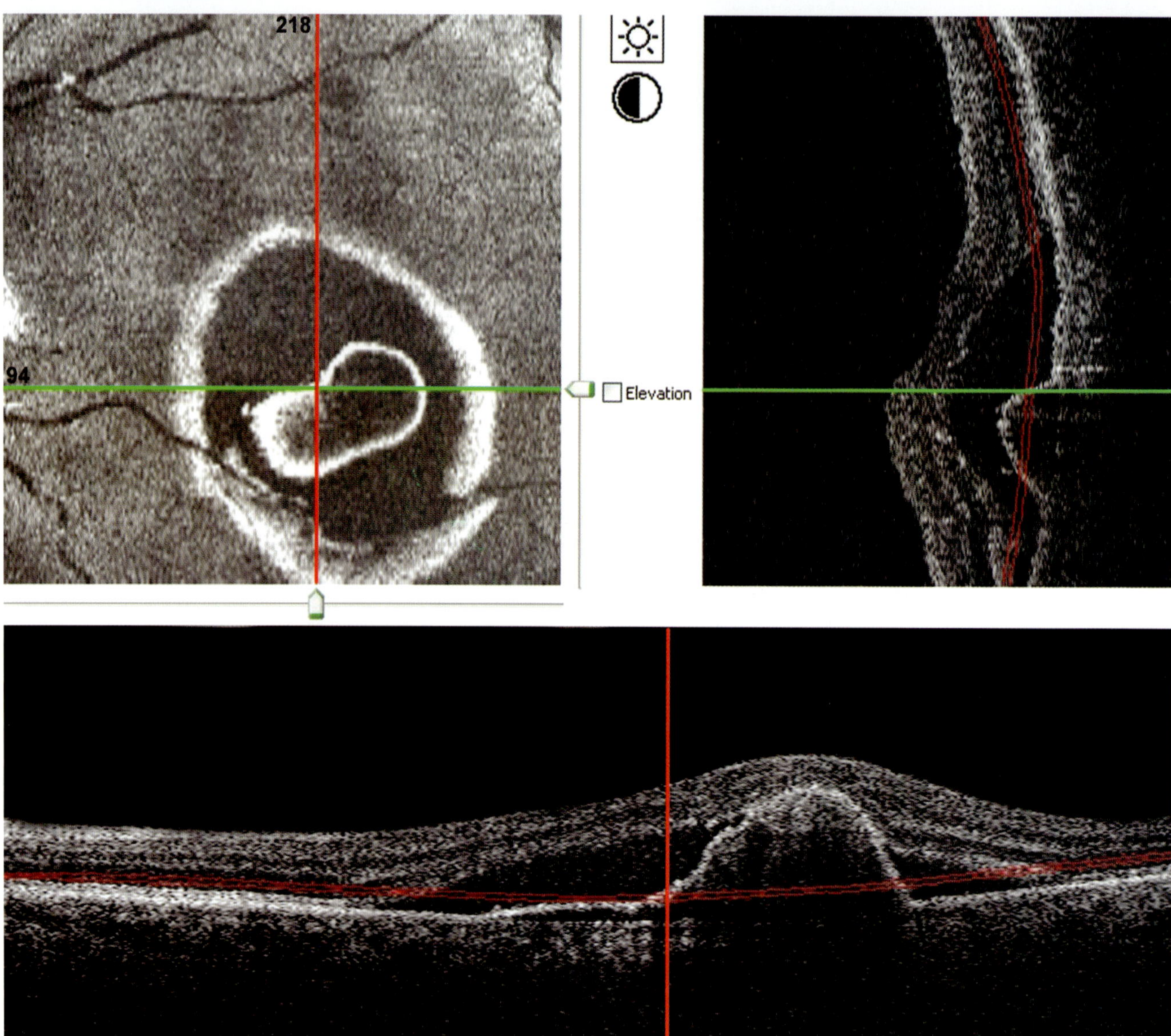

Figure 5D: PED in polypoidal choroidal vasculopathy

Age-related Macular Degeneration

En face scans allow an in-depth study of the shape of PEDs and a precise assessment of their walls. It enables to assess different features, shape, thickness, dimensions, etc. PED shape can be regular or irregular. It is important to measure its diameter if rounded and its dimensions if shape is irregular or multilobular.

In a study published by the authors, in Retina in 2011, in AMD, PEDs shape shows distinctive features. PED shape can be irregular, irregularly ovoid (29%), multilobular (24%) and multilobular and cluster (24%). Retinal PED dimensions are bigger in AMD than in other considered diseases. PED walls are thick, rough and irregular. Inner silhouette is granular (62%) or lightly granular (38%). Walls are lightly irregular (67%) or irregular (33%). Retinal PED wall thickness is larger in AMD than in other diseases **(Figures 7 to 9)**.

Nonvascularized Retinal Pigment Epithelium Detachment Contents

In case of nonvascularized retinal PED, the contents are clear (67%) or contain flare (33%) **(Figures 9E and F).**

Vascularized Retinal Pigment Epithelium Detachment Contents

In case of vascularized retinal PED with occult neovascularization the contents are generally set in two levels:
- *Inferior level:* Hazy close to the Bruch's membrane
- *Superior level:* Dense hyper-reflective tissue towards detachment cupola **(Figure 9G).**

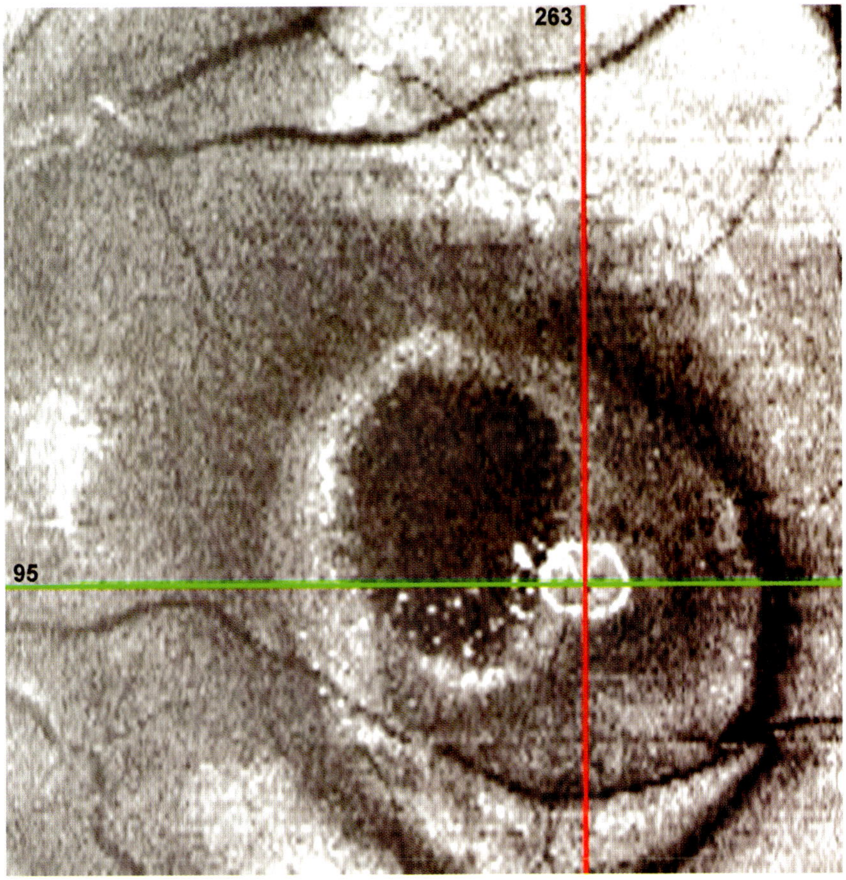

Figure 5E: PED in polypoidal choroidal vasculopathy

Figures 5A to E: Pigment epithelium detachments (PEDs) as seen in polypoidal choroidal vasculopathy. (A) Three-dimensional PED scan showing the slightly irregular structure and dimensions of PEDs, similar to chronic diffuse epitheliopathy (Optovue RTVue); (B) Cross-section scan showing the shape is elongated and slightly irregular. A small serous retinal detachment is associated, showing alterations of the photoreceptors. Inside PED, retinal PED shows clear contents in the inferior part with presence of dense hyper-reflective vascular tissue (angioma) towards detachment cupola (Optovue RTVue); (C) *En face* PED scan showing the shape in polypoidal choroidal vasculopathy is irregularly circular (it never acquires multilobular or cluster aspects). PED dimensions are smaller than in age-related macular degeneration (AMD), presence of dense hyper-reflective tissue towards detachment cupola. Close to it, irregularities of the retinal pigment epithelium (RPE) can be seen, related to the subepithelial vascular net. A small serous retinal detachment surrounds the PED (Optovue RTVue); (D) *En face* PED scan showing the wall features at the RPE level. Inner silhouette in polypoidal choroidal vasculopathy is mostly smooth. Wall aspects are light irregular or irregular. Wall thickness is larger than in the other considered diseases except AMD. A small serous retinal detachment surrounds the PED. Contents are mostly clear at the section level. Contents in polypoidal choroidal vasculopathy retinal PED are clear with presence of dense hyper-reflective tissue towards detachment cupola (Optovue RTVue); (E) PED *En face* scan at detachment dome level (Optovue RTVue)

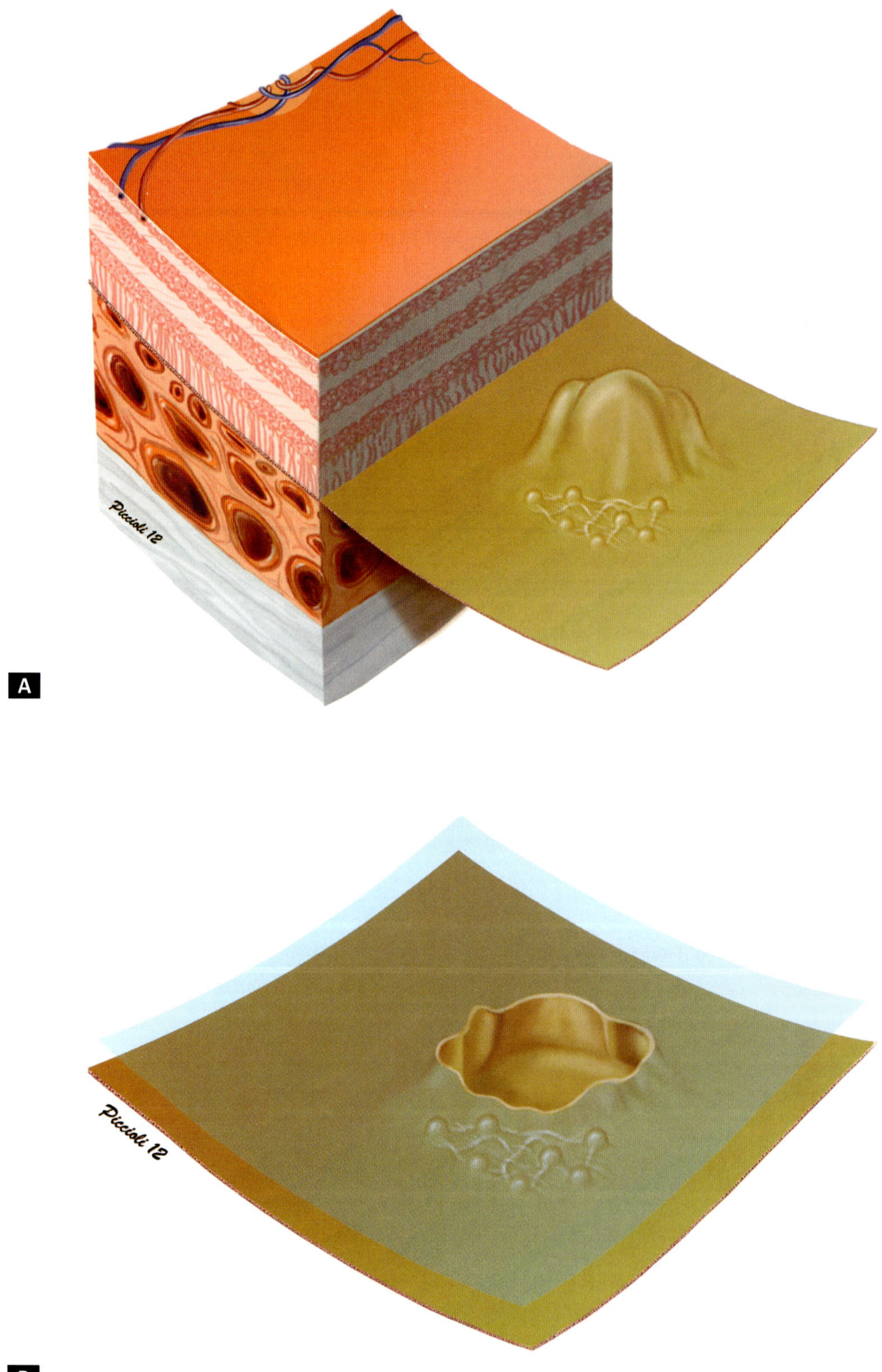

Figures 6A and B: In polypoidal choroidal vasculopathy, lightly irregular dimensions of pigment epithelium detachments are bigger than central serous chorioretinopathy, smaller than age-related macular detachments, similar to chronic diffuse epitheliopathy. The vascular angiomatous net is seen under the Bruch's membrane

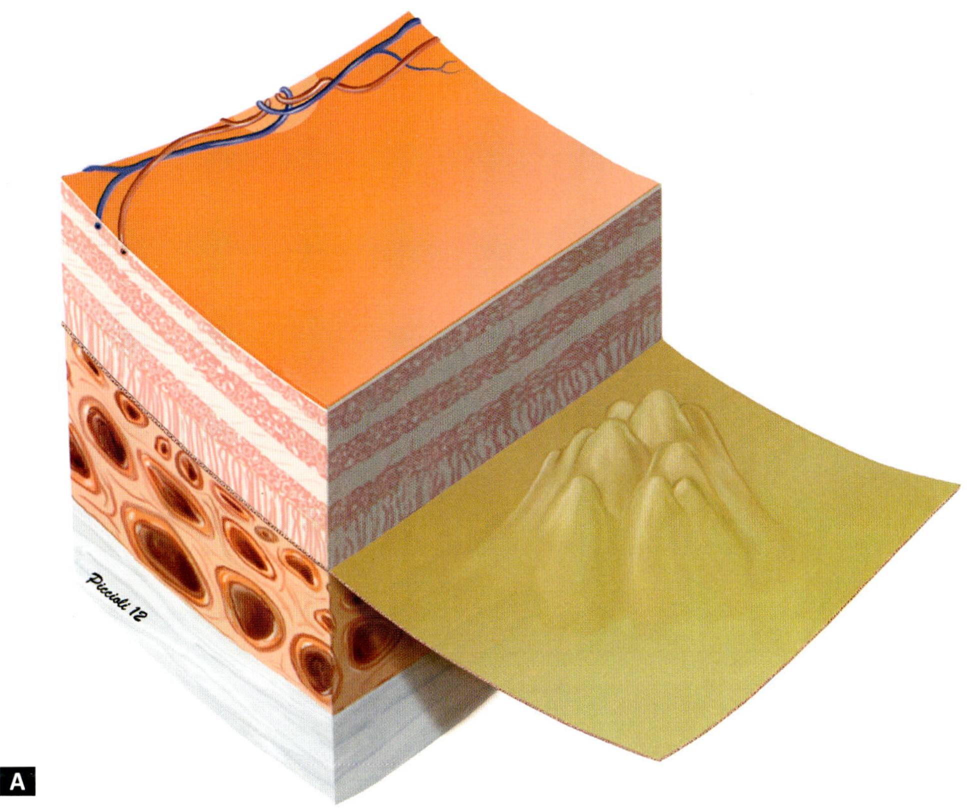

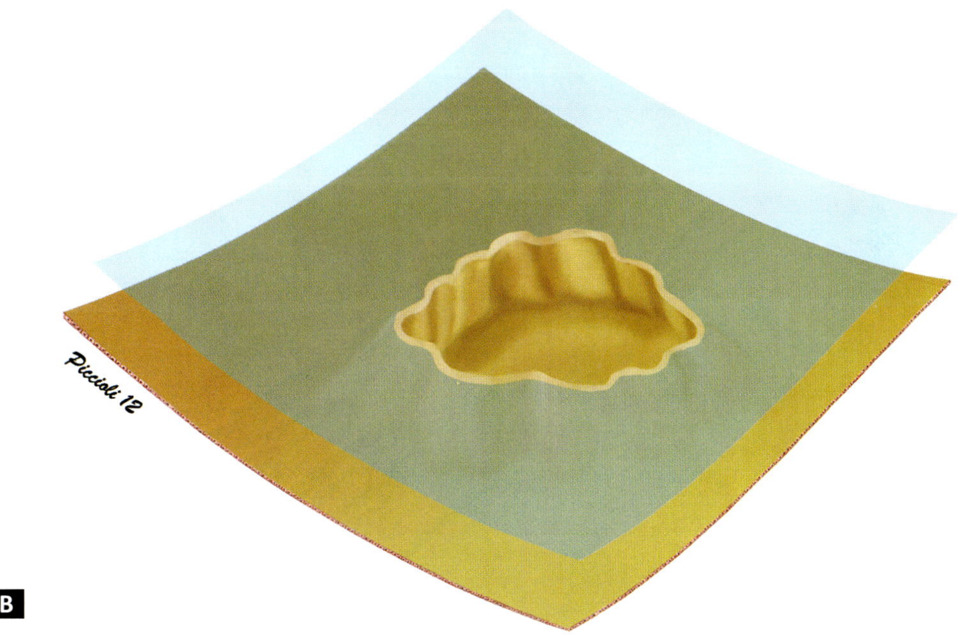

Figures 7A and B: Age-related macular degeneration, irregular structure and dimensions of pigment epithelium detachments. Cupolas or domes are neatly seen

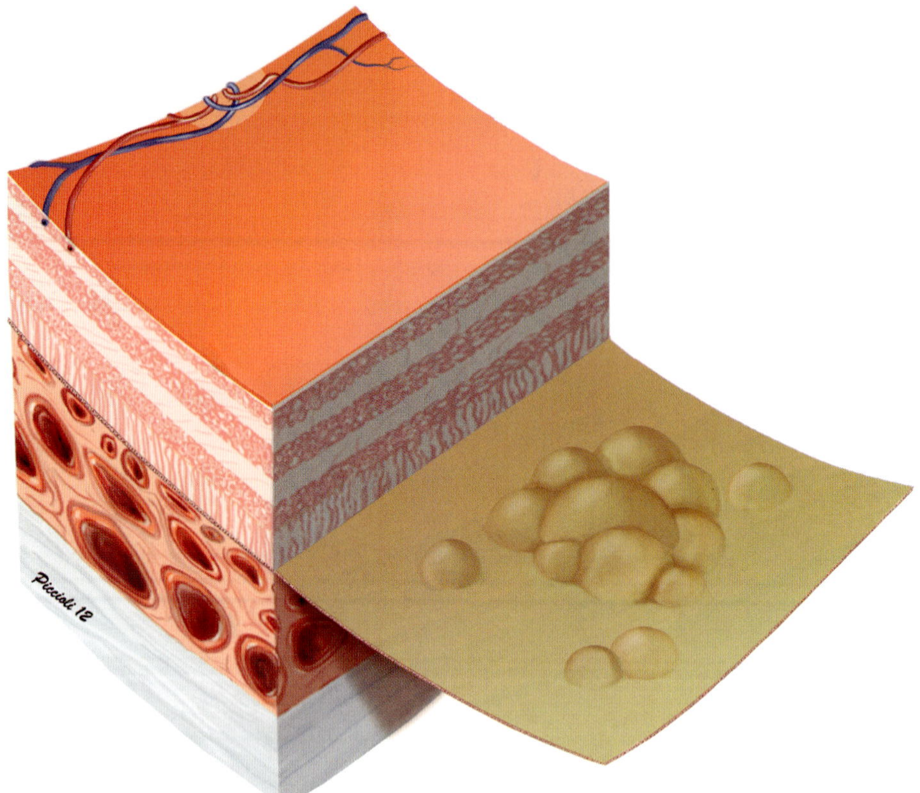

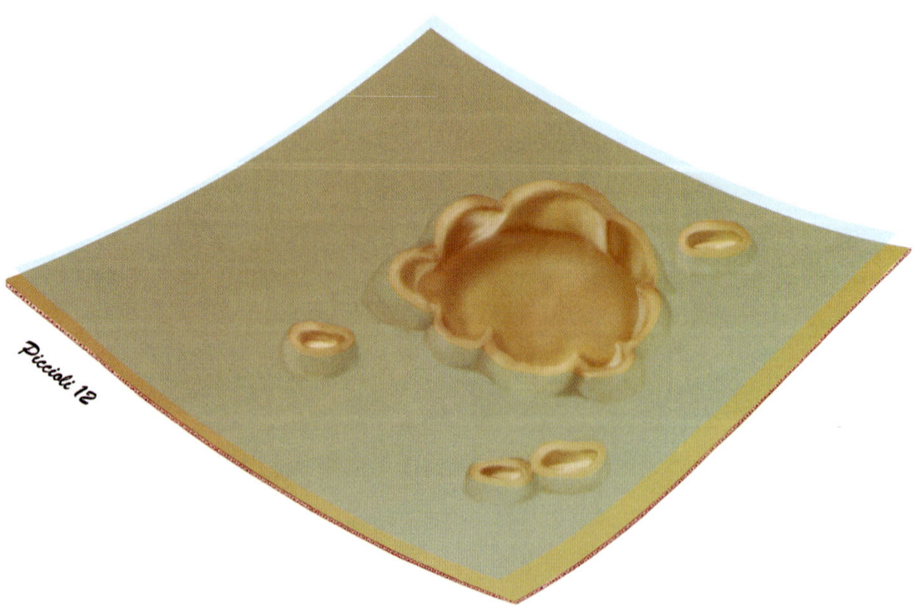

Figures 8A and B: Age-related macular degeneration, irregular structure and polylobular and cluster appearance of pigment epithelium detachments. Many clusters of cupolas or domes are neatly seen

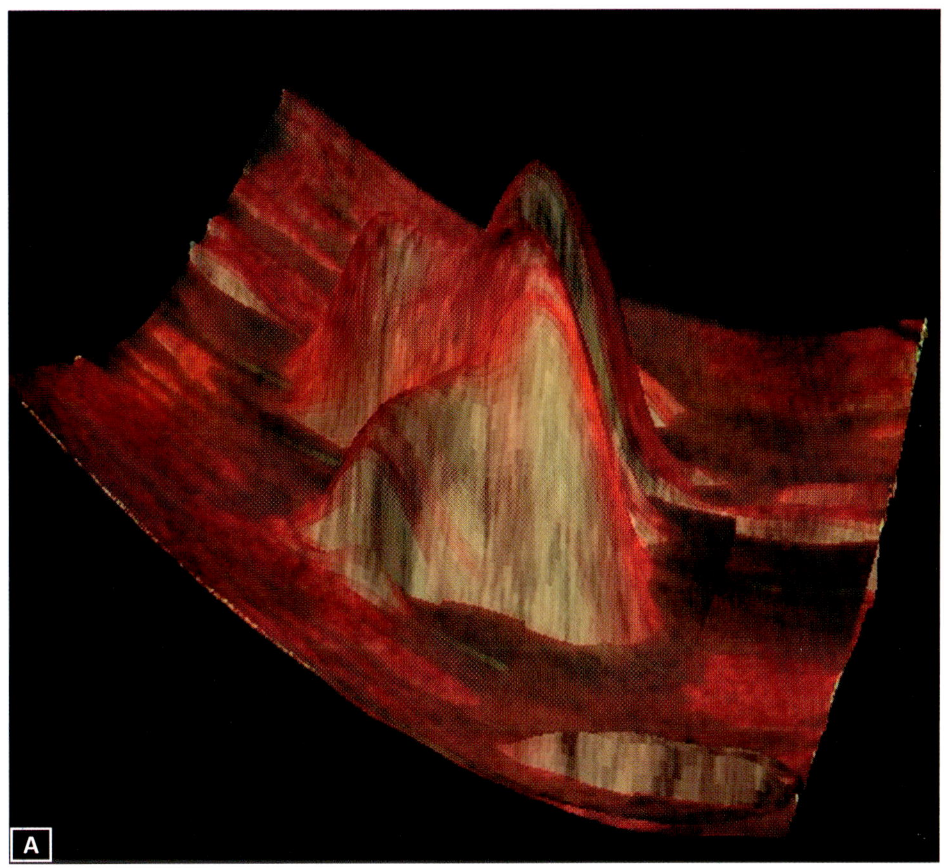

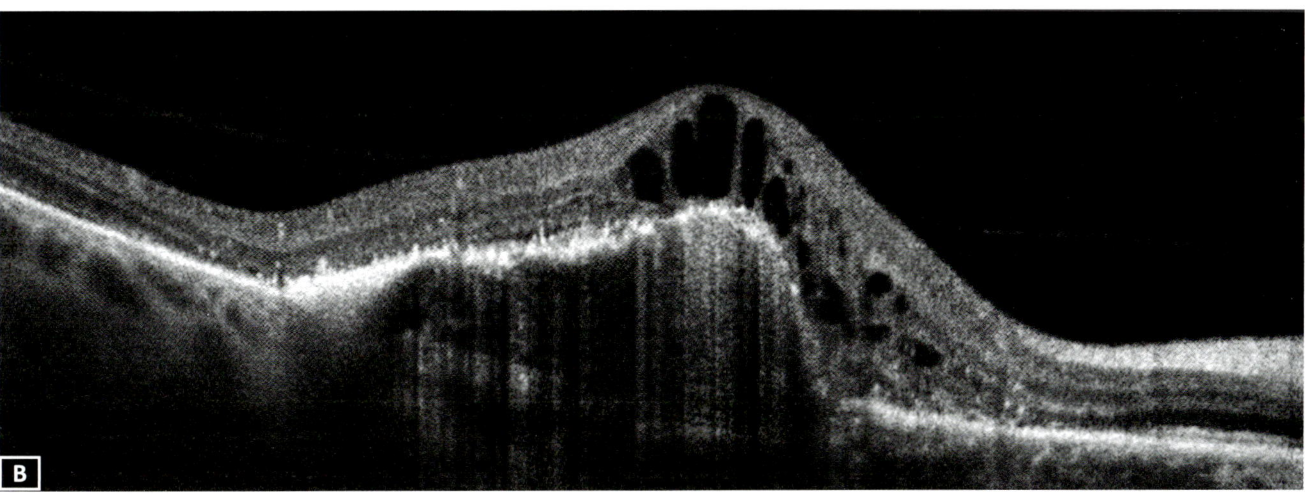

Figures 9A and B: PED in age-related macular degeneration

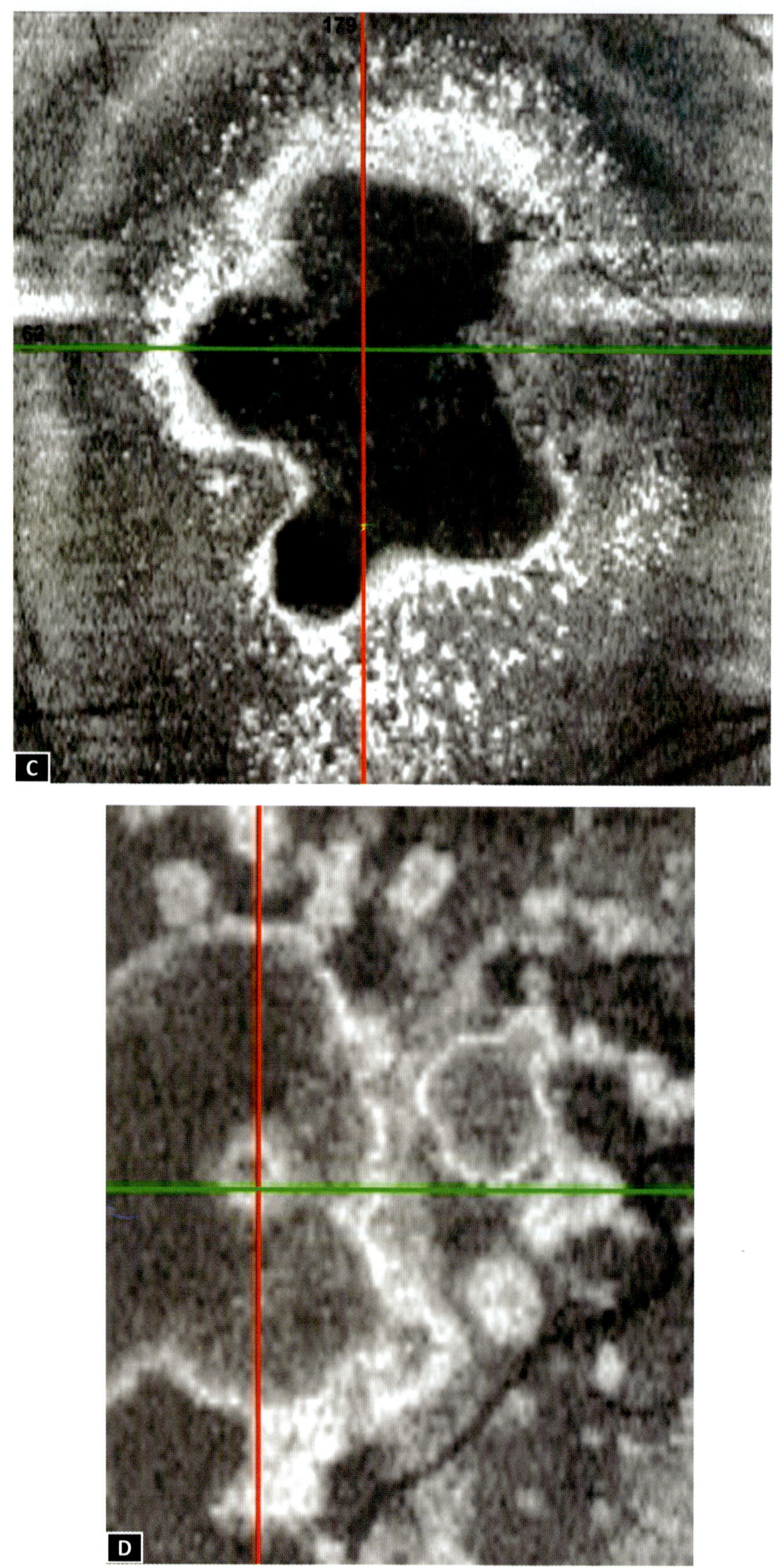

Figures 9C and D: PED in age-related macular degeneration

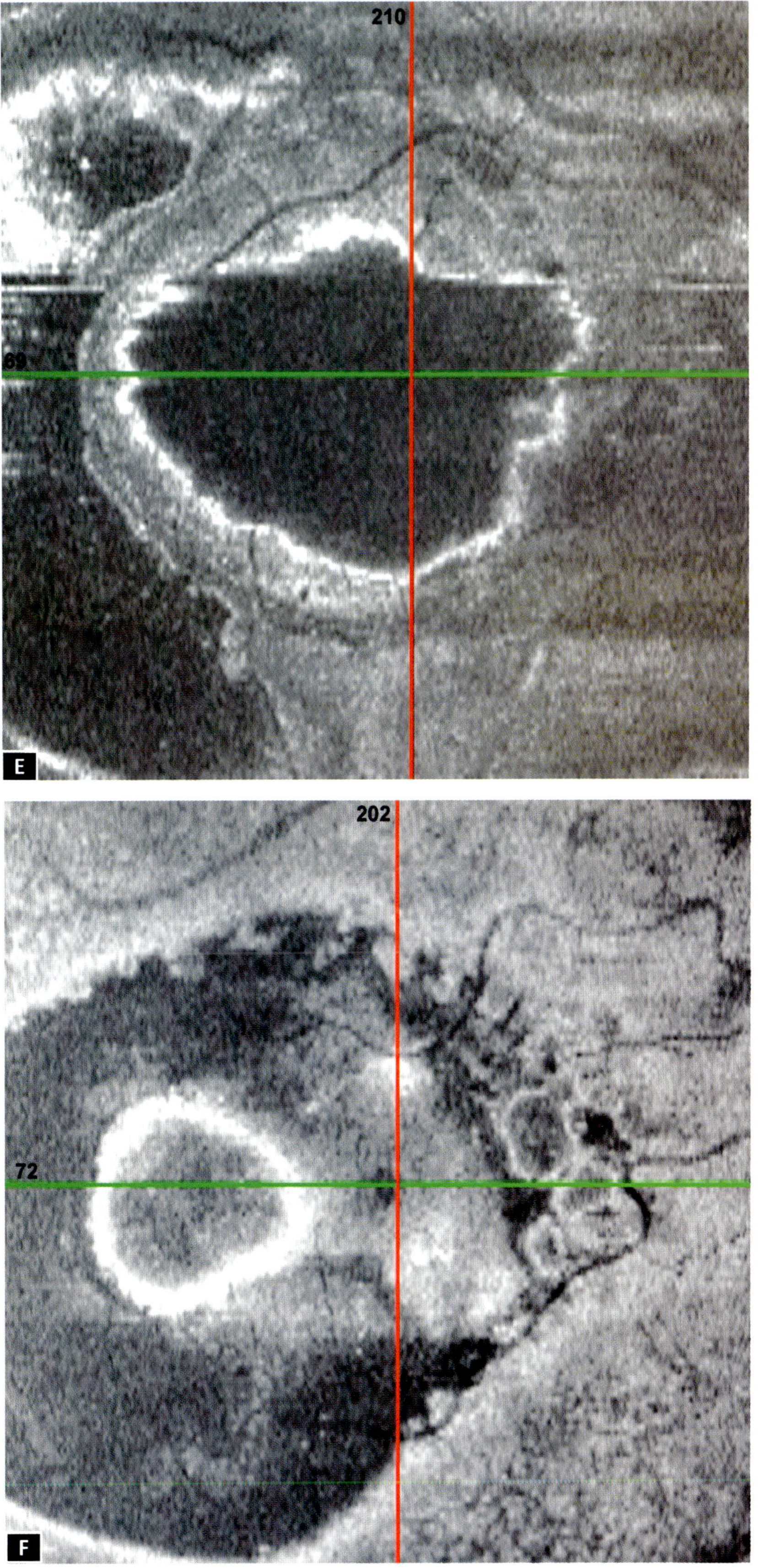

Figures 9E and F: PED in age-related macular degeneration

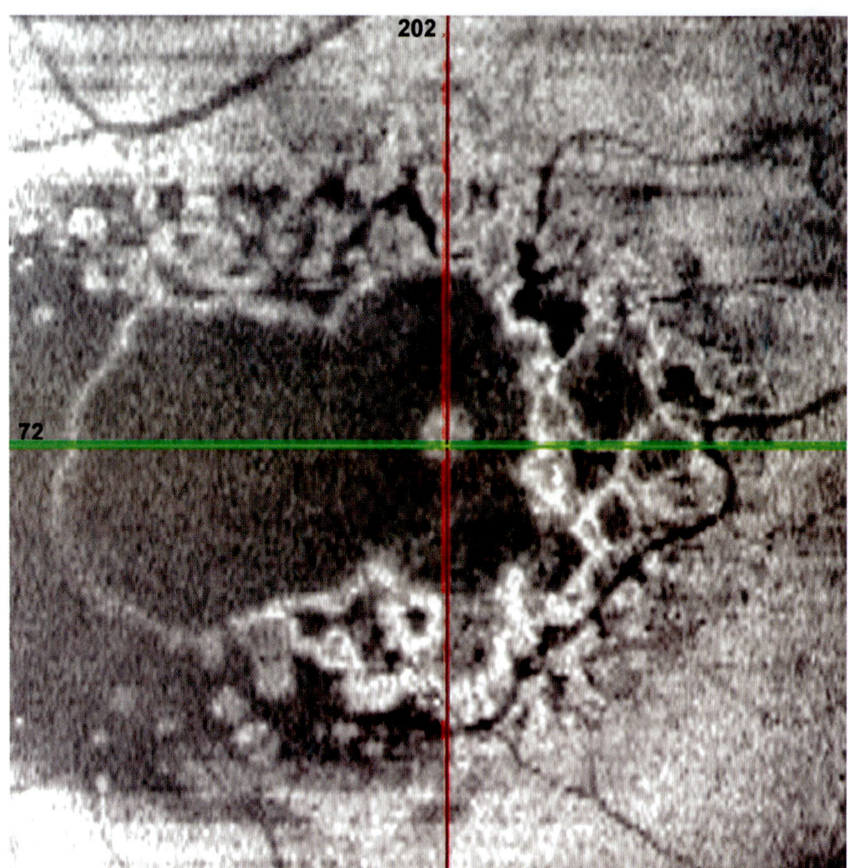

Figure 9G: PED in age-related macular degeneration

Figures 9A to G: Pigment epithelium detachments (PEDs) as seen in age-related macular degeneration (AMD). (A) Three-dimensional PED scan showing the irregular structure and dimensions of PEDs. Many cupolas or domes are neatly seen (Optovue RTVue); (B) Cross-section scan showing the retinal PED shape is irregular with dense, nonhomogenous contents. Retina above the PED is thickened by cystoid edema in the inner and outer nuclear layers and a small retinal elevation is seen. PED walls are thick and irregular, and the contents are dense, hazy (Optovue RTVue); (C) *En face* scan showing shape of PED in AMD. Retinal PED shape shows distinctive features and is irregular with some multilobular features. In this case we do not observe cluster appearance, walls are thick, rough and irregular. PED dimensions are bigger than in the other etiologies (Optovue RTVue); (D) *En face* scan showing multiple detachments. PED walls are thick, rough and irregular. Inner silhouette is granular, wall is irregular, retinal PED wall thickness is thicker in AMD than in the other considered diseases. In this case we observe a cluster of PEDs (Optovue RTVue); (E) Nonvascularized PED, *en face* scan carried out at pigment epithelium level showing the contents to be clear. Contents are clear in this case, but they can be sometimes hazy. PED walls are thick, rough and irregular. Inner silhouette is granular (Optovue RTVue); (F) Vascularized PED, cross-section scan. *En face* scans carried out at cupola level showing the contents as dense hyper-reflective tissue seem as it is normally found in the dome of vascularized PEDs. The fibrovascular tissue can be found filling all the retinal elevation or filling only a part of the detachment, immediately above and in contact with its walls. A serous retinal detachment with hyper-reflective deposits surrounds the PED. PED walls are thick, rough and irregular (Optovue RTVue); (G) Vascularized PED *en face* scan carried out at pigment epithelium level showing the contents to be clear. In vascularized retinal PED with occult neovascularization we can observe that its contents are clear at the inferior level. Dense hyper-reflective tissue will be found towards detachment cupola. *En face* scans carried out at pigment epithelium level may show the contents to be clear. Retinal PED wall thickness is thick and irregular. In this case we observe cluster appearance (Optovue RTVue)

The vascular and fibrovascular tissue can be found filling all the retinal elevation or filling only the superior part of the detachment, immediately above clear fluid and in contact with PED walls. *En face* scans carried out at lower pigment epithelium level may show the contents to be hazy or clear. *En face* scans carried out at cupola level show the contents to be a dense hyper-reflective fibrovascular tissue. The most recent OCT devices allow studying the structure of the vascular tissue. Sometimes the neovascularization is seen on the detachment dome, above the pigment epithelium **(Figures 10 to 13)**.

Evolution of vascularized pigment epithelium detachment with occult neovascularization after anti-VEGF treatment: After antivascular endothelial growth factor (VEGF) treatment vascularized retinal PED with occult neovascularization shows critical change and alteration. A few days after treatment the detachment appears to be more compact and is much less elevated. The cupola is deflated and no more evident while the detachment appears to be flattened. Walls get to be thinner. Contents are more dense and homogeneous. The fibrovascular tissue, it contains more compact, less reflective; it seems less vascularized and more fibrous. PED

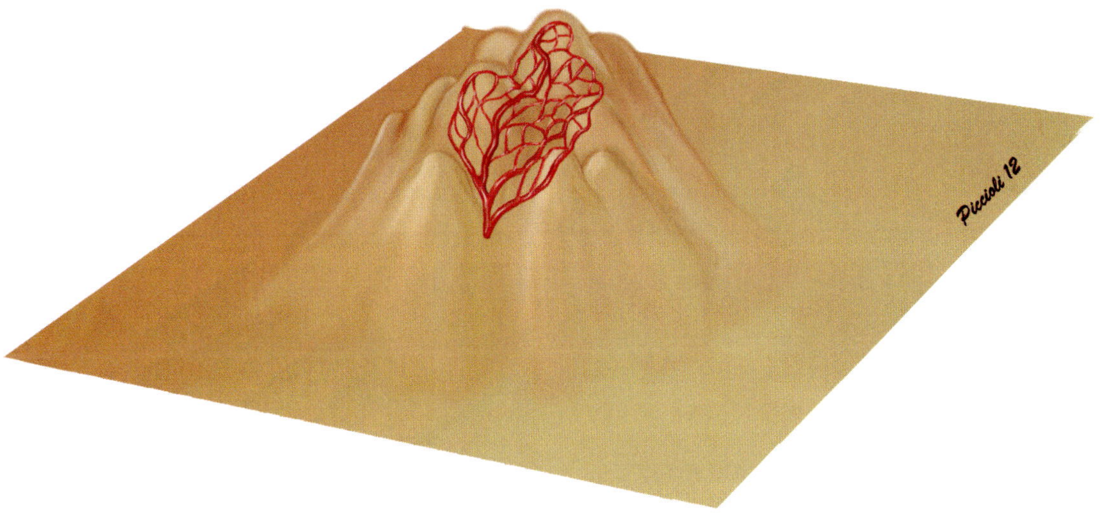

Figure 10: Age-related macular degeneration, classic choroidal neovascularization, irregular structure and dimensions of pigment epithelium detachments (PEDs). Many cupolas or domes are clearly seen. The new vessels grow above and outside the PED

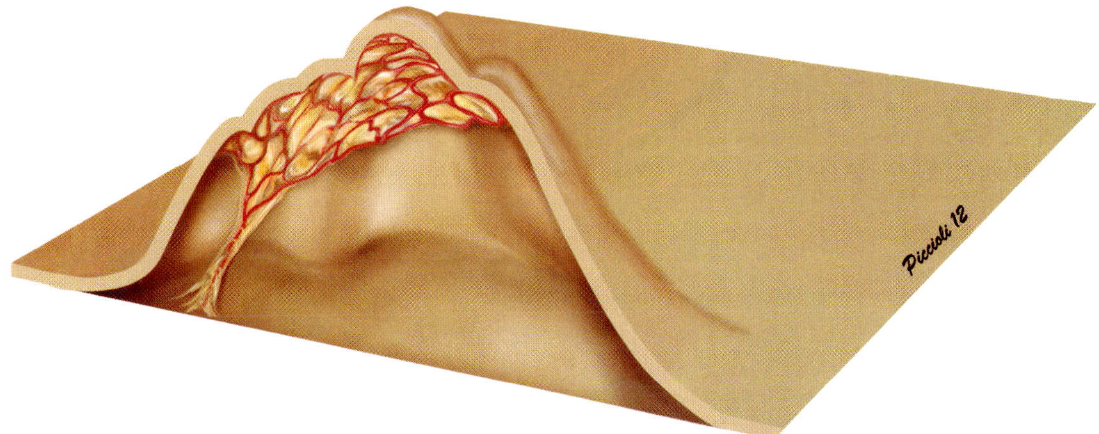

Figure 11: Age-related macular degeneration vascularized pigment epithelium detachments (PEDs), occult choroidal neovascularization, PED is irregular. Many cupolas or domes are visible. The new vessels are located inside the pigment epithelium detachment. At cupola level the fibrovascular tissue fills only a part of the detachment. Serous fluid is seen below the fibrovascular tissue. The artist has drawn a stalk originating from choriocapillaris and perforating the Bruch's membrane. Vascular tissue is always found close or against the detachment dome

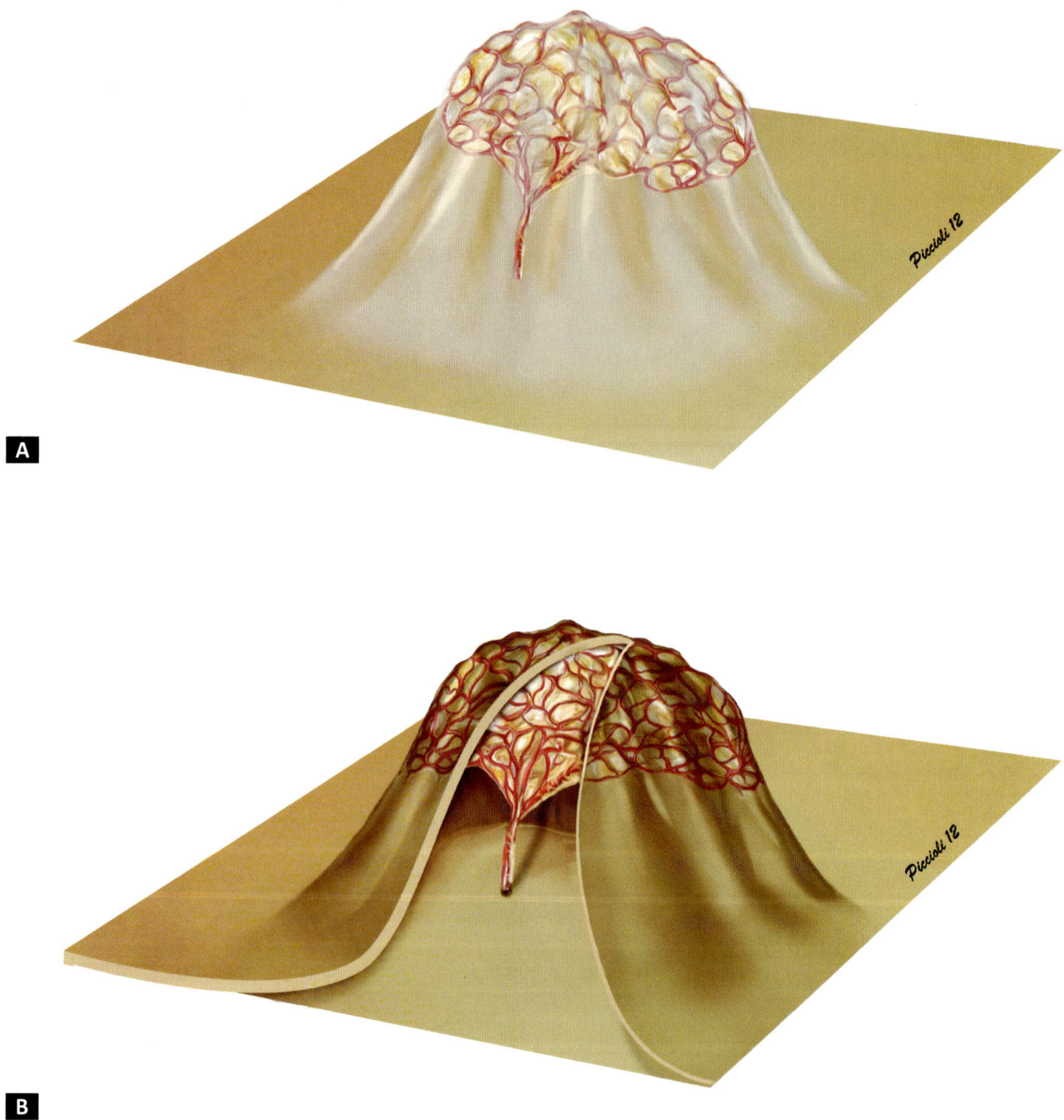

Figures 12A and B: (A) Age-related macular degeneration vascularized pigment epithelium detachment (PED), occult choroidal neovascularization (CNV), many domes are present. The occult new vessels are located inside the PED under the detachment cupola, in contact with the superior walls. At cupola level the fibrovascular tissue fills most of the superior part of the PED. Serous fluid is located below the fibrovascular tissue. Contents are clear at the inferior level. The artist has drawn a stalk originating from choriocapillaris, perforating the Bruch's membrane to bring blood to the fibrovascular membrane; (B) Age-related macular degeneration, vascularized PED, occult CNV, showing PED contents. At cupola level the fibrovascular tissue fills most of the superior part of the pigment epithelium detachment. Serous fluid is located below the fibrovascular tissue. Vascular tissue is always found close or against the detachment dome

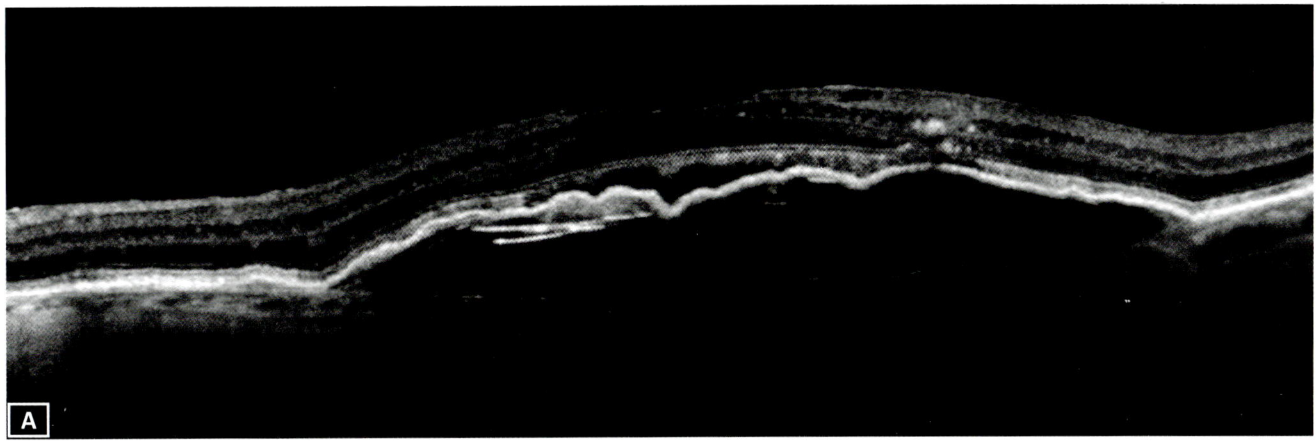

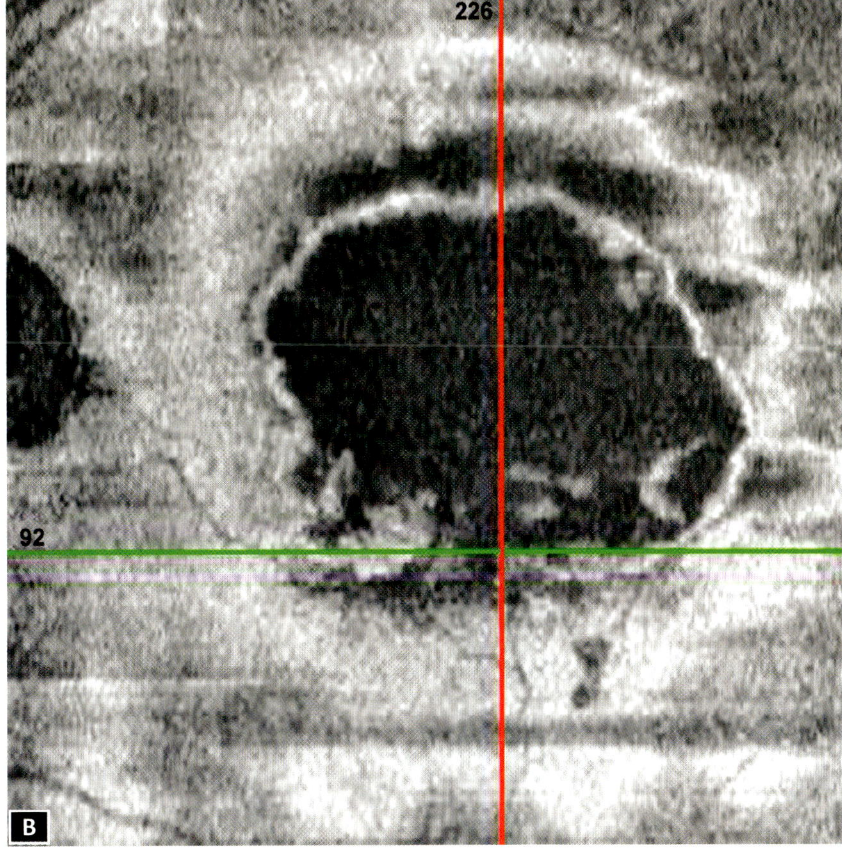

Figures 13A and B: Vascularized PED in age-related macular degeneration with occult CNV

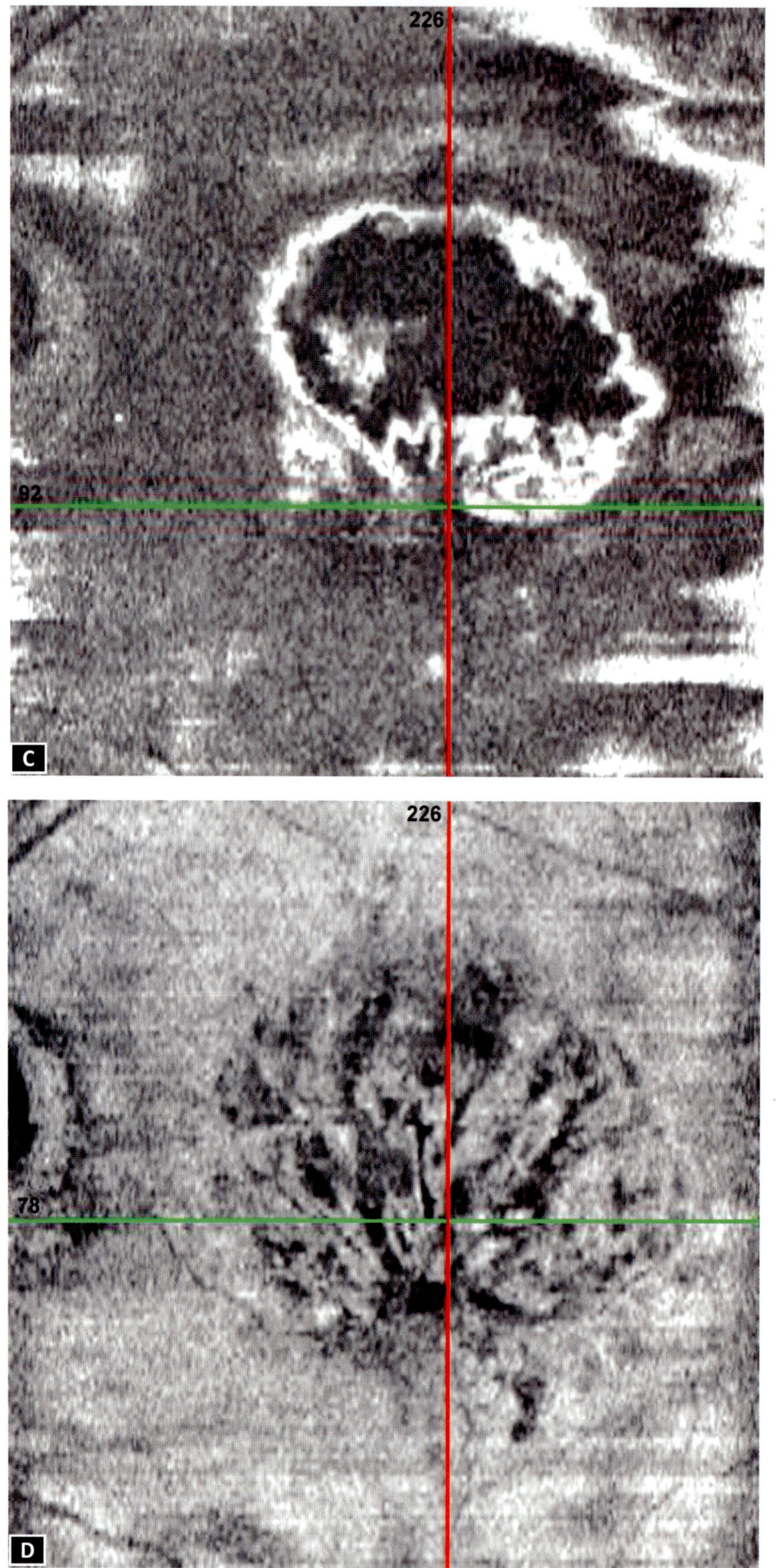

Figures 13C and D: Vascularized PED in age-related macular degeneration with occult CNV

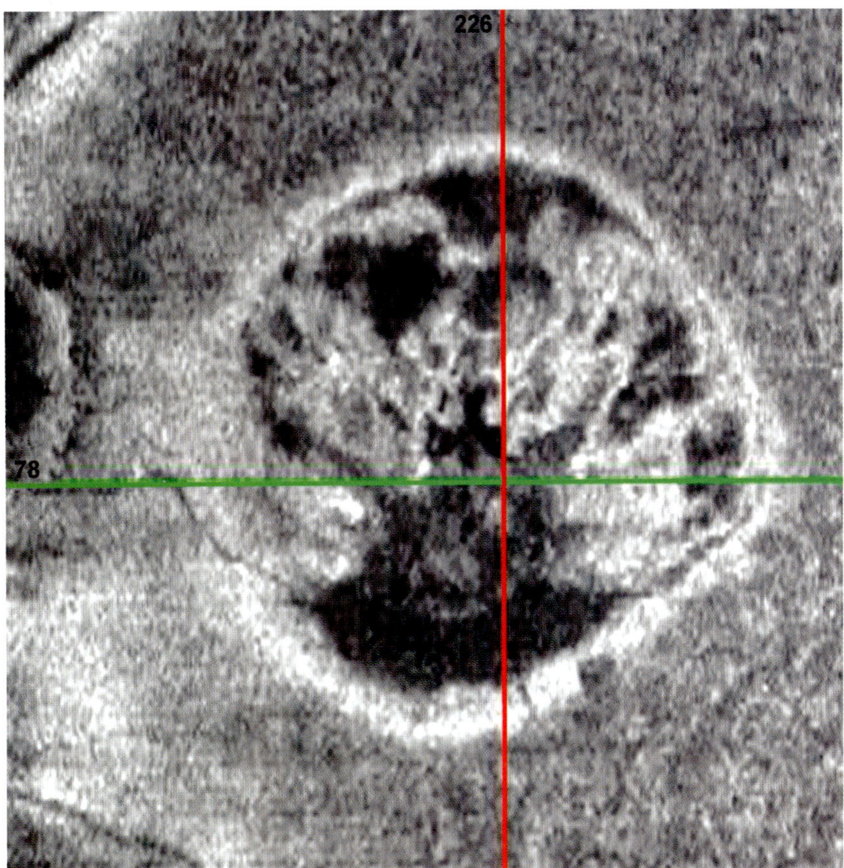

Figure 13E: Vascularized PED in age-related macular degeneration with occult CNV

Figures 13A to E: Vascularized pigment epithelium detachment (PED) with occult choroidal neovascularization (CNV) in age-related macular degeneration (AMD). (A) Cross-section scan showing irregular structure and dimensions of PEDs. The new vessels are located inside the PED. At cupola level the fibrovascular tissue can be found filling only a part of the detachment. Serous fluid is seen below the fibrovascular tissue (Optovue RTVue); (B) *En face* scan at the retinal pigment epithelium (RPE) level. At RPE level fibrovascular tissue is not seen. Serous fluid is located below the fibrovascular tissue (Optovue RTVue); (C) *En face* scan at mid-detachment level. Some fibrovascular tissue is seen close to PED wall. Serous fluid is located below the fibrovascular tissue (Optovue RTVue); (D) *En face* scan at the cupola level. The *en face* scan is generated following a natural surface contour, in this case the PED, the frontal scan follows the detachment convexity in contact with the dome walls. The fibrovascular tissue is clearly seen with the vascular ramification and branching close to PED wall. Serous fluid is located below the fibrovascular tissue (Optovue RTVue); (E) Fibrovascular tissue in contact with the PED dome. Vascular tissue is always found close or against the detachment dome (Optovue RTVue)

contents are generally less clear than before treatment with presence of denser hyper-reflective tissue towards detachment cupola. The fibrovascular tissue can be found inside the retinal elevation or immediately above and in contact with it.[10] Retinal folds around the detachment are less evident (**Figures 14 and 15**).

Outer Retinal Tubulations

In patients with AMD and in some patients with other maculopathies after a long evolution, the doctors observed another type of cavities in the outer retina—*tube shaped lesions*.[11] These are apparently common in advanced diseases affecting the outer retina and RPE (**Figure 16A**).

They appear as rounded or ovoid hyporeflective spaces with dense hyper-reflective borders on cross scans. In frontal scans they range from single, straight or branching tubules or forked tubules to a complex irregular tangled web of tubulations and tubular networks, usually overlying areas of pigment epithelial alteration or subretinal fibrosis. These structures generally remain stable over time (**Figure 16B**).

Conclusion

En face OCT is important in imaging analysis and essential to detect the tiny alterations of RPE and retinal PED in many retinal disorders. Conventional longitudinal OCT scan

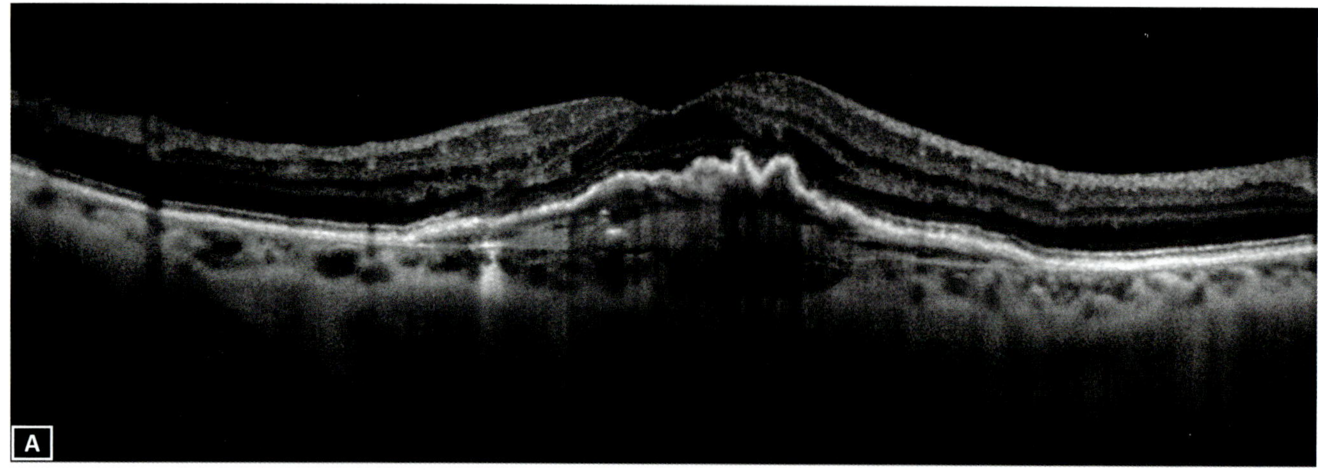

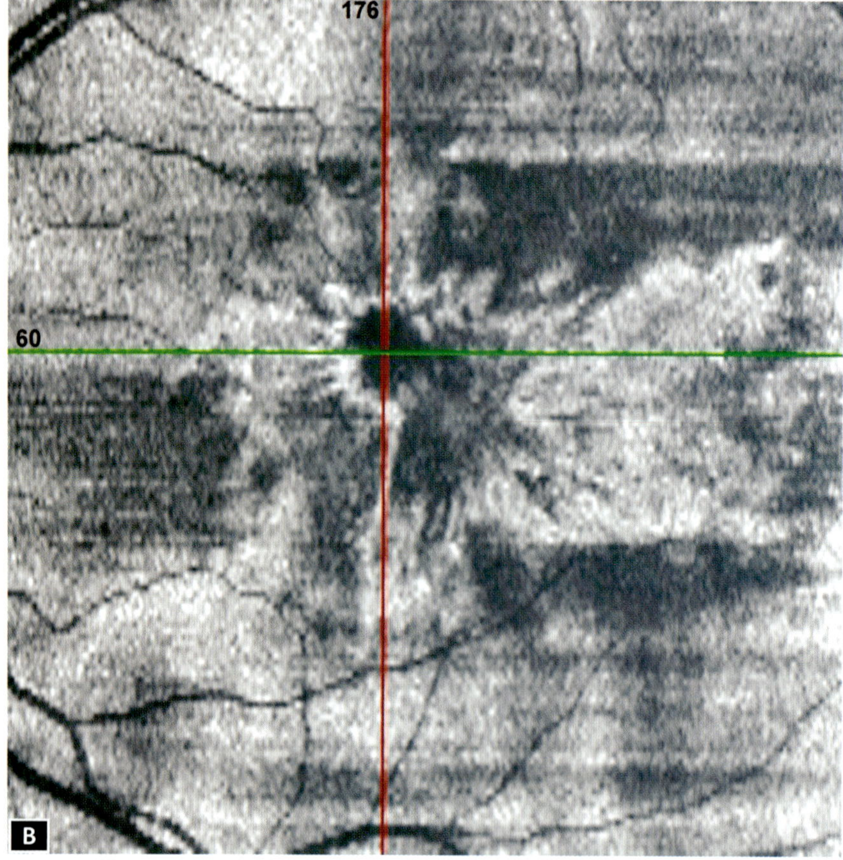

Figures 14A and B: Vascularized PED in age-related macular degeneration with occult CNV before treatment

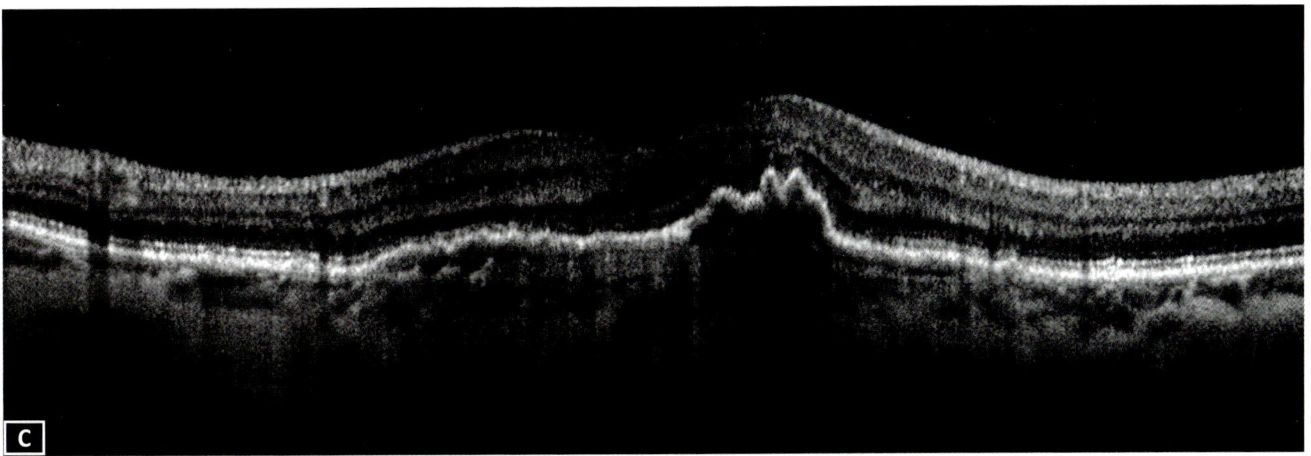

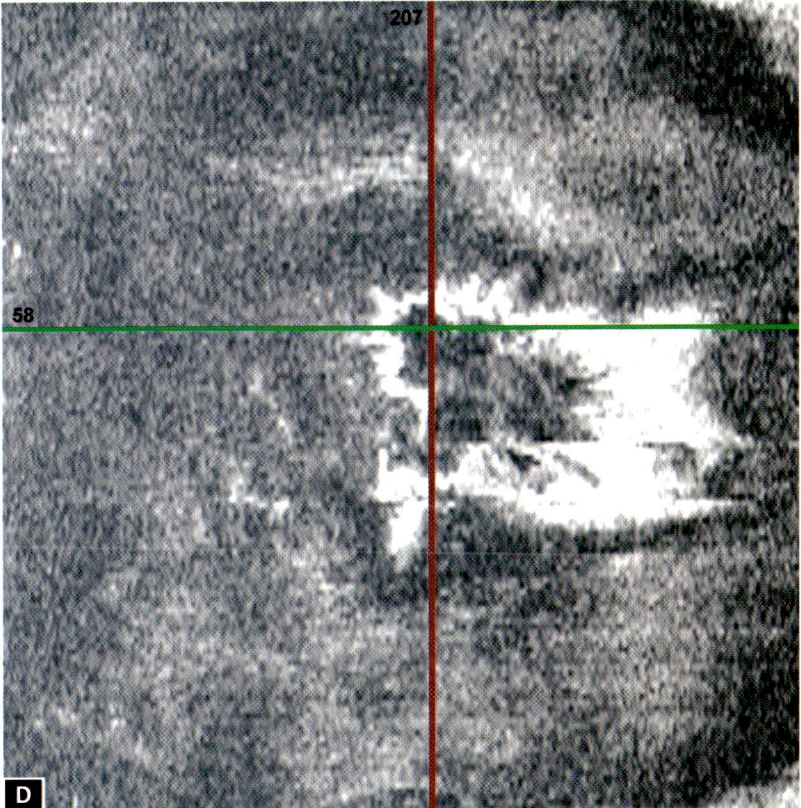

Figures 14C and D: Vascularized PED in age-related macular degeneration with occult CNV treated by anti-VEGF

Figures 14A to D: Age-related macular degeneration, vascularized pigment epithelium detachment (PED) with occult neovascularization treated by anti-VEGF. (A) Cross-section scan before anti-vascular endothelial growth factor (VEGF) treatment. Retina is thickened by diffuse edema and rare cystoid cells. The PED shape is very irregular, contents are dense and Bruch's membrane is seen (Optovue RTVue); (B) *En face* scan before anti-VEGF treatment. Retina is thickened by diffuse edema and rare cystoid cells. The PED shape is very irregular, contents are dense, radial folds can be seen (Optovue RTVue); (C) Cross-section scan after anti-VEGF treatment. Retina has less edema. The pigment epithelium detachment shape is still very irregular but walls are thinner. Contents are denser. Bruch's membrane is seen (Optovue RTVue); (D) *En face* scan after anti-VEGF treatment. After anti-VEGF treatment vascularized PED with occult neovascularization shows important change pigment alteration. After a few days the detachment appears to be more compact and is much less elevated. The cupola is flattened and less evident; the detachment appears to be deflated. Walls are thinner, contents are more dense and homogeneous. The fibrovascular tissue it contains get to be more compact, less reflective. It is less vascularized and more fibrous. Contents are less clear than before treatment with presence of denser hyper-reflective tissue towards detachment cupola. The fibrovascular tissue can be found inside the retinal elevation or immediately above and in contact with it. Retinal folds around the detachment are less evident (Optovue RTVue)

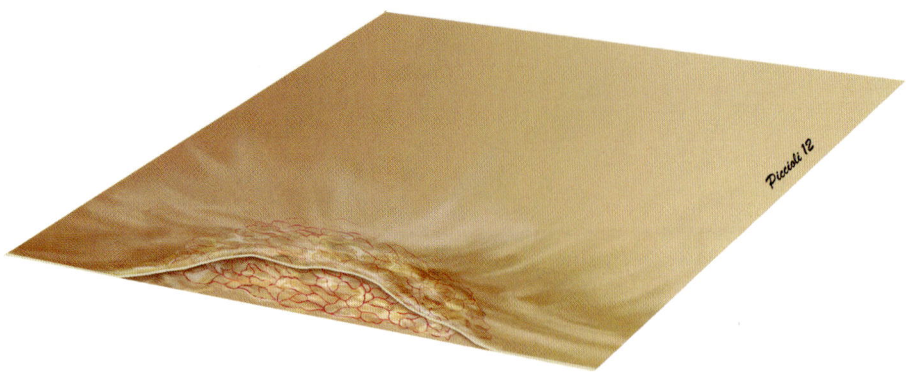

Figure 15: Age-related macular degeneration, vascularized pigment epithelium detachment (PED) with occult neovascularization after anti-vascular endothelial growth factor (VEGF) treatment. After anti-VEGF treatment vascularized pigment epithelium detachment with occult neovascularization shows important change and alteration. The detachment appears to be deflated, walls are thinner. Contents are more dense and homogeneous. The fibrovascular tissue is less vascularized and more fibrous

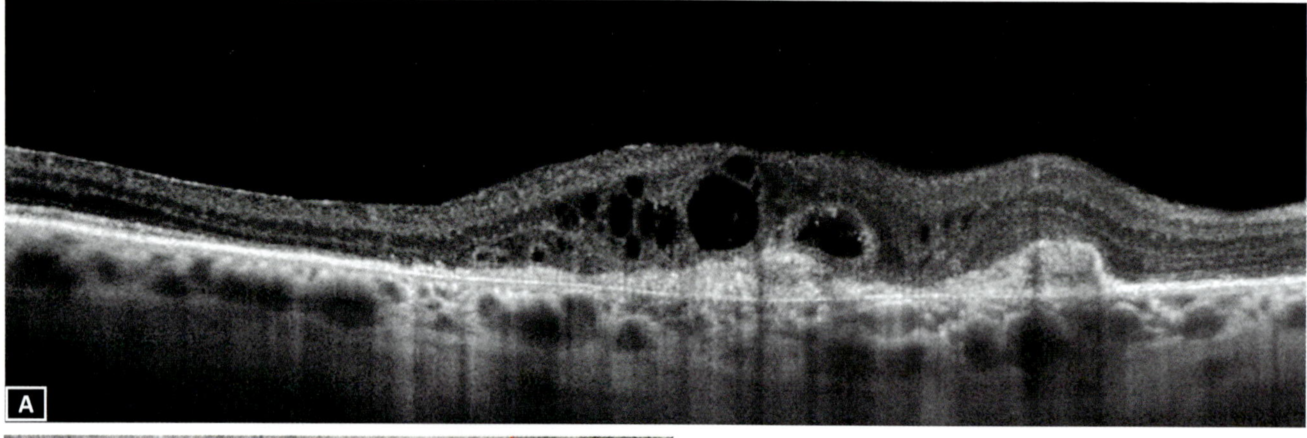

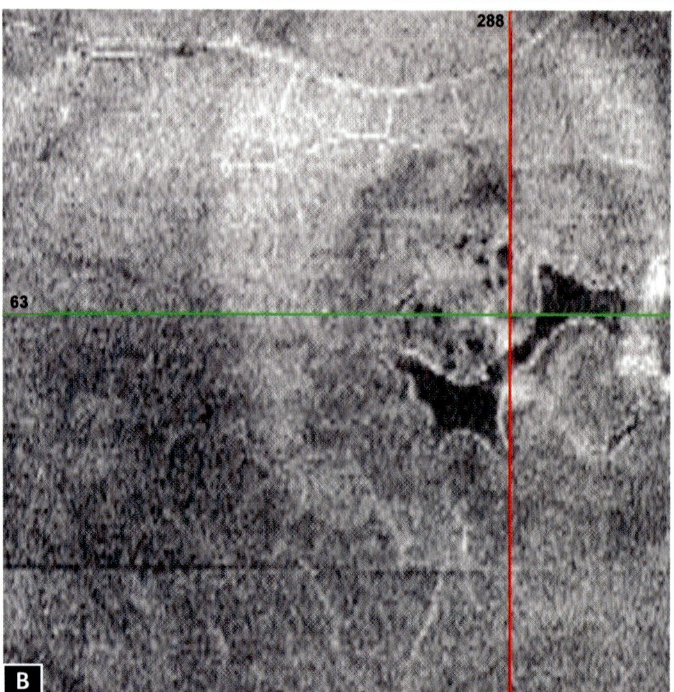

Figures 16A and B: Outer retinal tubulations. (A) Cross-section scan. In some patients with age-related macular degeneration or other long standing macular disease we can observe a peculiar type of cavities in the outer retina—tube shaped lesions. In B scans they are rounded or ovoid hyporeflective spaces with dense hyper-reflective borders (Optovue RTVue); (B) Outer retinal tubulations in *en face* scans range from single straight or branching tubules or forked tubule to complex irregular tangled web of tubulations and tubular networks, usually overlying areas of pigment epithelial alteration or subretinal fibrosis. These structures generally remain stable over time (Optovue RTVue)

gives only fragmental information about retinal PED and could induce diagnosis errors and software-related artifacts during the analysis of the images.[7,9] OCT *en face* scan, instead, is able to localize smallest retinal PED detachment and to detect clinically useful morphological characteristics. Vascular tissue is always found close or against the detachment dome.

The authors believe that three important factors may have a part shaping the retinal PED. Chronic disease, longer disease duration associated to the age of the patients could take part in forming the aspect of the RPE in these cases. It would be very interesting finding the functional factors that give these anatomical aspects.

References

1. Murphy RP, Yeo JH, Green WR, et al. Dehiscences of the pigment epithelium. Trans Am Ophthalmol Soc. 1985;83: 63-81.
2. Green WR, McDonnell PJ, Yeo JH. Pathologic features of senile macular degeneration. Ophthalmology. 1985;92: 615-27.
3. Bird AC, Marshall J. Retinal pigment epithelial detachments in the elderly. Trans Ophthalmol Soc, UK. 1986; 105:674-82.
4. Mitarai K, Gomi F, Tano Y. Three-dimensional optical coherence tomographic findings in central serous chorioretinopathy. Graefes Arch Clin Exp Ophthalmol. 2006;244:1415-20.
5. Hirami Y, Tsujikawa A, Sasahara M, et al. Alterations of retinal pigment epithelium in central serous chorioretinopathy. Clin Experiment Ophthalmol. 2007;35:225-30.
6. Montero JA, Ruiz-Moreno JM. Optical coherence tomography characterisation of idiopathic central serous chorioretinopathy. Br J Ophthalmol. 2005;89:562-4.
7. Karam EZ, Ramirez E, Arreaza PL, et al. Optical coherence tomographic artefacts in diseases of the retinal pigment epithelium. Br J Ophthalmol. 2007;91:1139-42.
8. Lumbroso B, Savastano MC, Rispoli M, et al. Morphologic differences, according to etiology, in pigment epithelial detachments by means of *en face* optical coherence tomography. Retina. 2011;31:553-8.
9. Hee MR. Artifacts in optical coherence tomography topographic maps. Am J Ophthalmol. 2005;139:154-5.
10. Coscas F, Coscas G, Querques G, Massamba N, Querques, L, Bandello F, Souied EH. En face enhanced depth imaging OCT of fibrovascular PED. IOVS, 2012;53(7): 4147-51.
11. Wolff B, Matet A, Vasseur V, Sahel JA, Mauget-Faÿsse M. En Face OCT Imaging for the Diagnosis of Outer Retinal Tubulations in Age-Related Macular Degeneration.J Ophthalmol. 2012;2012:542417. E-pub August 2012.

chapter 9

Cystoid Macular Edema

Bruno Lumbroso, Marco Rispoli

Introduction

The possibility to use *en face* C scan allows us to highlight specific aspects and patterns of cystoid macular edema (**Table 1**). *En face* scans are essential in studying diffuse and cystoid macular edema, allowing identification of the extension and evolutive stage of the retinal swelling. Optical coherence tomography (OCT) *en face* scans show that the anteroposterior and radial structure of Henle fibers and Müller cells are basic in shaping the layout of pseudocystic cavities.[1-3]

Correlations have been made between OCT and fluorescein angiography aspects.[4,5]

Retinal edema evolution can be classified in the following phases:

- Focal and diffuse noncystoid edema
- Early cystoid edema
- Advanced cystoid edema
- Regressed cystoid edema.

To understand edema's extension and evolutive stage series of cross-sectional OCT scans and series of *en face* scans are necessary to study edema progression and its evolution. One single *en face* scan is not enough to have a good understanding of the cystoid cells layout.

En face scans should be made at least at three retinal levels, and even more in case of in depth study:

- The first *en face* scan should be placed at the internal limiting membrane (ILM), to show epiretinal and retinal membranes, plaques, macular retinal surface alterations and minute or important folds and vitreomacular interface relations. Scan thickness should be 30 micron.
- The second scan is parallel to the ILM, but placed 40 micron inside the retina. *It will show inner nuclear layer cystoid cells.*
- The third scan is parallel to the ILM but placed deeper inside the retina. *It will show outer nuclear layer cystoid cells.* Second and third scan thickness should be 30 micron thick.
- The fourth scan is parallel to the pigment epithelium but placed 50 micron in front of it. *It will show a double row of inner and outer nuclear layer cystoid cells.* Thickness should be 30 micron thick. A deeper section frequently shows a small retinal serous detachment.

The two intraretinal scans show edema cells at their onset in the inner and outer nuclear layers and, later in evolution, the bigger central cells.

The different scans must be confronted against one another.

En face OCT is very helpful in the study and assessment of the cystoid cavity shape and dimension and helps follow cystoid edema progression and allows differential diagnosis between early, advanced and regressive cystoid macular edema (**Figures 1A to F).**

Table 1: Causes of cystoid macular edema

Most frequent
• Diabetic retinopathy
• Venous occlusions
• Age-related macular degeneration
• Postsurgery syndrome (Irvine-Gass)

Frequent
• Traction by epiretinal membrane
• Macular pucker
• Chronic diffuse retinal epitheliopathy
• Retinitis pigmentosa
• Uveitis, pars planitis and choroiditis

Less frequent
• Birdshot retinopathy
• Epinephrine

Rare	
• Telangiectasis	• Coats' disease
• Leber's disease	• Retinal and choroidal
• Retinal angioma	neoformations
• Hamartoma	• Osteoma
• Choroidal nevus	• Melanoma
• Metastatic tumor	• Radiation retinopathy

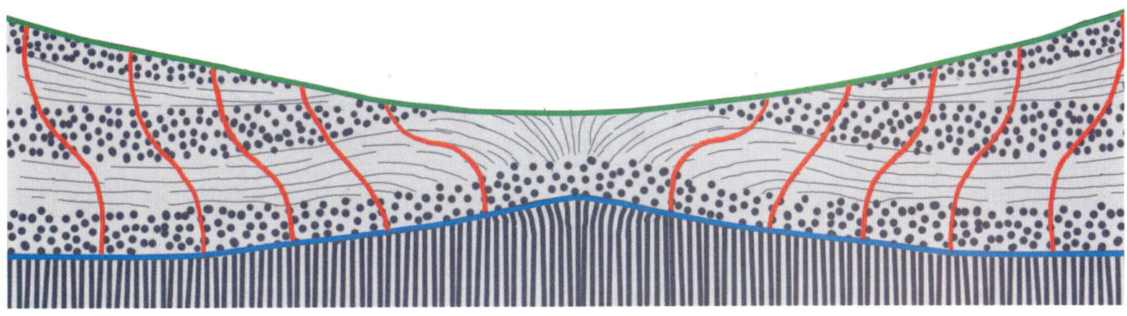

Figure 1A: Normal retina showing Muller cells

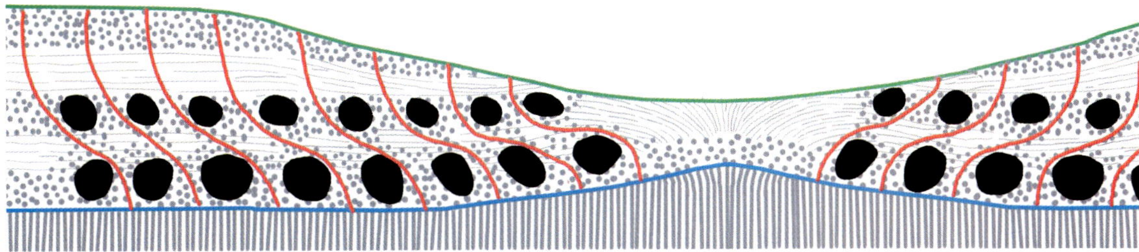

Figure 1B: Early cystoid edema

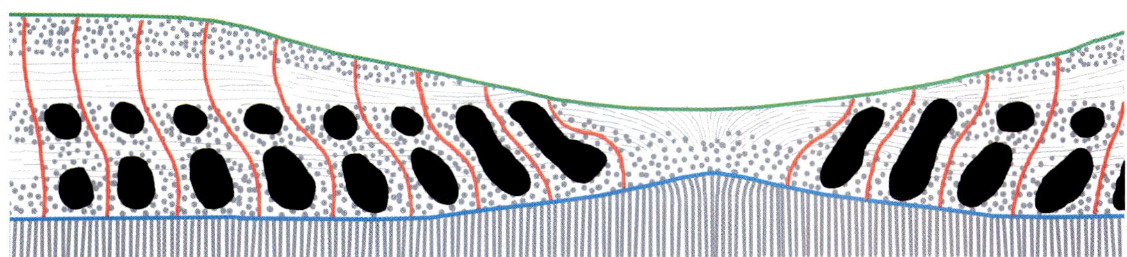

Figure 1C: Early cystoid edema

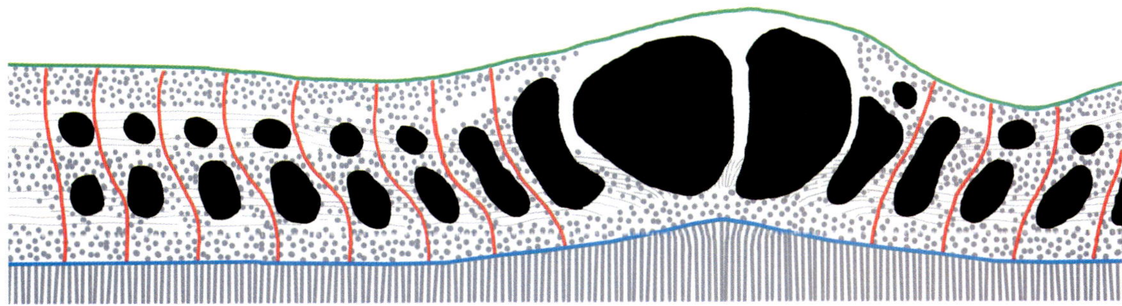

Figure 1D: Advanced cystoid edema

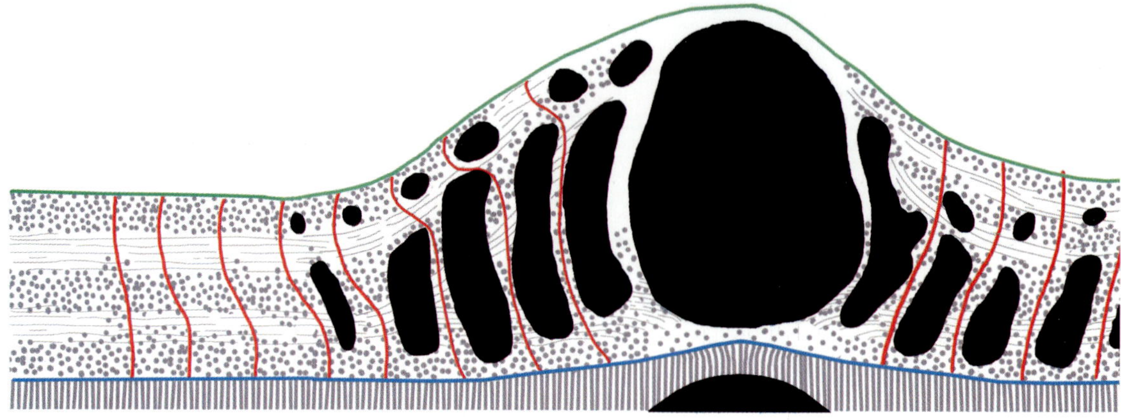

Figure 1E: Advanced cystoid edema

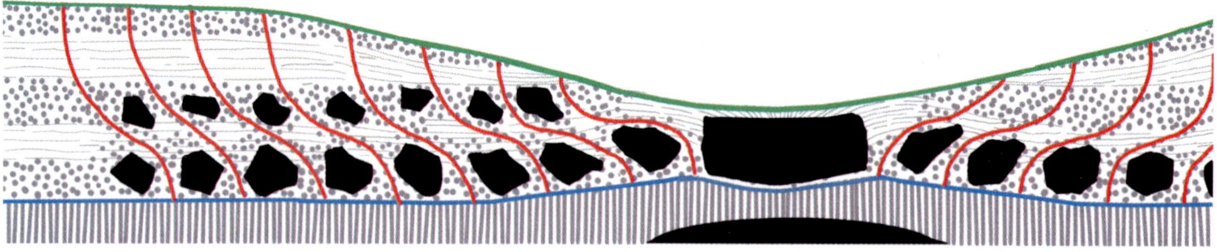

Figure 1F: Regressed cystoid edema

Figures 1A to F: These drawings show the evolution of the cystoid macular edema from early (A and B) to advanced (C to E) to regressed (F)

Focal edema frontal scans show only a localized thickening of the retina with a spongy appearance. *Diffuse noncystoid edema* cross-section scans show a thickening of the retina close to the fovea; *en face* scans show spongy aspect. It is seen as a diffuse decrease in retinal reflectivity due to a reduced density of optical backscattering within the retina **(Figures 2A and B)**.

Early Cystoid Edema

Optical coherence tomography (OCT) cross-sectional scans show areas of intraretinal fluid accumulation in cystic spaces. Lesion morphology and structure are influenced by the architectural macular framework of the horizontal and vertical structures of the retina. Henle fibers and Muller cells framework form the basis for shape and evolution of cystoid cells.

Accumulation of fluid is seen in small intraretinal cavities located at the onset around the fovea in the *outer and inner nuclear layers*. Nuclear layers are involved first and then gradually the entire thickness of the retina.

Later the pseudo cell number increase. Cavities are separated from each other by thick walls that appear regular, smooth and rounded.

En face OCT scans parallel to the ILM but placed 40 micron inside the retina show inner nuclear layer cystoid cells. These cells are petal shaped centrally, bigger than peripheral cavities. Around it are placed numerous smaller rounded cavities.

Deeper *en face* scans placed in the outer nuclear later show regular, bigger cystoid cells, their shape is grossly ovoid, polygonal converging toward the fovea, flower shaped **(Figure 3)**.

Advanced Cystoid Edema

After a longer evolution, edema cavity dimensions increase. Cells first merge vertically: cells in the inner layer grow toward cells in the outer nuclear layer, forming larger vertically ovoid cavities. The walls get thinner, but the cystoid cell shape remains smooth, regular, globular and spherical.

Cell enlargement leads to first to vertical merging between cells in the inner nuclear and the outer nuclear layers. Lateral merging between neighboring cavities comes later.

Cavity merging results in large chambers or crypts supported by pillars formed by residual tissue, vertical cell

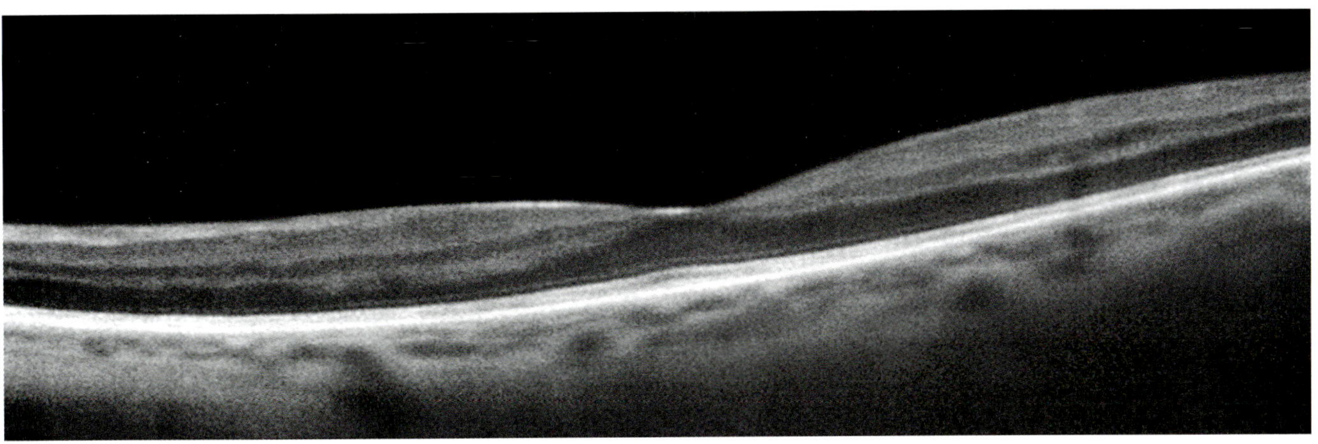

Figure 2A: Focal edema, diffuse noncystoid edema, cross-section scans show only localized, focal thickening of the retina with a spongy appearance (Optovue RTVue)

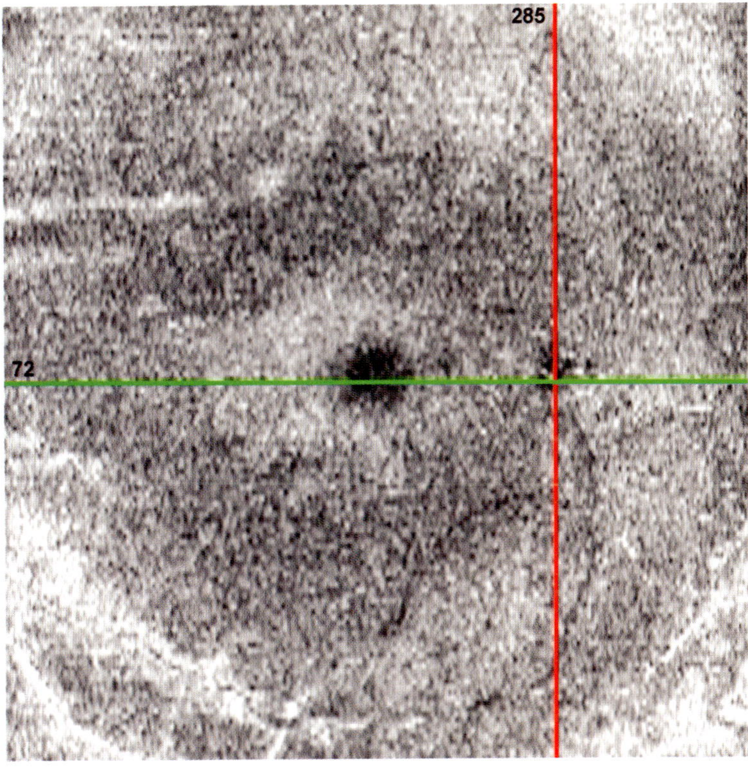

Figure 2B: Focal edema, diffuse noncystoid edema, frontal scans show only localized spongy appearance (Optovue RTVue)

chains and Müller cells. During evolution a big central foveal cell may appear, due to lesser microstructure rigidity at the fovea **(Figures 4A and B)**.[6,7]

The largest cystic spaces are found centrally, forming one or more bulging chambers. The longer the evolution, the larger the cystoid cavities. Their partitions gradually disappear leading to larger and more irregular chambers. Finally, cystoid edema evolution leads to large vaults sustained by vertical pillars of residual tissue similar to columns in a cathedral or tree trunks in a forest.

En face OCT: The frontal scan placed inside the retina shows at the inner nuclear layer level numerous petal shaped cystoid cells. The frontal or coronal flower or honeycomb pattern is caused by the Henle fibers stellate structure **(Figures 4C and D)**. Cells are grossly ovoid with tips converging toward the fovea, flower or clover shaped.

In the outer nuclear layer we see regular, bigger cystoid cells, their shape is more polygonal than ovoid converging toward the fovea **(Figure 4E)**.

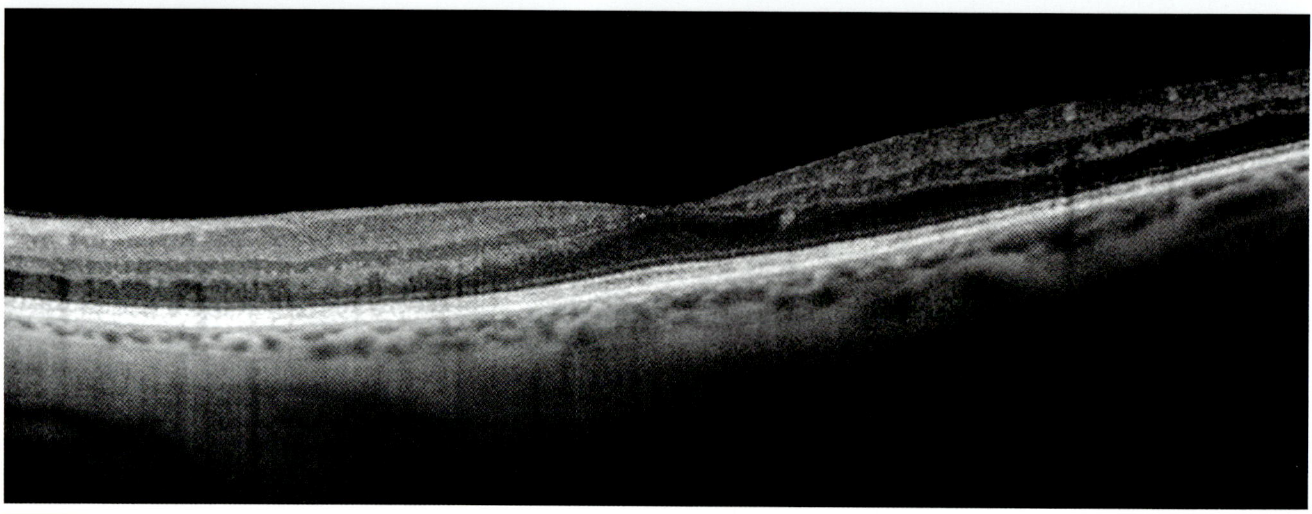

Figure 3: Early cystoid edema, cross-section scan showing location of the first cystoid cells: Three small cavities in the inner nuclear layer (Optovue RTVue)

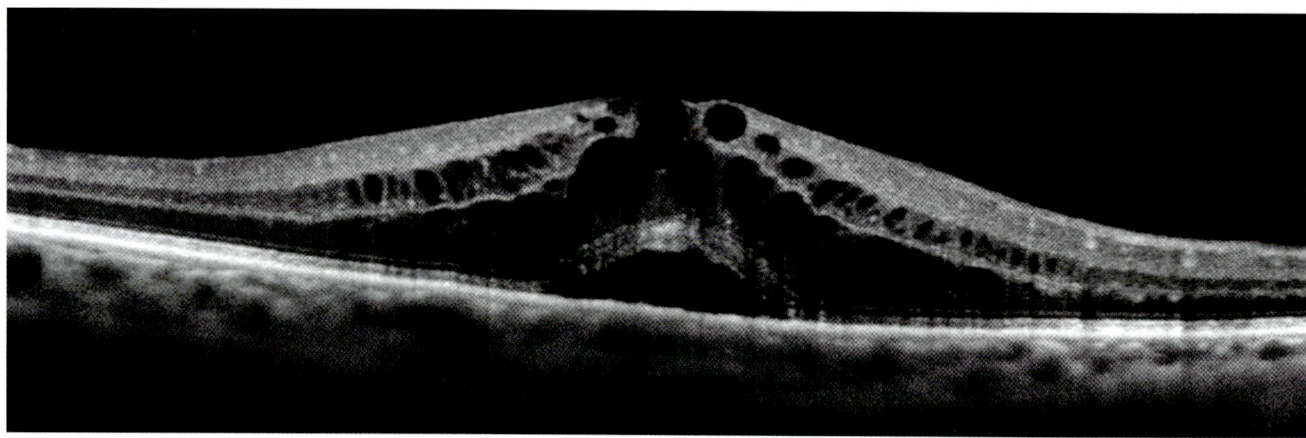

Figure 4A: Advanced cystoid edema, cross-section scan showing location of the rows of cystoid cells and a small retinal serous elevation at the fovea (Optovue RTVue)

Later in the evolution walls between cells disappear leading to large irregular chambers sustained by rare columns of residual retinal (**Figure 4F**).

Regressed Cystoid Edema

After a long evolution and repeated intravitreal and laser treatments, cystoid cells dimension decrease. Cystoid cavities shrink and get to be irregular, with thinner walls. They take a distorted, twisted appearance. Their shape get to be irregularly rectangular, their main dimension horizontal. Walls are thinner with sharp bends. Plexiform layers tend to disappear or to be very thin and irregular. The outer limiting membrane and the IS/OS junction are fragmented and interrupted (**Figure 5A**). Cavity contents become hazy.

Retinal tissue around regressive edema shows disruption of the normal structure (**Table 2**). Retinal layers disappear and in their place we see two pathological layers, one

Table 2: Causes of regressive cystoid edema

- Long-standing diabetic retinopathy, age-related macular degeneration (AMD), venous occlusion nontreated
- Diabetic retinopathy treated by laser for more than 5 years
- Diabetic retinopathy repeatedly treated by antivascular endothelial growth factor (VEGF)
- Venous occlusion repeatedly treated by anti-VEGF
- Age-related macular degeneration repeatedly treated by anti-VEGF
- Retinal telangiectasis

corresponding to the block of inner retina, and the other corresponding to the photoreceptors layer.

En face OCT: The frontal scan parallel to the ILM but placed inside the retina shows very irregular large chambers (**Figure 5B**). Their shape is frequently irregularly rectangular. Sometimes the cavities form a labyrinth, a maze of long rectangular cavities with intersections. The walls take a

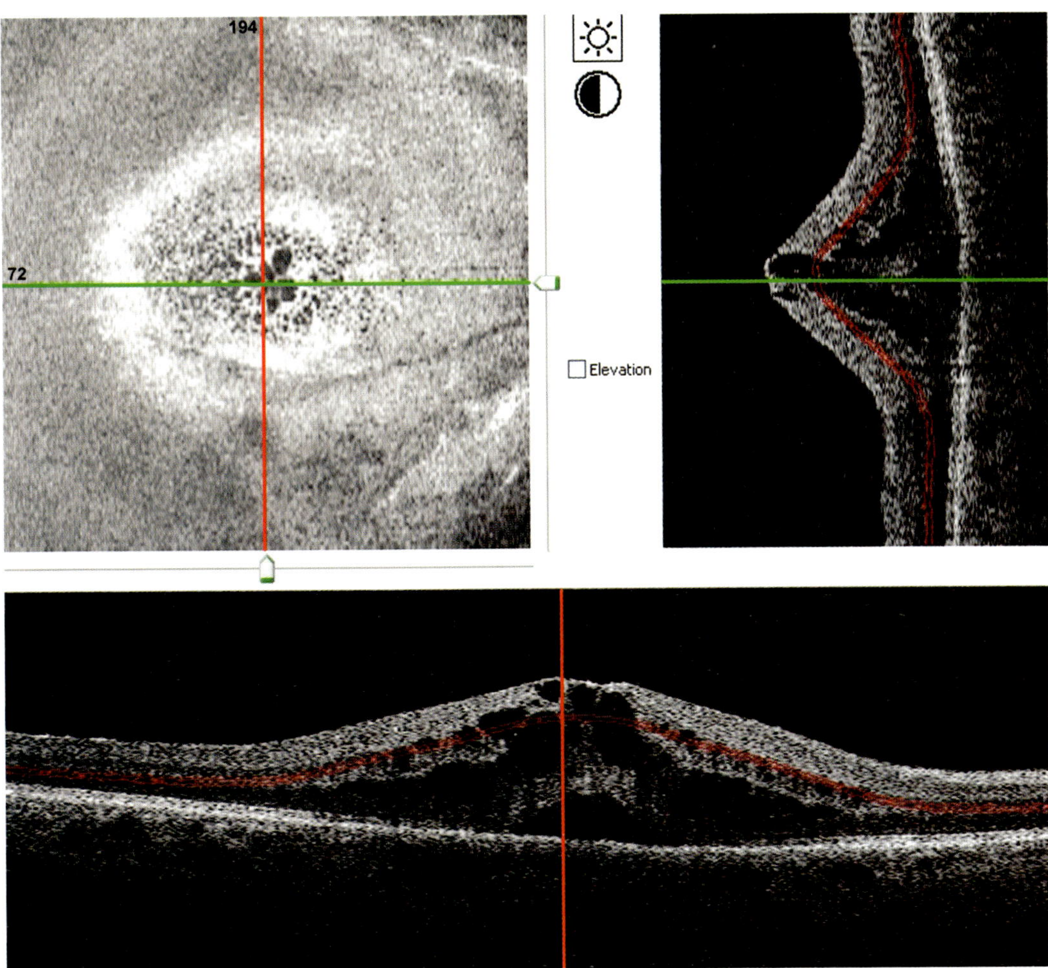

Figure 4B: Advanced cystoid edema, *en face* scan inner nuclear layer level. The frontal scan placed at the inner nuclear layer level shows numerous small cavities at the periphery. At the center petal shaped cystoid cells can be seen. The frontal or coronal flower or honeycomb pattern is caused by the Henle fibers stellate structure. The lateral cross scans show the level of the frontal section adapted to the inner nuclear layer convexity (Optovue RTVue)

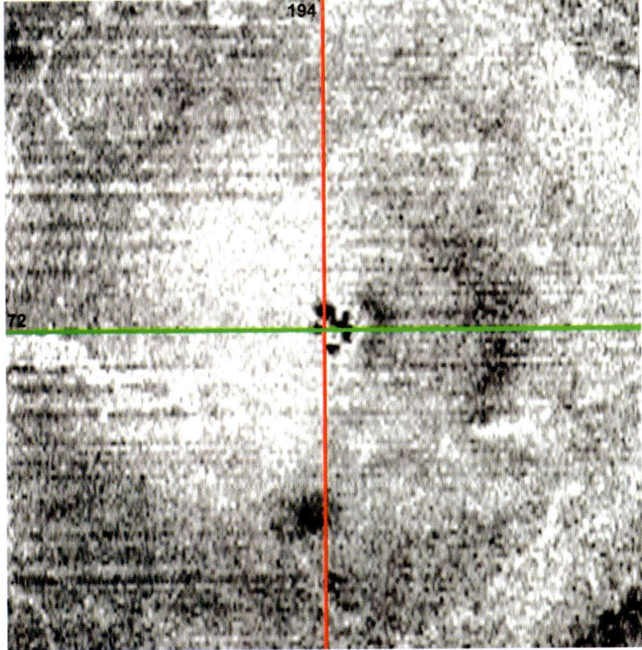

Figure 4C: Advanced cystoid edema, *en face* scan, at inner limiting membrane level. The *en face* scan follows the ILM elevation at the level of the macular edema. At the center of the ILM elevation we can see a few small cavities where the scan has cut a few cystoid cells (Optovue RTVue)

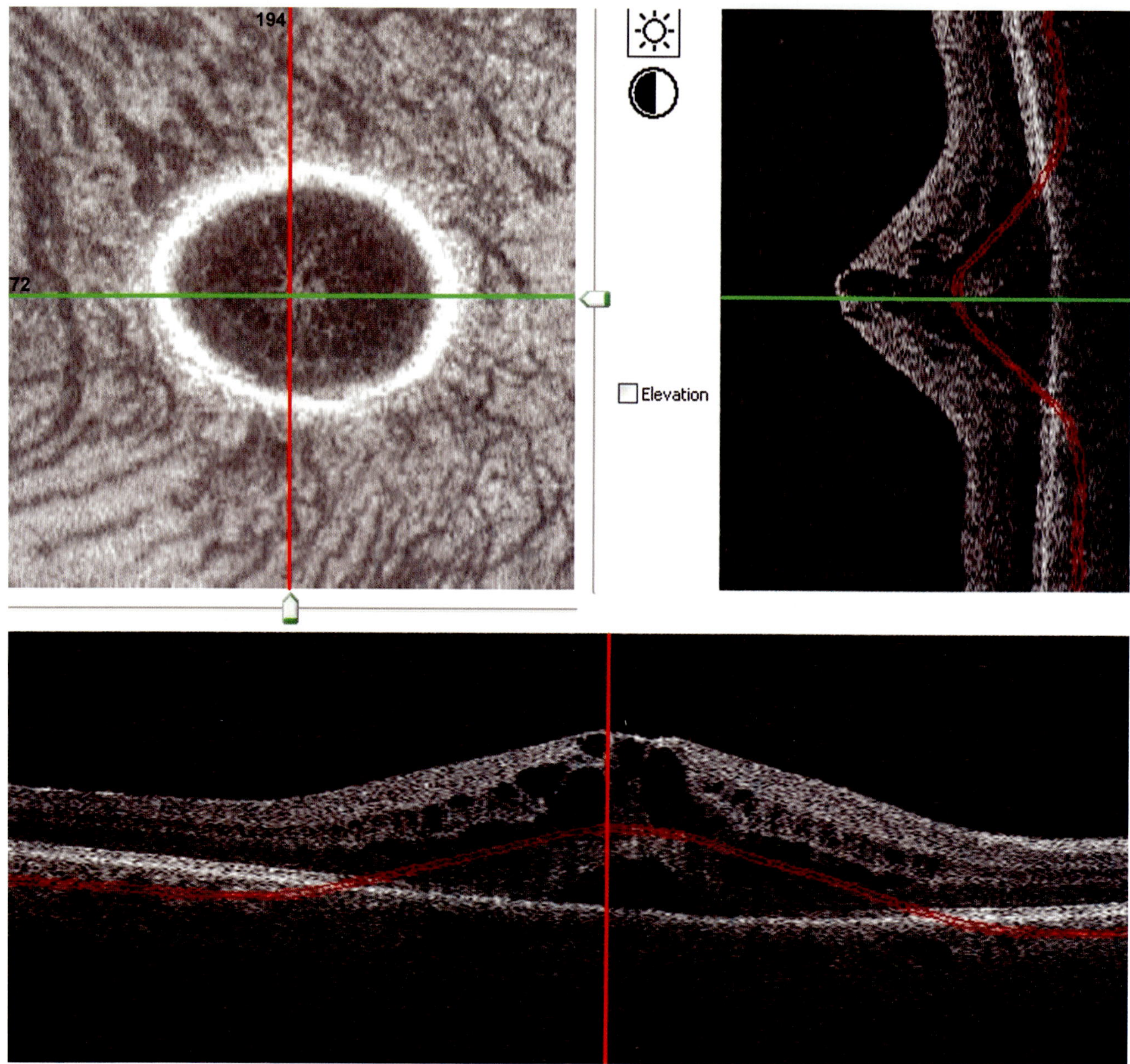

Figure 4D: Advanced cystoid edema, *en face* scan outer nuclear layer. In the outer nuclear layer we see regular, bigger cystoid cells. Their shape is more polygonal than ovoid converging toward the fovea. The frontal or coronal flower or honeycomb pattern is caused by the Henle fibers stellate structure. The cross scans show the level of the frontal section adapted to the outer nuclear layer convexity. Later in the evolution the walls between cells will disappear leading to large irregular chambers sustained by rare columns of residual retinal (Optovue RTVue)

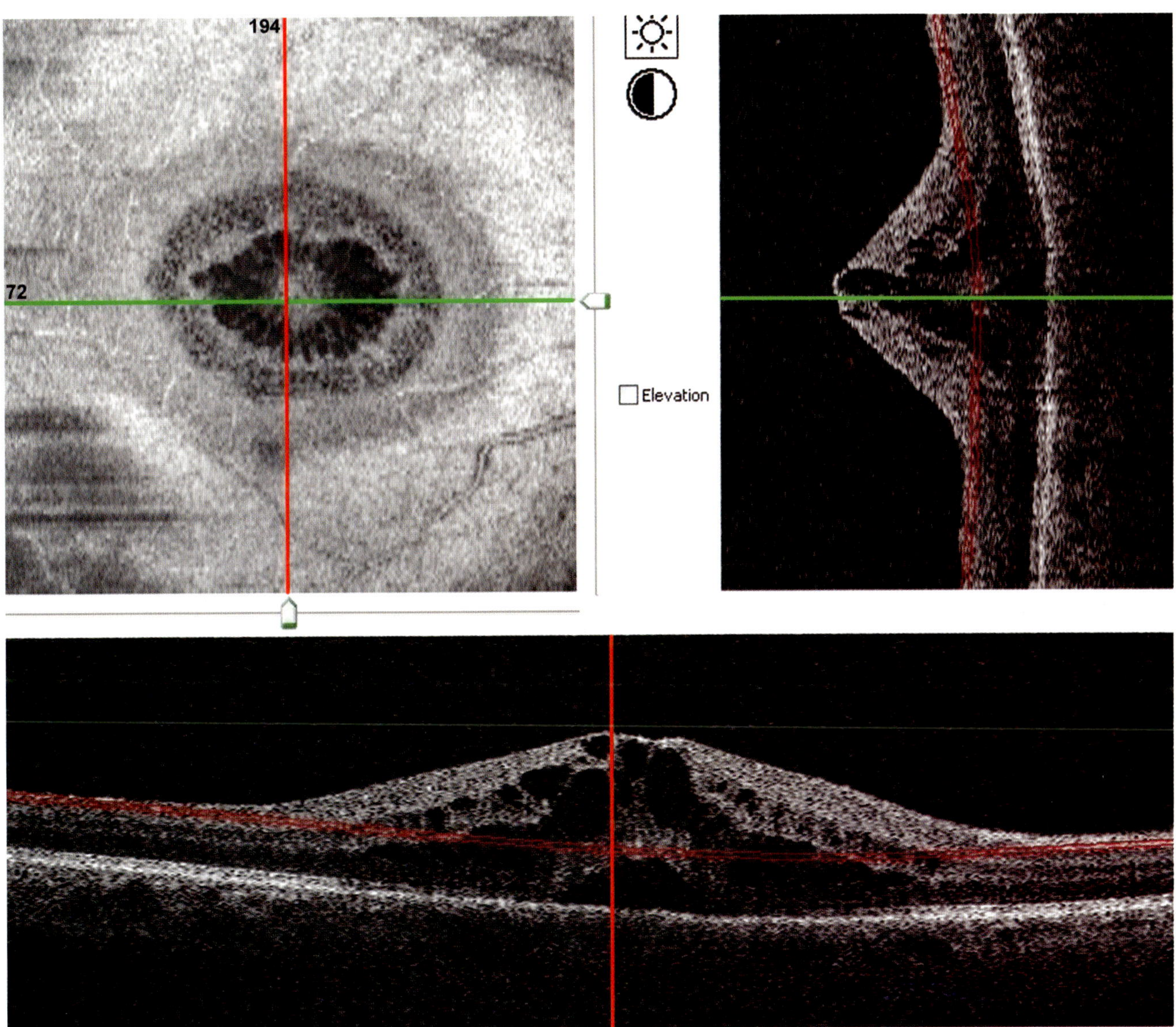

Figure 4E: Advanced cystoid edema, flat *en face* scan showing a double ring of inner and outer nuclear layer cystoid cells. The scan is parallel to the pigment epithelium and placed 50 micron in front of it. It cuts through inner and outer nuclear layers and shows a double ring of inner and outer nuclear layer cystoid cells. Scan thickness is 30 micron thick. The lateral cross scans show the location of the flat frontal section (Optovue RTVue)

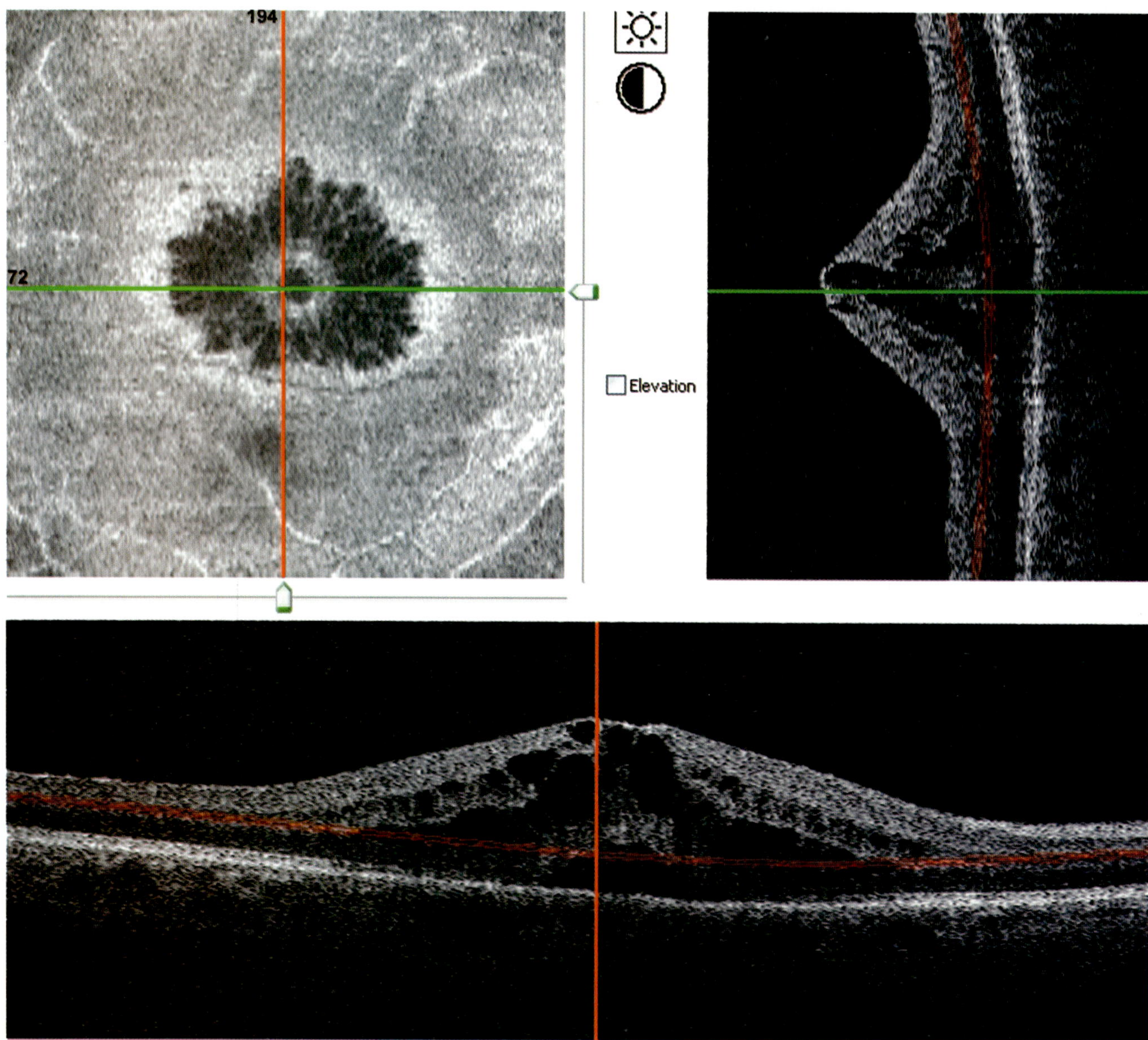

Figure 4F: Advanced cystoid edema, flat *en face* scan cutting through outer nuclear layer and also the central rounded small retinal detachment. The scan is parallel to the pigment epithelium but placed only at 20 micron in front of it. It cuts through outer nuclear layer and also the central rounded small retinal detachment. Scan thickness is 30 micron thick. The lateral cross scans show the location of the flat frontal section (Optovue RTVue)

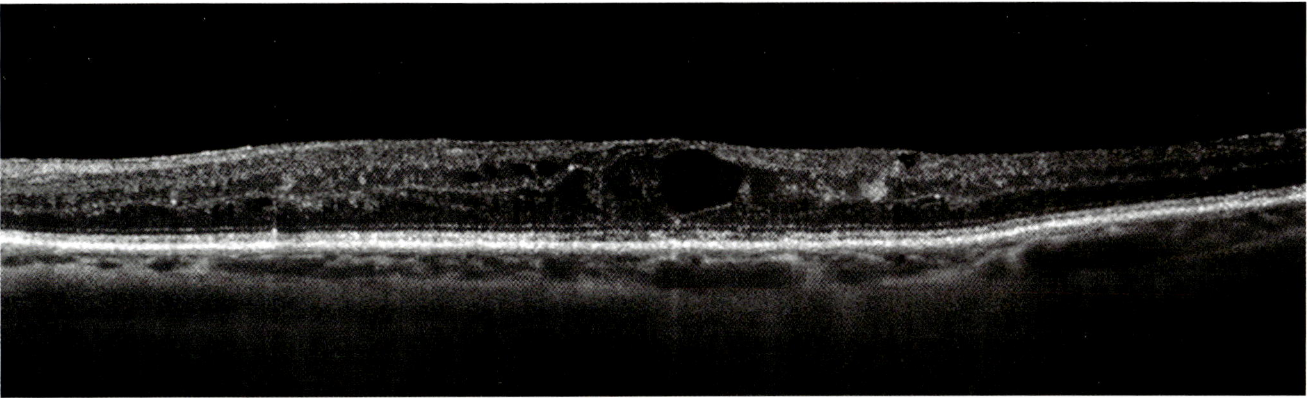

Figure 5A: Regressed cystoid edema, cross-section scan showing location of the shape of the regressed cystoid cells. They take a distorted, twisted appearance. Their shape get to be irregularly rectangular, their main dimension's horizontal. Walls are thinner with sharp bends. Plexiform layers tend to disappear or to be very thin and irregular (Optovue RTVue)

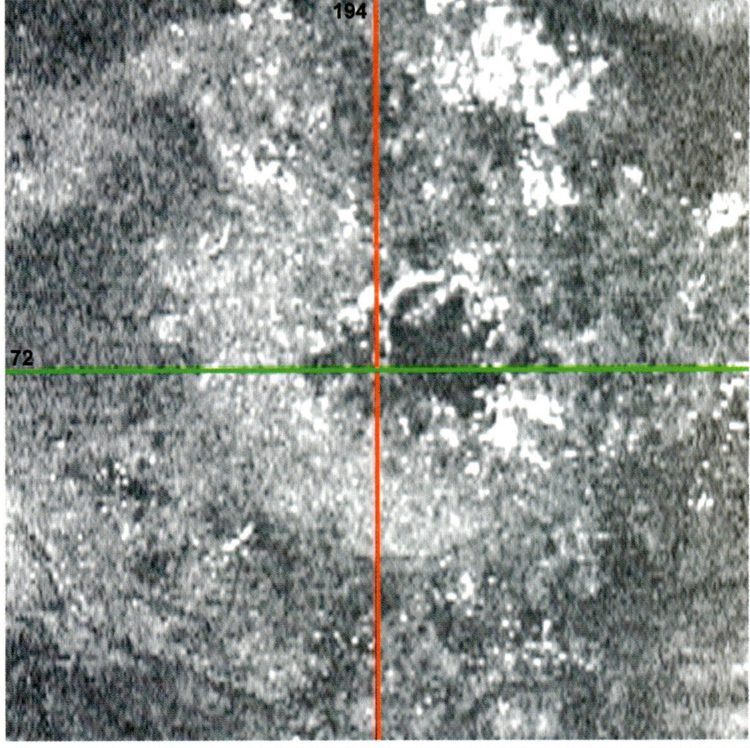

Figure 5B: Regressed cystoid edema, *en face* scan. The frontal scan parallel to the ILM but placed inside the retina shows very irregular large chambers. Their shape is frequently irregularly rectangular. Sometimes the cavities form a labyrinth, a maze of long rectangular cavities with intersections. The walls take a distorted, twisted appearance (Optovue RTVue)

distorted, twisted appearance. At the macula they are square or cubic in shape, occupying all the thickness of the fovea (**Figures 5C and D**). It is not rare at this stage to see outer retinal tubulations coexisting with regressed edema.

Postoperative Edema (Irvine-Gass Syndrome)

Cystoid macular edema shows generally a very regular layout of the pseudocystic cavities, much more evenly arranged than in diabetic retinopathy or in venous occlusion. Postoperative edema is developed in the next chapter.

Venous Branch Occlusion Edema

En face scans are essential in studying diffuse and cystoid macular edema, allowing identification of the extension and evolutive stage (**Figure 6**).

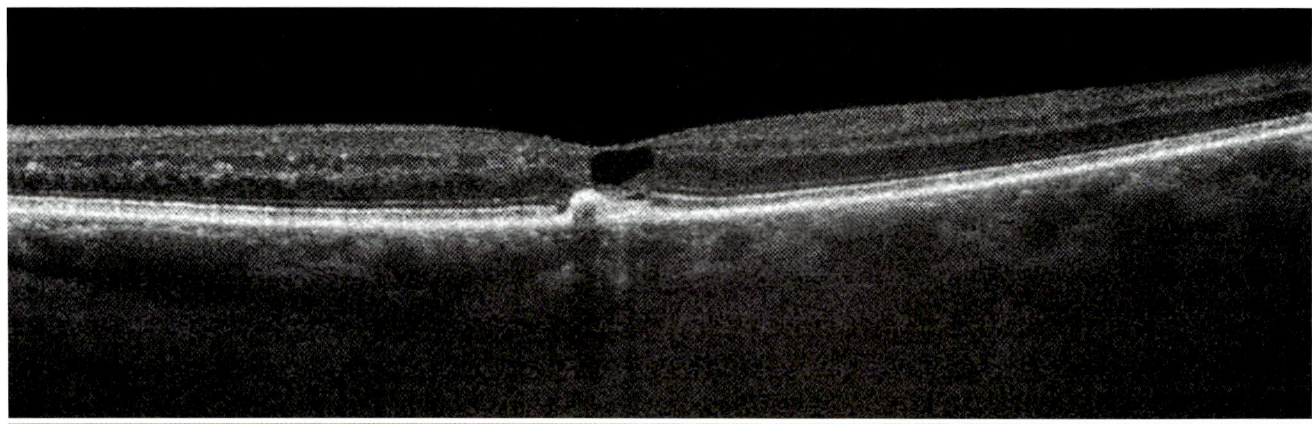

Figure 5C: Regressed cystoid edema, cross-section scan. At the macula one single pseudocyst is square or cubic in shape, occupying almost all the thickness of the fovea (Optovue RTVue)

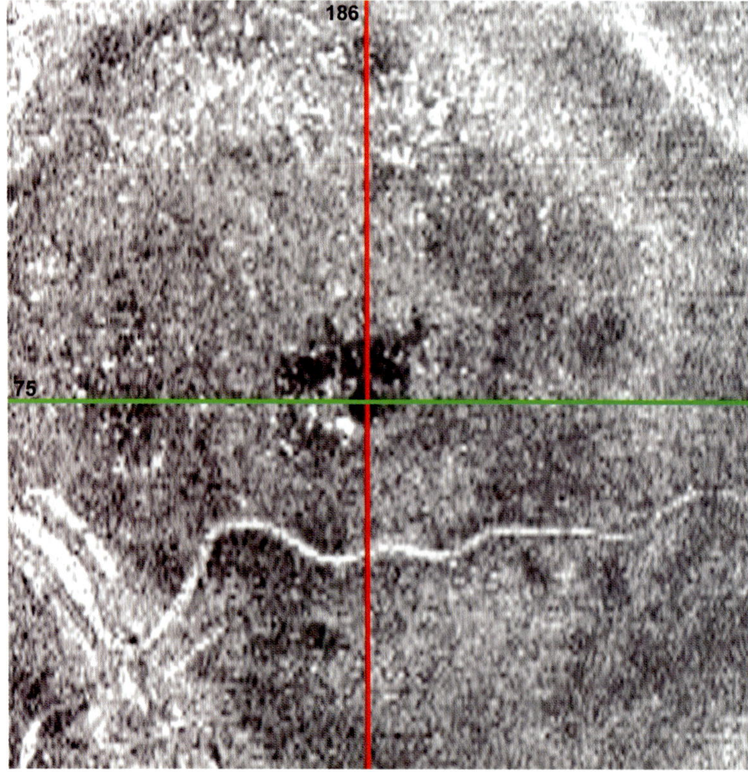

Figure 5D: Regressed cystoid edema, macular *en face* scan. The single central foveal cavity is cubic in shape, occupying the full thickness of the fovea (Optovue RTVue)

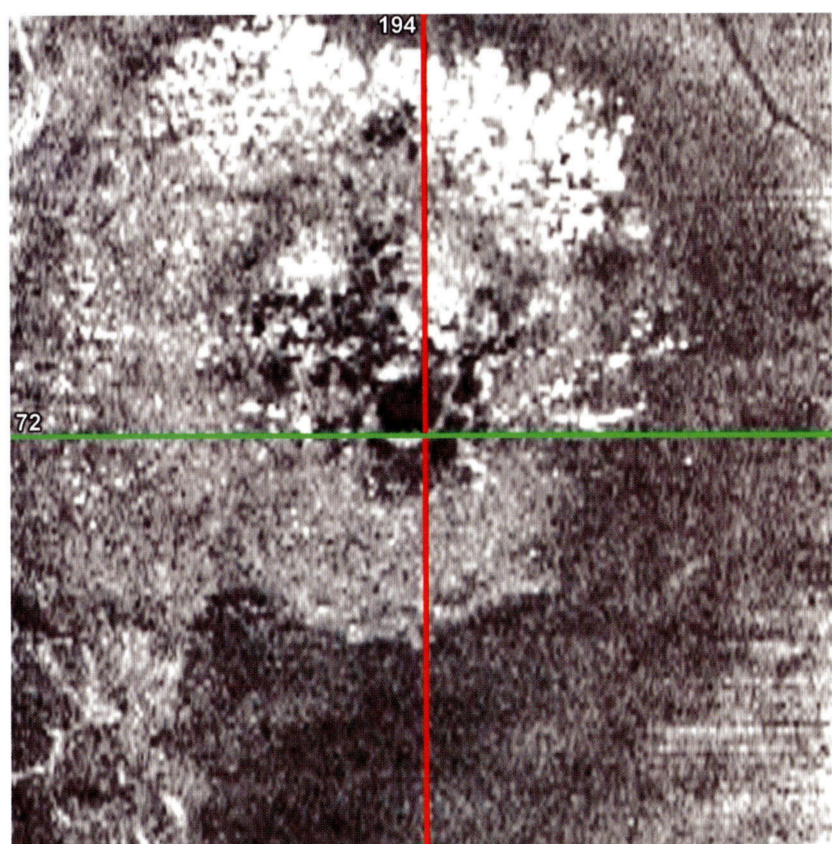

Figure 6: Venous branch occlusion edema, macular *en face* scan. *En face* scans are essential assessing cystoid macular edema, allowing identification of the extension and evolutive stage in venous branch occlusion. Retinal edema shows an irregular layout of the pseudocystic cavities, much less evenly arranged than in Irvine-Gass syndrome. Hyper-reflective hemorrhages and hard exudates can be seen (Optovue RTVue)

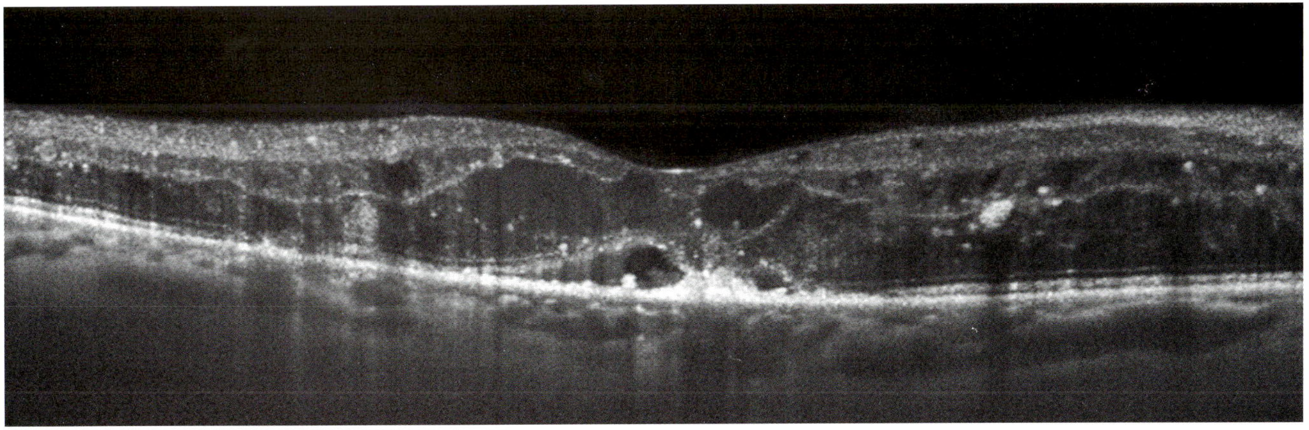

Figure 7: Cystoid edema in choroiditis and uveitis cross-section scan. Cystoid cells and cavities are bigger and rarer more irregular in uveitis than in noninflammatory diseases. Their content is hazy. Their walls are thicker than normally and highly reflective. Their inner surface may show granular irregularities. Hard exudates can be seen (Optovue RTVue)

Cystoid Edema in Choroiditis and Uveitis

Cystoid cells and cavities are generally bigger and rarer and more irregular in uveitis than in non-inflammatory diseases (**Figure 7**). Their walls are thicker and highly reflective. Walls surface shows granular irregularities. Their content is hazy and reflective (**Figure 8**).

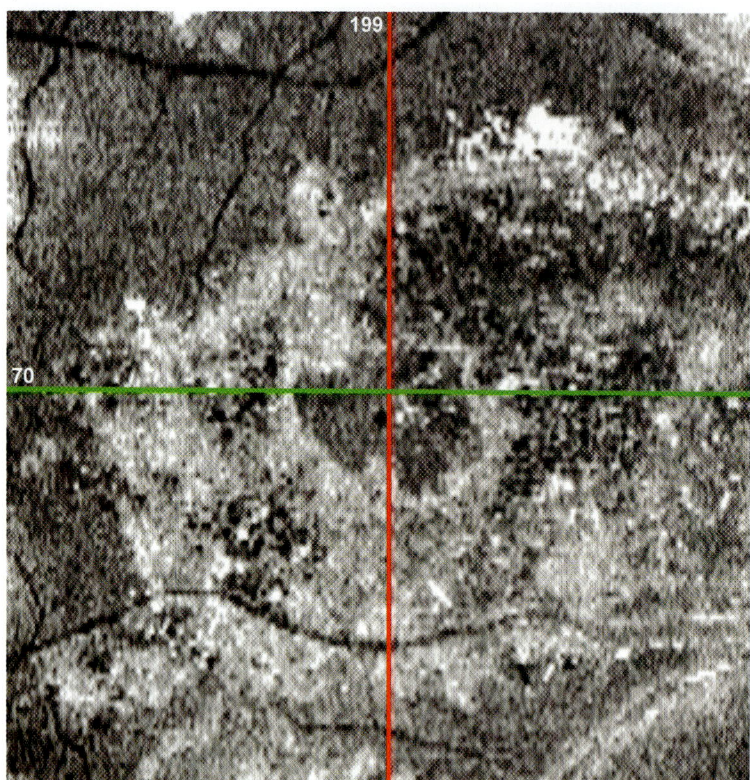

Figure 8: Cystoid edema in choroiditis and uveitis *en face* scan. Cavities are bigger and more irregular than in uveitis. Their walls are thicker and highly reflective. Their content is hazy. Hard exudates can be seen (Optovue RTVue)

References

1. Bringmann A, Pannicke T, Grosche J, et al. Müller cells in the healthy and diseased retina. Prog Retin Eye Res. 2006;25(4):397-424.

2. Tout S, Chan-Ling T, Holländer H, et al. The role of Müller cells in the formation of the blood-retinal barrier. Neuroscience. 1993;55(1):291-301.

3. Bringmann A, Pannicke T, Biedermann B, et al. Role of retinal glial cells in neurotransmitter uptake and metabolism. Neurochem Int. 2009;54:143-60.

4. Bolz M, Ritter M, Schneider M, et al. A systematic correlation of angiography and high-resolution optical coherence tomography in diabetic macular edema. Ophthalmology. 2009;116(1):66-72.

5. Yeung L, Lima VC, Garcia P, et al. Correlation between Spectral Domain Optical Coherence Tomography Findings and Fluorescein Angiography Patterns in Diabetic Macular Edema. Ophthalmology. 2009;116(6):1158-67.

6. Gass JD. Muller cell cone, an overlooked part of the anatomy of the fovea centralis: hypotheses concerning its role in the pathogenesis of macular hole and foveo-macular retinoschisis. Arch Ophthalmol. 1999;117(6): 821-3.

7. Yamada E. Some structural features of the fovea centralis in the human retina. Arch Ophthalmol. 1969;82(2): 151-9.

chapter 10

Postoperative Macular Edema

Marco Rispoli, Bruno Lumbroso, Vanessa Pala

Postoperative cystoid macular edema (CME) is the most common cause of visual loss after cataract surgery. Angiographic postoperative CME is observed in 20–30% of patients after uneventful cataract surgery and vision decreases approximately 6–8 weeks after cataract surgery. Postoperative CME disappears spontaneously within 6 months in 50–75% of patients. However, permanent CME with severe vision loss has been reported in 2.35% of cases. Postoperative CME after cataract surgery results from two main causes, both of which could coexist.[1,2]

According to the inflammatory theory,[3] inflammatory mediators (e.g. prostaglandins) and vascular endothelial growth factor are upregulated in the aqueous and vitreous humors after surgical manipulation. Inflammation breaks down the blood-retinal barrier with resultant edema in the inner nuclear and plexiform layers of the retina **(Figure 1)**.

According to the mechanical theory, the posterior pole inflammatory reaction is triggered by tractional forces caused by transient ocular hypotony and vitreous movements subsequent to surgical procedures on the anterior segment.

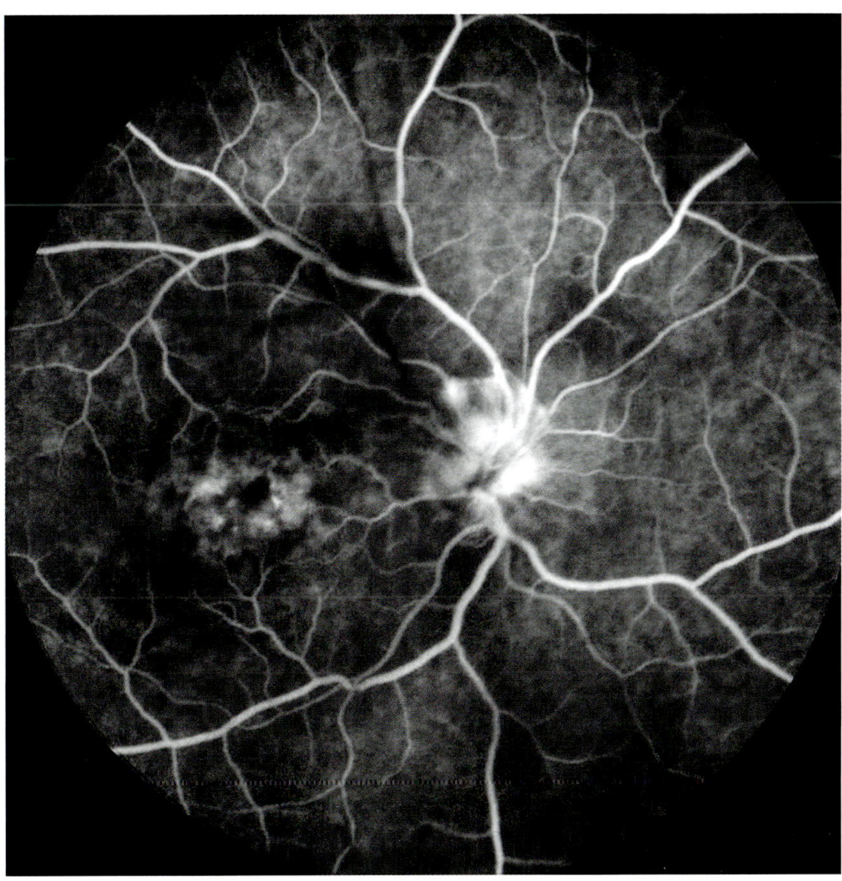

Figure 1: Angiography in Irvine-Gass syndrome. Macular and optic nerve head staining and pooling expression of inflammation

The mechanical stress can be increased in patients with pathological vitreous-retinal adherences at the posterior pole.

Postoperative CME has a characteristic aspect in optical coherence tomography (OCT). B scan shows a relevant macular thickening associated with absence of the physiological foveal pit. The superficial and nuclear layers of the retina are chiefly compromised. Sometimes a serous neuroepithelium foveal detachment appears **(Figure 2A)**.[4,5]

The analysis of vitreoretinal interface can show thin folds (more evident in horizontal scans) and hypertrophy of the internal limiting membrane (ILM) may be present. Inner nuclear layer shows pseudocysts appearing as an optically empty space that is square-shaped. These cystoid spaces tend to be smaller peripherally and larger centrally **(Figure 2B)**.

The outer nuclear layer is more affected by inflammation with large and drop-shaped cavities with the apex directed toward fovea. Their aspect follows the distribution of the Henle's fibers which radiate away from the foveal pit. The rapid onset edema can cause an optically empty detachment

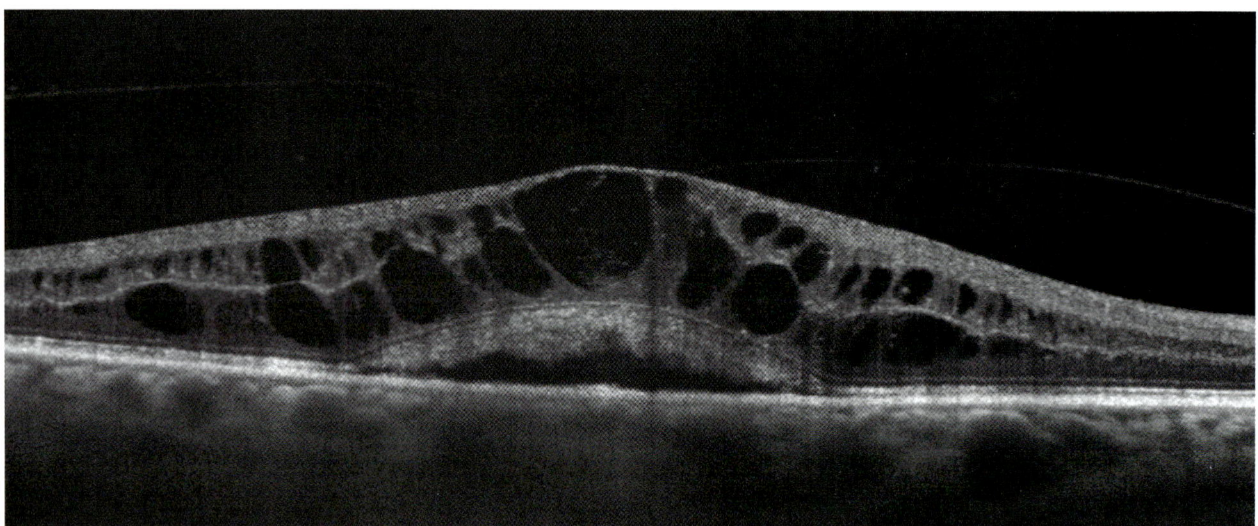

Figure 2A: OCT B scan of an Irvine-Gass syndrome case. Both nuclear layers are affected by cystoid edema. A serous foveal neuroepithelium detachment appears when the edema stimulus strenght is high (Optovue, RTVue)

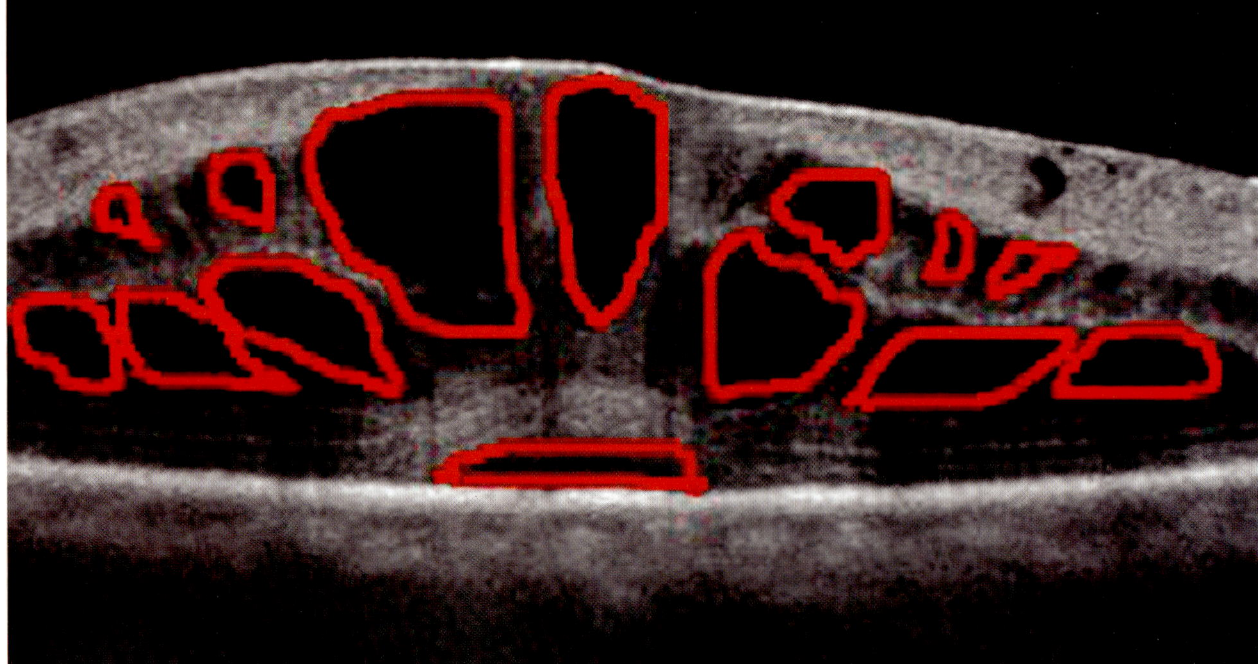

Figure 2B: Pseudocystoid cells shape in the inner and outer nuclear layer. Cystoid cells are square shaped in the inner nuclear layer, drop shape in the outer nuclear layer (Optovue, RTVue)

of the sensory retina in the macula associated with thickening of the outer segments of photoreceptors **(Figure 2A)**.[6]

The *en face* study of postoperative CME requires three different approaches:

- First, the evaluation of vitreoretinal interface by a scan thinner than 20 microns could show the macular thickening characterized by perimacular folds and ILM retraction causing vitreoretinal traction **(Figure 3A)**. These phenomena are more evident in patients with long-lasting edema **(Figure 3B)**.
- Second, the evaluation of the inner nuclear layer is performed by ILM parallel scans due to the parallelism of these layers in CME. The recommended cut thickness ranges in between 20 microns and 25 microns according to the pseudocyst dimensions. These rounded irregular cavities have a sponge-like aspect with thick septa **(Figure 4)**.
- Third, the evaluation of the outer nuclear layer is performed by RPE adapted scans, up to 30 microns of thickness. The edematous cavities have an orange slice aspect with very thin and long septa. The length of the cavities is proportional to the foveal distance because they follow Henle's fibers pathway (vertical in the fovea and horizontal peripherally). The edema severity in the outer nuclear layer is usually greater than the one observed in the inner nuclear layer **(Figure 5A)**.

The possible presence of a sensory retinal detachment could appear as a ring with thickened, irregular and hyper-reflective edges, optically empty, fovea-centered **(Figure 5B)**.

When diagnosis is developed early and treatment starts properly, the OCT shows frequent *restitutio ad integrum* **(Figures 6A to C)**.[7,8] When there is a significative edema and in the cases of vitreous adherence, ILM *en face* analysis can show several folds and retractions **(Figure 7)**.

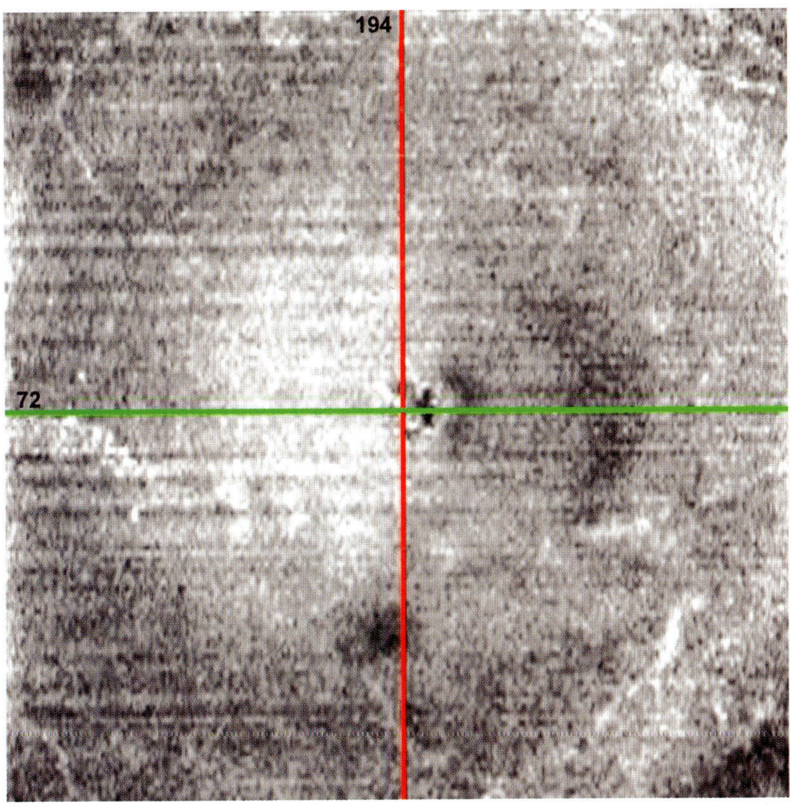

Figure 3A: Surface *en face* section performed by ILM parallel scan. This scan shows all surface alterations due to macula thickening (Optovue, RTVue)

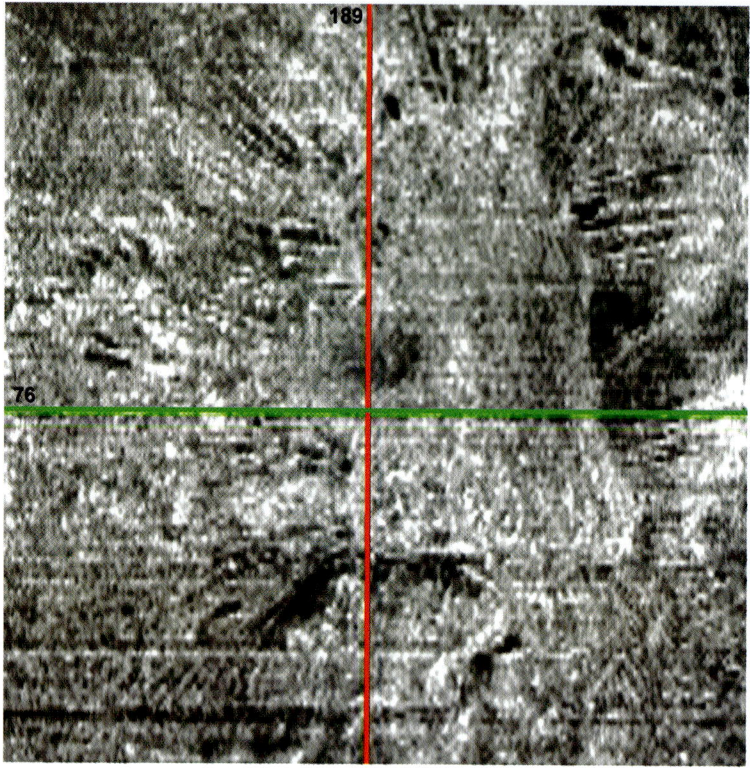

Figure 3B: Surface *en face* section on long lasting CME in Irvine-Gass syndrome. We can appreciate some vitreoretinal plaques and relative retinal folds (Optovue, RTVue)

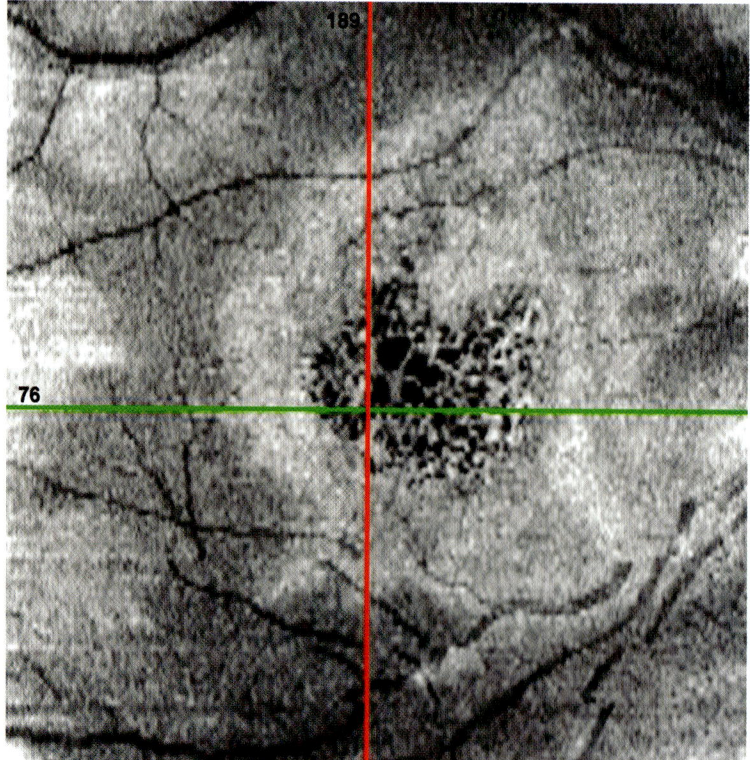

Figure 4: Pseudocystic cavities in the inner nuclear layer appear on *en face* view rounded, sponge like, regular, optically empty. Septa are thicker than the outer nuclear layer (Optovue, RTVue)

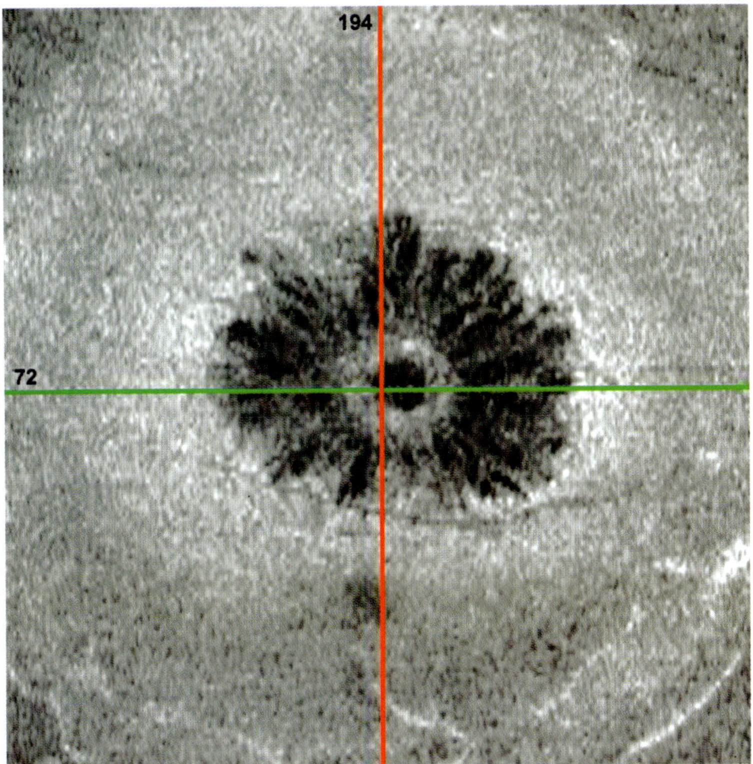

Figure 5A: Pseudocystic cavities in the outer nuclear layers appear drop shaped, with thin and stretched out septa. Their distribution is centered on the fovea (Optovue, RTVue)

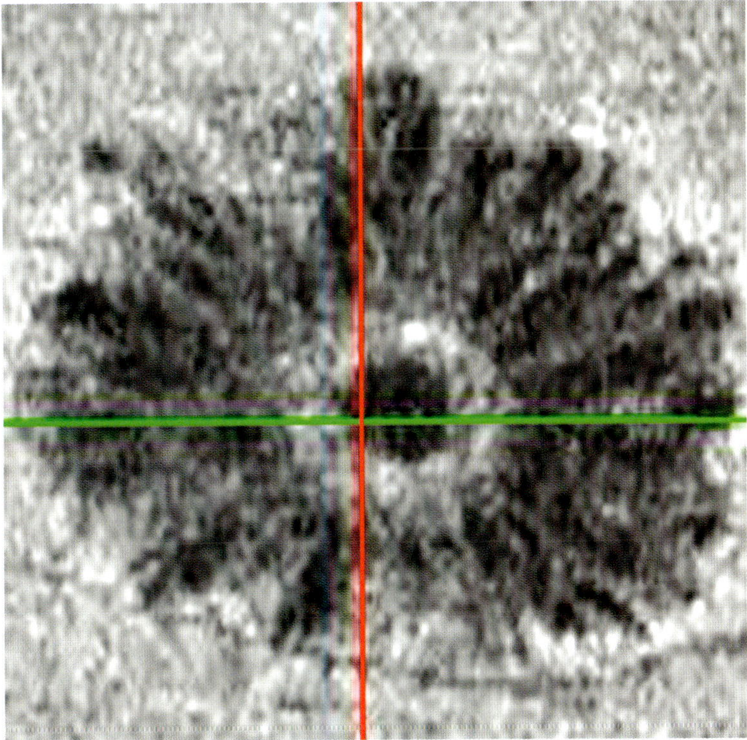

Figure 5B: *En face* view of the serous foveal detachment. The detachment appears like a ring on a section parallel to RPE centered on the fovea. Walls are thick, irregular and the contents optically empty (Optovue, RTVue)

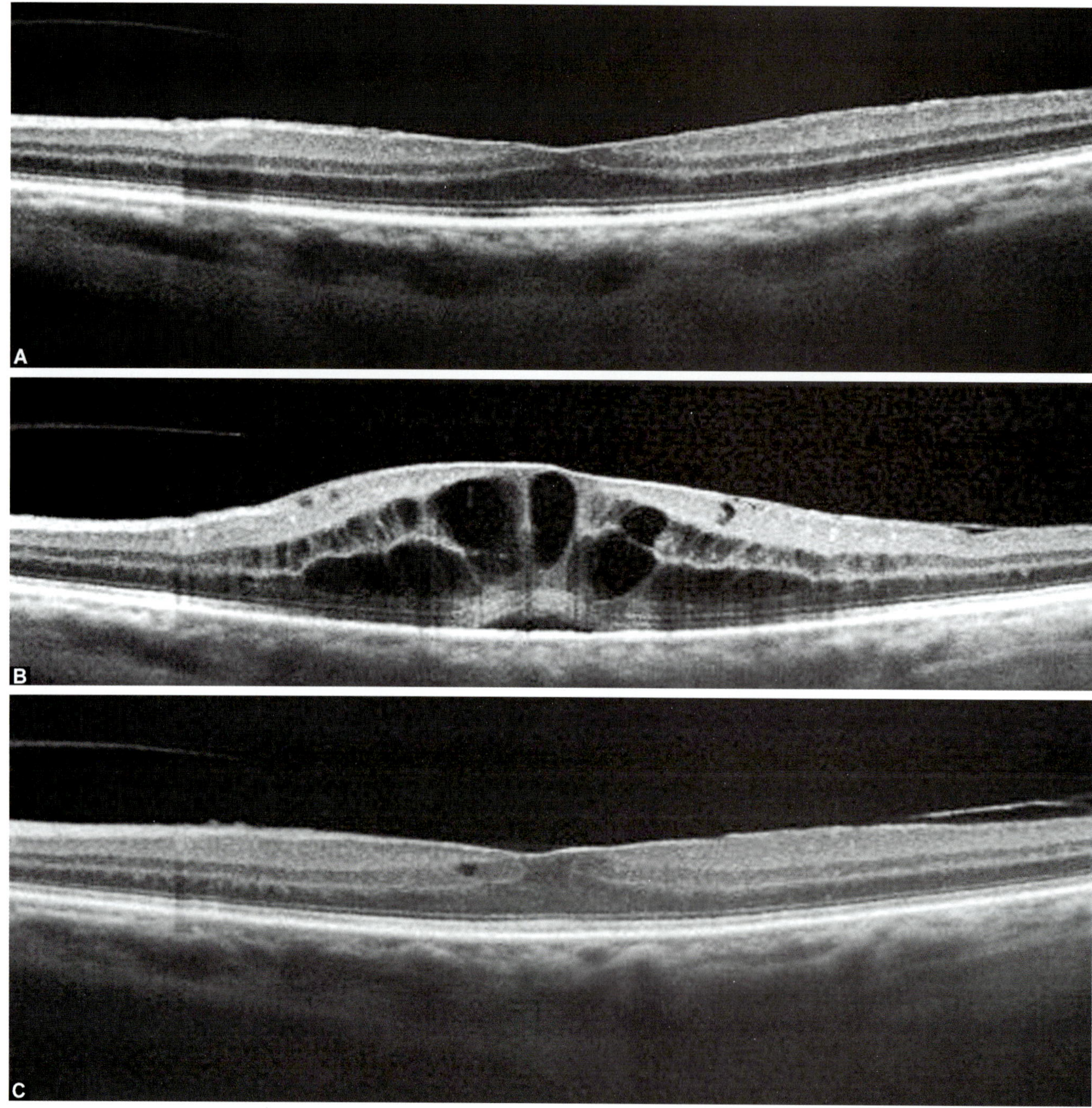

Figures 6A to C: B scan evolution of an Irvine-Gass syndrome. Before surgery, after one week and four weeks after treatment with local FANS and systemic steroids (Optovue, RTVue)

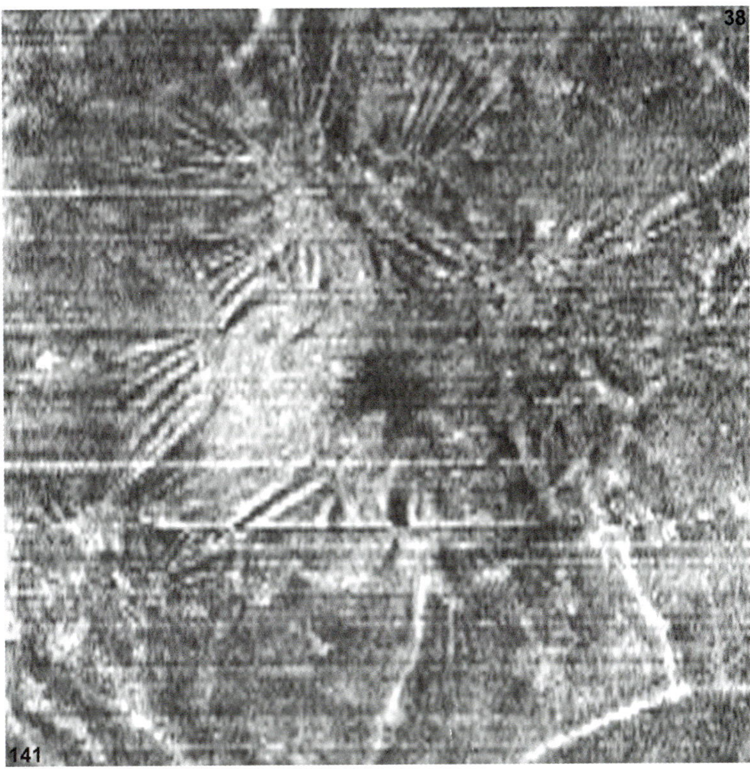

Figure 7: *En face* internal limiting membrane adapted scan on chronic postsurgical cystoid macular edema. Internal limiting membrane shows some perimacular retractions, probably due to chronic inflammation (Optovue, RTVue)

References

1. Minnella AM, Savastano MC, Zinzanella G, et al. Spectral-domain optical coherence tomography in Irvine-Gass syndrome. Retina. 2012;32(3):581-7.
2. Scarpa G. Bilateral cystoid macular edema after cataract surgery resolved by vitrectomy. Eur J Ophthalmol. 2011; 21(5):677-9.
3. Metge P, Bonnefoy-Mandirac C, Chauvet G. Hemato-aqueous barrier and the Irvine-Gass syndrome. Bull Soc Ophtalmol Fr. 1983;83(1):145-8.
4. Katsimpris JM, Petropoulos IK, Zoukas G, et al. Central foveal thickness before and after cataract surgery in normal and in diabetic patients without retinopathy. Klin Monbl Augenheilkd. 2012;229(4):331-7.
5. Kusbeci T, Eryigit L, Yavas G, et al. Evaluation of cystoid macular edema using optical coherence tomography and fundus fluorescein angiography after uncomplicated phacoemulsification surgery. Curr Eye Res. 2012;37(4): 327-33.
6. Haut J, Larricart P, Van Effenterre G, et al. Physiopathology of the Irvine-Gass syndrome and the role of posterior detachment of the vitreous body. Apropos of 2 cases. Bull Soc Ophtalmol Fr. 1984;84(3):243-4.
7. Randazzo A, Vinciguerra P. Chronic macular edema medical treatment in Irvine-Gass syndrome: case report. Eur J Ophthalmol. 2010;20(2):462-5.
8. Boulanger G, Weber M. Irvine-Gass syndrome and central serous chorioretinopathy, pure coincidence or non-fortuitous association? Report of three cases. J Fr Ophtalmol. 2009;32(8):566-71.

chapter 11

Macular Retinoschisis

Bruno Lumbroso, Marco Rispoli

Introduction

Optical coherence tomography (OCT) *en face* scans show that the radial structure of Henle fibers and Müller cells are basic in shaping the pattern of macular retinoschisis cavities.

Juvenile Macular Retinoschisis

Juvenile X-linked macular retinoschisis is a bilateral evolutive hereditary maculopathy, seen in young patients. Diagnosis is generally made at the age of 12–15 years. Clinically, slit lamp examination shows stellate spoke-like cystic maculopathy and sometimes atrophic foveal lesion in some eyes.

Optical coherence tomography cross-sections show cavities and slits splitting the inner nuclear layer and less frequently the outer plexiform layer in some patients. Schisis cavities on cross-section scans are always more regular and uniform than cystoid edema cells that tend to be irregular and asymmetrical. Frequently schisis cells are not only present at the macula but there are also latent peripheral areas of retinoschisis. Small cysts can be seen in the outer nuclear layer and in the ganglion cell layer.

Optical coherence tomography *en face* scans' typical retinoschisis images are very different from cystoid edema cells; their pattern is not flower-shaped but wheel-shaped. At the fovea cavities, they are star-shaped or wheel-shaped, following the radial structure of Henle fibers and Müller cells.[1] *En face* OCT shows areas of stereotyped, harmonious, regular, uniform cystoid cells corresponding to schisis cavities in the inner and outer nuclear layer and in the inner plexiform layer. Around the fovea and on midperiphery cavity walls form parallel harmonious curves centering the fovea. These lesions are symmetrical, and are located in the nuclear and in the inner plexiform layers. *En face* OCT allows differential diagnosis between cystoid macular edema and juvenile retinoschisis (**Figures 1 to 3**).[2,3]

Other Macular and Retinal Retinoschisis

En face and cross-section OCT scans are very helpful in the diagnosis of other forms of schisis such as peripheral retinoschisis of the adult, Goldmann-Favre vitreo-tapetoretinal degeneration, retinoschisis secondary to traction, impending hole, Wagner vitreoretinopathy and optic pit.

In the Goldmann-Favre vitreo-tapetoretinal degeneration OCT, cross-sections show cells and slits splitting the outer nuclear layer, and the outer plexiform layer. Schisis cavities appear regular and uniform; more so than the cystoid edema cells that are irregular and asymmetrical. In Goldmann-Favre, patients' OCT shows schisis cavities around the macula and midperiphery, and there are peripheral areas of retinoschisis also (**Figures 4 and 5**).

In eyes with optic pit it is very frequent to see areas of retinoschisis around the fovea and between fovea and optic disk. OCT cross-sections show cells and slits generally splitting the outer nuclear layer.

Macular Schisis in Myopia

Adult macular schisis is not unique to myopia but it is in the high myopia that this condition is most frequently seen. Schisis features in myopia differ completely from juvenile schisis features. Ocular elongation, myopic staphyloma and epimacular membrane traction are the main factors in retinal splitting in myopia. In more advanced cases, the schisis may fill the posterior staphyloma giving the appearance of a posterior pole retinal detachment. Retinal thickness is sometimes very increased.

The OCT will easily detect a complex intraretinal splitting. The retinal tissue is delaminated in strips and strands, forming with each other angles of not more than 10 degrees. The various layers separate from each other, while still preserving some connections. Acute angles are formed by the retinal layers at the delamination points. The delamination of the

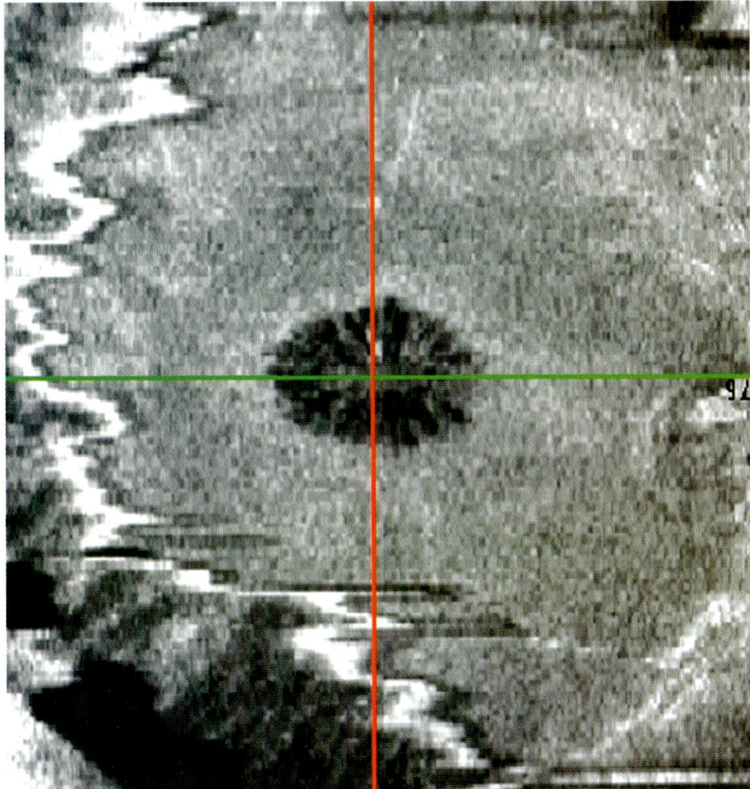

Figure 1: Early juvenile X-linked retinoschisis. On *en face* scans typical retinoschisis optical coherence tomography images show star-shaped or wheel-shaped, elongated cavities following the radial structure of Henle fibers and Müller cells

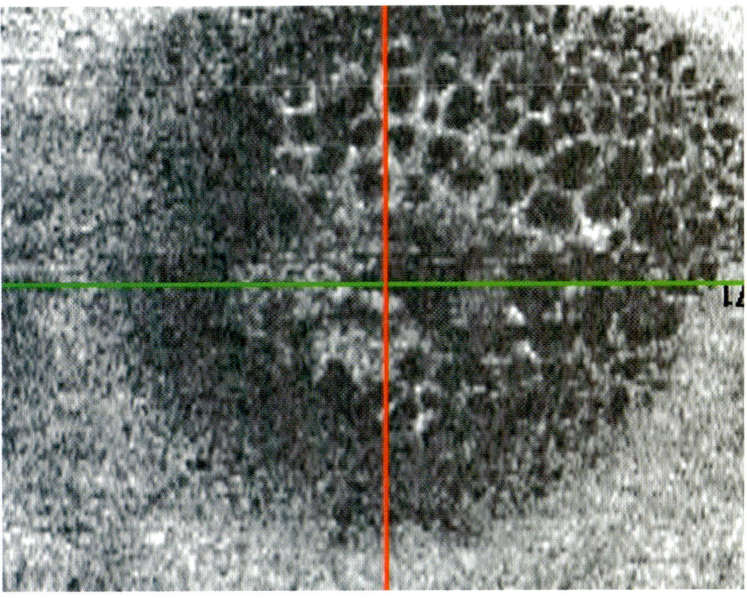

Figure 2: Advanced juvenile X-linked retinoschisis *en face* scan. *En face* optical coherence tomography (OCT) shows areas of harmonious, regular, uniform cystoid cells corresponding to schisis cavities in the inner and outer nuclear layer. *En face* OCT scans help in the differential diagnosis between cystoid macular edema and juvenile X-linked retinoschisis

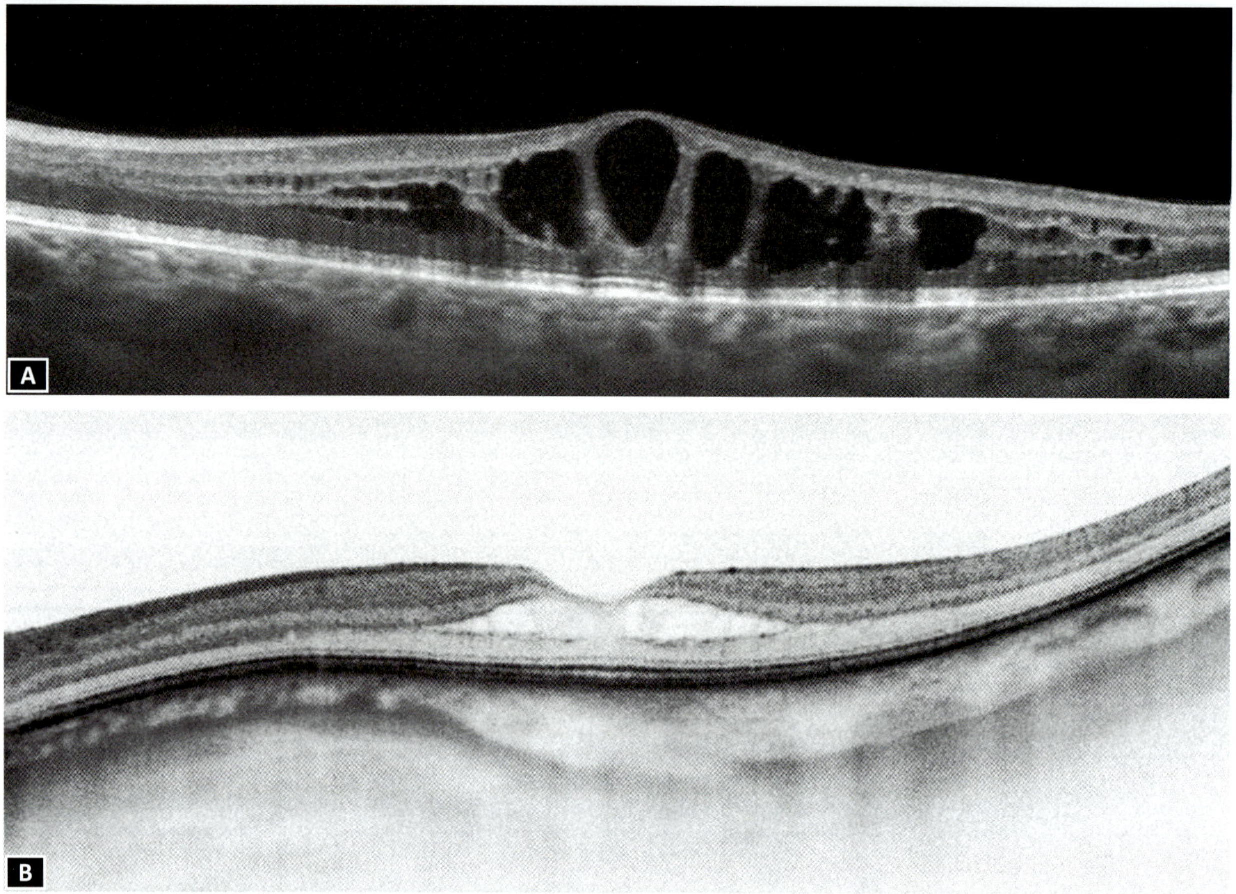

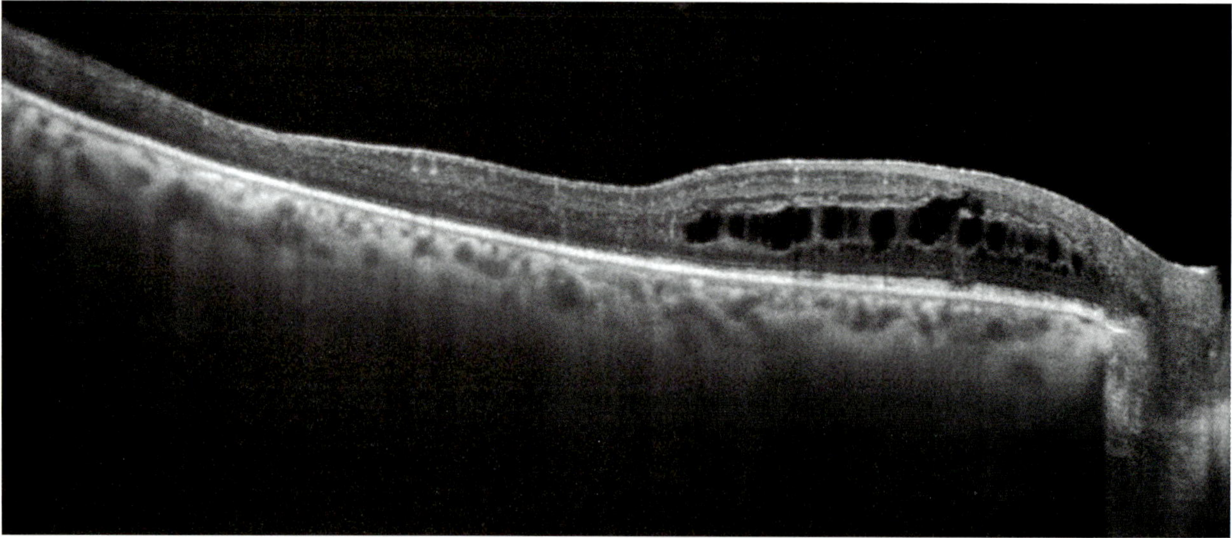

Figures 3A and B: Juvenile X-linked retinoschisis cross-section scan. Optical coherence tomography (OCT) cross-sections show cavities and slits splitting mainly the inner nuclear layer, but also the outer plexiform layer. Schisis cavities on cross-section scans are always more regular and uniform than cystoid edema cells that tend to be irregular and asymmetrical. OCT reveals that schisis cells are not present only at the macula but there are latent peripheral areas of retinoschisis. Small cysts, can be seen in the outer nuclear layer and in the ganglion cells

Figure 4: Advanced Goldmann-Favre retinoschisis cross-section scans. In the Goldmann-Favre vitreo-tapetoretinal degeneration optical coherence tomography cross-sections show cells and slits splitting the outer nuclear layer, and the outer plexiform layer. Schisis cavities on cross-section scans appear regular and uniform; more so than the cystoid edema cells that are irregular and asymmetrical

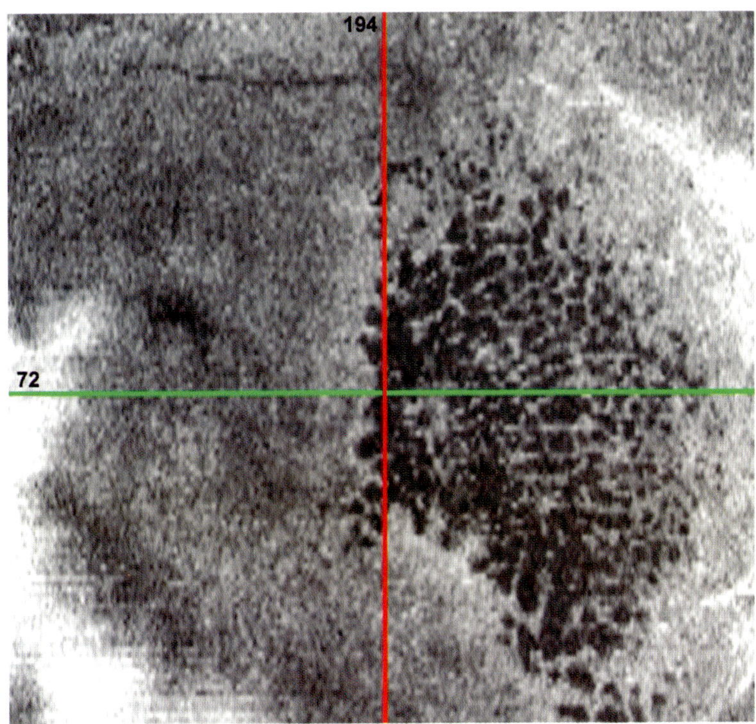

Figure 5: Advanced Goldmann-Favre retinoschisis *en face* scans. In Goldmann-Favre patients *en face* optical coherence tomography (OCT) reveals that schisis cells are present around the macula and midperiphery and that there are also peripheral areas of retinoschisis. Around the fovea and on midperiphery cavity walls form parallel harmonious curves centring the fovea. *En face* OCT shows areas of harmonious, regular, uniform cystoid cells corresponding to schisis cavities in the inner and outer nuclear layer and in the inner plexiform

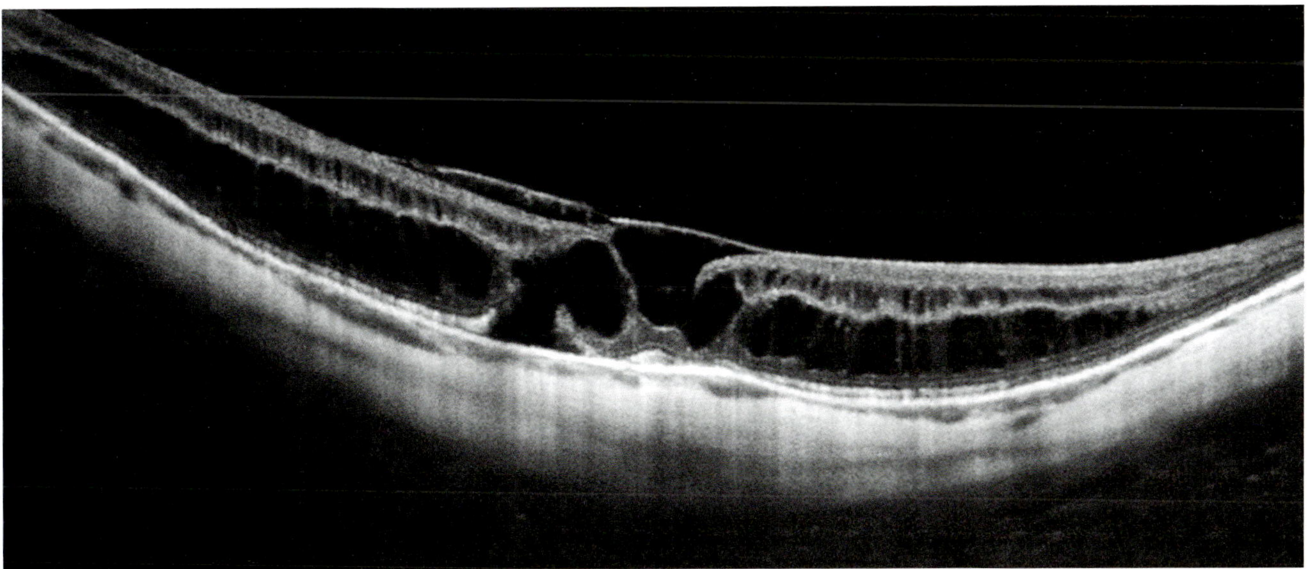

Figure 6A: Myopic retinoschisis: Cross-section scan

retinal layers usually occurs first at the level of the outer plexiform layer. The retinal layers are thin and regular.[4-7]

The aspect is very different from juvenile schisis edema or retinal detachments as the angle formed between the separated retinal layers are regular.

In some other cases of acute onset schisis two retinal layers may move abruptly away from each other remaining connected by regular parallel strands.

The myopic macular schisis can be very stable and show no evolution for a long time (more than a few years).

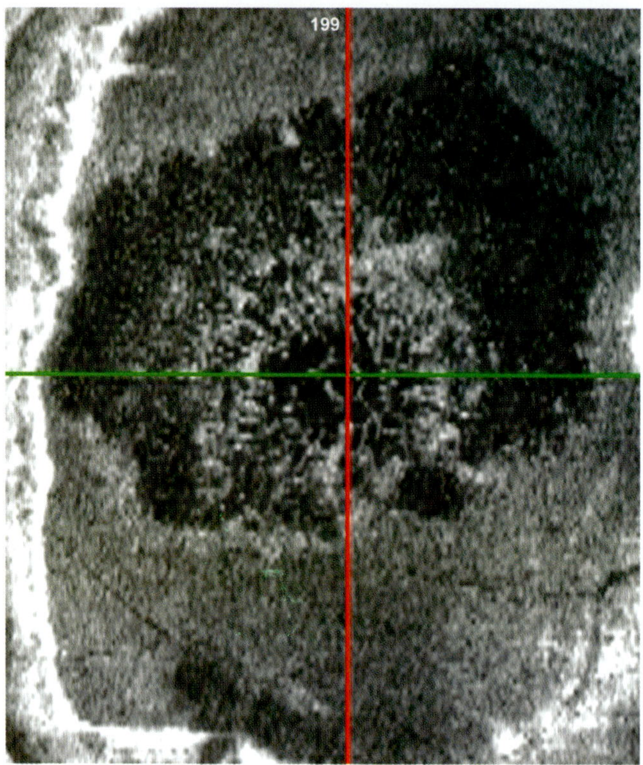

Figure 6B: Myopic retinoschisis: *En face* scan

Figures 6A and B: (A) Macular schisis in myopia, cross-section scan. The aspect is very different from juvenile schisis edema or retinal detachments. The angles formed between split retinal layers are regular. In some cases two retinal layers split abruptly away and distance from each other remaining connected by regular parallel strands; (B) Macular schisis in myopia, *en face* scans. The angles formed between split retinal layers are regular

Posterior pole retinoschisis can often lead to macular lamellar hole formation and vision loss. Macular detachment can happen with or without retinal hole (**Figures 6A and B**).[7-11]

References

1. Gregori NZ, Berrocal AM, Gregori G, et al. Macular spectral-domain optical coherence tomography in patients with X-linked retinoschisis. Br J Ophthalmol. 2009;93(3): 373-8.
2. Hayashi T, Omoto S, Takeuchi T, et al. Four Japanese male patients with juvenile retinoschisis; only three have mutations in the RS1 gene. Am J Ophthalmol. 2004;138 (5):788-98.
3. Mooy CM, Van Den Born LI, Baarsma S, et al. Hereditary X-linked juvenile retinoschisis: a review of the role of Müller cells. Arch Ophthalmol. 2002;120(7):979-84.
4. Forte R, Cennamo G, Pascotto F, et al. *En face* optical coherence tomography of the posterior pole in high myopia. Am J Ophthalmol. 2008;145(2):281-8.
5. Shimada N, Ohno-Matsui K, Baba T, et al. Natural course of macular retinoschisis in highly myopic eyes without macular hole or retinal detachment. Am J Ophthalmol. 2006;142(3):497-500.
6. Benhamou N, Massin P, Haouchine B, et al. Macular retinoschisis in highly myopic eyes. Am J Ophthalmol. 2002;133(6):794-800.
7. Forte R, Manzi G, Gallo O, et al. Three-dimensional visualization of vitreoretinal abnormalities in high myopia. Ophthalmic Surg Lasers Imaging. 2009;40(3):304-7.
8. Tammewar AM, Bartsch DU, Kozak I, et al. Imaging vitreomacular interface abnormalities in the coronal plane by simultaneous combined scanning laser and optical coherence tomography. Br J Ophthalmol. 2009;93(3):366-72.
9. Baba T, Ohno-Matsui K, Futagami S, et al. Prevalence and characteristics of foveal retinal detachment without macular hole in high myopia. Am J Ophthalmol. 2003;135(3):338-42.
10. Wu PC, Chen YJ, Chen YH, et al. Factors associated with foveoschisis and foveal detachment without macular hole in high myopia. Eye (Lond). 2009;23(2):356-61.
11. Ripandelli G, Coppé AM, Parisi V, et al. Fellow eye findings of highly myopic subjects operated for retinal detachment associated with a macular hole. Ophthalmology. 2008;115(9):1489-93.

chapter 12

Outer Retinal Tubulations

Benjamin Wolff, Alexandre Matet, Vivien Vasseur
José-Alain Sahel, Martine Mauget-Faÿsse

Introduction

Outer retinal tubulations (ORTs) have recently been identified in age-related macular degeneration (AMD) thanks to technological improvements in spectral domain optical coherence tomography (SD-OCT).[1] They usually have a characteristic presentation and thus can be easily diagnosed. They are frequently observed in AMD (56% of exudative and 21% of atrophic forms).[2] It is of clinical significance to recognize them since they do not indicate ongoing exudative process and, therefore, do not require treatment. ORTs have also been observed in other degenerative retinal diseases, including Bietti's crystalline dystrophy[3] and Best's disease.

Methods of Acquisition

The following description of *en face* OCT imaging of ORT was obtained with SD-OCT (Spectralis® Heidelberg Engineering, Heidelberg, Germany).

Outer retinal tubulations on B scan OCT, are round hyporeflective lesions which may contain a few focal hyper-reflective spots and are always delineated by an hyper-reflective ring, in contrast to the wholly hyporeflective retinal cystoid lesions. They are always located at the level of the outer nuclear layer and in AMD are classically found very close to areas of neovascular fibrosis or retinal atrophy **(Figure 1)**. These lesions have been named "tubulations" because they exhibit a tubular morphology when observed in frontal sections using *en face* OCT scans (C scan). *En face* SD-OCT is very useful in evaluating the extent of structural damage observed in cases of ORT.

Outer Retinal Tubulation Patterns

Outer retinal tubulations exhibit two main patterns according to their location, either above a fibrovascular scar or next to an area of retinal atrophy **(Table 1 and Figure 2)**.

Table 1: Outer retinal tubulations pattern

Location	Pattern
Fibrotic scar	Pseudodendritic pattern
Geographic atrophy	Perilesional pattern

Outer Retinal Tubulation Pattern Above a Fibrovascular Scar

The most frequent finding is a branching network emanating from a fibrovascular scar with numerous ramifications (or digitations) resulting in a pseudodendritic pattern **(Figure 3A)**. The fibrotic neovascular choroidal network is identified as a hyper-reflective lesion above the level of the retinal pigment epithelium. Associated intraretinal cystoid cavities related to neovascular reactivation or the progression of retinal degeneration may be observed **(Figure 3B)**.

Outer Retinal Tubulation Pattern in Cases of Geographic Atrophy

Outer retinal tubulation have a perilesional pattern stretched along the margins of the chorioretinal atrophic area. Autofluorescence imaging usually demonstrates that ORT does not extend beyond the hyper-reflective border of the atrophic area. Invaginations of ORT inside the atrophic zone may be observed.

The observation of ORT, using *en face* OCT, indicates the size of these lesions inside the retina **(Figure 4)**. The combination of SD-OCT B scan with *en face* OCT enhances its sensitivity, allowing earlier diagnosis and more reliable follow-up. This technique also improves the distinction between ORT and their main differential diagnoses; cystoid cavities and forms of serous retinal detachments **(Figure 5)**.

Physiopathogenic mechanisms leading to ORT remain poorly understood. According to Zweifel et al,[1] these lesions

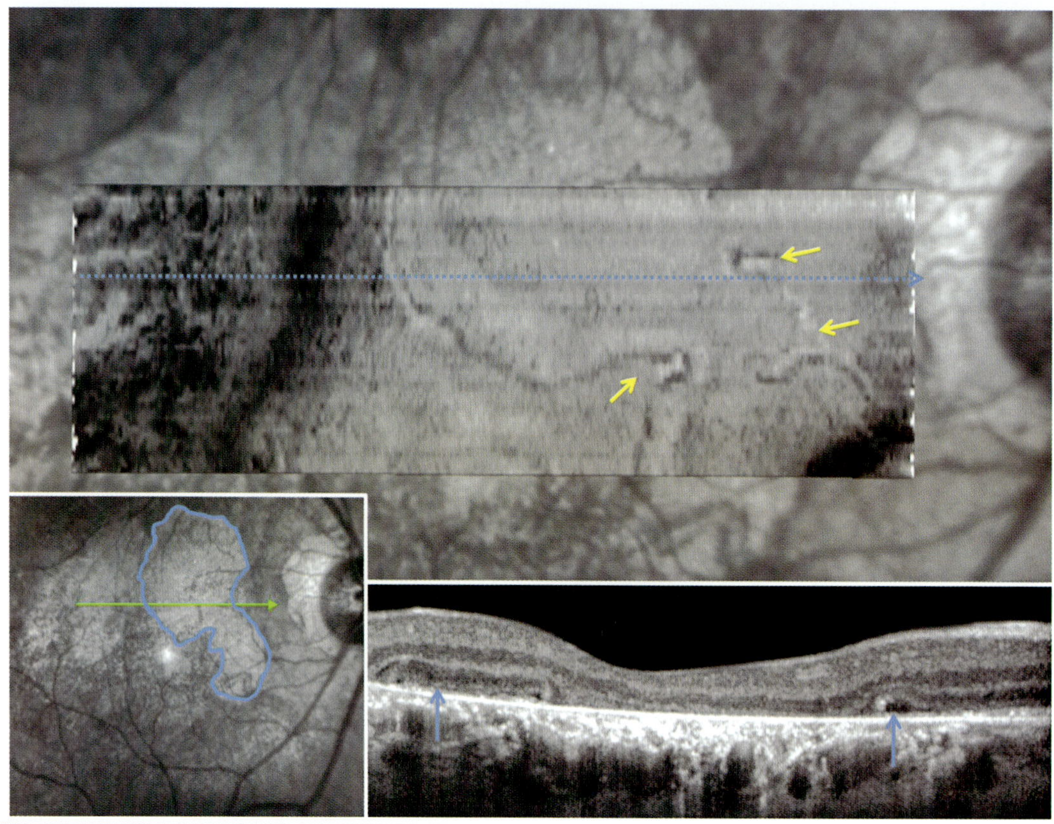

Figure 1: Perilesional pattern of outer retinal tubulations along the margins of an atrophic area. Digitations of the tubular network inside the atrophic area are visible (yellow arrows). Blue arrows represent outer retinal tubulations on B scan

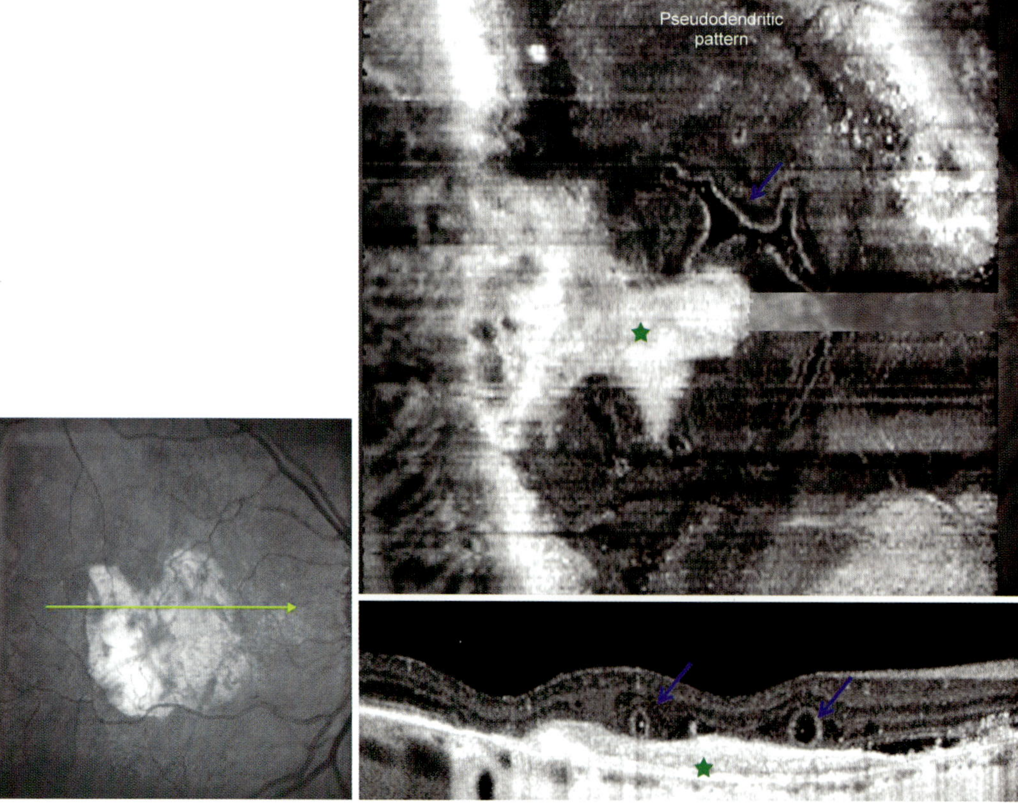

Figure 2: Outer retinal tubulations (blue arrows) with pseudodendritic pattern surrounding a subretinal fibrotic scar (green star)

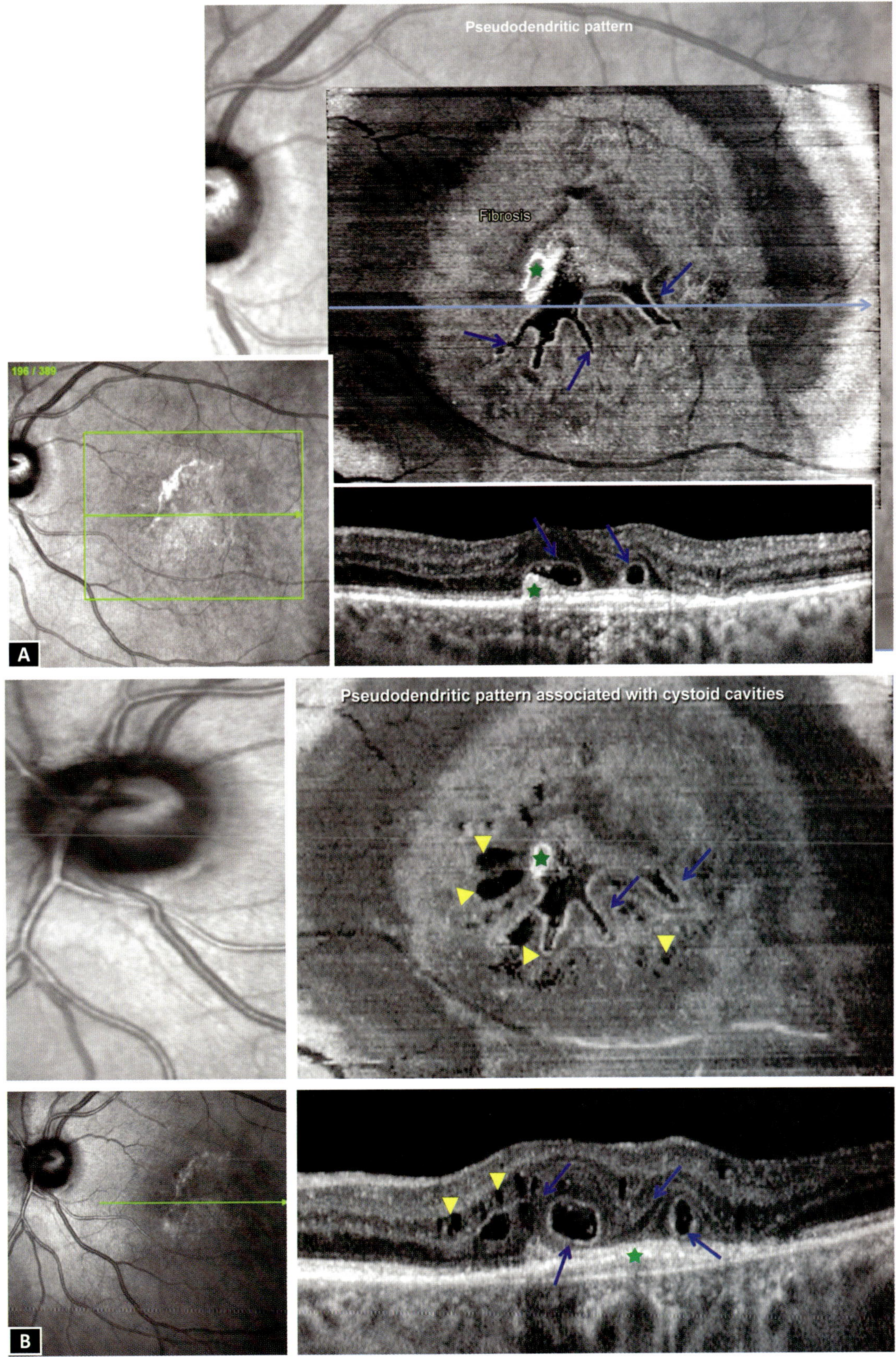

Figures 3A and B: (A) Pseudodendritic pattern of outer retinal tubulations (blue arrows) next to a hyper-reflective fibrotic scar (green star); (B) During follow-up, recurrent exudation was observed. *En face* optical coherence tomography evidenced hyporeflective intraretinal cystoid cavities without hyper-reflective border (yellow arrow heads), close to the tubular pseudodendritic lesion

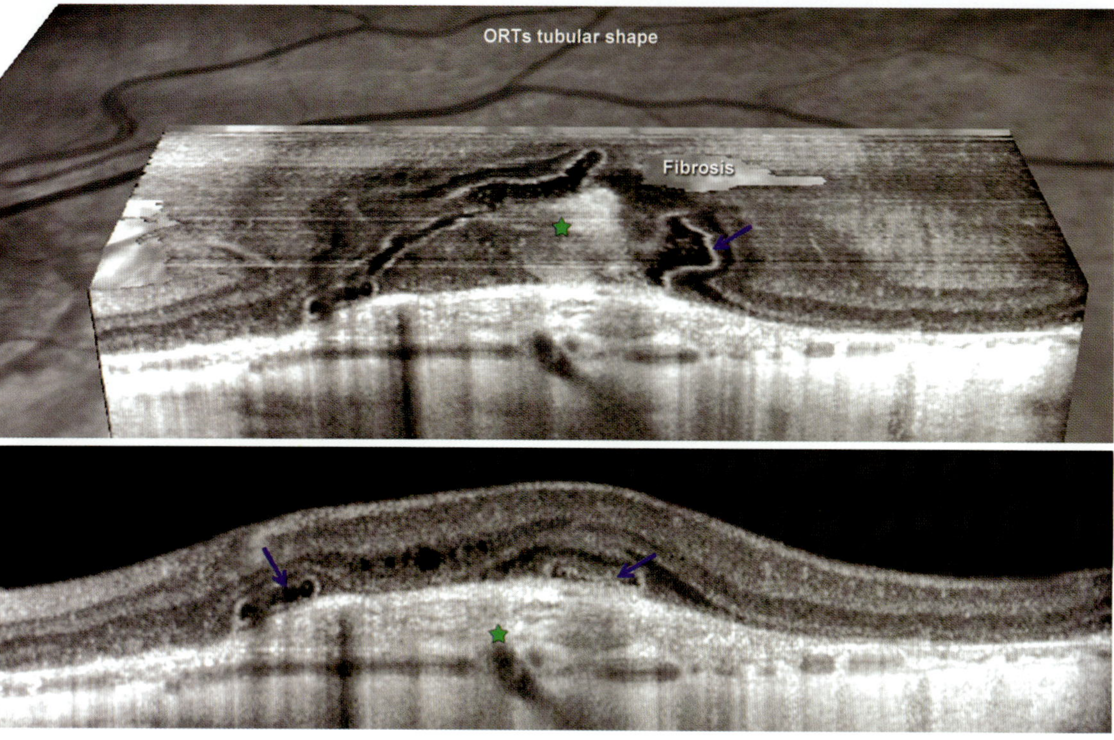

Figure 4: Typical tubular intraretinal lesion (blue arrows) extending deeply into the external retina next to a subretinal fibrotic scar (green star)

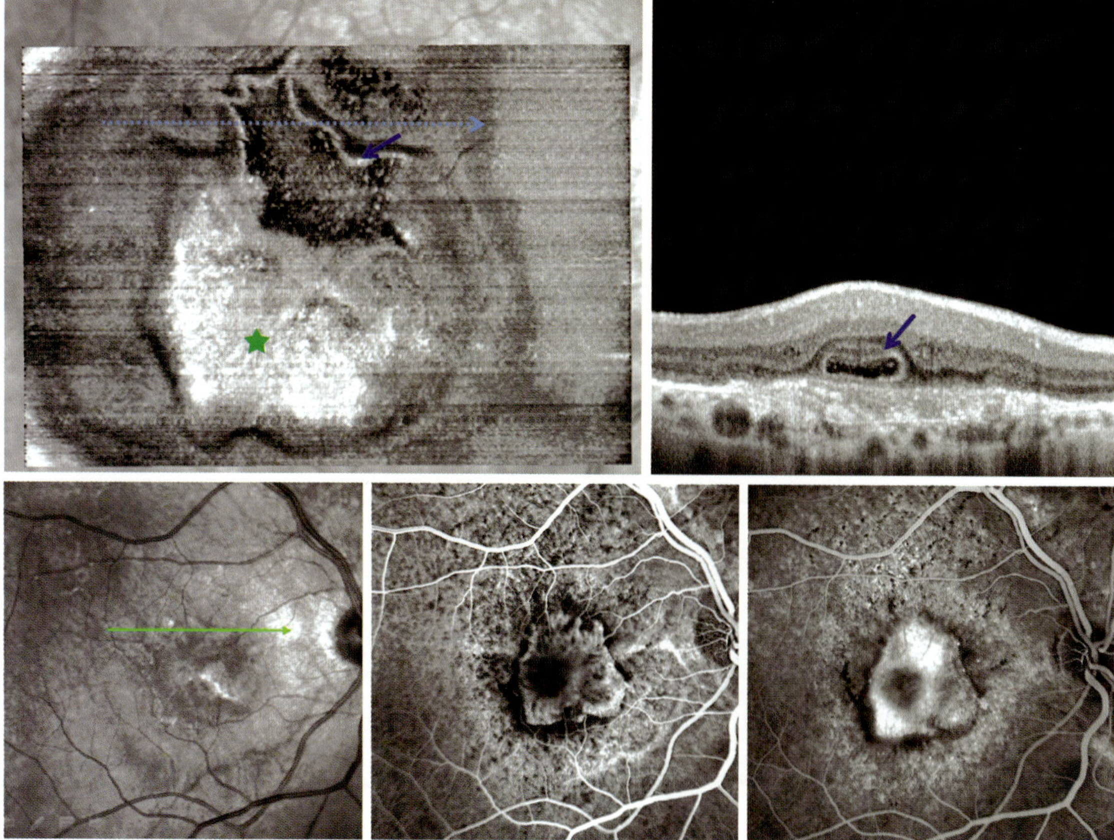

Figure 5: Giant outer retinal tubulations (blue arrows) mimicking serous retinal detachment. The pseudodendritic pattern and the hyper-reflective border lead to the diagnosis of outer retinal tubulations next to a hyper-reflective fibrotic scar (green star)

may result from the outward folding of the photoreceptor layer. Tissue damage associated with retinal degeneration may produce a loss of interdigitations of the photoreceptors with the retinal pigmentary epithelium, and a disruption of tight junctions between the outer segments and adjacent glial elements. Upon repeated microscopic injury, the photoreceptor layer may fold into tubular structures limited to the outer retina. This type of degeneration has been histologically described under the term "rosette formations" in retinitis pigmentosa.[4]

Conclusion

In conclusion, *en face* OCT has allowed the characterization of the two main subtypes of tubular formations in AMD— pseudodendritic forms that develop next to fibrotic scars and perilesional forms that develop in the periphery of atrophic areas.

References

1. Zweifel SA, Engelbert M, Laud K, et al. Outer retinal tubulation: a novel optical coherence tomography finding. Arch Ophthalmol. 2009;127:1596-602.
2. Wolff B, Maftouhi MQ, Mateo-Montoya A, et al. Outer retinal cysts in age-related macular degeneration. Acta Ophthalmol. 2011;89:496-9.
3. Yannuzi LA. Hereditary chorioretinal dystrophy. The Retinal Atlas. Elsevier; 2010. pp.158-60.
4. Wolter JR. A case of advanced retinitis pigmentosa with rosette-shaped formations on the retina. Klin Monbl Augenheilkd Augenarztl Fortbild. 1955;127:687-94.

chapter 13

Localized Lesions of Outer Retina Layers

Bruno Lumbroso, Marco Rispoli

Introduction

In some cases of localized disruption of the photoreceptors and of limited lesions of the junction between inner and outer segment of the photoreceptors cross-section scans and *en face* optical coherence tomography (OCT) scans show very dark areas simulating cavities.

En face OCT scans adapted to the concavity of the posterior pole and passing exactly through the level of the junction between inner and outer segment of the photoreceptors normally show only a gray uniform sheet.

In case of localized lesions they allow to exactly pinpoint and map the lesions of the photoreceptors as dark areas. They show the lesion shape, extension, surface and localization. *The study and mapping of photoreceptor lesions constitute one of the major achievements of en face OCT.* These limited dark areas are not fluid containing cavities but tiny defects of the photoreceptors. OCT reveals limited disorganization of the outer segments.

In cross-section scans the dark areas appear as rectangular, horizontal pseudo-cavities. Their dimensions range from very small, to small, to medium. They are located in outer retina close to pigment epithelium at the junction between inner and outer segment of the photoreceptors. Their limits are smooth and contents hyporeflective. These lesions are very well seen in *en face* scans passing exactly through the level of the junction between inner and outer segment of the photoreceptors.

En face scans allow us to see if the lesion is single or multiple. Frequently frontal sections show that the lesions are not single but part of a wider disease. Residual tissue can be seen inside the disrupted area.

These defects can be seen in cases of acute retinitis, acute epitheliitis, eclipse (solar) retinopathy, multiple evanescent white dot syndrome (MEWDS), acute zonal occult outer retinopathy and tamoxiphen lesions. Photoreceptors localized lesions frequently simulate an outer retinal cavity and are sometimes denominated *outer lamellar holes* or lesions. They include a wide range of disorders.

White Dot Syndromes

Chorioretinal multifocal inflammations that present scattered multiple choroiditis foci are not infrequent. They include birdshot chorioretinopathy, MEWDS, acute posterior multifocal placoid pigment epitheliopathy, punctate inner choroidopathy, multifocal choroiditis, acute retinal pigment epitheliitis or acute retinitis present more frequently a single focus. Fundus examination shows white dots in the retina. They form a wide chapter of retinal inflammations. Sometimes, serpiginous choroiditis is associated in this group of retinal diseases. Symptoms in all cases include a prodromal flu-like episode, photopsia, scotoma, and decreased and blurred vision.

Multiple evanescent white dot syndrome is a retinal syndrome that usually affects young women and appears a few days after a viral influenza fever. Clinically it is unilateral, multifocal retinitis. Fundus examination shows multiple yellowish or whitish spots of various sizes at the posterior pole out to the midperiphery. Patients report unilateral blurred vision and visual field defects. There is an acute visual loss that varies from minimal to 200/100. The visual fields frequently show enlarged blind spots and scotomas. Some cases are unilateral, some are bilateral. Frequently vitritis is present.

Fluorescein angiography, indocyanine green (ICG) angiography, microperimetry confirm the diagnosis. Generally the episode is followed by complete morphologic and functional recovery, but retinal scars may persist. Multiple evanescent white dot syndrome seems to disrupt the photoreceptor outer segments, as confirmed by OCT scans.

Etiology remains unknown but it could be an autoimmune disease. ICG generally shows scattered hypofluorescent dots.

Optical coherence tomography cross-section scans show one or more areas of disrupted photoreceptors or irregular photoreceptor inner/outer segment junction line of varied extent in all affected eyes and some fellow eyes. Disrupted photoreceptor areas correspond with hypofluorescent areas in the late phase of ICG. Retinal profile is normal; there is no swelling of the retina and no edema. The outer limiting membrane is normal.

After 1–6 months follow-up the vision returns to normal along with resolution of the white dots in all eyes. The inner/outer segment junction line is restored in most eyes, but sometimes some degree of focal disruption persists.

Optical coherence tomography cross scan shows that the alterations at the level of the inner segment/outer segment junction and outer segment of the photoreceptors can persist for some time.

En face OCT scans adapted to the concavity of the posterior pole and passing exactly through the level of the photoreceptors and junction show areas of alteration and give an exact map of the lesions.

These disrupted areas appear as patchy dark areas scattered in the posterior pole. The lesions are more precisely delimited than with ICG angiography. Areas of decreased retinal sensitivity on microperimetry match areas of junction disruption on OCT images[1] (**Figures 1 and 2**).

Solar Retinopathy

Solar (eclipse) lesions are seen after the subject looked directly to the sun, on occasion of an eclipse, or for religious reasons (waiting for saint apparition), or under the influence of drugs.

Optical coherence tomography cross-section scan show rectangular, horizontal, localized lesions of the photoreceptors. Their dimensions vary from very small to small. They are located in the outer retina close to the pigment epithelium. They appear immediately and will last for life. No edema is seen.[2-4]

En face OCT scans adapted to the concavity of the posterior pole and passing exactly through the level of the photoreceptors show small irregular dark areas of alteration, and give an exact map of the lesions. Disrupted photoreceptor patches are sharply delimited. Residual tissue granulations can be seen inside the disrupted area (**Figures 3 and 4**).

Idiopathic Outer Lamellar Defects

Some patients may show outer lamellar defects at the fovea seen as lesions of 50–100 micron in size located at the level of the outer retina showing, on cross-section and *en face* OCT scans, sharp interruption of the inner/outer segments junction of photoreceptors and to the complex retinal pigment epithelium-choriocapillaris. As in solar retinopathy *en face* OCT scans adapted to the concavity of the posterior pole and passing exactly through the level of the photoreceptors show small irregular dark areas of alteration, and give an exact map of the lesions. Disrupted photoreceptor patches are sharply delimited. Residual tissue granulations can be seen inside the disrupted area.

Ocular history does not find episodes of looking at the sun, fluorescein angiography may show window like defects. Autofluorescence may show hypoautofluorescent area patches that are sharply delimited and surrounded by an irregular area of increased fluorescence[4] (**Figures 5 and 6**).

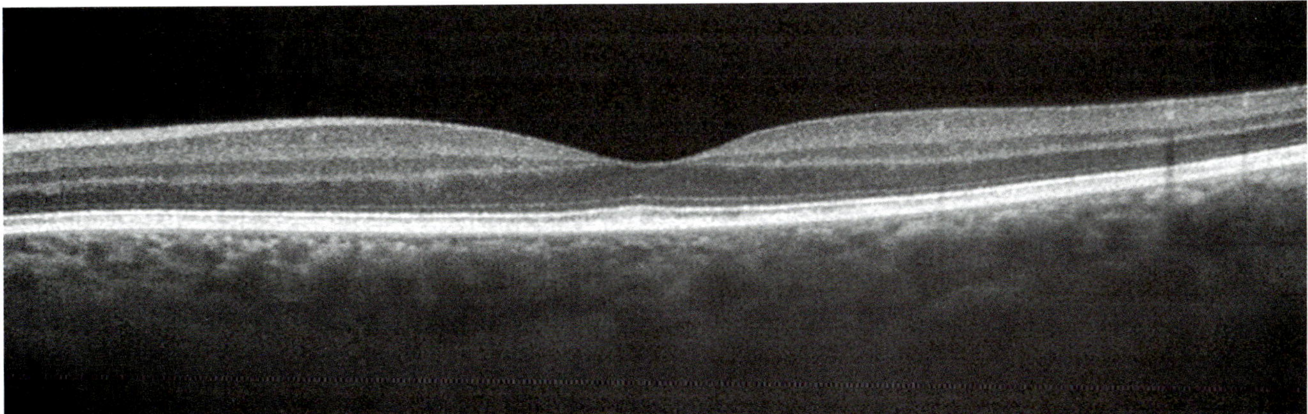

Figure 1: Multiple evanescent white dot syndrome (MEWDS) B scan. Lesions of the photoreceptors appear as localized disruption of the IS/OS junction. Their dimensions range from very small, to small, to medium. They are located in outer retina close to pigment epithelium at the junction between inner and outer segment of the photoreceptors. Walls are smooth and contents hyporeflective (Optovue RTVue)

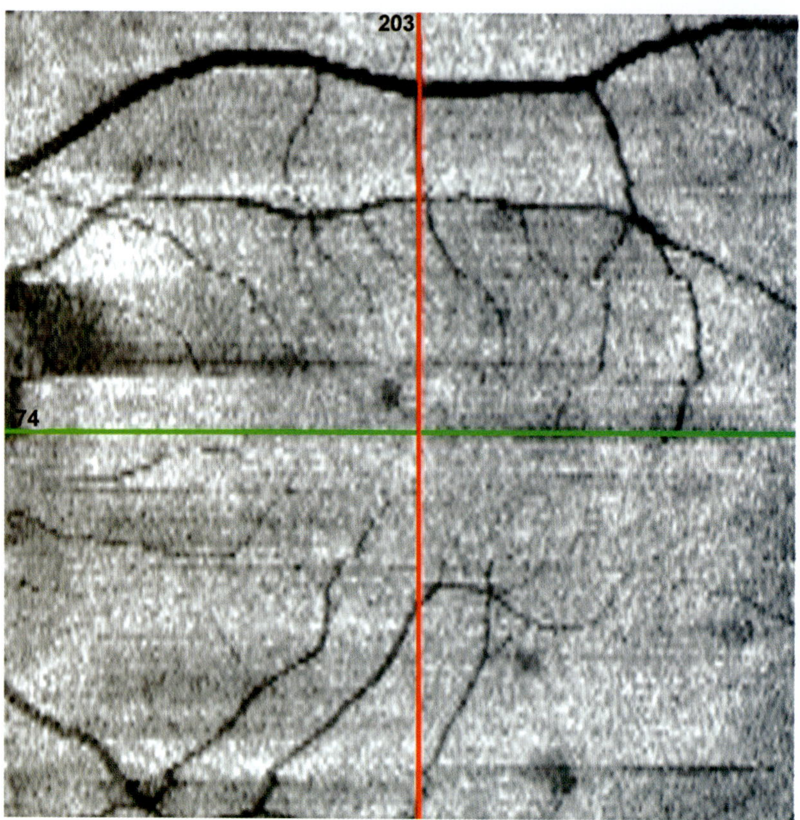

Figure 2: Multiple evanescent white dot syndrome (MEWDS) *en face* scan. Lesion of the photoreceptors simulating a cavity. MEWDS lesions are very well seen in *en face* scans passing exactly through the level of the junction between inner and outer segment of the photoreceptors. They give an exact map of the lesions. These disrupted photoreceptor areas appear as patchy dark areas scattered in the posterior pole. The lesions are more precisely delimited than with indocyanine green angiography. Areas of decreased retinal sensitivity on microperimetry match areas of junction disruption on optical coherence tomography images (Optovue RTVue)

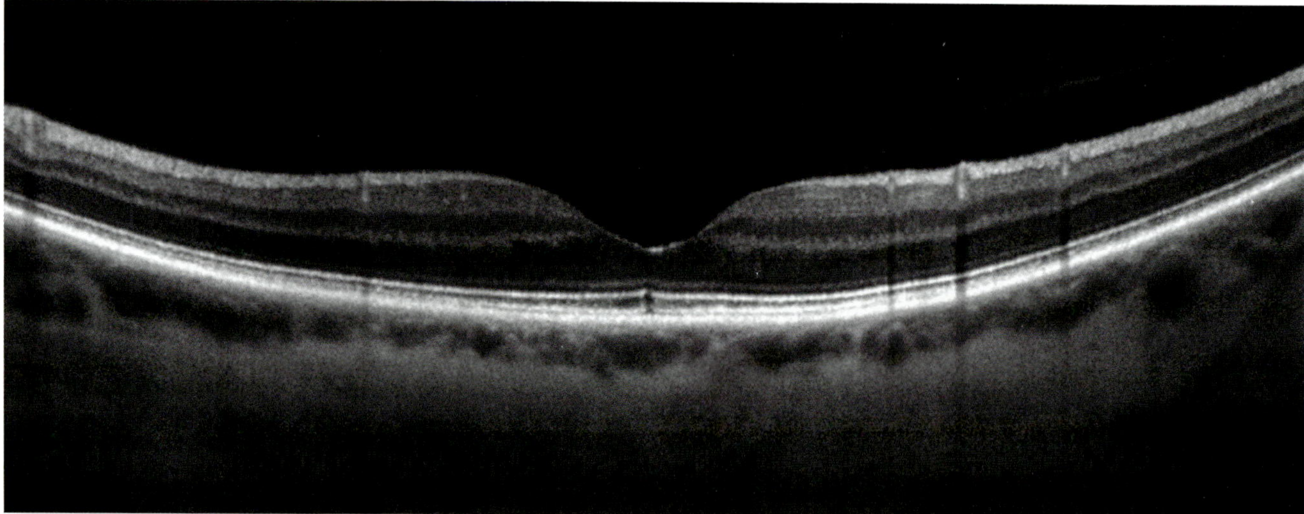

Figure 3: Eclipse lesion of the photoreceptors simulating a cavity. B scan phototraumatism. Optical coherence tomography cross-section scans show rectangular, horizontal, localized lesions of the photoreceptors. Their dimensions vary from very small to small. No edema is seen. They are located in the outer retina close to pigment epithelium. They appear immediately after sunburn and will last for life (Optovue RTVue)

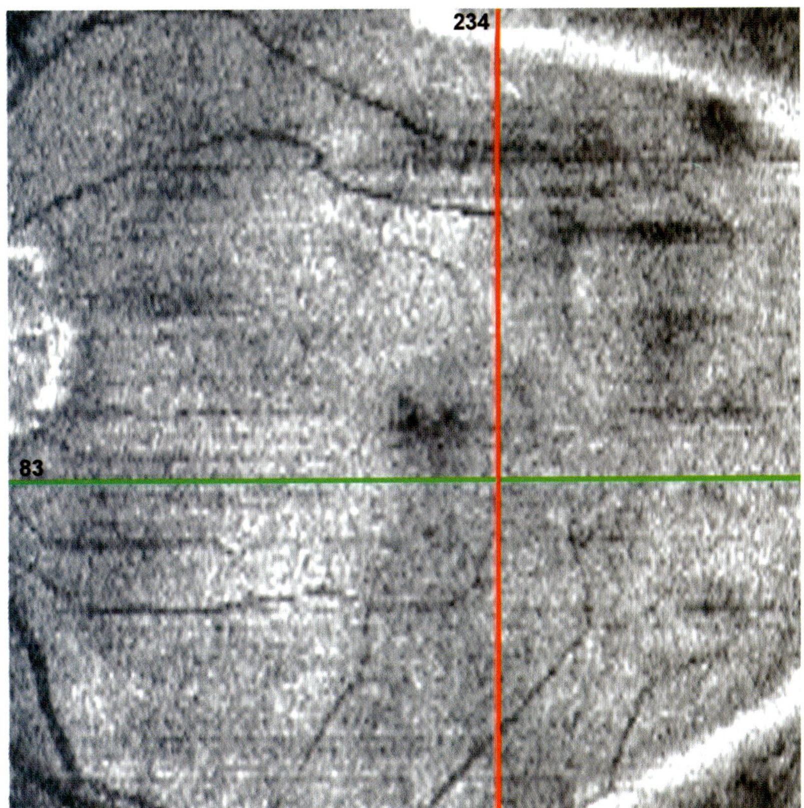

Figure 4: Eclipse lesion of the photoreceptors simulating a cavity. *En face* scan phototraumatism. *En face* optical coherence tomography scans adapted to the concavity of the posterior pole and passing exactly through the level of the photoreceptors show small irregular dark areas of alteration and give an exact map of the lesions. Disrupted photoreceptor patches are sharply delimited. Residual tissue granulations can be seen inside the disrupted area (Optovue RTVue)

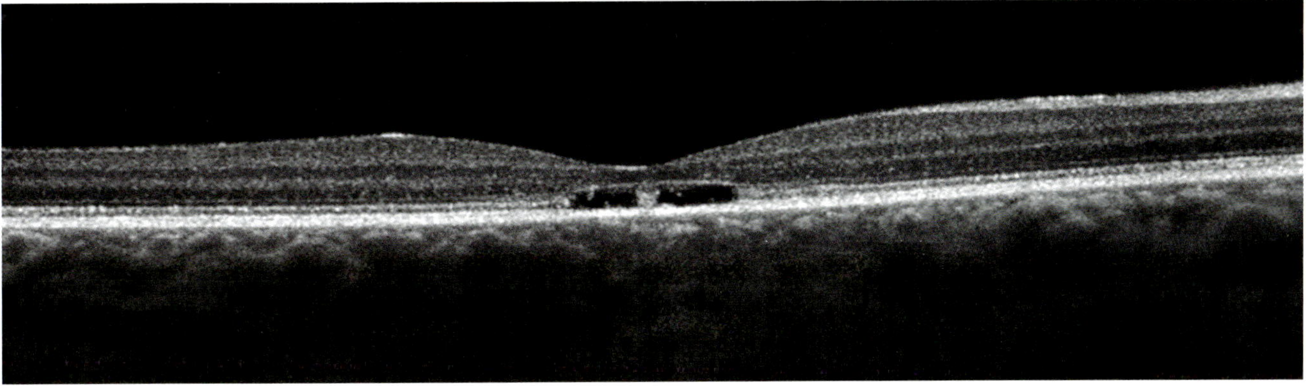

Figure 5: Idiopathic outer lamellar defects. Cross section-scan show outer lamellar defects at the fovea seen as lesions of 50–100 micron in size located at the level of the outer retina with sharp interruption of the inner/outer segments junction of photoreceptors and to the complex retinal pigment epithelium-choriocapillaris. Residual tissue granulations can be seen inside the disrupted area (Optovue RTVue)

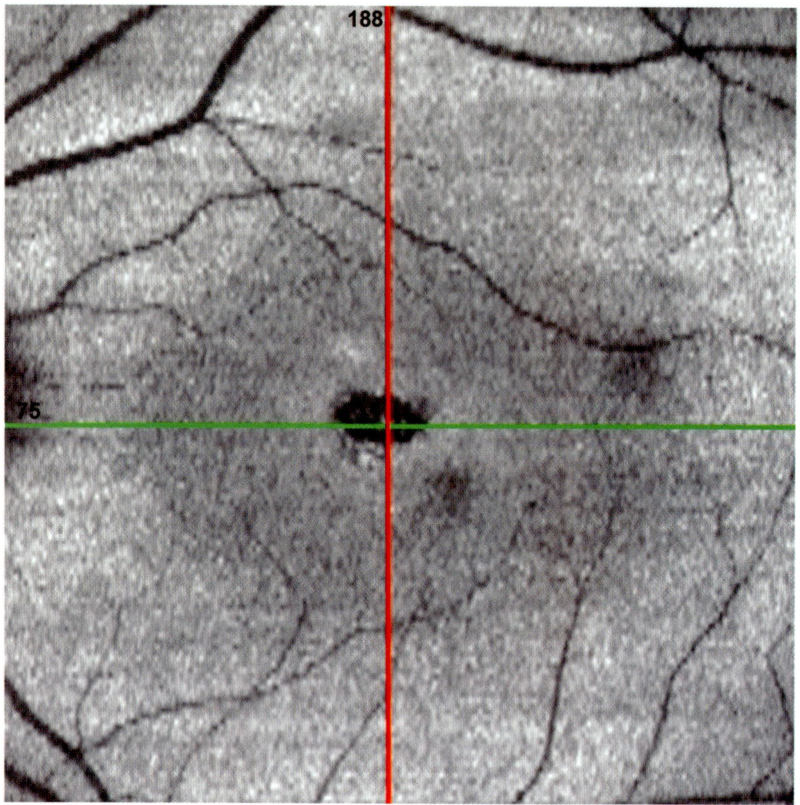

Figure 6: Idiopathic outer lamellar defects. *En face* optical coherence tomography scans adapted to the concavity of the posterior pole and passing exactly through the level of the photoreceptors show small irregular dark areas of alteration and give an exact map of the lesions. Disrupted photoreceptor patches are sharply delimited. Residual tissue granulations can be seen inside the disrupted area (Optovue RTVue)

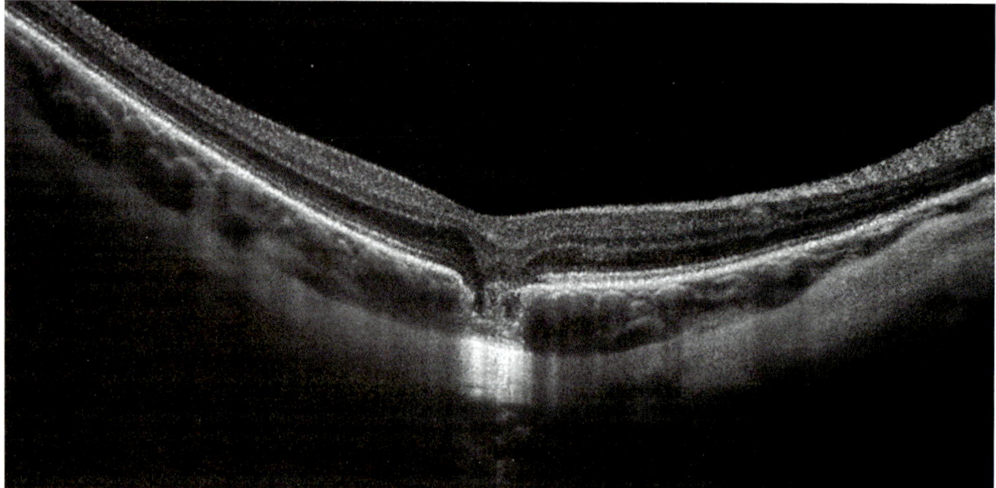

Figure 7: Epitheliitis lesion of the pigment epithelium showing a limited cavity B scan. A cross-section scan placed parallel to the pigment epithelium and passing exactly through its level shows a small sharply limited lesion of the pigment epithelium (Optovue RTVue)

Epitheliitis

Rarely lesion of the pigment epithelium showing a limited cavity B scan and *en face* scans can be seen. They can follow flu like episode or Epstein-Barr virus infection. A cross-section scan shows a small sharply limited lesion. *En face* scan, placed parallel to the pigment epithelium and passing exactly through its level, shows a small rounded sharply limited lesion.[5-7] In some cases lesions of the outer retina layers are seen close to the RPE alteration (**Figures 7 and 8**).

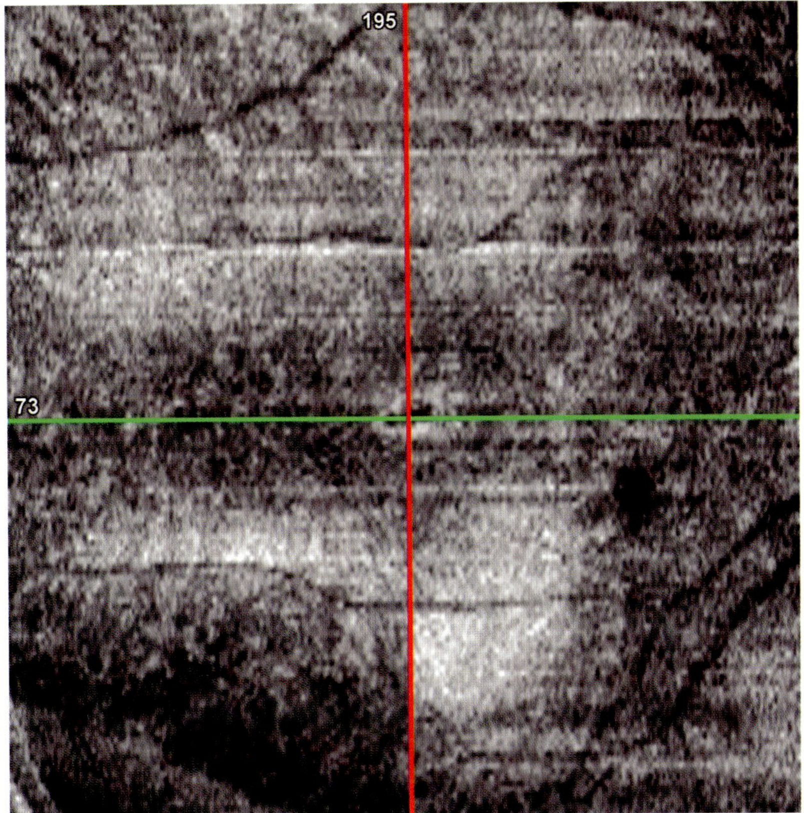

Figure 8: Epitheliitis *en face* lesion of the pigment epithelium simulating a cavity. *En face* scan placed parallel to the pigment epithelium and passing exactly through its level of the shows a small rounded sharply limited lesion (Optovue RTVue)

Extensive Lesions of the Photoreceptors

More extensive photoreceptors lesions can be seen in diabetic retinopathy, hypertensive retinopathy, macular degeneration, retinal detachment, vitreoretinal surgery, venous occlusions, macular telangiectasis, radiation retinopathy.

Lymphoma

In some cases of retinal lymphoma, fundus examination shows white dots in the retina. These disseminated *retinal deposits* can be seen on *en face* scans.

Optical coherence tomography images demonstrate hyper-reflective nodules at the RPE level. OCT cross-section scans show areas of disrupted photoreceptors and pigment epithelium deposits all over retina. These areas correspond with hyperfluorescent areas in the late phase of fluorescein angiography. Retinal profile is normal; there is no swelling of the retina and no edema. The outer limiting membrane is normal.

En face OCT scans adapted to the concavity of the posterior pole and passing exactly through the level of the pigment epithelium show areas of alteration and nodules, and give an exact map of the lesions **(Figures 9 and 10)**.

References

1. Li D, Kishi S. Restored photoreceptor outer segment damage in multiple evanescent white dot syndrome. Ophthalmology. 2009;116:762-70.
2. Jain A, Desai RU, Charalel RA, et al. Solar retinopathy: comparison of optical coherence tomography (OCT) and fluorescein angiography (FA). Retina. 2009;29: 1340-5.
3. dell'omo R, Konstantopoulou K, Wong R, et al. Presumed idiopathic outer lamellar defects of the fovea and chronic solar retinopathy: an OCT and fundus autofluorescence study. Br J Ophthalmol. 2009;93:1483-7.
4. Comander J, Gardiner M, Loewenstein J. High-resolution optical coherence tomography findings in solar maculo-pathy and the differential diagnosis of outer retinal holes. Am J Ophthalmol. 2011;152:413-9.

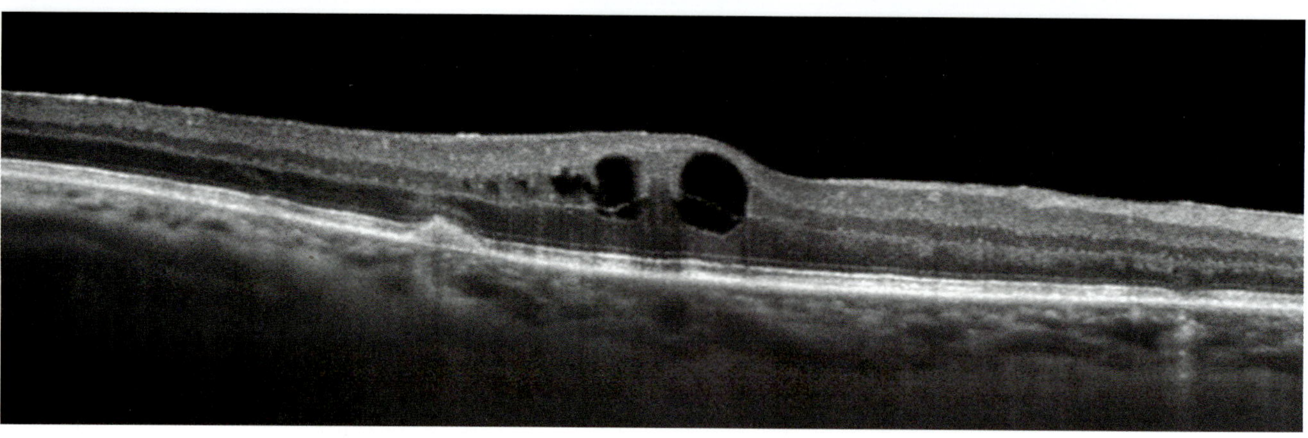

Figure 9: Lymphoma B scan lesion of the photoreceptors. Optical coherence tomography cross-section scans show areas of disrupted photoreceptors and pigment epithelium and other deposits all over retina. These areas correspond with hyperfluorescent areas in the late phase of fluorescein angiography. Retinal profile is normal; there is no swelling of the retina and no edema. The outer limiting membrane is normal (Optovue RTVue)

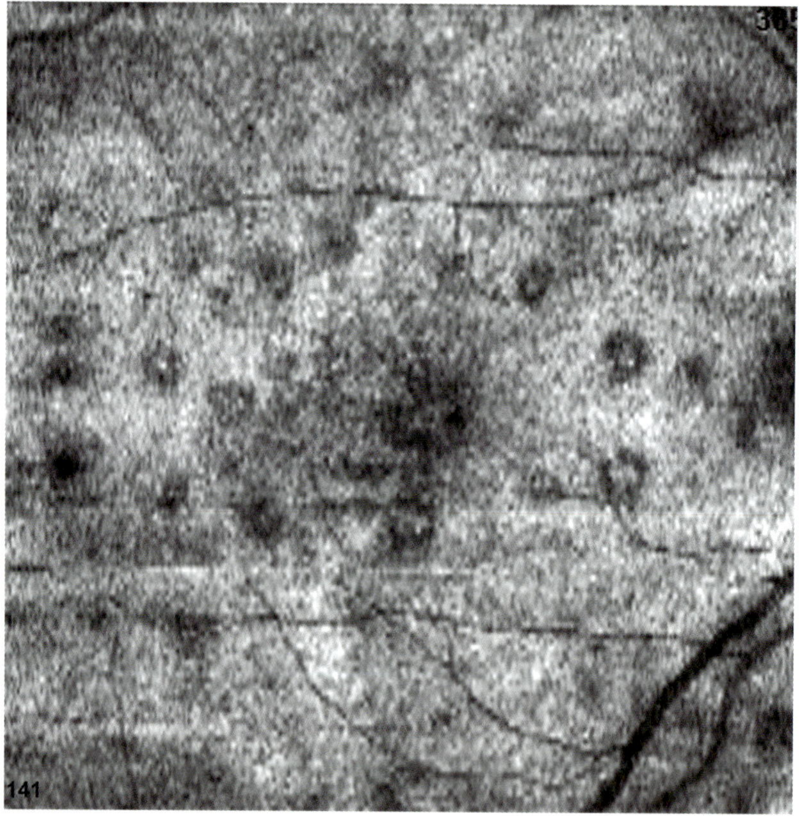

Figure 10: Lymphoma *en face* lesion of the photoreceptors. *En face* optical coherence tomography scans adapted to the concavity of the posterior pole and passing exactly through the level of the pigment epithelium show areas of alteration and nodules and give an exact map of the lesions (Optovue RTVue)

5. Cho HJ, Lee DW, Kim CG, et al. Spectral domain optical coherence tomography findings in acute retinal pigment epitheliitis. Can J Ophthalmol. 2011;46(6):498-500.
6. Kim JW, Jang SY, Park TK, et al. Short-term clinical observation of acute retinal pigment epitheliitis using spectral-domain optical coherence tomography. Korean J Ophthalmol. 2011;25:222-4.
7. Hsu J, Fineman MS, Kaiser RS. Optical coherence tomography findings in acute retinal pigment epitheliitis. Am J Ophthalmol. 2007;143:163-5.

Section 5

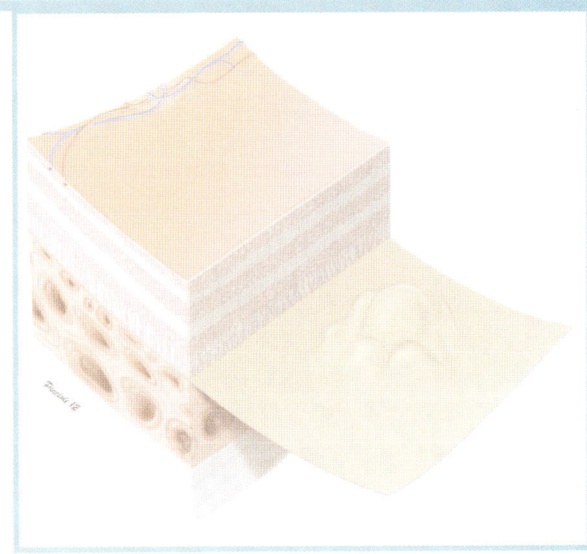

Retinal *En Face* Optical Coherence Tomography Examination: Macular Degenerations

En Face Spectral Domain Optical Coherence Tomography Imaging of Non-exudative Age-related Macular Degeneration

Zohar Yehoshua, Giovanni Gregori, Philip J Rosenfeld

Age-related macular degeneration (AMD) is the leading cause of severe vision loss in developed countries.[1] Geographic atrophy (GA) is a significant cause of both moderate and severe central vision loss, and is bilateral in most patients with advanced AMD.[2-5] GA is characterized by loss of retinal pigment epithelium (RPE), photoreceptor cells and the choriocapillaris layer. The natural history of GA has been described as a progressive condition that often develops as one or several small parafoveal lesions, which enlarge and coalesce over time, often sparing the fovea until late in the disease, with vision loss occurring over years.[5-7]

Spectral domain optical coherence tomography (SD-OCT) can be used to image and measure the area of GA.[8,9] Several studies have used SD-OCT to describe a wide spectrum of morphologic alterations that appear within the atrophic area, as well as within the adjacent and surrounding retinal tissue.[10-14] GA is associated with retinal atrophy which is seen as thinning or loss of outer nuclear layer and the absence of the external limiting membrane (ELM) and inner-segment/outer-segment (IS/OS) layer.[11,15] Distinct morphologic alterations have been identified at the junction between GA and the intact RPE where the outer retinal layers display a loss of normal architecture. The loss of photoreceptors often extends beyond the margins of GA with the ELM and IS/OS junctions disappearing while bridging across the GA margins.[10] Brar et al looked at the margins of GA using SD-OCT and correlated those changes with fundus autofluorescence (FAF) imaging. They found a statistically significant correlation between the pattern of FAF and the type of OCT changes found at the margins of GA.[16] Schmitz-Valckenberg et al showed that the mean length of an atrophic lesion measured on the FAF image had the closest agreement

with the appearance of choroidal hyper-reflectivity on the SD-OCT B scan, and the area of GA seen on FAF is spatially correlated with the abrupt transition on the SD-OCT B scan from a hyporeflective choroid to a hyper-reflective choroid.[15] This increased penetration of light below the Bruch's membrane is presumably due to the loss of the RPE and choriocapillaris.[9,10]

Optical coherence tomography imaging can also provide an *en face* image of GA that complements the B scan cross-sectional images. An *en face* image can generated from the 200 × 200 and 512 × 128 raster scan patterns from the Cirrus HD-OCT instrument (Carl Zeiss Meditec, Inc., Dublin, CA). This OCT fundus image (OFI) is generated by summing the signal of each of the A scans and viewing their relative values *en face*.[10,17,18] GA appears as a bright area on the *en face* OFI due to increased penetration of light into the choroid. In areas with GA, the RPE and choriocapillaris are absent[19] and these two layers of the eye normally cause a large percentage of the incident light to scatter, preventing deeper transmission of light into the choroid. The brightness of GA on the OFI results from the summation of this increased light penetration relative to the surrounding tissue, which still has intact RPE and choriocapillaris. This OFI correlates well with the GA appreciated on clinical examination, fundus photography and autofluorescence imaging **(Figures 1 to 3)**.[8,9]

A new approach for imaging GA recently introduced in the Cirrus HD-OCT advanced RPE analysis software and known as the sub-RPE slab creates the *en face* image only from the light reflected from beneath the RPE. The sub-RPE slab is formed by axially projecting only the OCT image data from a region below the contour of a robust polynomial

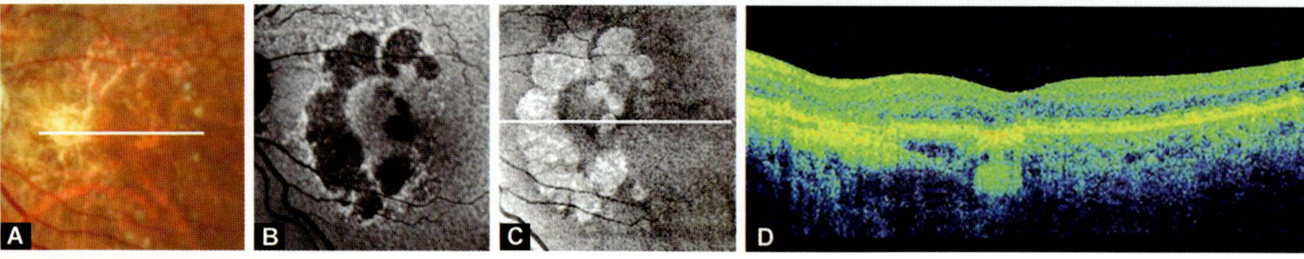

Figures 1A to D: Left eye of an 80-year-old woman with multifocal geographic atrophy imaged using different modalities. (A) The multifocal area of GA is shown on color fundus imaging with line representing the location of the B scan; (B) fundus autofluorescence imaging; (C) OCT fundus imaging with the line representing the location of the B scan; (D) OCT B scan

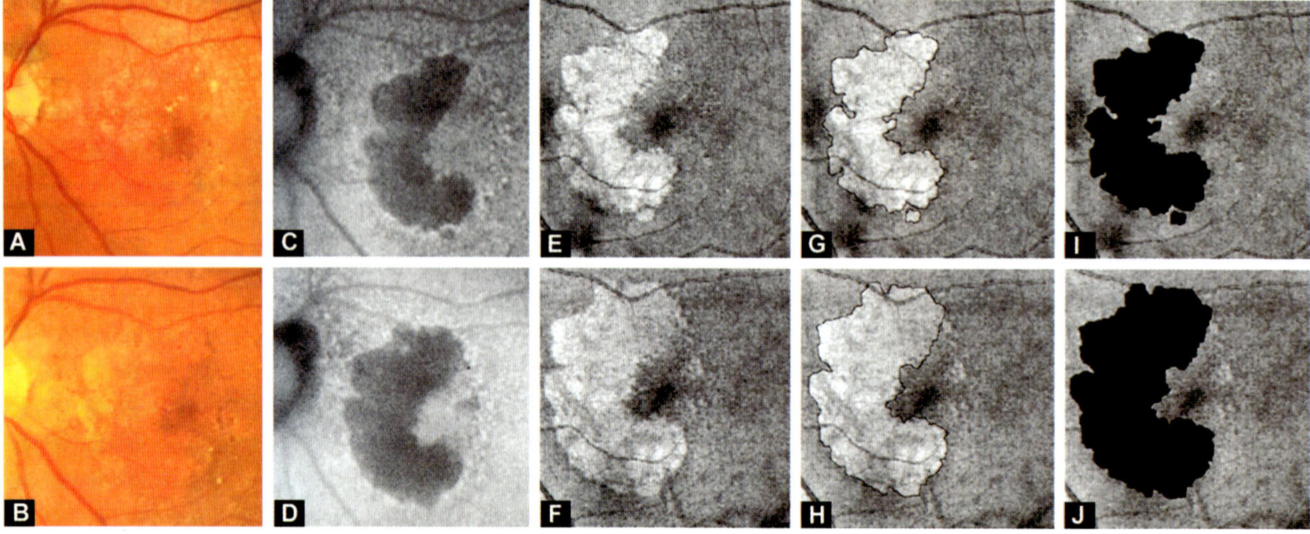

Figures 2A to J: (A and B) Unifocal area of geographic atrophy as seen by fundus photography; (C and D) autofluorescence and (E and F) OCT fundus imaging at baseline (A to I) and at the end of a 12 months follow-up period (B to J). The boundaries of GA were manually outlined on the OCT fundus image at baseline (G) and at the end of the follow up period (H). Areas of GA were calculated as 7.2 mm^2 (I) and 9.8 mm^2 (J)

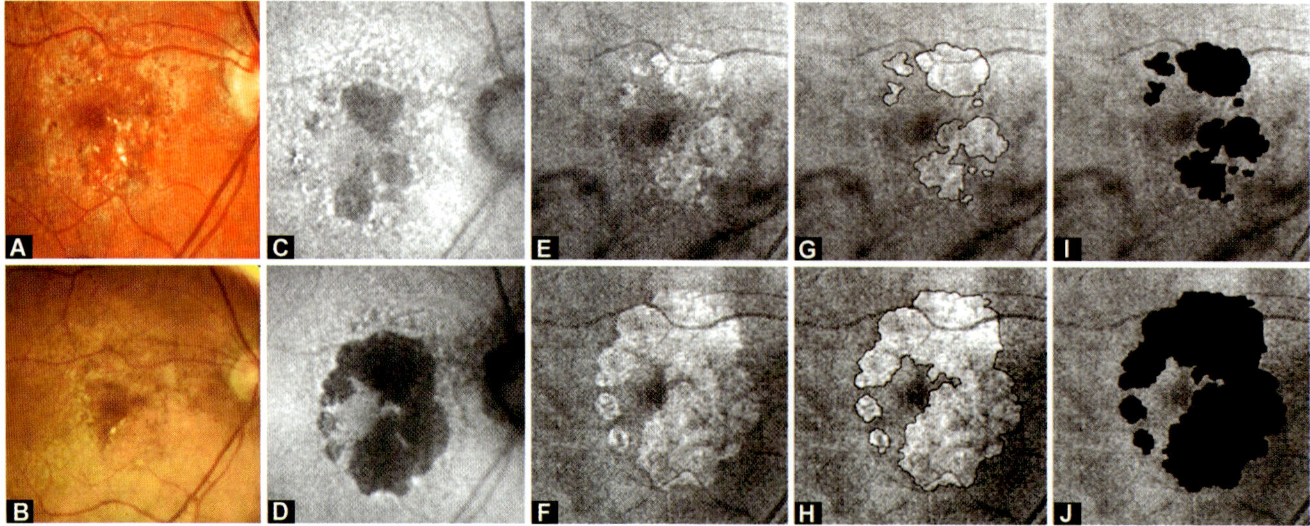

Figures 3A to J: (A and B) Multifocal area of geographic atrophy as seen by fundus photography; (C and D) autofluorescence and (E and F) OCT fundus imaging at baseline (A to I) and at the end of 18 months follow-up period (B to J). The boundaries of GA were manually outlined on the OCT fundus image at baseline (G) and at the end of the follow-up period (H). Areas of GA were calculated as 4.1 mm^2 (I) and 9.9 mm^2 (J)

fit to the RPE segmentation. This region extends from 65 to 400 microns below the robust RPE fit. By only using the light that penetrates into the choroid, the sub-RPE slab has the advantage of higher contrast at the borders of GA and the GA appears more distinct **(Figure 4)**. Also this approach might eliminate hyperreflective areas on the OFI possibly due to other effects. The three-dimensional (3D) dataset from the Cirrus SD-OCT (version 6.0) is used to generate both the *en face* fundus image and the sub-RPE slab. These *en face* virtual fundus images can be used to measure the area of GA **(Figures 2, 3 and 5)**.[8] A proprietary algorithm included in the Cirrus OCT software can automatically quantitate the area of GA from the sub-RPE slab image **(Figure 5)**.

C scans enable a better appreciation of the topographic relationships of intraretinal structures in a manner that cannot be readily appreciated from conventional B scan sections alone. Using a C scan, authors can view branching tubular structures that are located in the outer nuclear layer of the retina and appear as round or ovoid hyporeflective spaces with hyper-reflective borders on conventional B scan OCT sections. These structures were given the name outer retinal tubulation (ORT)[20] **(Figures 6A to D)**. ORT was first described in patients with neovascular AMD. These tubules can simulate

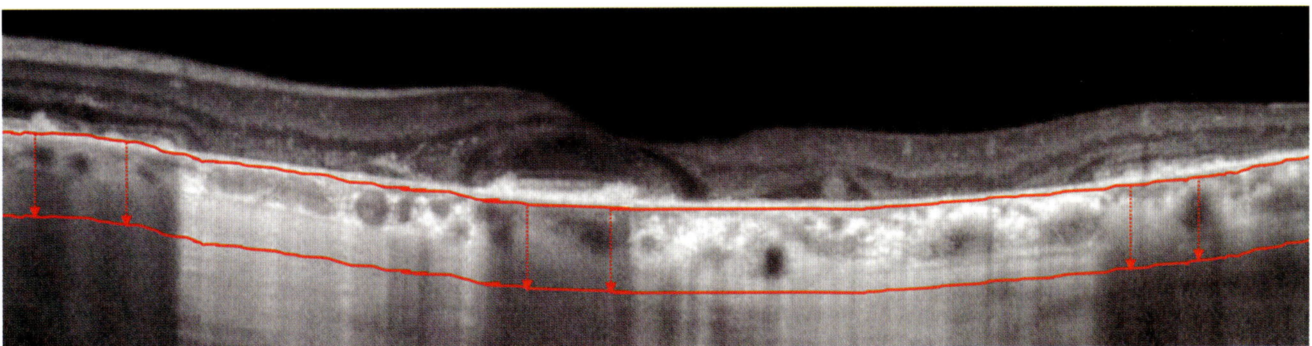

Figure 4: B scan with representation of the area that was used to generate the sub-RPE slab (between the red lines)

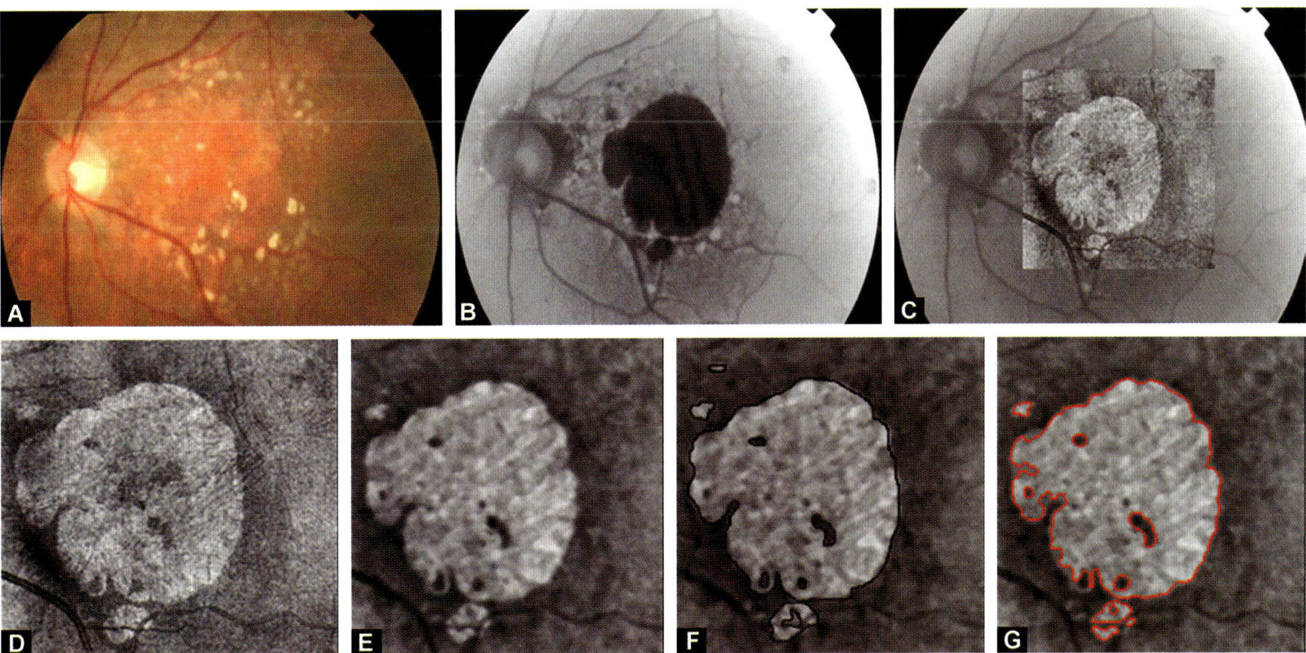

Figures 5A to G: Left eye of a 75 year old woman with multifocal geographic atrophy imaged using different modalities and measured using both manual and automated techniques. (A) The multifocal area of GA is shown on color fundus imaging, (B) autofluorescence imaging, (C) OCT fundus imaging with the OCT fundus image superimposed on the autofluorescence image, (D) OCT fundus image (area = 10.73 mm^2) and (E) Sub-RPE slab image. (F) The boundaries of GA were manually outlined on the sub-RPE slab image with the area of GA measured to be 10.8 mm^2. (G) The automatic algorithm measured the area of GA to be 10.65 mm^2

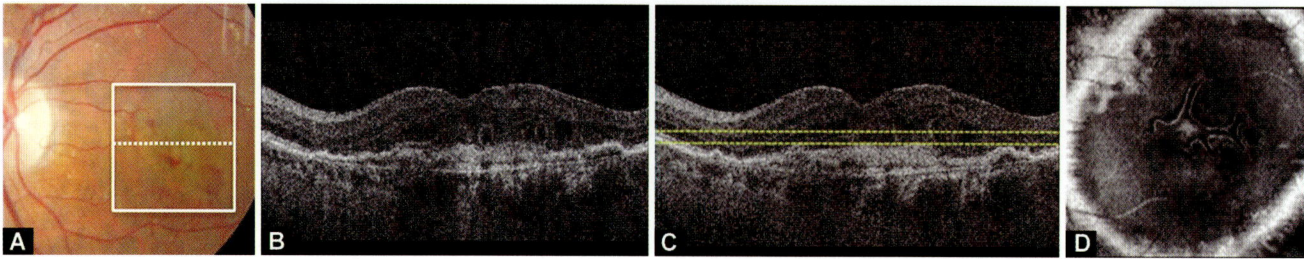

Figures 6A to D: Schematic representation of the method used to identify outer retinal tubulation in the retina using *en face* image. Left eye of a 74-year-old man with history of multiple anti-VEGF treatments (last injection one year ago). (A) Color fundus image with a square representing the 6 X 6 mm imaged area with a dashed white line representing the location of the B scan; (B) Foveal horizontal B scan; (C) Foveal horizontal B scan with two yellow dashed lines representing the slab with a thickness of 90 μm used to generate the *en face* image; (D) *En face* image showing the outer retinal tubulation

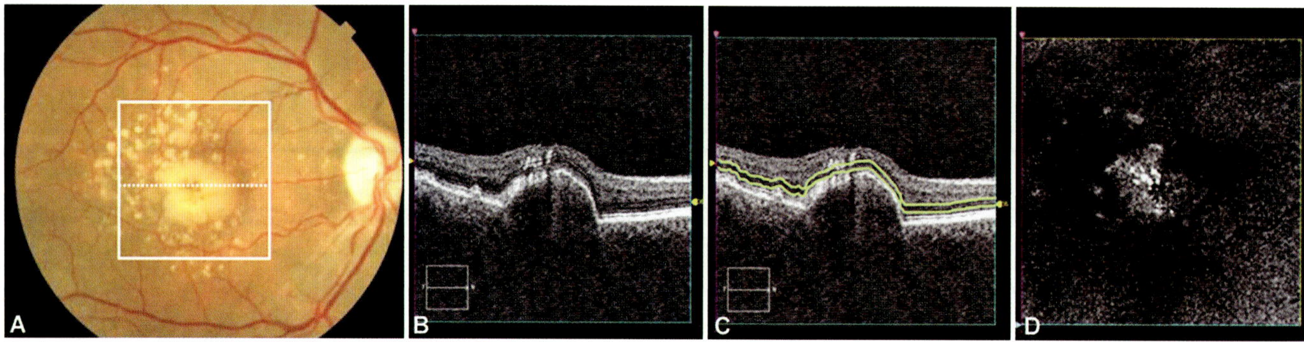

Figures 7A to D: Schematic representation of the method used to identify RPE pigment clumping in the retina using *en face* image. (A) Right eye of a 78-year-old man with a drusenoid PED. Color fundus image with line representing the location of the B scan; (B) foveal horizontal B scan; (C) foveal B scan with two lines with the RPE segmentation contour located at 20 μm and 60 μm above the RPE; (D) *En face* image which can be used to identify pigment clumps which are seen as bright spots on the image

the appearance of macular edema and subretinal fluid on single B scan sections, so their recognition may help to prevent unnecessary treatments since ORT does not respond to treatments for neovascular AMD. Compared with conventional B scan images, C scan images provide better recognition of the more complex tubular and branching networks associated with ORT. Unlike the cystic spaces associated with macular edema, which are mostly found in the inner nuclear layer and may resemble the round or ovoid structures of ORT on individual B scan sections, ORT is located exclusively in the outer nuclear layer, which makes C scan imaging ideal for its detection. In addition, ORT structures are surrounded by a hyper-reflective border, which is thought to be composed of the connecting cilia (IS/OS junctions) of the photoreceptor cells and possibly other glial cells. Furthermore, unlike the cysts of cystoid macular edema (CME), the lumens of ORT typically contain varying amounts of hyper-reflective material, which likely representing malformed and degenerating photoreceptor outer segments. Moreover, unlike the cysts in CME which are arranged in a petaloid fashion, ORT is distributed randomly over the macula.[20]

Previous reports have described the presence of small hyper-reflective lesions within the retina in patients with dry AMD, which were considered as intraretinal aggregations of migrating RPE cells.[11, 21-23] Ho et al found a high incidence of intraretinal RPE cell migration in patients with dry AMD (61.4% of patients or 54.5% of eyes). In addition, all eyes with documented intraretinal hyper-reflective lesions on SD-OCT imaging had corresponding areas of pigment clumping on color fundus photographs. Ninety-seven percent of the eyes showed correlation between pigment clumping on color fundus photography and intraretinal hyper-reflective lesions on SD-OCT imaging.[21] Areas of intraretinal RPE pigment migration on OCT were located directly above drusen in the majority of the eyes which may suggest that drusen may play a role in stimulating intraretinal migration of the RPE cells. Pigment clumping on color fundus photography may be mistaken for RPE pigment hypertrophy or choroidal hyperpigmentation, but by using SD-OCT *en face* imaging, authors can clearly differentiate between these entities. **Figures 7A to D** show the use of slab above the RPE, which demonstrate the pigment clumps.

Spectral domain optical coherence tomography is capable of documenting both *en face* and cross-sectional images of the macula and following patients with dry AMD. This imaging approach ensures that the area of perceived GA actually corresponds to the loss of photoreceptors and RPE, which correlates with the loss of visual function. Another advantage using *en face* and C scan imaging is differentiating retinal tubulation from intraretinal fluid and identifying pigment clumps in the outer retina.

References

1. van Leeuwen R, Klaver CC, Vingerling JR, et al. Epidemiology of age-related maculopathy: a review. Eur J Epidemiol. 2003;18(9):845-54.
2. Schatz H, McDonald HR. Atrophic macular degeneration. Rate of spread of geographic atrophy and visual loss. Ophthalmology. 1989;96(10):1541-51.
3. Potter JW, Thallemer JM. Geographic atrophy of the retinal pigment epithelium: diagnosis and vision rehabilitation. J Am Optom Assoc. 1981;52(6):503-8.
4. Sunness JS, Bressler NM, Tian Y, et al. Measuring geographic atrophy in advanced age-related macular degeneration. Invest Ophthalmol Vis Sci. 1999;40(8): 1761-9.
5. Maguire P, Vine AK. Geographic atrophy of the retinal pigment epithelium. Am J Ophthalmol. 1986;102(5): 621-5.
6. Sarks JP, Sarks SH, Killingsworth MC. Evolution of geographic atrophy of the retinal pigment epithelium. Eye (Lond). 1988;2(Pt 5):552-77.
7. Sunness JS, Gonzalez-Baron J, Applegate CA, et al. Enlargement of atrophy and visual acuity loss in the geographic atrophy form of age-related macular degeneration. Ophthalmology. 1999;106(9):1768-79.
8. Yehoshua Z, Rosenfeld PJ, Gregori G, et al. Progression of geographic atrophy in age related macular degeneration imaged with spectral domain optical coherence tomography. Ophthalmology. 2010;In press.
9. Lujan Bj, Rosenfeld PJ, Giovanni G, et al. Spectral domain optical coherence tomographic imaging of geographic atrophy. Ophthalmic Surg Lasers Imaging. 2008;39(4 Suppl):S8-S14.
10. Bearelly S, Chau FY, Koreishi A, et al. Spectral domain optical coherence tomography imaging of geographic atrophy margins. Ophthalmology. 2009;116(9):1762-9.
11. Fleckenstein M, Charbel Issa P, Helb HM, et al. High-resolution spectral domain-OCT imaging in geographic atrophy associated with age-related macular degeneration. Invest Ophthalmol Vis Sci. 2008;49(9):4137-44.
12. Fleckenstein M, Schmitz-Valckenberg S, Adrion C, et al. Tracking progression with spectral-domain optical coherence tomography in geographic atrophy caused by age-related macular degeneration. Invest Ophthalmol Vis Sci. 2010;51(8):3846-52.
13. Helb HM, Charbel Issa P, Fleckenstein M, et al. Clinical evaluation of simultaneous confocal scanning laser ophthalmoscopy imaging combined with high-resolution, spectral-domain optical coherence tomography. Acta Ophthalmol. 2010;88(8):842-9.
14. Fleckenstein M, Schmitz-Valckenberg S, Martens C, et al. Fundus autofluorescence and spectral-domain optical coherence tomography characteristics in a rapidly progressing form of geographic atrophy. Invest Ophthalmol Vis Sci. 2011;52(6):3761-6.
15. Schmitz-Valckenberg S, Fleckenstein M, Gobel AP, et al. Optical coherence tomography and autofluorescence findings in areas with geographic atrophy due to age-related macular degeneration. Invest Ophthalmol Vis Sci. 2009;50:3915-21.
16. Brar M, Kozak I, Cheng L, et al. Correlation between spectral-domain optical coherence tomography and fundus autofluorescence at the margins of geographic atrophy. Am J Ophthalmol. 2009;148(3):439-44.
17. Jiao S, Knighton RW, Huang X, et al. Simultaneous acquisition of sectional and fundus ophthalmic images with spectral-domain optical coherence tomography. Opt Express. 2005;13(2):444-52.
18. Wojtkowski M, Srinivasan V, Fujimoto JG, et al. Three-dimensional retinal imaging with high-speed ultrahigh-resolution optical coherence tomography. Ophthalmology. 2005;112(10):1734-46.
19. Drexler W, Sattmann H, Hermann B, et al. Enhanced visualization of macular pathology with the use of ultrahigh-resolution optical coherence tomography. Arch Ophthalmol. 2003;121(5):695-706.
20. Zweifel SA, Engelbert M, Laud K, et al. Outer retinal tubulation: a novel optical coherence tomography finding. Arch Ophthalmol. 2009;127(12):1596-602.
21. Ho J, Witkin AJ, Liu J, et al. Documentation of intraretinal retinal pigment epithelium migration via high-speed ultrahigh-resolution optical coherence tomography. Ophthalmology. 2011;118(4):687-93.
22. Pieroni CG, Witkin AJ, Ko TH, et al. Ultrahigh resolution optical coherence tomography in non-exudative age related macular degeneration. Br J Ophthalmol. 2006; 90(2):191-7.
23. Schuman SG, Koreishi AF, Farsiu S, et al. Photoreceptor layer thinning over drusen in eyes with age-related macular degeneration imaged in vivo with spectral-domain optical coherence tomography. Ophthalmology. 2009; 116(3):488-96 e2.

chapter 15

Geographic Atrophy

Nalin J Mehta

Introduction

Geographic atrophy (GA) of the macula has been found to commence most commonly from areas of soft drusen and RPE mottling; as these areas progress to GA, the risk of CNV decreases.[1] SD-OCT *en face* imaging should be particularly useful in monitoring the extent and progression of GA of the RPE and choriocapillaris. In addition, hyperfluorescence from subretinal neovascular membranes (SRNVM) may be difficult to discern from underlying GA, whereas OCT can demonstrate exudative changes in this instance.

Geographic atrophy (**Figures 1 and 2**) results in an increased throughput of the OCT signal secondary to decreased light scatter through areas of attenuation of both RPE and choriocapillaris, resulting in greater signal penetration to, and therefore better visualization of, the deeper choroidal vessels and sclera.

This also results in the *en face* macular image noted in the high density/3D OCT scan to outline a hyper-reflective signal in areas of GA. Since there is less light scatter from the OCT laser light source in areas of RPE attenuation, with corresponding loss of melanin (which is known to strongly scatter light)[2] and blood, there is increased signal throughput to the deeper choroidal and scleral layers. This in turn increases the light reflected directly back to the OCT's spectrometer resulting in a bright signal corresponding to the area of GA.

This *en face* image not only correlates well with GA histopathologically,[1] but also psychophysically with preferential hyperacuity (vernier acuity) perimetry (PHP) (**Figure 3**), a measure of distortion which is superior to Amsler grid testing.[3,4]

This area of GA outlined on *en face* imagery (**Figure 4A**) has been found to have a 97% correlation with macular fundus auto-fluorescence (FAF) studies (**Figure 4B**), which

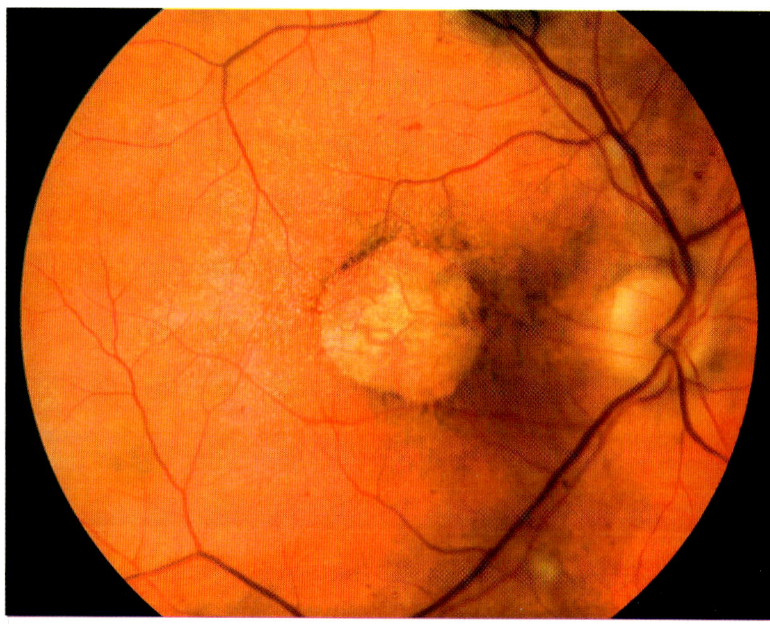

Figure 1: Fundus photograph demonstrating geographic macular atrophy (GA)

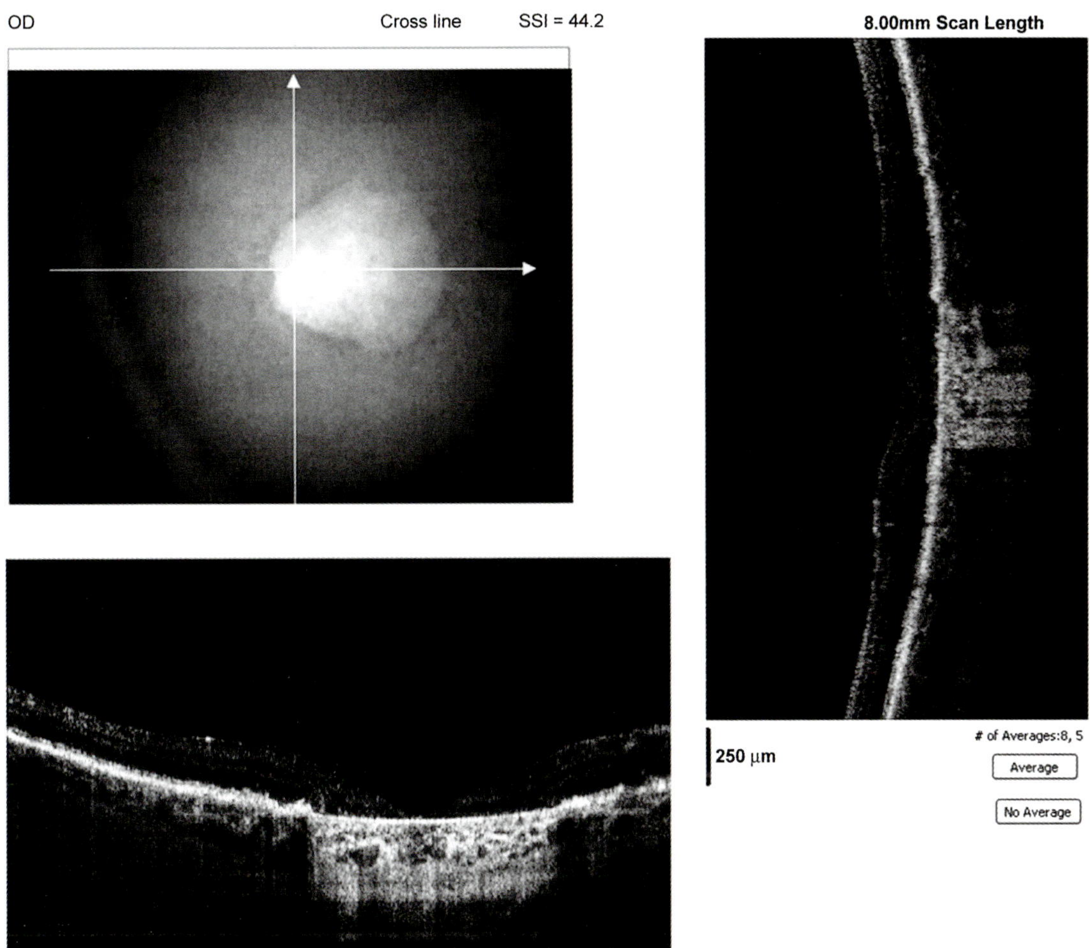

Figure 2: Cross-sectional B scan images of GA

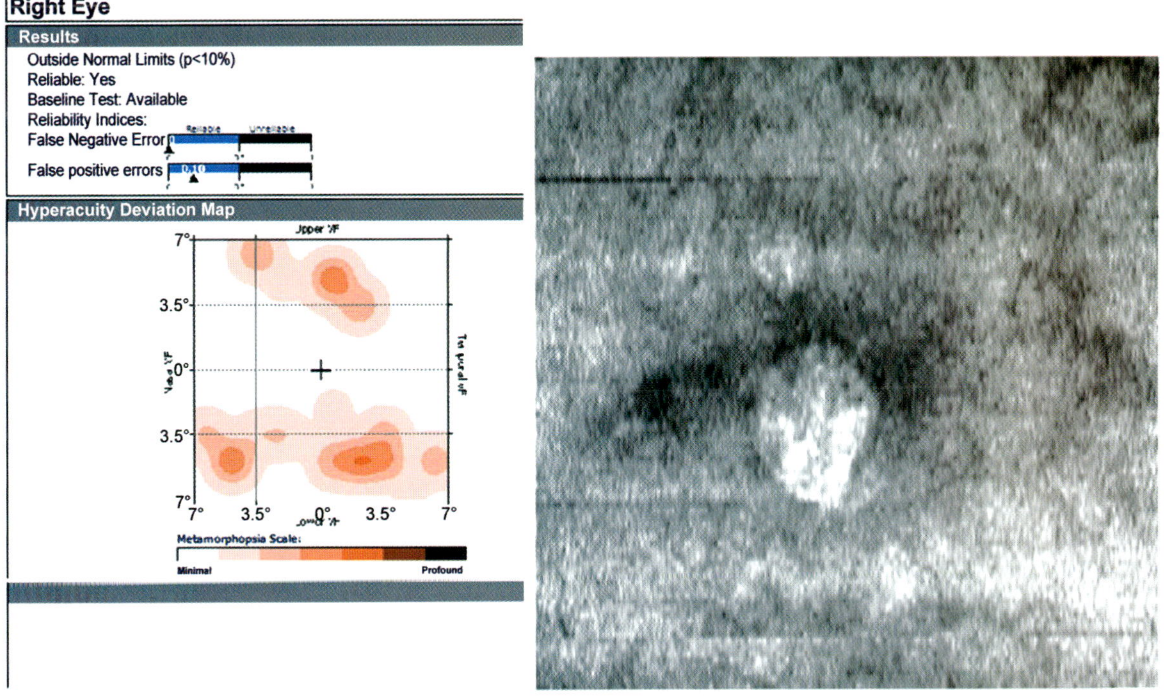

Figure 3: Correlation of preferential hyperacuity perimetry (left) and *en face* OCT (right) of GA

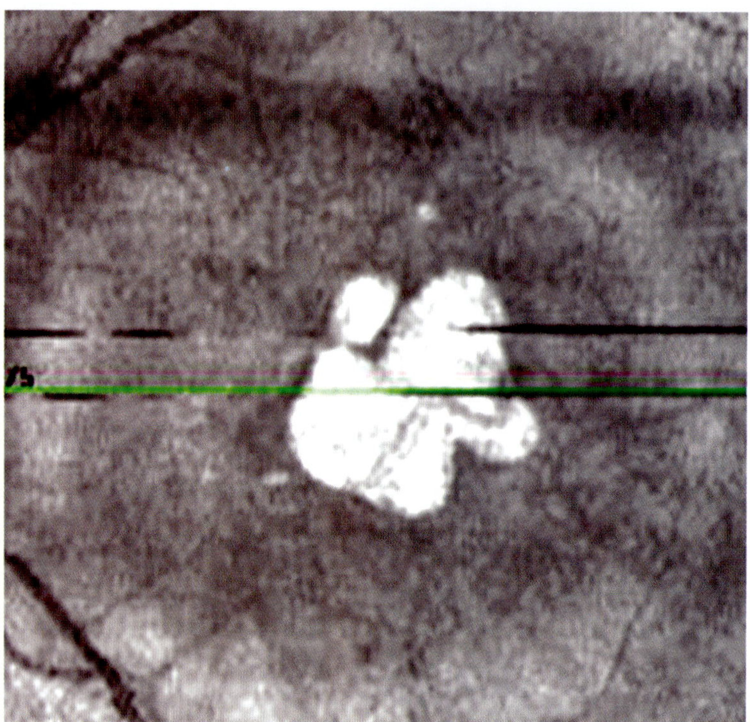

Figure 4A: *En face* OCT of GA

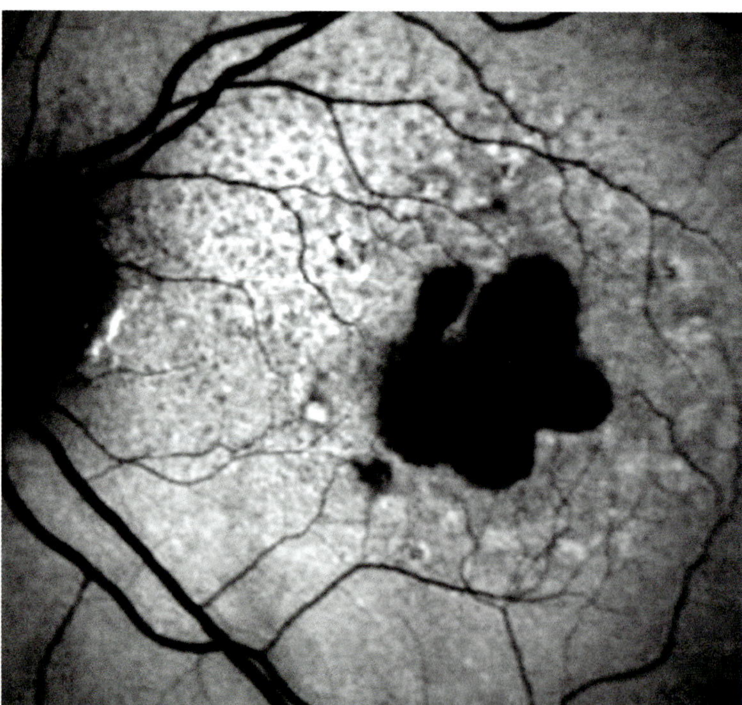

Figure 4B: Fundus autofluorescence (FAF) image of GA in Figure 4A

show an inverse, darker-colored signal given the lack of lipofuscin in the areas of RPE attenuation, which is responsible for the auto-fluorescence phenomenon.[5] More recent studies furthermore indicate that SD-OCT may be superior to FAF studies in the detection of GA.[6]

Numerous studies are now looking at the role of pharmacologic agents in decreasing the progression of GA in AMD,[7,8] and the ability to quantify the area of the same may prove beneficial in monitoring the effects of these treatment strategies.

References

1. Sarks JP, Sarks SH, Killingsworth MC. Evolution of geographic atrophy of the retinal pigment epithelium. Eye. 1988;2(Pt 5):552-77.
2. Wolbarsht ML, Walsh AW, George G. Melanin. A unique biological absorber. Appl Opt. 1981;20:2184-6.
3. Alster Y, Bressler NM, Bressler SB. Preferential Hyperacuity Perimeter (PreView PHP) for detecting choroidal neovascularization study. Ophthalmology. 2005;112(10): 1758-65.
4. Goldstein M, Loewenstein A, Barak A, et al. Results of a multicenter clinical trial to evaluate the preferential hyperacuity perimeter for detection of age-related macular degeneration. Retina. 2005;25(3):296-303.
5. Lujan BJ, Rosenfeld PJ, Gregori G, et al. Spectral domain optical coherence tomographic imaging of geographic atrophy. Ophthalmic Surgery, Lasers & Imaging. 2008;39(4)(supplement): S8-S14.
6. Sayegh RG, Simader C, Scheschy U, et al. A systematic comparison of spectral-domain optical coherence tomography and fundus autofluorescence in patients with geographic atrophy. Ophthalmology. 2011;118:1844-51.
7. Petrukhin K. New therapeutic targets in atrophic age-related macular degeneration. Expert Opin Ther Targets. 2007;11:625-39.
8. Gehrs KM, Anderson DH, Johnson LV, et al. Age-related macular degeneration-emerging pathogenetic and therapeutic concepts. Ann Med. 2006;38:450-71.

chapter 16

Drusen and Retinal Pigment Epithelium Detachments

Nalin J Mehta

Drusen

Yellow-pigmented lesions at the level of retinal pigment epithelium (RPE) can have several etiologies, from hard and soft drusen to small retinal pigment epithelium detachments (RPEDs). Histologically, macular drusen are made up of cellular debris, modified proteins lipid and lipofuscin (lipid pigment), which accumulate under the aging RPE cells, in Bruch's membrane.[1-4]

Some drusen are so subtle as to only be seen histo-pathologically not clinically.[1] Studies suggest that drusen alter their consistency as age-related macular disease (AMD) progresses, resulting in a spectrum starting with hard drusen, then transforming to semi-solid, soft and regressing forms; softening of drusen is associated with early subretinal neovascularization.[3,5,6] It is important to be able to differentiate these lesions from one another, as management protocols and prognosis vary greatly.[7] *En face* spectral domain optical coherence tomography (SD-OCT) not only assists in identifying even the smallest drusen which may be obscured by nuclear sclerotic cataract or surrounding pigmented tissues, but also demonstrates unique characteristics in each of these subtypes which makes it possible to differentiate between these lesions.

Figures 1 and 2 represent a patient with moderate, hard drusen. Note the numerous, discrete punctate hyper-reflective lesions in the plane between the RPE and inner-segment/outer-segment (IS/OS) border (i.e. protruding into the outer segment). Note the shadows surrounding these lesions. These hyper-reflective foci are consistent with light reflecting off

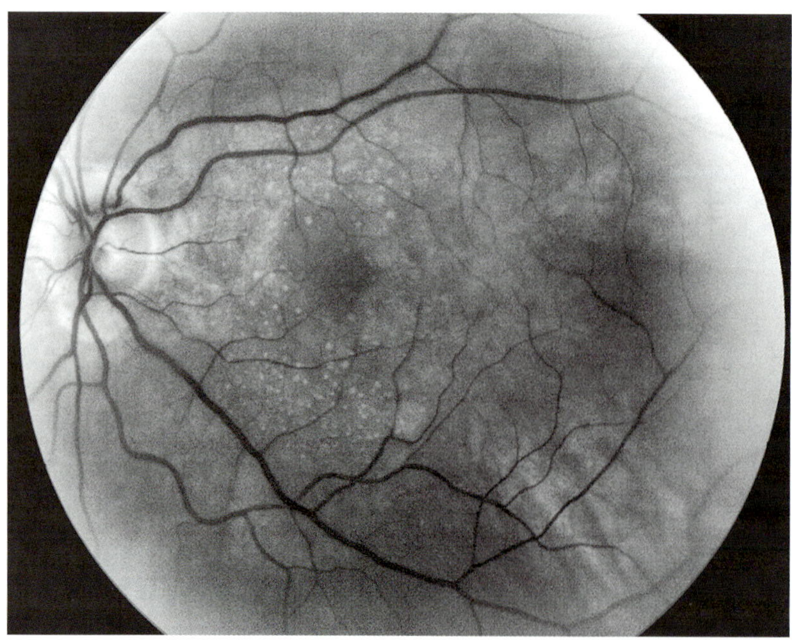

Figure 1: Red-free photograph of fine, hard macular drusen

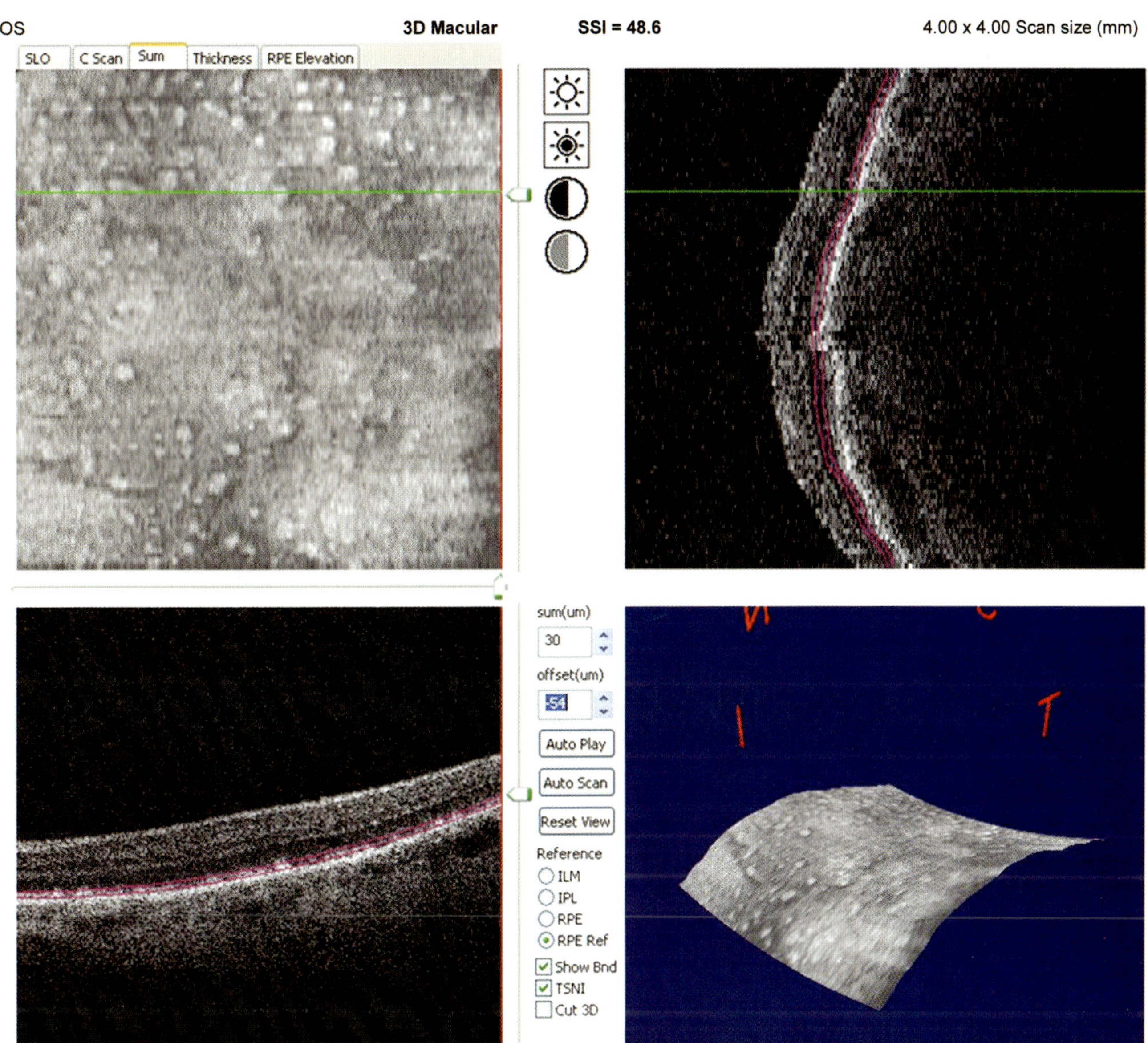

Figure 2: *En face* images of hard drusen in the plane between the RPE and IS/OS border

of the RPE protrusions. Such punctate lesions have been associated with lipoidal degeneration of individual RPE cells.[8] *En face* OCT imaging for drusen detection, furthermore, correlates well with fundus photographs.[9]

Figures 3 and 4 represent a patient with large, soft drusen. Soft drusen have been associated with overlying RPE hypopigmentation and focal atrophy, as well as a diffusely thickened Bruch's membrane, in pathologic studies.[8,10] Soft drusen have also been associated with RPE migration into the retina and have been shown to precede choroidal neovascularization (CNV).[5]

Analyzing the *en face* C scan image in the plane of the outer segment just above the RPE, the soft drusen appear relatively isoreflective when compared with surrounding areas, with hyper-reflective borders.

This relative isoreflectivity could be explained by light absorption by melanin remaining within the RPE overlying the soft drusen combined with increased light absorption and scatter from the semi-solid material within the drusen, negating the hyper-reflectivity expected from underlying tissues despite RPE hypopigmentation and atrophy. This could also explain why there is a subtle shadowing beneath the

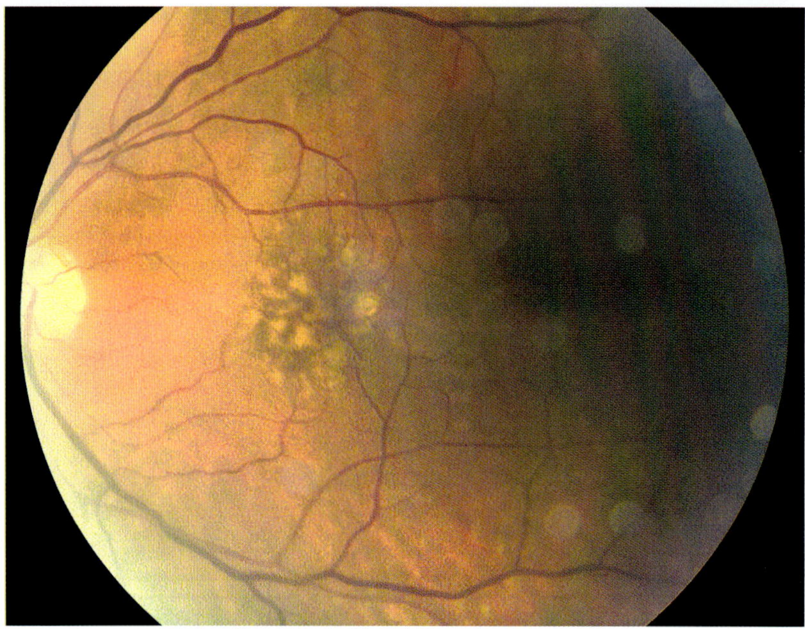

Figure 3: Fundus photograph of large, soft drusen

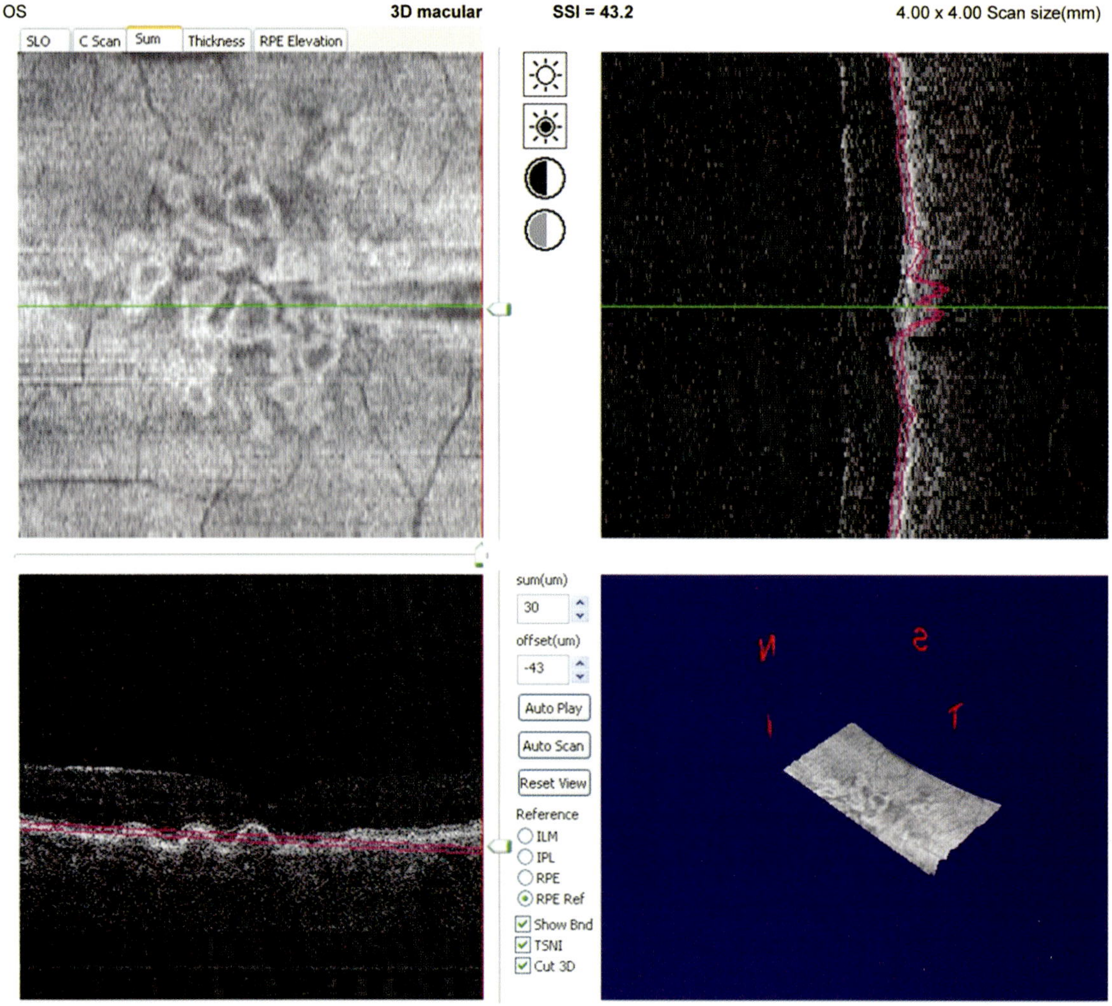

Figure 4: *En face* images of soft drusen in the plane between the RPE and IS/OS border

soft drusen on the B scan, rather than a hyper-reflective signal which would be expected with loss of melanin associated with focal atrophy.

The hyper-reflective borders may be explained by the relatively perpendicular orientation of the melanin-rich RPE walls surrounding the drusen with respect to the RPE plane, which in turn simulates the B scan RPE signal from this border.

Clear Serous Retinal Pigment Epithelium Detachment

Figures 5 and 6 denote the B scan and corresponding *en face* image of a serous RPED taken in the plane just above the RPE. Note the hyporeflective pocket correlating with low-density serous fluid and a strong overlying RPE signal.

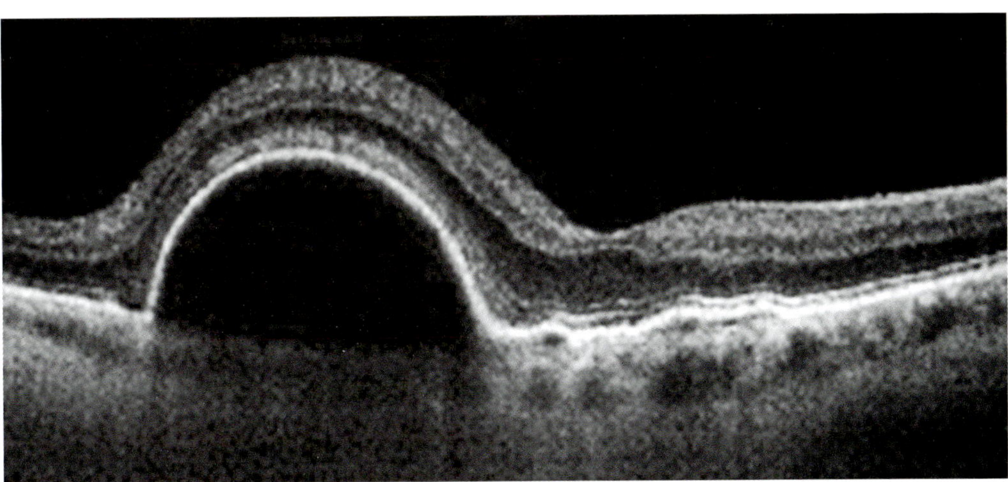

Figure 5: B scan of serous RPE detachment

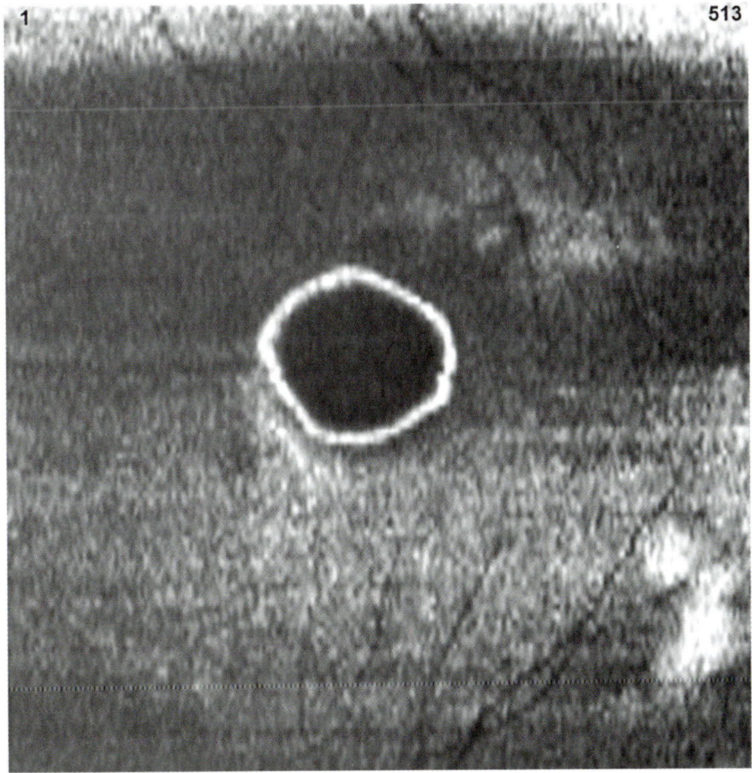

Figure 6: *En face* image of serous RPE detachment in the plane between the RPE and IS/OS border

Turbid Serous Retinal Pigment Epithelium Detachment

Figures 7 to 9 demonstrate the photo, fluorescein angiography (FA) and OCT of a patient with a relatively large, multi-lobed, turbid serous RPED. One can easily quantify the diameter and area of the RPED base with C scan *en face* imagery; note the isodense nature of the RPED when compared to surrounding retinal tissue. Recall a similar pattern is noted with soft drusen, sometimes making it difficult to

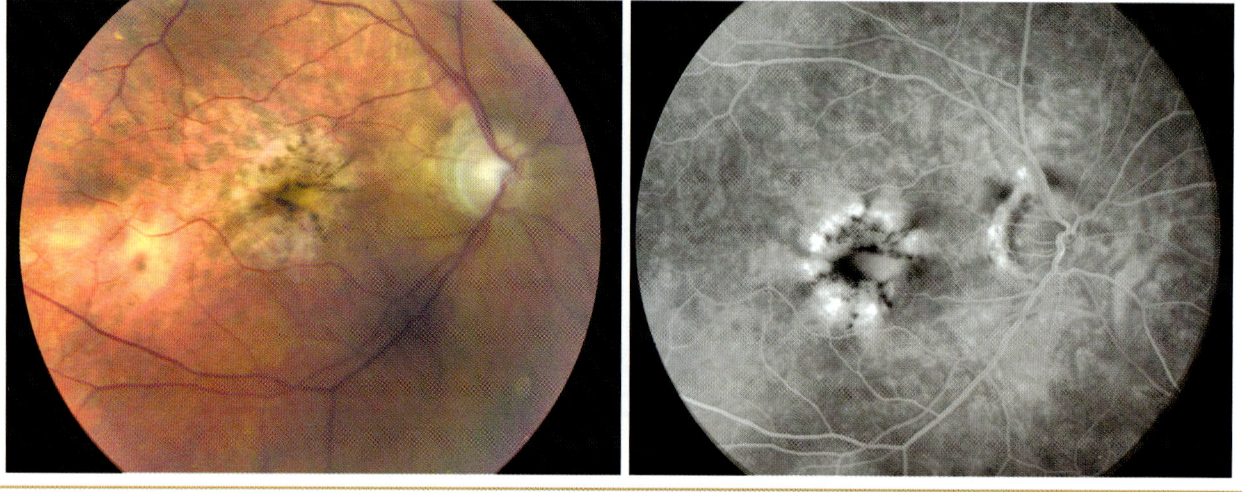

Figure 7: Fundus photograph (left) and fluorescein angiogram (right) of turbid (drusenoid) RPE detachment

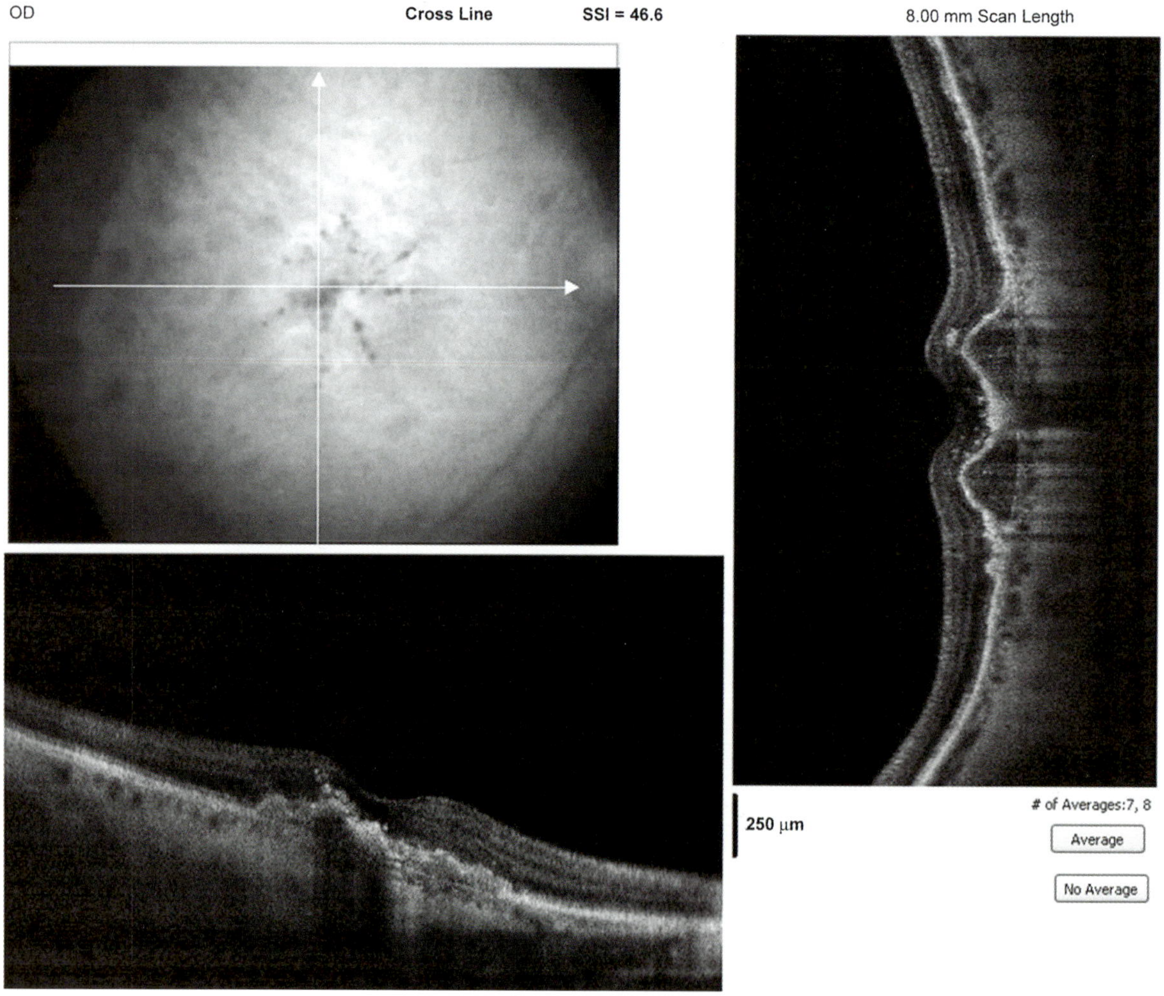

Figure 8: Cross-sectional B scan of turbid (drusenoid) RPE detachment

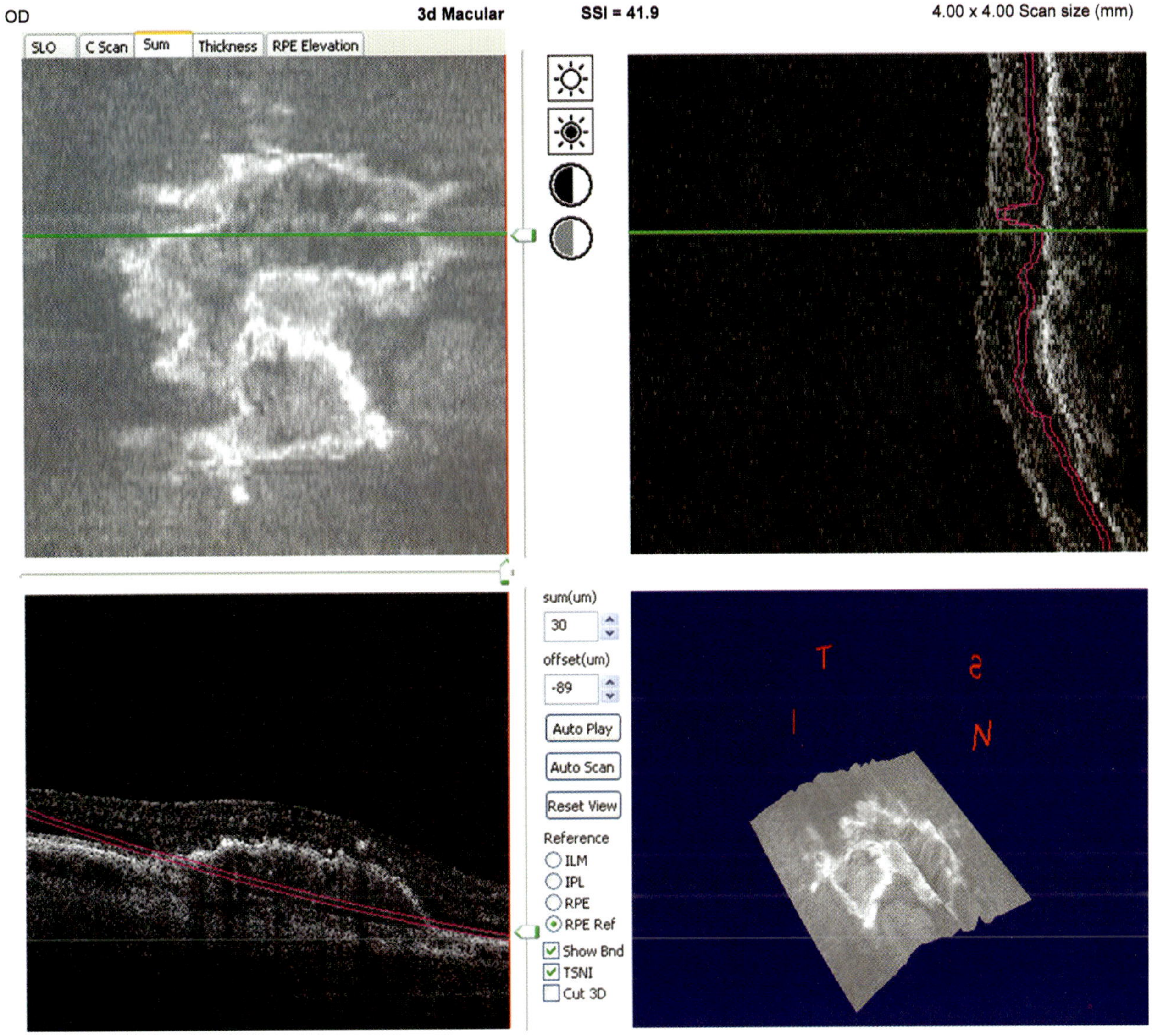

Figure 9: *En face* images of turbid (drusenoid) RPE detachment in the plane between the RPE and IS/OS border

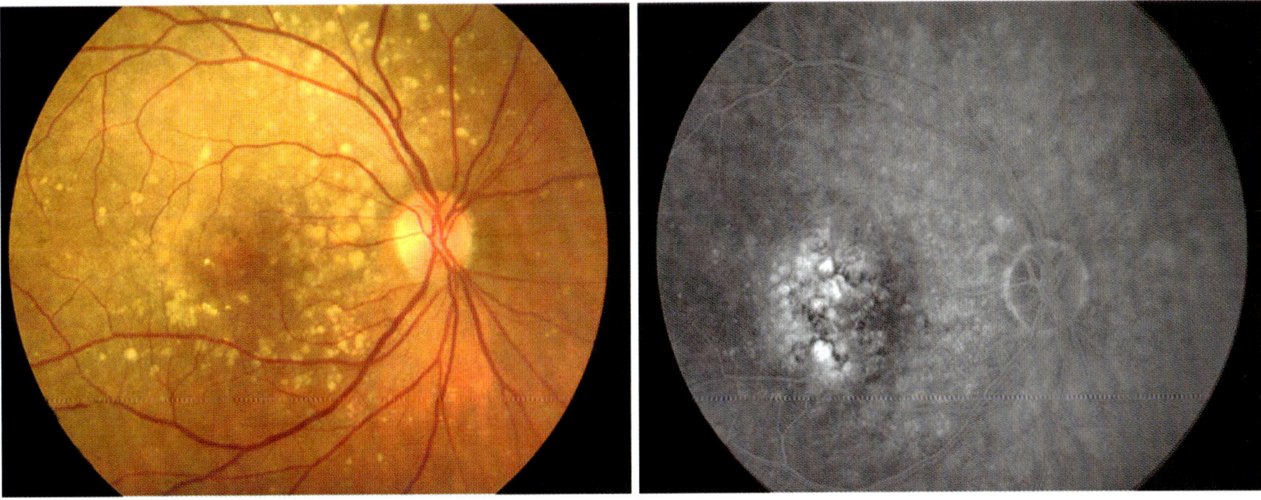

Figure 10: Fundus photograph (left) and fluorescein angiogram (right) containing a mixture of drusen and multiple RPE detachments

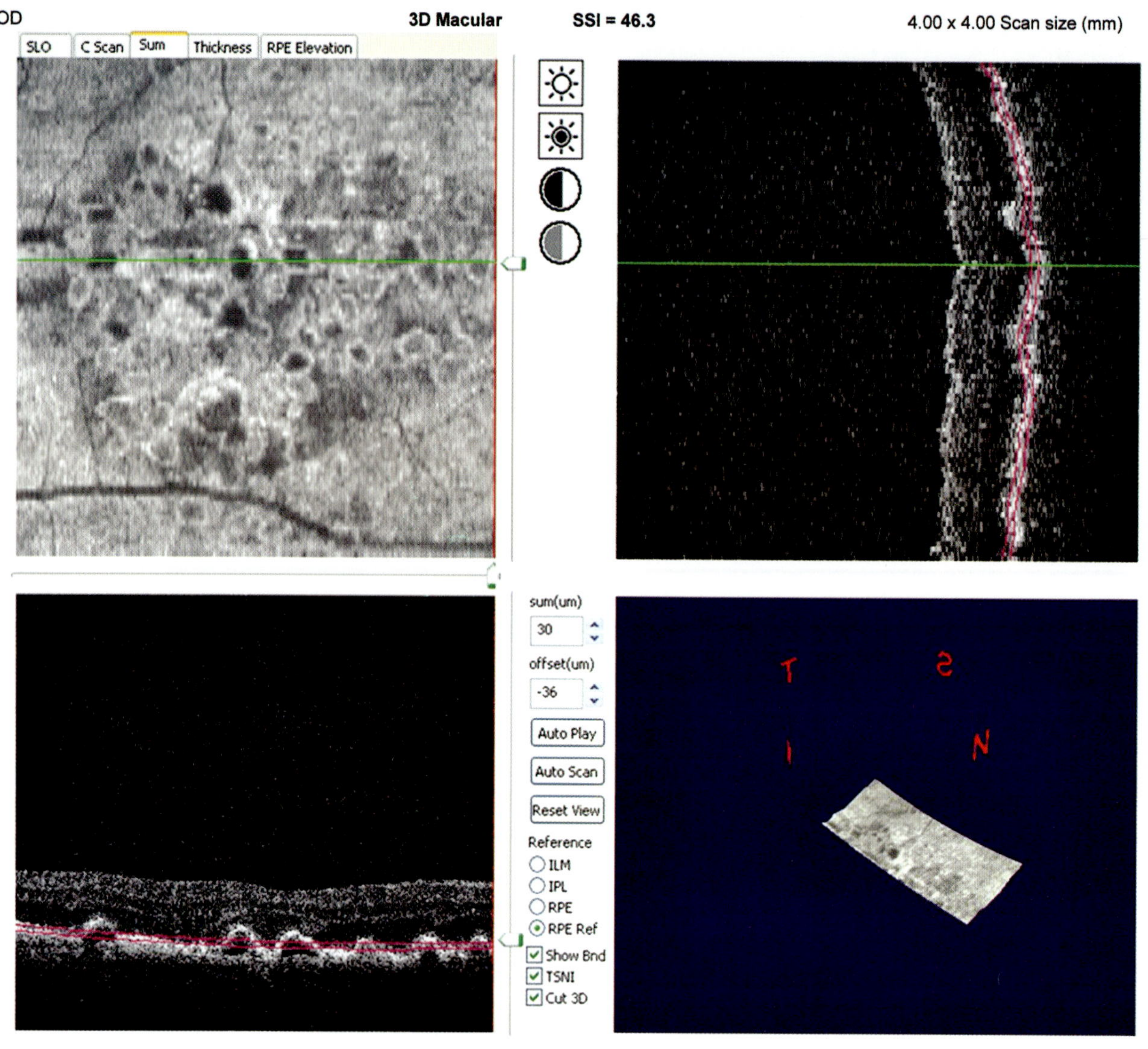

Figure 11: *En face* images showing a combination of drusen and RPEDs

differentiate between the two. Investigators have noted that a notch in the PED on OCT separating the lesion into multiple mounds may be an indication of underlying CNV.[11]

Figures 10 and 11 denote a patient with mixed drusen and multiple small RPEDs. Given that evolution of RPED may be part of a spectrum between hard drusen and exudative changes,[3,5,6] it is common to see a variegated picture such as this.

References

1. Sarks SH, Arnold JJ, Killingsworth MC, et al. Early drusen formation in the normal and aging eye and their relationship to age related maculopathy: a clinicopathological study. Br J Ophthalmol. 1999;83:358-68.
2. Sarks SH. Drusen and their relationship to senile macular degeneration. Aust J Ophthalmol. 1980;8:117-30.
3. Sarks JP, Sarks SH, Killingsworth MC. Evolution of soft drusen in age-related macular degeneration. Eye. 1994;8: 269-83.
4. Young RW. Pathophysiology of age-related macular degeneration. Surv Ophthalmol. 1987;31(5):291-306.
5. Sarks SH, Van Driel D, Maxwell L, et al. Softening of drusen and subretinal neovascularization. Trans Ophthalmol Soc UK. 1980;100(3):414-22.
6. Sarks SH. Council lecture. Drusen and their relationship to senile macular degeneration. Aust J Ophthalmol. 1980;8(2):117-30.
7. Morse PH, Torczynski E, Kumar M. Drusen and drusenoid macular lesions. Ann Ophthalmol. 1988;20(9):327-31.
8. El Baba F, Green WR, Fleischmann J, et al. Clinicopathologic correlation of lipidization and detachment of

the retinal pigment epithelium. Am J Ophthalmol. 1986;101(5):576-83.

9. Jain N, Farsiu S, Khanifar AA, et al. Quantitative comparison of drusen segmented on SD-OCT versus drusen delineated on color fundus photographs. Invest Ophthalmol Vis Sci. 2010;51(10):4875-83.

10. Bressler NM, Silva JC, Bressler SB, et al. Clinicopathologic correlation of drusen and retinal pigment epithelial abnormalities in age-related macular degeneration. Retina. 1994;14(2):130-42.

11. Sato T, Iida T, Hagimura N, et al. Correlation of optical coherence tomography with angiography in retinal pigment epithelial detachment associated with age-related macular degeneration. Retina. 2004;24(6):910-14.

Spectral Domain Optical Coherence Tomography and Drusen: The *En Face* Modality

Chiara M Eandi, Camilla Alovisi,
Federico Tridico, Federico M Grignolo

Introduction

Drusen are focal deposits of extracellular substances located between the basal lamina of the retinal pigment epithelium (RPE) and the inner collagenous layer of the Bruch's membrane found in normal aged human eyes and in eyes with age-related macular degeneration (AMD).[1]

Various types of drusen have been described: small or large drusen, hard or soft drusen, cuticular or basal laminar drusen and reticular pseudodrusen. Hard and soft drusen are the hallmarks of dry age-related maculopathy. Cuticular or basal laminar drusen are frequently associated with pseudovitelliform detachment of the fovea.[2]

The reticular pseudodrusen are instead a particular type of drusen found above the RPE in the subretinal space. Therefore they are also called subretinal drusen or subretinal drusenoid deposits.[3,4]

The availability of spectral domain optical coherence tomography (SD-OCT) has improved visualization and delineation of retinal substructures in a noninvasive way. Recently, a new imaging ocular method was introduced by combining OCT with transverse confocal analysis.[5]

The coronal images or C scans can give to the operator an *en face* image of the retina and its abnormality. In particular, the cross section images (B scan) are generated from a sequence of A scans (depth reflectivity profiles), while the C scans are the sum of several T scans (transversal scans). The sum of the C scan planes forms an *en face* image. The SD-OCTs have been developed to simultaneously acquire *en face* images and corresponding confocal ophthalmoscopic images along with B scans at specifiable locations on the confocal image.[6,7]

Analysis of drusen is not only based on two-dimensional (2D) B scan, but also on 3D scan. This protocol of acquisition allows to measure the volume of the drusen giving a more reliable quantitative assessment of AMD. Moreover, with the *en face* modality it is possible to calculate both manually and automatically, the area of the RPE elevation.

Small or Hard Drusen

These are clearly visible on fundus biomicroscopy and fluorescein angiography in the mid-periphery. They appear as punctiform hyper-reflective spots on infra-red (IR) images, while are barely detected on fundus autofluorescence (FAF) and OCT. B scans demonstrate an irregular profile of the RPE layer and the outer nuclear layer and external limiting membrane (ELM) are slightly modified. The *en face* image shows punctiform hyper-reflective spots with lower reflectivity in the central portion corresponding to hard drusen (**Figures 1A to E**). They are generally stable and can transform into typical soft drusen after many years.

Large or Soft Drusen

In ophthalmoscopic examination soft drusen appear pale yellow with irregular and poorly demarcated contours. On fluorescein angiography they stain late without leakage, while on ICG angiography remain hypofluorescent throughout the examination. On SD-OCT, B scans demonstrate an elevation of the RPE with moderately reflective cavity corresponding to the soft drusen. Over the dome of the RPE elevation are visible irregularities, disruptions and thickening of the inner segment/outer segment (IS/OS) of the photoreceptors interface, leaving Bruch's membrane visible without

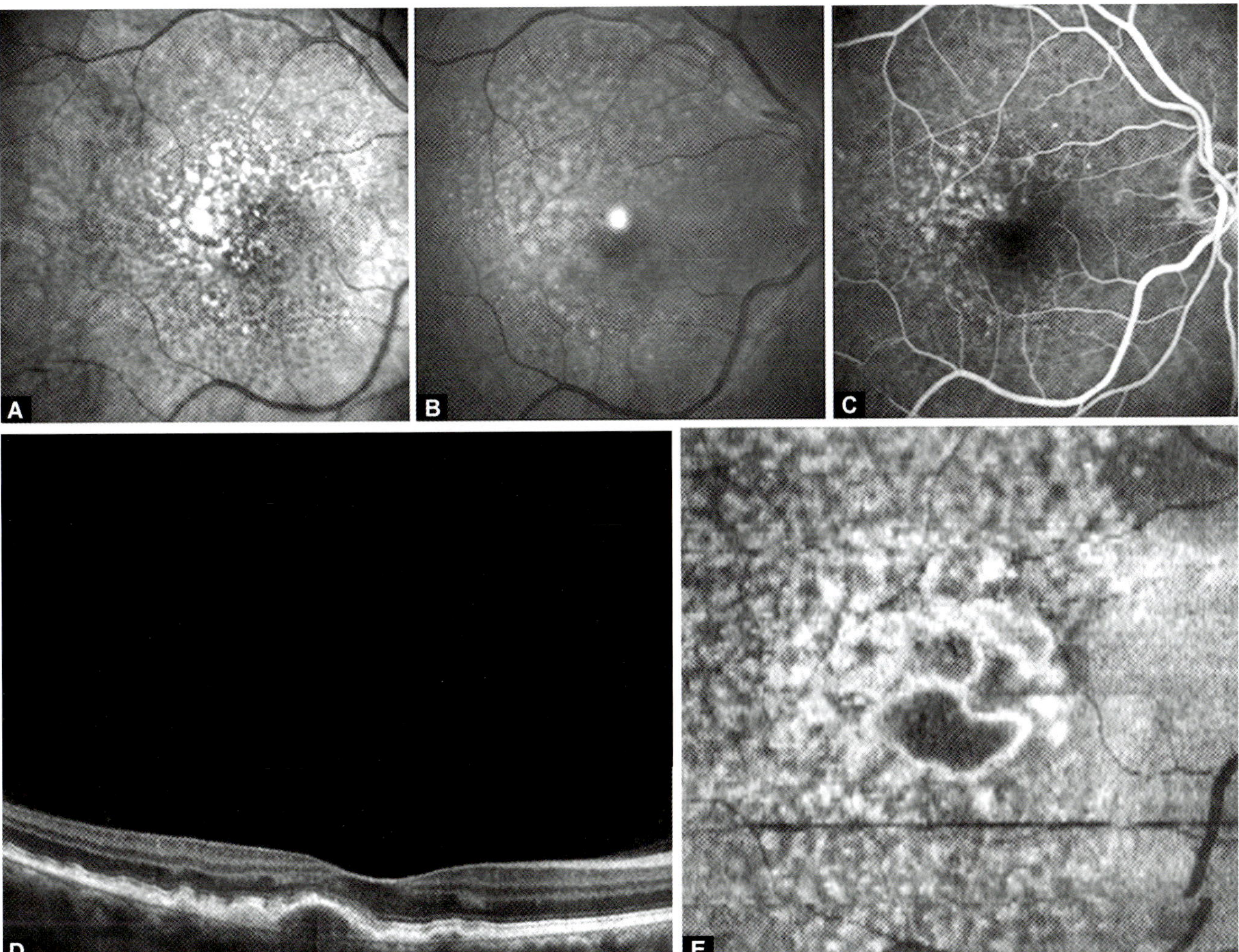

Figures 1A to E: A 68-year-old female with soft drusen in the center of the macula and hard drusen in the mid-periphery. (A) Infra-red, (B) blu light, and (C) fluorescein angiography show hyperfluorescent punctiform and larger spots in the macular area corresponding to hard and soft drusen, respectively. (D) B scan SD-OCT demonstrates dome-shaped elevations of the retinal pigment epithelium caused by underlying accumulation of material in the center of the macula corresponding to soft drusen, while in the mid-periphery is evident an altered profile of the retinal pigment epithelium, photoreceptor and external limiting membrane layers corresponding to hard drusen. (E) The *en face* SD-OCT image in the foveal area reveals the typical aspect of the RPE detachment with hyper-reflective circular and uniform contours and hypofluorescent central area, while in the mid-periphery are evident hyper-reflective punctiform spots at the level of the RPE corresponding to hard drusen

shadowing. Their dimensions can vary and often can become confluent. The IS/OS junction and ELM remain visible and continuous, but the outer nuclear layer appears to be displaced and thinned over the drusen with the typical jagged appearance/profile. *En face* scan shows the characteristic aspect of the RPE detachment with circular shape, uniform aspect of the wall, smooth inner silhouette, and slightly flare content. The boundaries are hyper-reflective, while the center is hypofluorescent or mild hyperfluorescent depending on the content (**Figures 1A to E**). Soft drusen are associated with an increasing risk of neovascular or atrophic AMD.

Cuticular or Basal Laminar Drusen

These are mainly composed of lipoproteins located between the RPE basement membrane and the inner collagenous layer of Bruch's membrane. Localization and composition of cuticular drusen seem to be similar to hard drusen in AMD. Clinically, they appear as numerous, small, uniformly sized, round, yellow, subretinal lesions. On fluorescein angiography they have the characteristic stars-in-the-sky appearance with early fluorescence.[8] B scans SD-OCT reveal hyper-reflectivity and a sawtooth appearance.[9] The overlying retina has a

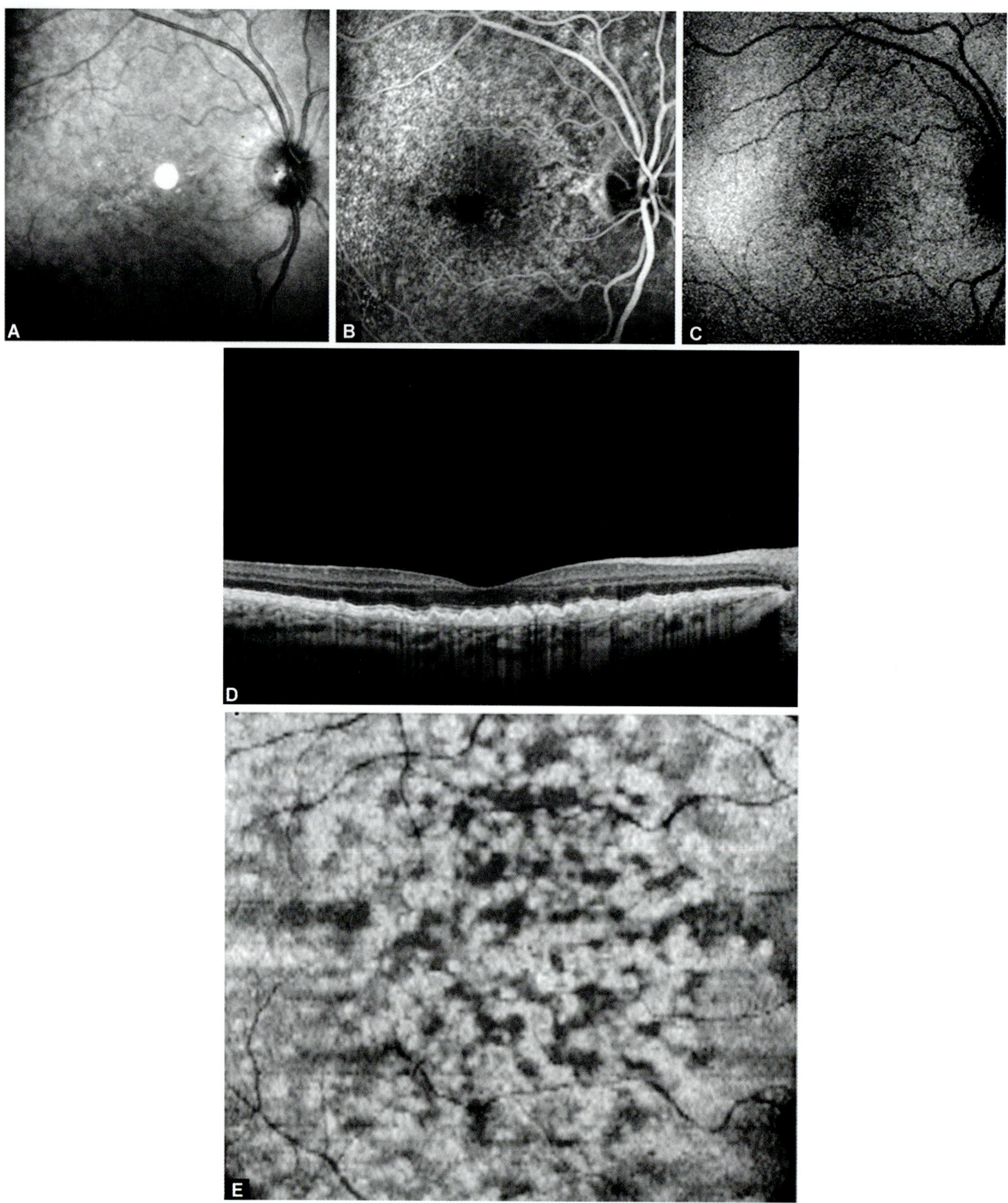

Figures 2A to E: A 53-year-old female with cuticular drusen in the mid-periphery. (A) Infra-red, and (B) fluorescein angiography show hyperfluorescent punctiform spots in the mid-periphery corresponding to cuticular drusen, while fundus autofluorescence (FAF) (C) reveals fine granular alterations. (D) B scan SD-OCT demonstrates an altered profile of the retinal pigment epithelium, photoreceptor and external limiting membrane layers with a "sawtooth" appearance corresponding to cuticular drusen. (E) The *en face* OCT reveals the characteristic aspect of hyper-reflective spots at the level of the retinal pigment epithelium on a "stars-like pattern" similar to the fluorangiographic and IR pattern

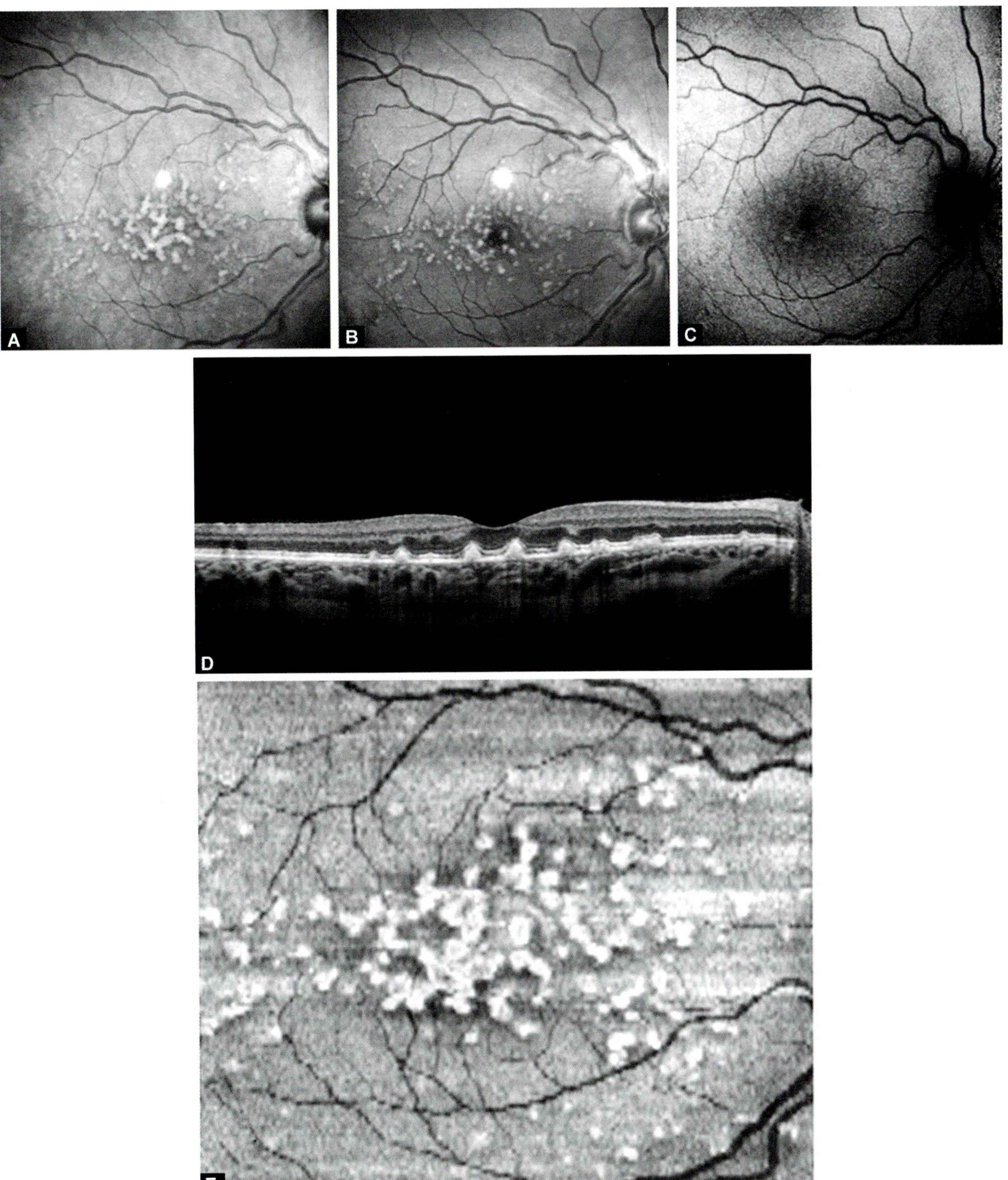

Figures 3A to E: A 33-year-old female presents subretinal drusenoid deposits in the macular area. (A) Infra-red and (B) blu light images show hyper-reflective small areas corresponding to pseudodrusen. (C) Fundus autofluorescence cannot visualize these alterations. (D) B scan SD-OCT is typical and demonstrates the presence of hyper-reflective material above the RPE in the subretinal space. (E) _En face_ OCT image shows hyper-reflective spots similar to infra-red pattern

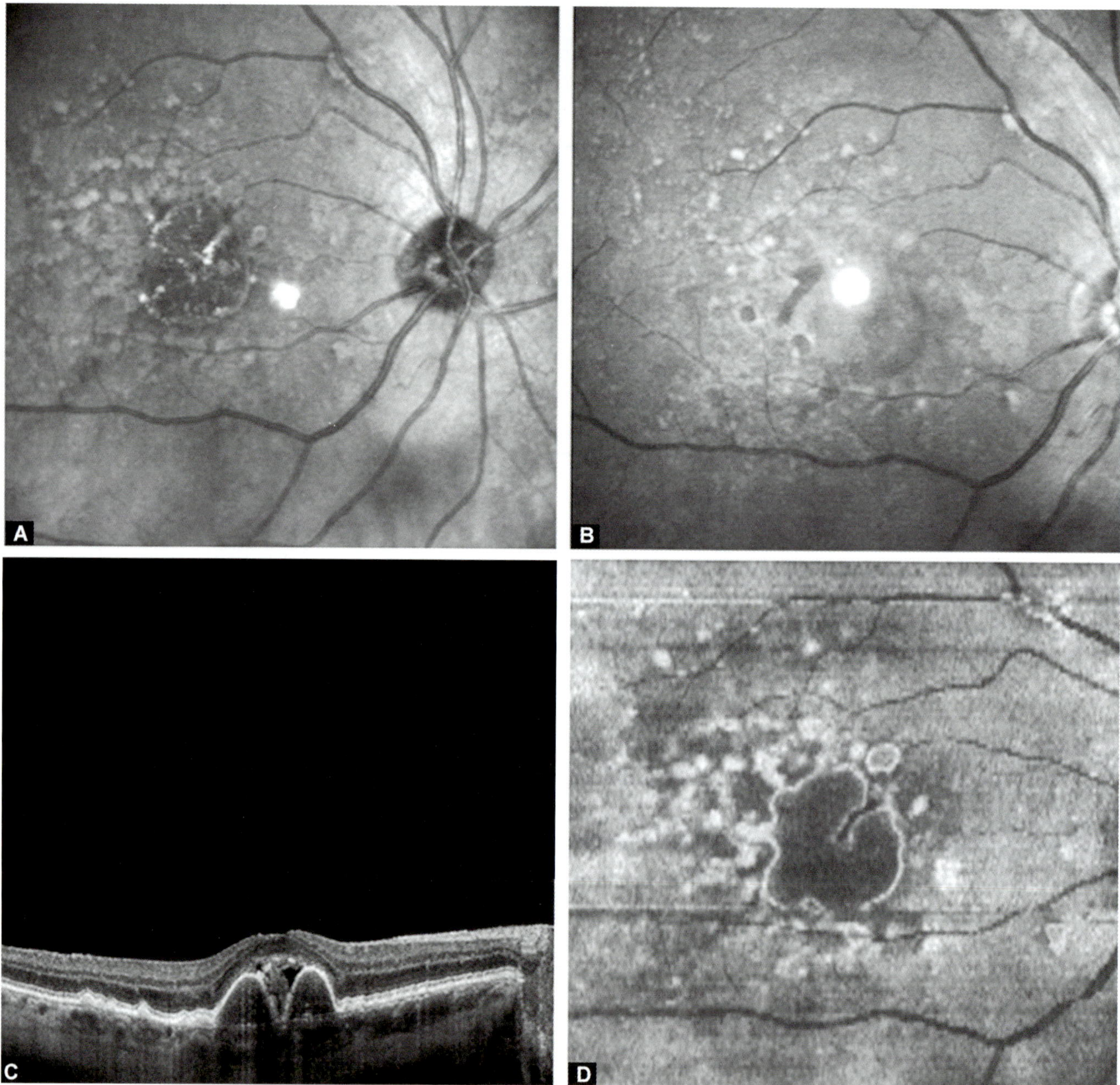

Figures 4A to D: A 74-year-old male presents drusenoid retinal pigment epithelial (RPE) detachment in the macular area. (A) Infra-red and (B) blu light images show drusenoid RPE detachment with hyper-reflective boundaries and hypofluorescent central portion. (C) B scan SD-OCT demonstrates dome-shaped elevations of the RPE secondary to accumulation of material. In the subretinal space above the RPE detachment is also evident hyper-reflective foci and alterations at the level of the outer retina layers. Irregularities of the RPE, IS/OS junction are present in the temporal portion of the macular region. (D) *En face* SD-OCT image shows the typical aspect of the RPE detachment with hyper-reflective circular and uniform contours and hypofluorescent central area. Hyper-reflective punctiform spots are visible in the adjacent area corresponding to drusen decreased thickness. The *en face* images show the same stars-in-the-sky pattern with multiple hyper-reflective spots (**Figures 2A to E**). These lesions are more frequently associated with adult onset vitelliform dystrophy.[9]

Reticular Pseudodrusen

These are usually adjacent to the temporal vascular arcade and easily visible on blue light. However, SD-OCT can detect the reticular pseudodrusen more frequently than the blu channel of color photographs.[3] SD-OCT shows the deposit material above the level of the RPE in the subretinal space, and not under the RPE as characteristic of the small drusen. Moreover, on SD-OCT is visible a thickening and undulation at the level of the RPE, but with no alteration of the outer nuclear layer. *En face* SD-OCT image shows hyper-reflective spots corresponding to the deposit material of pseudodrusen similar to the fluorangiographic and IR pattern (**Figures 3A to E**). Reticular pseudodrusen represent an additional risk factor for wet AMD.

Drusenoid Retinal Pigment Epithelium Detachment (Figures 4A to D)

As drusen increase in size, not only the RPE layer, IS/OS interface and ELM can appear irregular, thinned, and disrupted, but also the outer nuclear layer. They might represent a sign of photoreceptor damage. *En face* SD-OCT shows similar findings of soft drusen with larger dimension

of the RPE elevation. With this modality the extension of the RPE detachment is more clearly delineated than with other imaging techniques.

References

1. Spaide RF, Curcio CA. Drusen characterization with multimodal imaging. Retina. 2010;30(9):1441-54.
2. Yannuzzi LA. The Retinal Atlas. Saunders Elsevier 2010.
3. Zweifel SA, Spaide RF, Curcio CA. Reticular pseudodrusen and subretinal drusenoid deposits. Ophthalmology. 2010;117(2):303-12.e1.
4. Querques G, Querques L, Martinelli D, et al. Pathologic insights from integrated imaging of reticular pseudodrusen in Age-Related Macular Degeneration. Retina. 2011;31(3):518-26.
5. Podoleanu AG, Dobre GM, Cucu RC, et al. Combined multiplanar optical coherence tomography and confocal scanning ophthalmoscopy. J Biomed Opt. 2004;9:86-93.
6. Wanek J, Zelkha R, Lim JI, et al. Feasibility of a method for *en face* imaging of photoreceptor cell integrity. Am J Ophthalmol. 2011;152(5):807-14e1. Epub 2011 Jul 20.
7. Srinivasan VJ, Adler DC, Chen Y. Ultrahigh-speed optical coherence tomography for three-dimensional and en-face imaging of the retina and optic nerve head. Invest Ophthalmol Vis Sci. 2008;49(11):5103-10. Epub 2008 Jul 24.
8. Leng T, Rosenfeld PJ, Gregari G, et al. Spectral domain optical coherence tomography characteristics of cuticular drusen. Retina. 2009;29:988-93.
9. Finger RP, Charbel Issa P, et al. Spectral domain optical coherence tomography in adult-onset vitelliform macular dystrophy with cuticular drusen. Retina. 2010;30: 1455-64.

chapter 18

En Face Imaging of Reticular Pseudodrusen

Mahsa Sohrab, Srinivas R Sadda, Amani A Fawzi

Introduction

Reticular pseudodrusen, first identified on blue-light fundus photography,[1] are yellow, faint, interlacing networks originally associated with the development of neovascular age-related macular degeneration (AMD),[2-5] but subsequently found to confer an increased risk of developing both atrophic and neovascular AMD.[6] Given the association of reticular pseudodrusen with poor prognosis in AMD and with higher mortality overall as compared to other AMD patients,[6] an improved understanding of the pathogenesis of these deposits is critical. The origin of these deposits remains unclear, with original histopathology localizing these changes to the choroid,[2] though newer optical coherence tomography (OCT) studies have described subretinal deposits.[7,8]

Advances in retinal imaging have led to improvements in surgeons understanding of AMD, with current techniques allowing improved visualization of the choroid.[9] In this chapter, authors review the multimodal imaging characteristics of reticular pseudodrusen and the use of *en face* OCT imaging to study choroidal changes in association with the development and progression of reticular pseudodrusen.

Multimodal Imaging of Reticular Pseudodrusen

Early characterizations of reticular pseudodrusen (RPD) relied on color fundus and red-free photography, where they were identified as indistinct, interlacing, yellowish or light lesions in the outer macula.[2,4] However, the more peripheral location of RPD, in contrast to the typical central soft drusen associated with AMD, as well as their faint appearance on color fundus imaging, led to diagnostic challenges. The advent of scanning laser ophthalmoscopic imaging allowed for improved identification of RPD, which appeared as groupings of hypofluorescent or hyporeflective lesions on autofluorescence (AF) and infra-red (IR) imaging, respectively.[4] Indocyanine green (ICG) angiography of RPD demonstrated hypofluorescent dots in the mid-to-late-phases of the angiogram.[3,4] Correlations of the multimodal imaging findings are associated with RPD using automated image registration related their presence to alterations in the retinal pigment epithelium (RPE) and inner choroid.[4]

Improved visualization of the RPE and choroid through OCT has led to better definitions of RPD. Studies using the Heidelberg Spectralis spectral-domain OCT (SD-OCT) have suggested that RPD may correlate with granular hyper-reflective deposits in the subretinal space.[7,8] Most recently, surgeons group developed a novel technique using *en face* cross-sections of the choroid (C scans) obtained on the Cirrus high definition OCT (HD-OCT) device (Carl Zeiss Meditec, Inc., Dublin, CA) to reveal choroidal changes associated with the presence of RPD, implicating the choroid in the pathogenesis of this disease process.[10]

En Face Imaging of Reticular Pseudodrusen

Image Acquisition

Patients identified as having reticular pseudodrusen on the basis of characteristic imaging findings described above were imaged on the Cirrus HD-OCT Model 4000 device, using superluminescent diode (SLD) light source at 840 nm, which achieves 5 µm of axial and 15 µm of transverse tissue resolution. The device captures 27,000 A scans per second at 2 mm of depth, and the images were viewed with the Cirrus HD-OCT software (v 5.0; Carl Zeiss Meditec Inc.). As part of authors standard Cirrus imaging protocol, all eyes underwent two scanning protocols: a five-line raster consisting

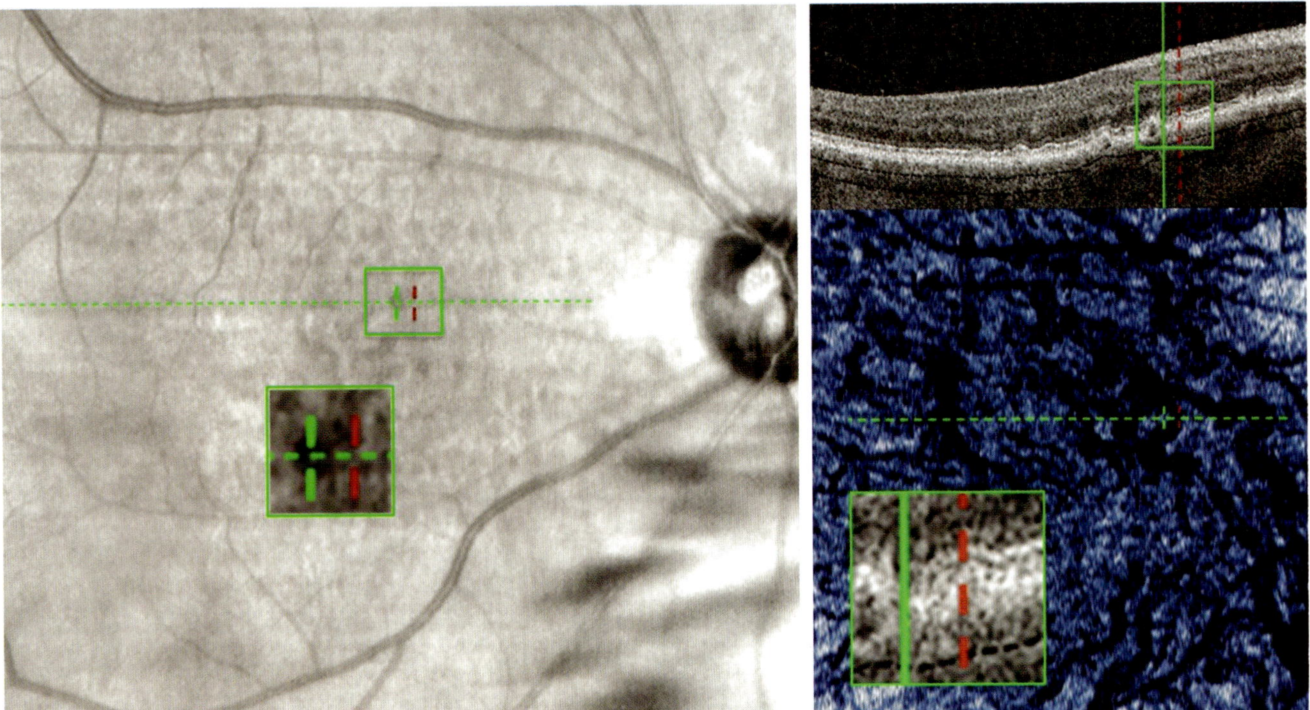

Figure 1: Individual RPD in the right eye of a patient correlates to the choroidal stroma on OCT *en face* imaging. Contrast-enhanced infrared (IR) image from the right eye of a patient with RPD (left), horizontal OCT B scan (top right), and *en face* pseudocolorized choroidal section (bottom right) are displayed. Dashed green horizontal line in the IR and choroidal sections are registered to the horizontal OCT B scan. The registered green vertical marker on IR overlies an individual RPD lesion, which in turn corresponds to an area adjacent to inner segment/outer segment (IS/OS) change on OCT (green vertical line, top right) and to choroidal stroma on *en face* imaging (green vertical marker, bottom right). The registered red vertical marker on IR lies adjacent to the selected RPD lesion, which in turn corresponds to IS/OS change on the horizontal OCT B scan (dashed red line, top right) and to a large choroidal vessel on *en face* imaging (red marker, bottom right). The areas of interest on the IR and OCT B scan are highlighted as magnified insets

of 4096 A scans for each of the five B scans and a 512 × 128 macular cube volume scan consisting of 128 equally spaced horizontal B scans (each composed of 512 A scans) over a 6 mm square grid. The line scanning laser ophthalmoscope (LSLO) feature also obtained a registered OCT fundus image for each data cube. The Cirrus OCT imaging protocol in surgeons imaging unit also required photographers to repeat OCT volume scans if the summed OCT projection image suggested that significant motion artifact was present, and those scans that were free of motion artifact were selected for the study.[10]

Image Analysis

Each OCT volume scan (512 × 128 macular cube) was reviewed on the Cirrus version 5.0 software using the advanced visualization feature. As previously described,[11,12] the RPE feature was used to obtain *en face* slices, or C scans, which were contoured based on each patient's RPE curvature. The horizontal section (slab thickness) was adjusted to ensure that the RPE band or sclera were not included in any of the C scan slabs. The inner aspect of the slab feature was placed at a fixed distance below the RPE band, and then *en face* choroidal slabs of variable thickness (ranging from 20–60 μm) were generated and reviewed for every patient. By using the RPE slice overlay feature, these slabs were reviewed as registered to the Cirrus IR fundus image. Additional *en face* sections including only the inner segment/outer segment (IS/OS) junction and outer nuclear layer were also obtained and overlaid onto the Cirrus IR image for review.[10]

Retinal vessel crossing points were used as invariant landmarks to allow manual registration of the OCT fundus (projection) image with the cSLO IR and AF and red-free images (obtained with either the Spectralis cSLO or Topcon camera). GIMP, a freely available GNU Image Manipulation Program (v 2.6; available from http://www.gimp.org) was used to align and register the images. New drawing layers were then created and the paint brush tool was used to manually segment individual RPD lesions on the IR images, which were then superimposed to the Cirrus OCT C scan slabs to look for correspondence between the RPD lesions on IR images and structures on the OCT.[10]

Findings

Sections of choroid of varying thickness evaluated *en face* (OCT cross-sections) were viewed as OCT slabs registered to IR images on Cirrus HD-OCT and were manually registered to fundus imaging. RPD lesions marked on registered IR,

AF and red-free images followed the pattern of the underlying choroidal stroma on *en face* OCT sections (**Figures 1 and 2**). Individual reticular lesions were found to overly choroidal stroma, closely abutting (but definitely not overlying) larger choroidal vessels. Areas of hyper-reflective subretinal deposits and associated IS/OS disruption frequently occurred directly adjacent to RPD lesions (**Figure 1**). *En face* OCT sections through the IS/OS junction and subretinal space yielded a map of the distribution of these small hyper-reflective deposits. By comparing this map to the IR image, it became

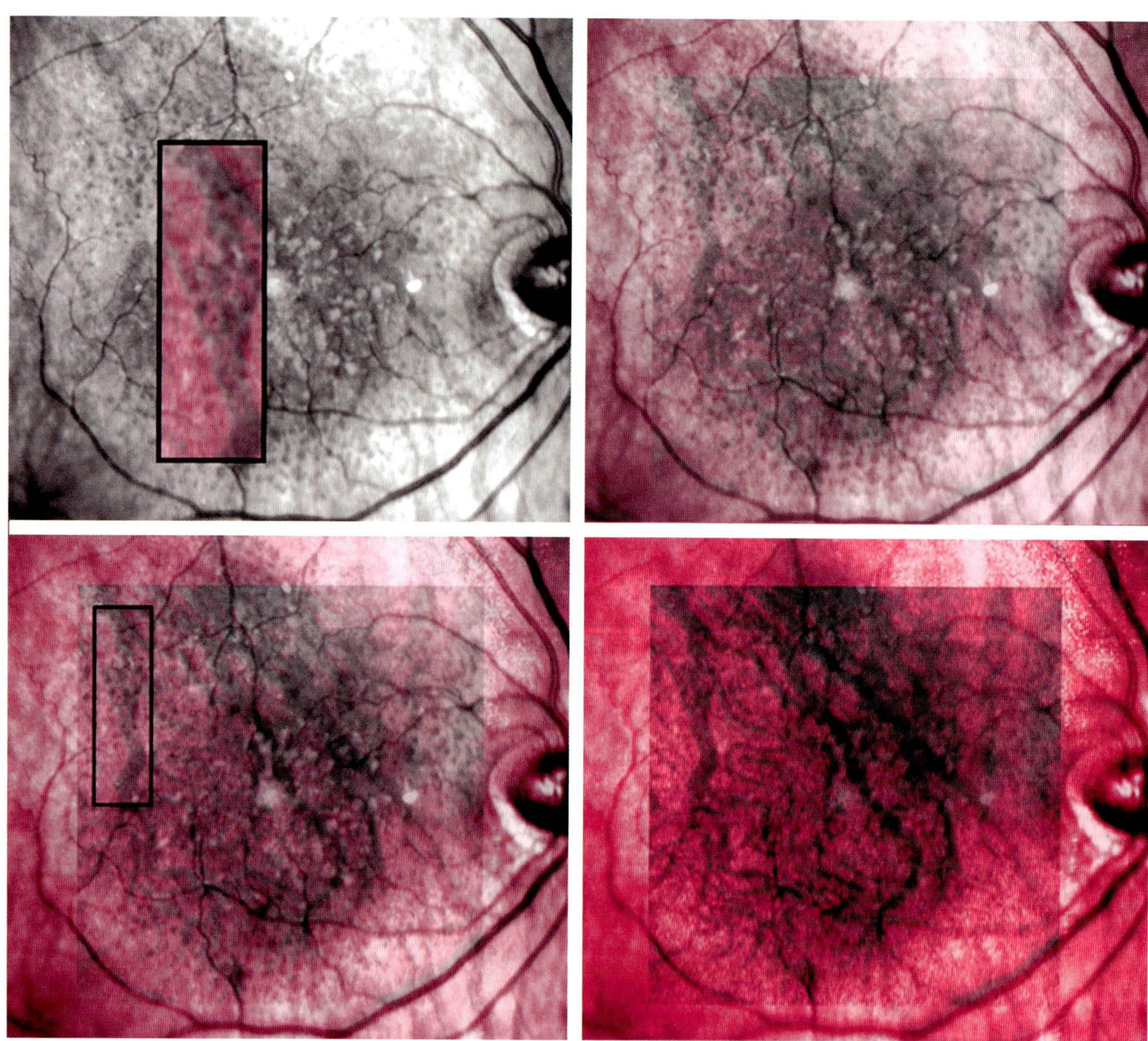

Figure 2: Transitional overlay of *choroidal en face* OCT scan onto the infrared image of the right eye of a patient with RPD shows the alignment of RPD lesions along choroidal vessels. Infrared image of a patient with RPD obtained on the Heidelberg Spectralis device (top left) was manually registered to the *en face* choroidal OCT section reconstructed on the Cirrus device (bottom right). The *en face* choroidal scan was pseudocolorized on GIMP. Transitional overlay of the *en face* OCT section onto the IR at increasing opacities (top right and bottom left, respectively) reveals alignment of RPD lesions with large choroidal vessels, as seen in the magnified inset (from bottom left)

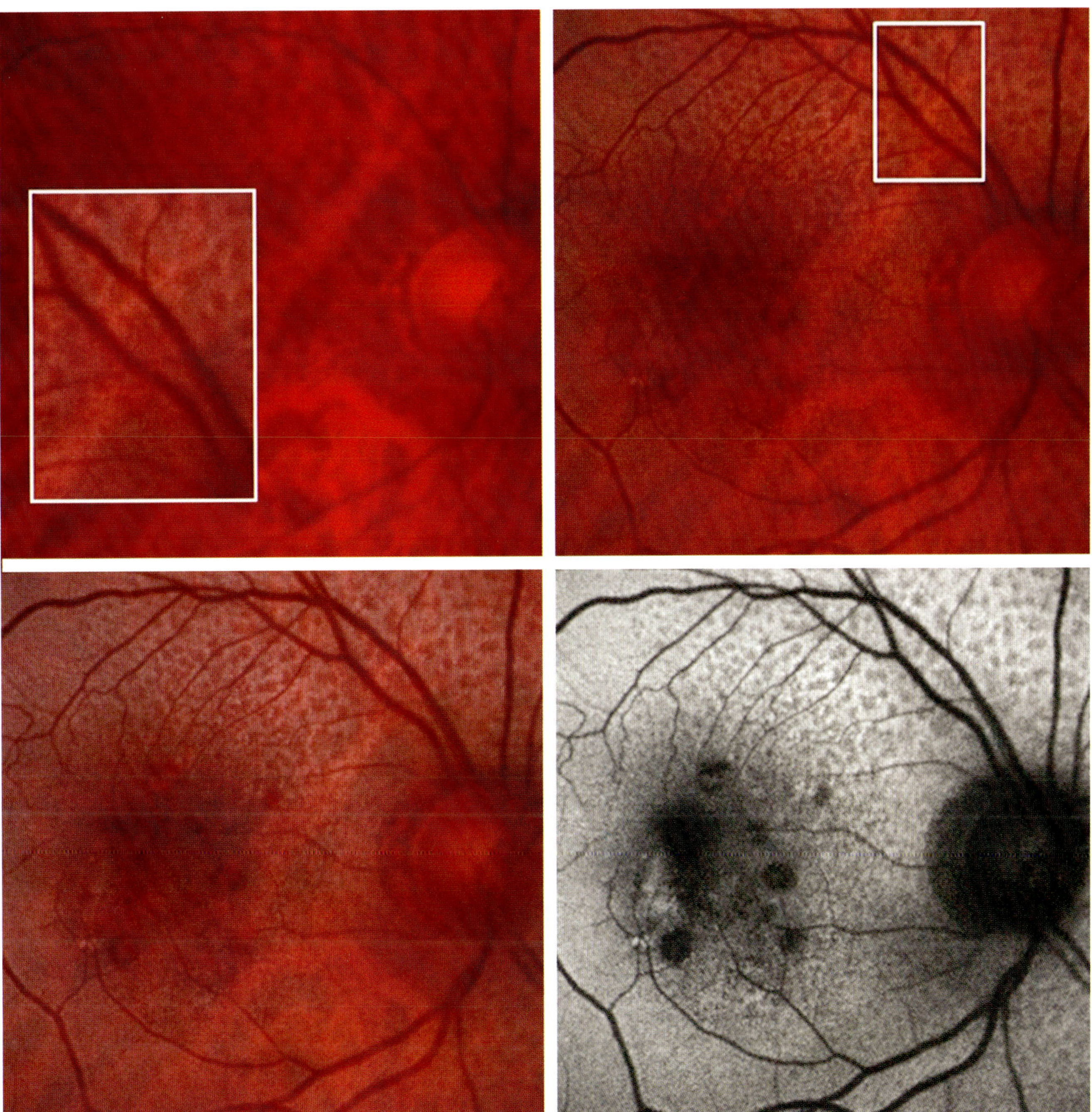

Figure 3: Transitional overlay of autofluorescence (AF) image onto color fundus (CF) image of the right eye of a patient with RPD shows the alignment of RPD lesions along choroidal vessels. CF image with prominent choroidal vasculature was obtained on TopCon 50 xl fundus camera (top left) and contrast-enhanced on GIMP. It was then manually registered to corresponding autofluorescence image (bottom right) obtained on the Heidelberg Spectralis device using retinal vessels as landmarks. Transitional overlay of the AF image onto the CF image at increasing opacities (top right and bottom left, respectively) reveals alignment of RPD lesions along large choroidal vessels, particularly notable superonasally. To better delineate this, the choroidal vessels in the superonasal quadrant of (bottom left) are highlighted with blue tracing. Magnified inset from (top right) further highlights this finding

clear that the subretinal lesions do not correspond to the entire RPD pattern.[10]

When reviewing transitional overlays of varying opacities of choroidal *en face* images obtained on OCT, and manually registered IR, AF and color fundus images, similar associations of reticular patterns with choroidal vessels were noted. These images revealed that groups of reticular lesions closely followed the outline of the large choroidal vessels **(Figures 2 and 3)**. Individual RPD lesions are abutted and appeared to line up along the edges of the choroidal vessels.[10]

Discussion

En face OCT sections of the posterior pole demonstrated that RPD lesions aligned with the choroidal stroma, while the previously reported subretinal hyper-reflective deposits[7,8] were on top of the large choroidal vessels. Surgeons approach uses a high-density map (Cirrus macular cube, 6 × 6 mm) to create an *en face* section of the outer retina and the choroidal vasculature in the entire macula. Authors findings suggest that the RPD lesions most consistently followed the choroidal stroma and that previously reported RPE derangements and subretinal deposits may be secondary pathologic changes.[10] Further studies are needed to correlate these observed choroidal changes to histopathologic findings in RPD.

References

1. Mimoun G, Soubrane G, Coscas G. Macular drusen. J Fr Ophthalmol. 1990;13:511-30.
2. Arnold JJ, Sarks SH, Killingsworth MC, et al. Reticular pseudodrusen: a risk factor in age-related maculopathy. Retina. 1995;15:183-91.
3. Arnold JJ, Quaranta M, Soubrane G, et al. Indocyanine green angiography of drusen. Am J Ophthalmol. 1997; 124:344-56.
4. Cohen SY, Dubois L, Tadayoni R, et al. Prevalence of reticular pseudodrusen in age-related macular degeneration with newly diagnose choroidal neovascularization. Br J Ophthalmol. 2007;91:354-9.
5. Smith RT, Sohrab MA, Busuioc M, et al. Reticular macular disease. Am J Ophthalmol. 2009;148:733-43.
6. Klein R, Davis MD, Magli K, et al. The Wisconsin age-related maculopathy grading system. Ophthalmology. 1991;98:1128-34.
7. Zweifel SA, Spaide RF, Carcio CA, et al. Reticular pseudodrusen are subretinal drusenoid deposits. Ophthalmology. 2010;117:303-12.
8. Schmitz-Valckenberg S, Steinberg JS, Fleckenstein M, et al. Combined confocal scanning laser ophthalmoscopy and spectral-domain optical coherence tomography imaging of reticular pseudodrusen associated with age-related macular degeneration. Opthalmology. 2010;117: 1169-76.
9. Sohrab MA, Wu K, Fawzi AA. Pilot Study of En Face Optical Coherence Tomography of Choroidal Vasculature *in vivo*. PLOS one, in press.
10. Sohrab MA, Smith RT, Salehi-Had H, et al. Image registration and multimodal imaging of reticular pseudodrusen. Invest Ophthalmol Vis Sci. 2011;52:5743-8.
11. Yasuno Y, Miura M, Kawan K, et al. Visualization of subretinal pigment epithelium morphologies of exudative macular diseases by high-penetration optical coherence tomography. Invest Ophthalmol Vis Sci. 2009;50:405-13.
12. Gupta V, Gupta P, Dogra MR, et al. A. Spontaneous closure of retinal pigment epithelium microrip in the natural course of central serous chorioretinopathy. Eye. 2010;24: 595-9.

chapter 19

En Face Optical Coherence Tomography in Age-related Macular Degeneration: Preliminary Results with Spectralis *En Face* Optical Coherence Tomography

Gabriel Coscas, Florence Coscas, Umberto De Benedetto, Eric Souied

What can be Expected from *En Face* Optical Coherence Tomography in Age-related Macular Degeneration?

As a result of progress in imaging, *multimodal* imaging should now be used to obtain maximum information with a minimum of difficulty for patients.

The advantages of *angiography* are well known: safety (millions of examinations have been performed), very widespread availability providing useful information that is easy to interpret.

Optical coherence tomography (OCT) and Spectral domain optical coherence tomography (SD-OCT) have very similar advantages: widespread availability and easy and effective post-treatment follow-up examination; moreover, they are non-invasive techniques.[1] *En face OCT* can probably provide even more information.

The development of *fluorescein angiography* 50 years ago identified various forms of AMD with a "precursor" phase (drusen and pigment changes) and a "degeneration" phase with atrophic (the most frequent) and exudative forms (Exudative forms are characterized by the development of choroidal neovascularization).

Angiography is irreplaceable to visualize the retinal macular capillary bed, to detect and monitor signs of ischemia (absence of macular and/or peripheral perfusion), detect, analyse and monitor "leaks" and compare them with staining or a window defect: it is therefore essential for the diagnosis and follow-up of "active" neovascularization.

Indocyanine green angiography, introduced in 1970, allows imaging through the retinal pigment epithelium (RPE) screen under even better safety conditions by means of infrared light, thereby allowing visualization of the subretinal neovascular membrane [type 1 or occult choroidal neovascularization (CNV)], which is poorly visible on fluorescein angiography, as well as chorioretinal anastomoses and polyps.

Correlations between these two complementary types of angiography are obviously very useful and effective.

Optical coherence tomography (OCT) is a rapidly growing technique that provides particularly detailed images of retinal structures. **Age-related macular degeneration (AMD)** is one of the diseases that have probably derived the greatest benefit from this progress, by defining the clinical features, clinical course and treatment.

Optical coherence tomography (OCT) is **essential** to detect, analyse and monitor the exudative reaction and evaluate the impact of AMD on photoreceptors. Two-dimensional or B-mode anterior-posterior images (Huang, 1991; Fercher and Swanson, 1993) demonstrate the successive retinal layers and RPE and any spaces between these layers, allowing a first approach that is often almost intuitive.

In routine clinical practice, OCT therefore allows evaluation of *variations of thickness* of the retina and analysis of certain *structural changes*.

In particular, these changes consist of fibrovascular pigment epithelium detachments (FVPED),[2,3] serous

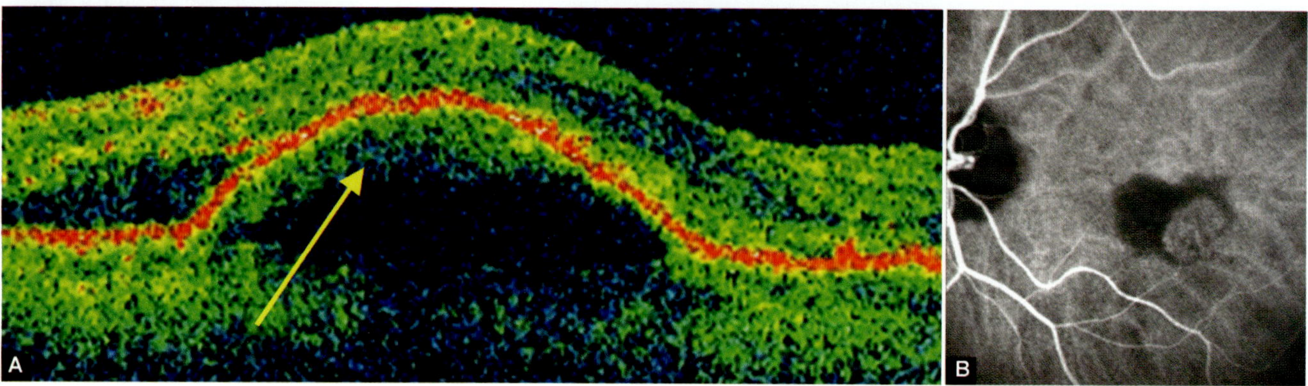

Figures 1A and B: TD-OCT: Fibrovascular pigment epithelium detachment (FVPED). Presence of a thin layer of hyper-reflective tissue posterior to the RPE, suggestive of type 1 occult CNV (*Courtesy:* Coscas F, et al: Am J Ophthalmol, 2007)

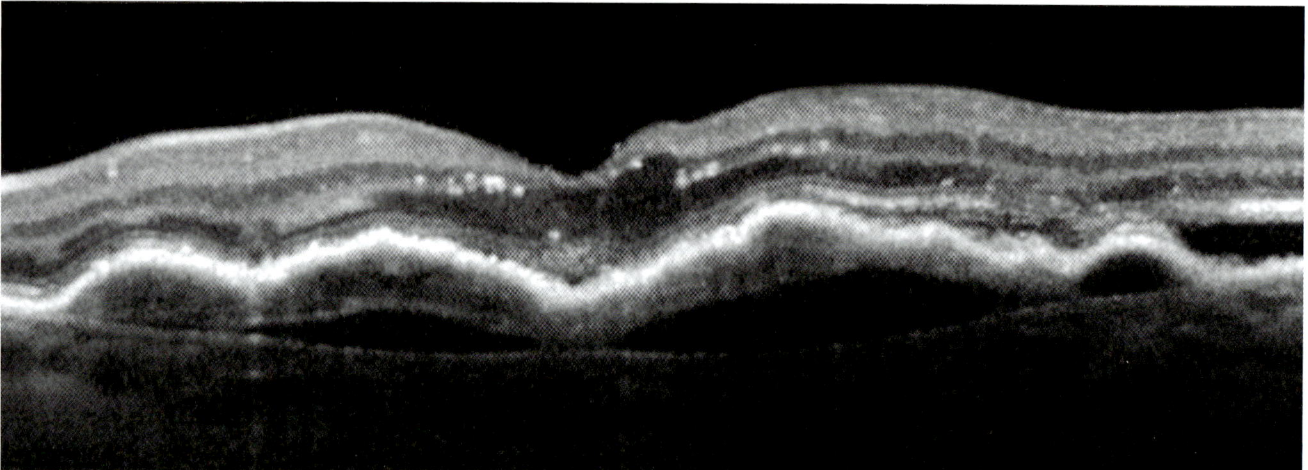

Figure 2: SD-OCT: Fibrovascular pigment epithelium detachment (FVPED) with a thin layer of hyper-reflective tissue posterior to the RPE. Note the hyper-reflective dots in different retinal layers, suggestive of active lesion with inflammatory reaction

detachment of the neurosensory retina (SRD), either isolated or associated with diffuse **fluid** accumulation or cystoid oedema, or **hyper-reflective dots** (suggesting an inflammatory reaction) or other hyper-reflective structures (pigment, fibrosis, exudation, material, etc.), **(Figures 1A and B and 2)** as well as pigment epithelium changes (irregularities and fragmentation).

A new method called *Enhanced Depth Imaging (EDI)*, has been proposed to improve depth imaging allowing visualization of all of the choroid.[2]

OCT is extremely useful to define modern treatment indications by intravitreous injections and especially for post-treatment follow-up in parallel with functional evaluation. Nevertheless, *CNV and the choroidal new vessels* have not been directly visible on OCT. *Time domain optical coherence tomography (TD-OCT)* can demonstrate the presence of a fine layer of hyper-reflective tissue posterior to the RPE, suggestive of type 1 occult CNV.[3]

This finding is also observed on *SD-OCT* and EDI[2] **(Figure 2)**.

However, this separate analysis of the various structures and changes observed on an OCT section is obviously *schematic* and somewhat arbitrary, as pathological lesions only very rarely involve a single layer or a single tissue.

Furthermore, interpretation of localized lesions *must take into account changes in adjacent structures and their interactions.*

En Face Optical Coherence Tomography

A new approach to OCT imaging, called En face OCT, combines OCT and monochromatic or angiographic confocal scanning Laser Ophthalmoscope (SLO) analysis.

En face OCT simultaneously provides longitudinal images (B-scans) and transverse images (C scans or frontal scans) of the macular region with very good pixel-to-pixel correspondence.

These *En face* images (C scans) reconstructed from EDI-OCT B scans allow *segmentation* of subretinal and preretinal changes associated with many retinal diseases such as AMD in the various planes of the retina, choroid and CNV.[4]

Authors' Experience

This study was based on a series of 157 patients with different patterns of AMD undergoing a complete assessment by fluorescein angiography and SLO-ICG as well as SD-OCT with eye tracking (Spectralis).[5]

This OCT examination comprised the acquisition, over 1 minute, of an adjustable volume of *97 horizontal B scans*, with a field of 20° × 15°, a slice increment of 30 μm and enhancement by fusion of 9 Automatic Real Time (ART) and EDI images (better visualization of the choroid).

This 3D volume generates *496 C scan frontal sections,* analysed either on a **video** or on still (frozen) images, that can be analysed either separately or by selecting a particular plane of section.

Complementary imaging was performed either on the reference infrared image or on SLO-ICG to confirm and compare the 2 types of imaging.

Interpretation *of frontal sections* of the retina must take into account the concavity of the eye and the fact that the layers of the retina all around a prominent or depressed lesion will be visualized as easily identifiable *concentric hypo- or hyper-reflective bands* **(Figure 3).**

Techniques allowing tracking of the **curvature of the posterior pole** are often used, but they are especially useful when the retina is flat, but less efficient in case of elevated lesions.

The use of *simple frontal sections* therefore comprises these concentric layers, which may initially appear to be unusual, but which can actually be used as **localization markers**.

Other segmentation techniques (Spectralis) using the *"flattened" RPE* as landmark can be used to recenter the images, when necessary, and avoid the disadvantages related to curvature of the eye **(Figures 4A and B).**

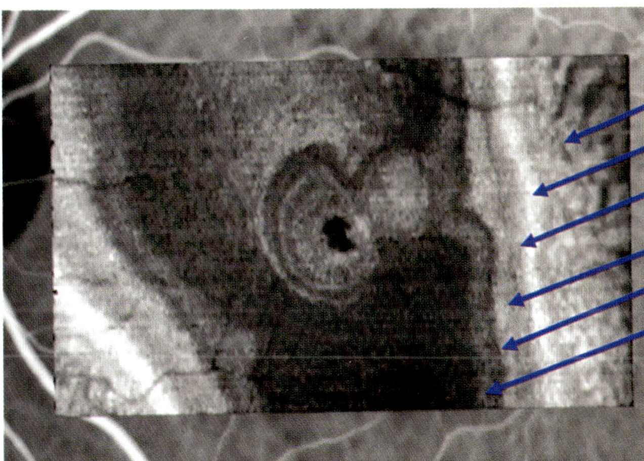

Figure 3: Interpretation of frontal sections of the retina (patient with juxtafoveolar classic CNV): The layers of the retina all around a prominent or depressed lesion are visualized as easily identifiable concentric hyporeflective or hyper-reflective bands

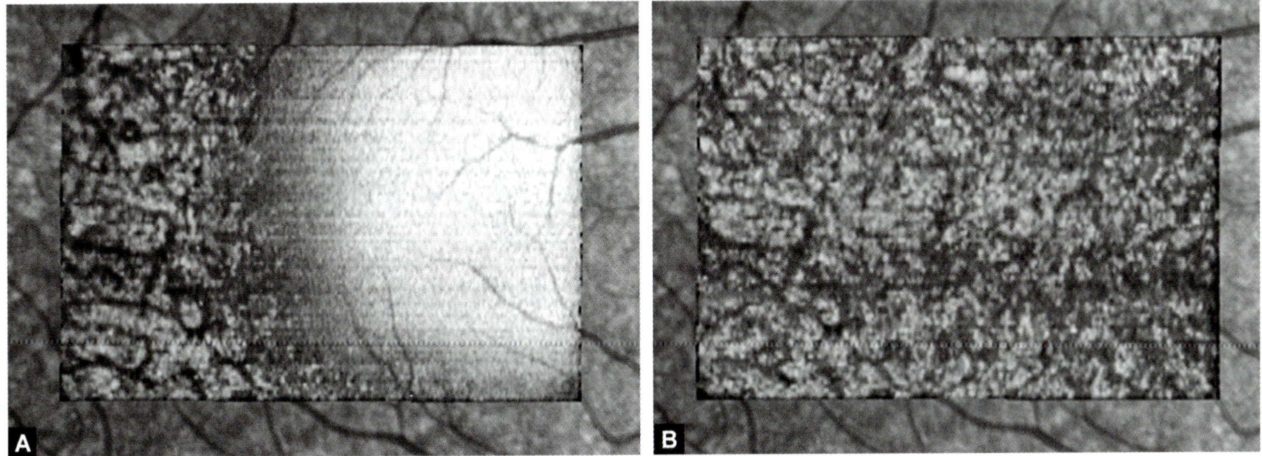

Figures 4A and B: Comparison of a simple frontal section and a section aligned on the plane of the RPE, in the choriocapillaris layer

However, this approach implies the preliminary choice of a plane of segmentation: either the RPE (or Bruch's membrane), or possibly the retina-vitreous interface.

This technique, still under development, will be useful to analyse the choriocapillaris and choroid. The analysis of selected frozen images from the video of any clinical case will be very helpful.

1. Drusen

Here is an example of clinical case with many, soft, large and confluent drusen will help to analyse the location, the shape and the contours of each drusen.

Soft drusen are usually ill-delimited with fuzzy borders, but will appear in *En face* OCT, with hyper-reflective and nicely visible limits that could allow easy analysis of their area and all changes during follow up.

The contents of each drusen is clearly visible as a homogenous (or not) material and the drusen location is in front of the Bruch's membrane.

During the video and on the frozen images, it is possible to *recognize successively* the optic fibers and the retinal vessels, the center of the fovea, the dome of different drusen, and their limits and content. Finally, the RPE layer, the Bruch's membrane and the choriocapillaris become visible **(Figures 5A to F)**.

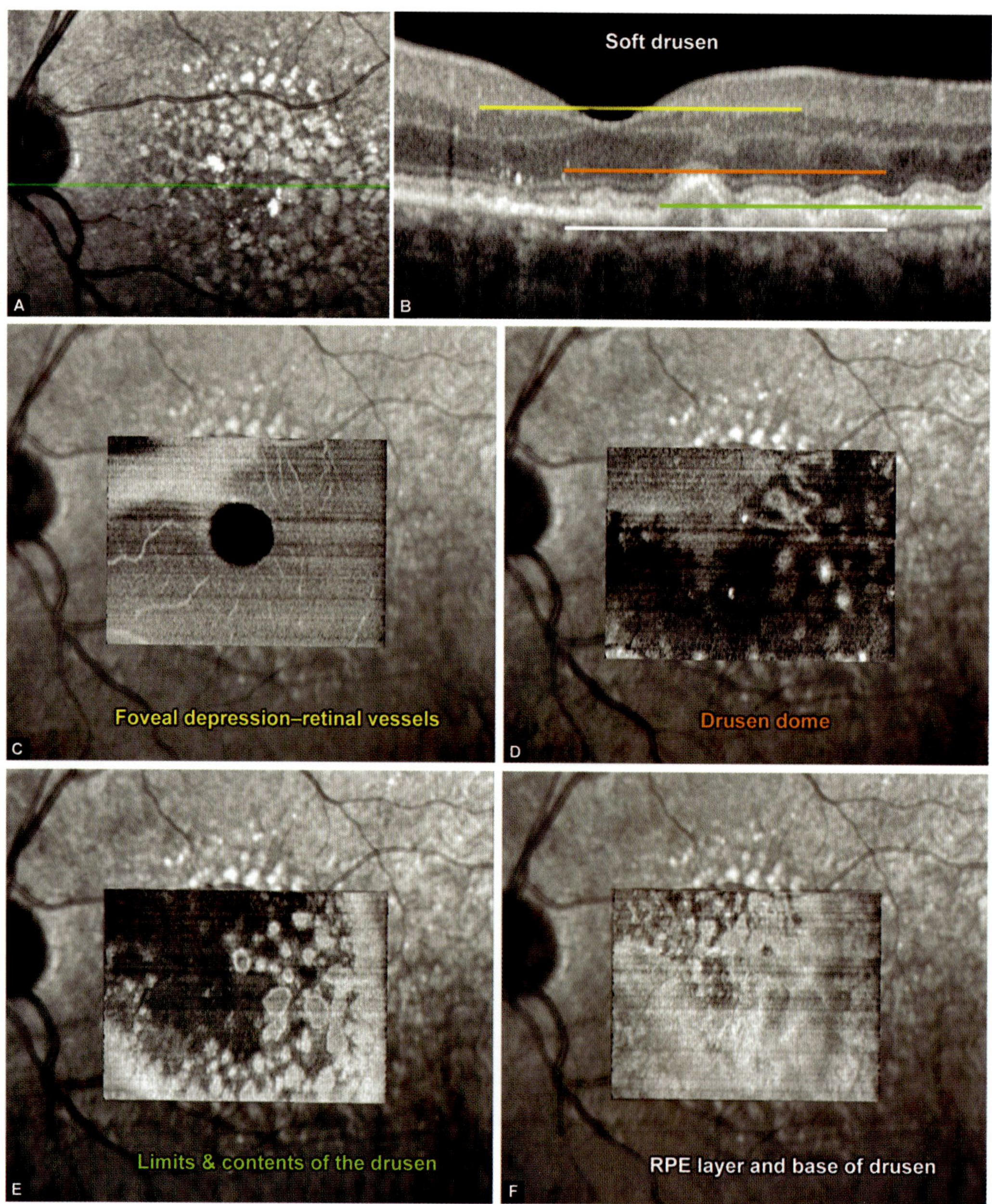

Figures 5A to F: Frozen images from the *en face* OCT video (intern to extern layers): Soft drusen. The "frozen" images in C, D, E and F correspond to the different section lines showed in (B)

2. Drusenoid PED

Drusenoid PED is a large lesion with confluent soft drusen, usually non homogenous, without fluid accumulation or neovascularization.

En face OCT will allow locating the lesion between Bruch's membrane and RPE layer and specific study of their shape and walls, assessing the dimension, and thickness. The limits can be regular or irregular, uni or multilobular.

The walls are thick and hyperreflective and precisely limited. There is no interruption or break at the level of RPE layer (**Figures 6A to F**).

During the video and on the frozen images, it is possible to *recognize successively* the retinal vessels, the dome of the detachment, the PED cavity, the non-homogenous contents of the drusenoid detachment, and finally; the RPE layer and the base of PED become visible

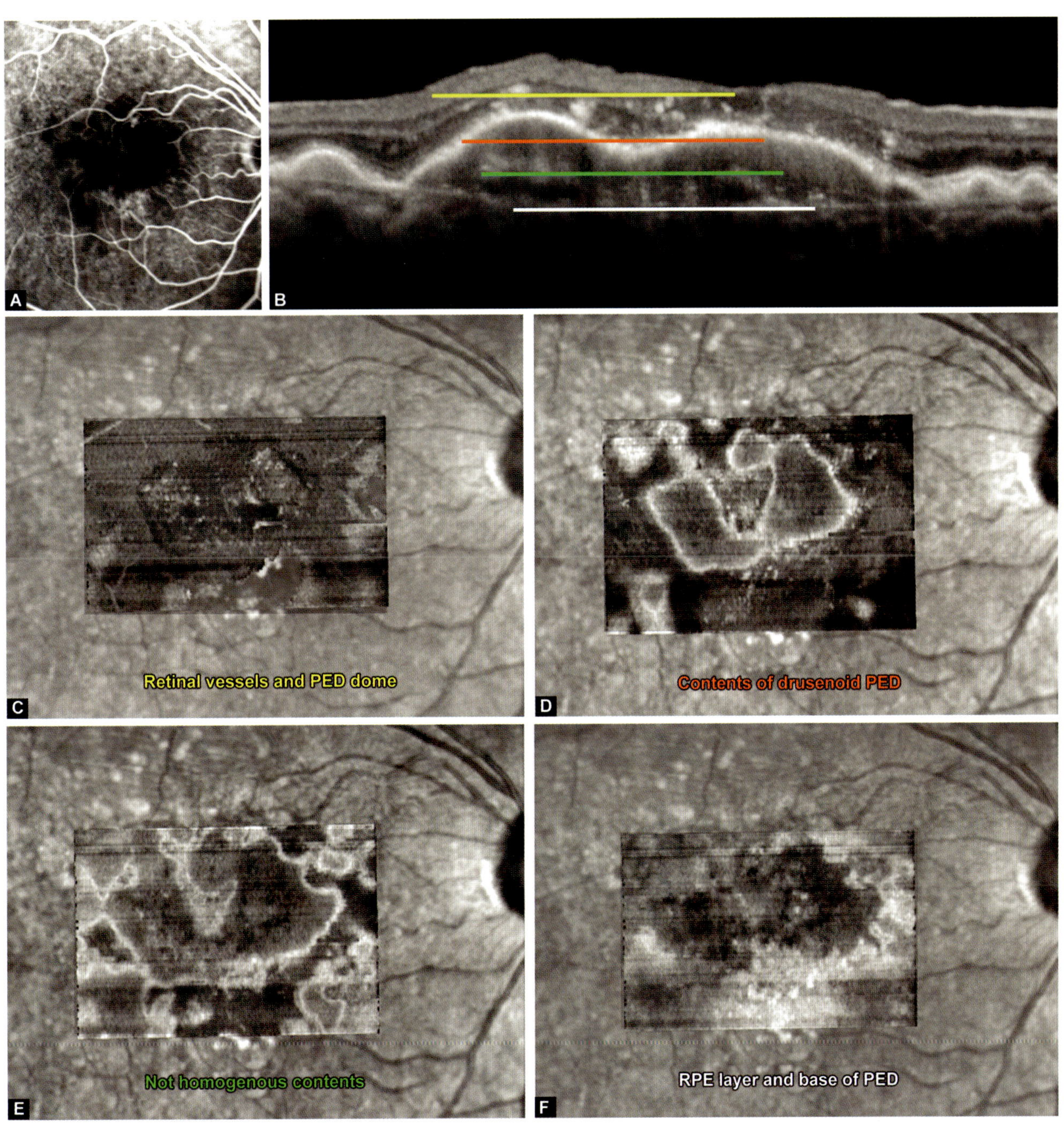

Figures 6A to F: *En face* optical coherence tomography of drusenoid PED in AMD. The "frozen" images in C, D, E and F correspond to the different section lines showed in (B)

3. Fibrovascular Pigment Epithelium Detachment (FV-PED) in AMD

The purpose of our recent study, was to develop a method of segmentation using *en face* C-scans to evaluate the choroidal neovascular network in *Fibrovascular-PED due to AMD.*[5,6]

The images were reconstructed to obtain *en face* cross-sections and then*, the images were superimposed* and compared on infrared and/or on SLO ICG images, to confirm the neovascularization.

A series of 38 consecutive patients (27 females and 11 males, mean age 76.7 ± 3 years) with type 1 CNV and FV-PED due to exudative AMD were recruited.

Twelve out of 38 eyes were treatment-naïve, while 17 out of 38 eyes had undergone previous intravitreal anti-vascular endothelial factor (VEGF) injections.

Diagnosis was made with: Fluorescein angiography (FA) + Indocyanine green angiography (ICGA) + SD-OCT (Spectralis, Heidelberg, Germany)

Results

Indocyanine green angiography (ICGA) allowed visualization of the entire choroidal neovascular membrane in the area occupied by FV-PED, in all 38 eyes (**Figure 7A**).

Enhanced depth imaging (EDI)-OCT B-scans showed, in 30/38 eyes the presence of *hyper-reflective lesions* within the FV-PED arranged along the back surface of the PED.

Hyporeflective fluid accumulation was seen beneath the hyper-reflective lesions (**Figure 7B**).

The remaining 8 eyes, showed only dense hyper-reflective collections consistent with fibrous tissue without fluid.

En Face OCT

In the En face OCT Video (intern to extern layers) the *hyper-reflective course of type 1 CNV* within the hyporeflective PED was revealed, in all 30 eyes [**Figure 8(B1)**].

The *branching network* was clearly visible in the upper part of the cavity of FV-PED, lying just beneath the under surface of the detached RPE [**Figure 8(B2)**].

Fluid accumulation was visible, deeper in the cavity as a hyporeflective area, optically empty, separating the CNV from the choroid [**Figure 8(B3)**].

Finally, normal choroid vessels became clearly visible, deeper and out of the PED [**Figure 8(B4)**].

The *En face* OCT *Video Imaging* of FV PED will allow to see successively, the retinal vessels (white and hyper-reflective), the foveal depression, later, the dome of FV-PED, the upper part of the cavity of FV-PED (with the hyper-reflective course of CNV).

Later again, the fluid beside the CNV and finally at a deeper level, the choroid, behind the FV-PED.

The hyper-reflective course of type 1 CNV was confirmed by comparative analysis on *en face* OCT and on ICGA, in all 30 eyes. Concordance between observers was very high: intraobserver: 97%; interobserver: 98% (**Figures 9A and B**).

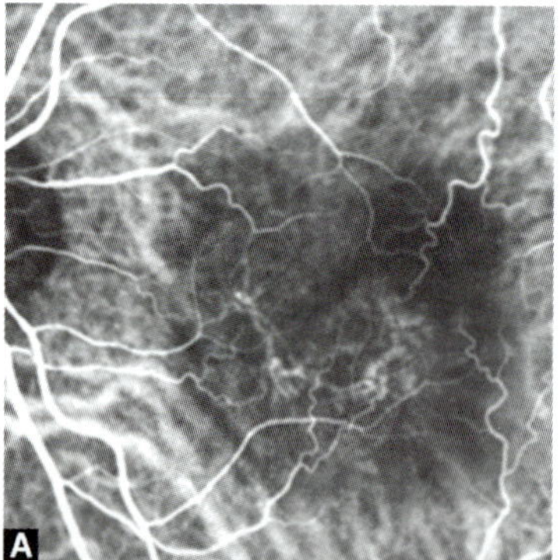

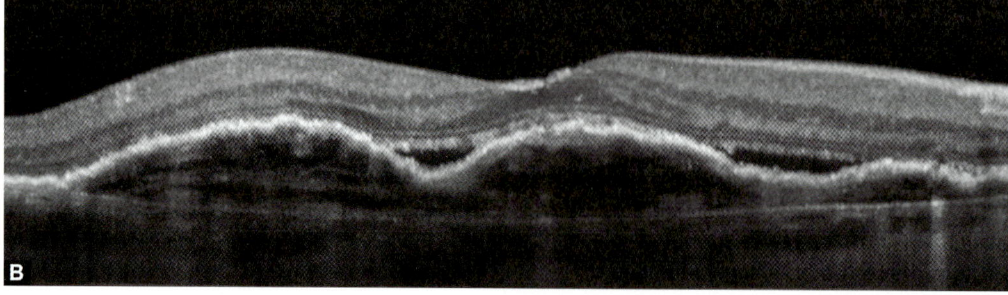

Figures 7A and B: (A) ICG angiography: Visualization of the entire CNV membrane in the FV-PED; (B) EDI-OCT B-scans: Presence of hyper-reflective lesions within the FV-PED. Hyporeflective fluid accumulation is seen beneath the hyper-reflective lesions

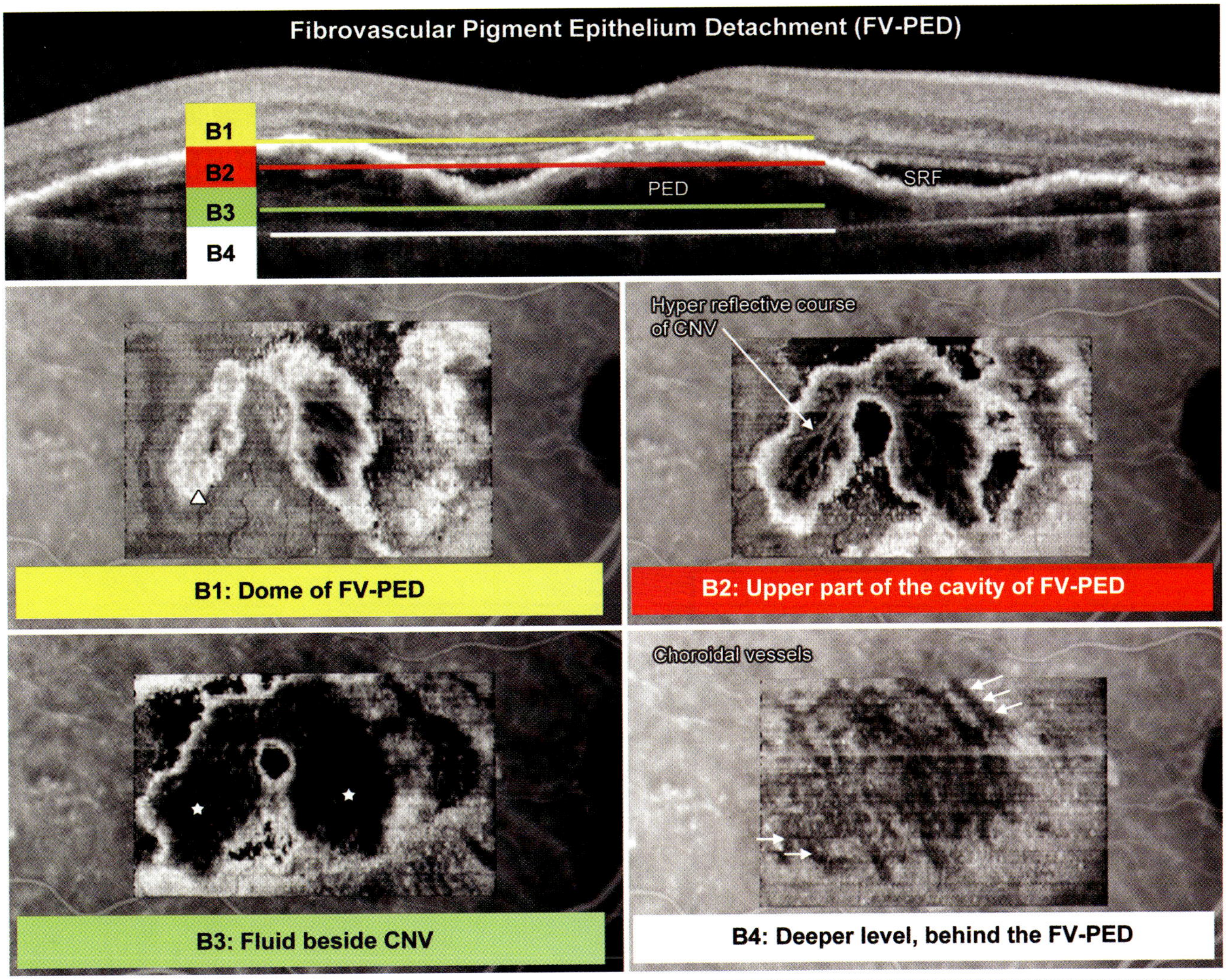

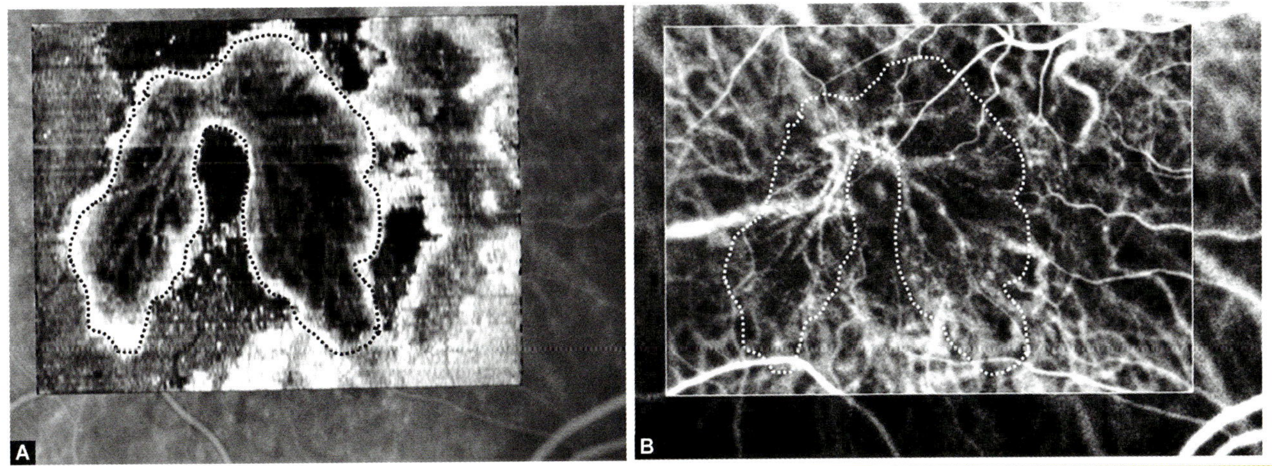

Figure 8: Fibrovascular pigment epithelium detachment (FV-PED). Frozen images from the *en face* OCT Video (intern to extern layers): B1—: Dome of FV-PED; B2—: Upper part of the cavity of FV-PED: hyper-reflective course of type 1 CNV within the hyporeflective PED; B3—: Fluid beside CNV; B4—Deeper level, behind the FV-PED
(*Source :* Coscas F, Coscas G, Querques G, Massamba N, Querques L, Bandello F, et al. En face enhanced depth imaging OCT of fibrovascular PED. IOVS. 2012;53(7):4147-51.)[5]

Figures 9A and B: The hyper-reflective course of type 1 CNV is confirmed by comparative analysis on en face OCT and on ICGA, in all 30 eyes

Another clinical case of FV-PED will show and confirm the same images on the video and on the different frozen images, successively from the internal layers to the most peripheral (**Figures 10A to F**).

It is easy to find the *different layers*: Retinal vessels; Sub retinal fluid; Dome of the PED; Cavity of the PED; CNV, clearly visible and well defined; Bottom of PED and finally the choroidal vessels.

Until now, CNV themselves were not precisely detectable in Conventional SD-OCT but only suggested by the exudative reaction.

This new *en face* **SD-OCT technology** with dynamic segmentation of the macula allows to visualize the contours and the shape of the FV-PED and   the choroid neovascular network in the FV-PED.

En face SD-OCT demonstrates for the first time direct signs of choroidal neovascularization, without any dye injection.

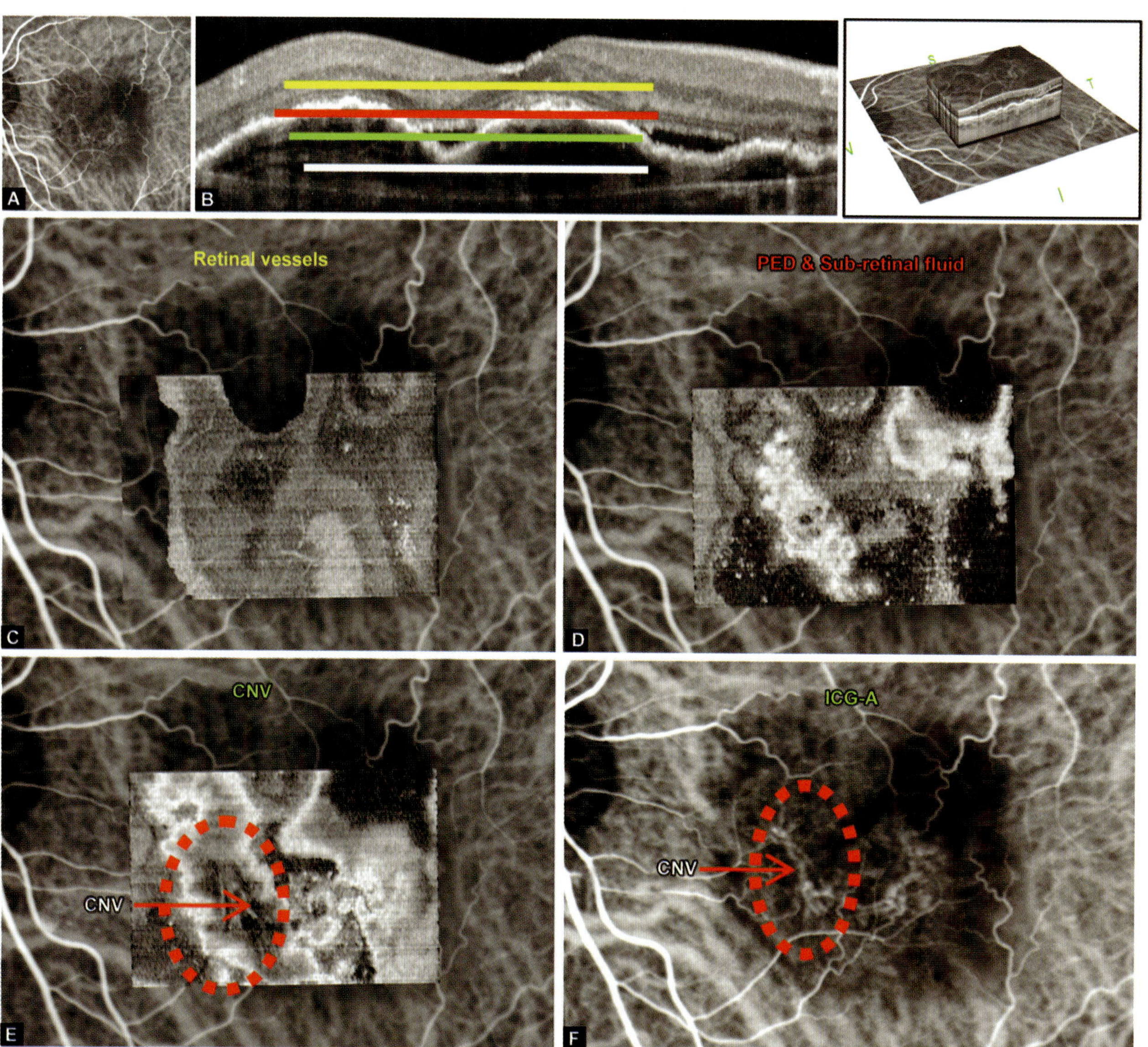

Figures 10A to F: Fibrovascular pigment epithelium detachment (FV-PED). Frozen images from the *en face* OCT video of a clinical case of FV-PED in AMD

4. Polypoidal Choroidal Vasculopathy

Polypoidal choroidal vasculopathy described in 1982 from Yannuzzi et al is characterized by a dilated abnormal choroidal network associated with Polypoidal lesions and multiple recurrent sero-sanguineous detachment of RPE with leakage, fluid accumulation and bleeding specifically coming from the polyps.

En face OCT examination has shown that the abnormal choroidal network is *located between Bruch's membrane and RPE layer*, very rarely extending above the RPE (**Figures 11A and B**).

During the video and on the frozen images, it is possible to recognize, the different elevated lesions in the macular area. Initially, the two different parts of the cavity of PED (optically empty) is very precisely limited by the RPE layer (**Figures 11C and D**). One active polyp is visible, adjacent and inside the PED and moderately hyperreflective.

A few sections deeper many other polyps become visible (**Figure 12C**); and, progressively the abnormal network (**Figure 12C**). And deeper, the hyperreflective RPE layer (**Figure 12D**). Finally, at the level of the choriocapillaris (**Figure 12E**) the polyps and the abnormal network are no more visible, suggesting that *the entire lesion is in front of Bruch's membrane* (**Figures 12A to F**).

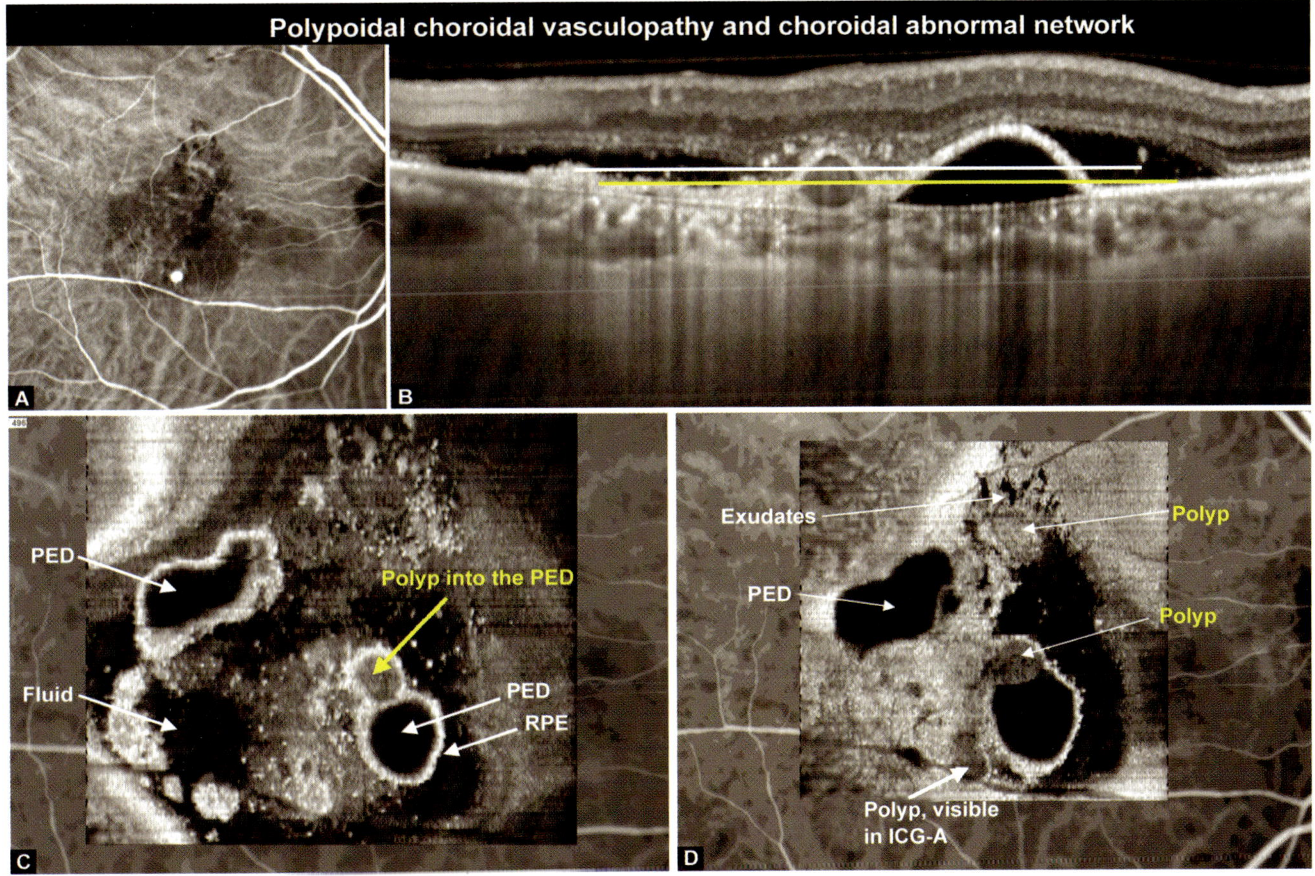

Figures 11A to D: Polypoidal choroidal vasculopathy and choroidal abnormal network: Frozen images from the *en face* OCT video: sections at the level of the PED and active polyp

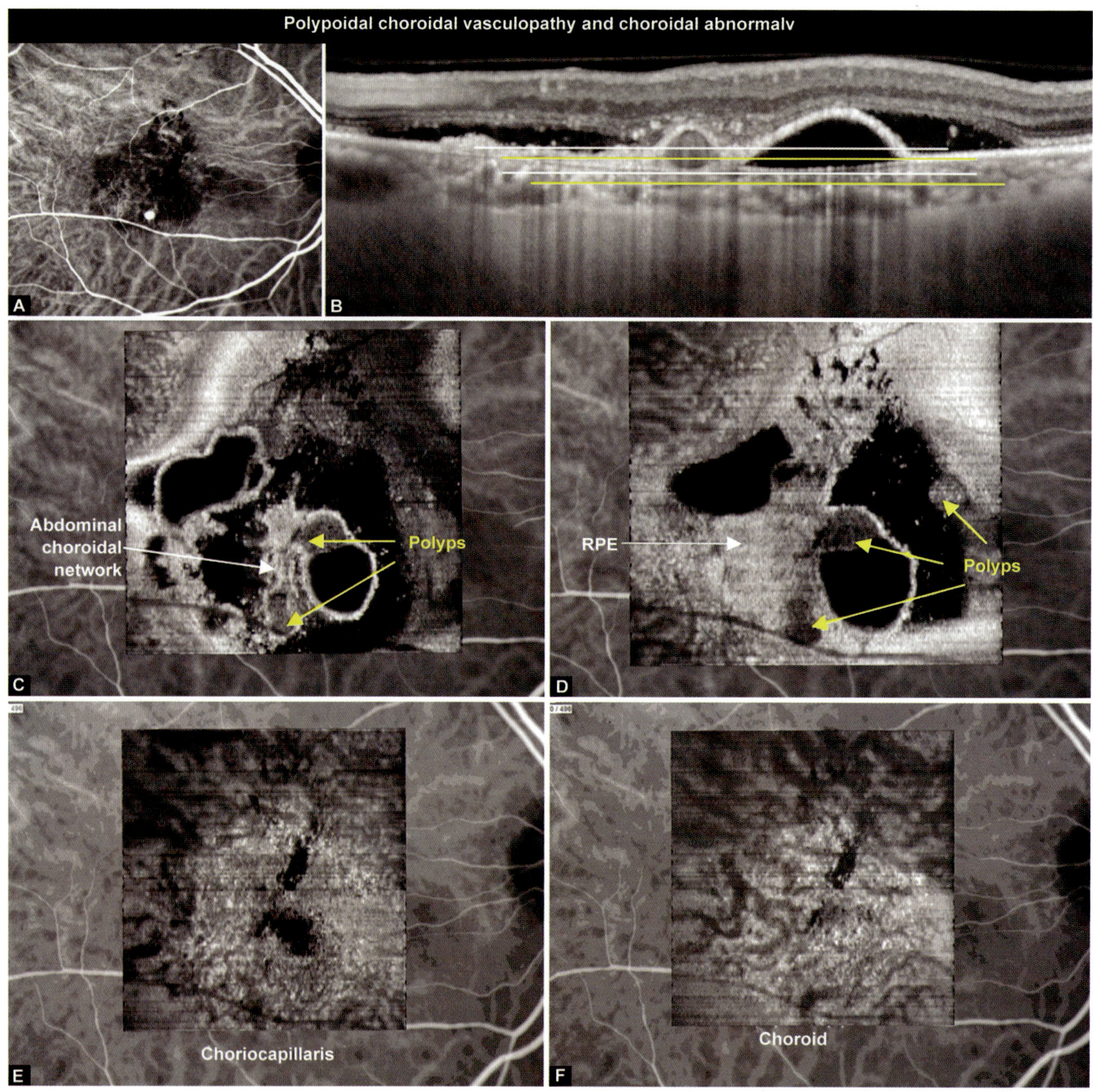

Figures 12A to F: Polypoidal choroidal vasculopathy and choroidal abnormal network: Sections at the level of the PED and active polyp and at the level of choriocapillaris

5. Classic CNV in AMD

This method of segmentation, using *en face* C scans allows evaluating the choroidal neovascular network in **Classic, type 2, CNV** due to AMD. Diagnosis was made with FA + ICGA + SD-OCT

In FA, pure classic CNV are well defined at early phase and then, profusely and progressively leaking. *In SLO-ICG*, the lesion is precisely delimited, confirming the diagnosis.

OCT B-scans showed the localized break in RPE layer. *The course of the hyper-reflective pedicle* (CNV) from inner choroid layers and choriocapillaris, through Bruch's membrane and RPE toward sub-retinal space, is visible toward the *intraretinal dense area* and serous *sub-retinal fluid*. **(Figures 13A to E).**

In all our series of 12 eyes, *the hyper-reflective area of the CNV* at the surface of the RPE was confirmed by exact *correspondence between* the ICGA images and *En face OCT*.[8]

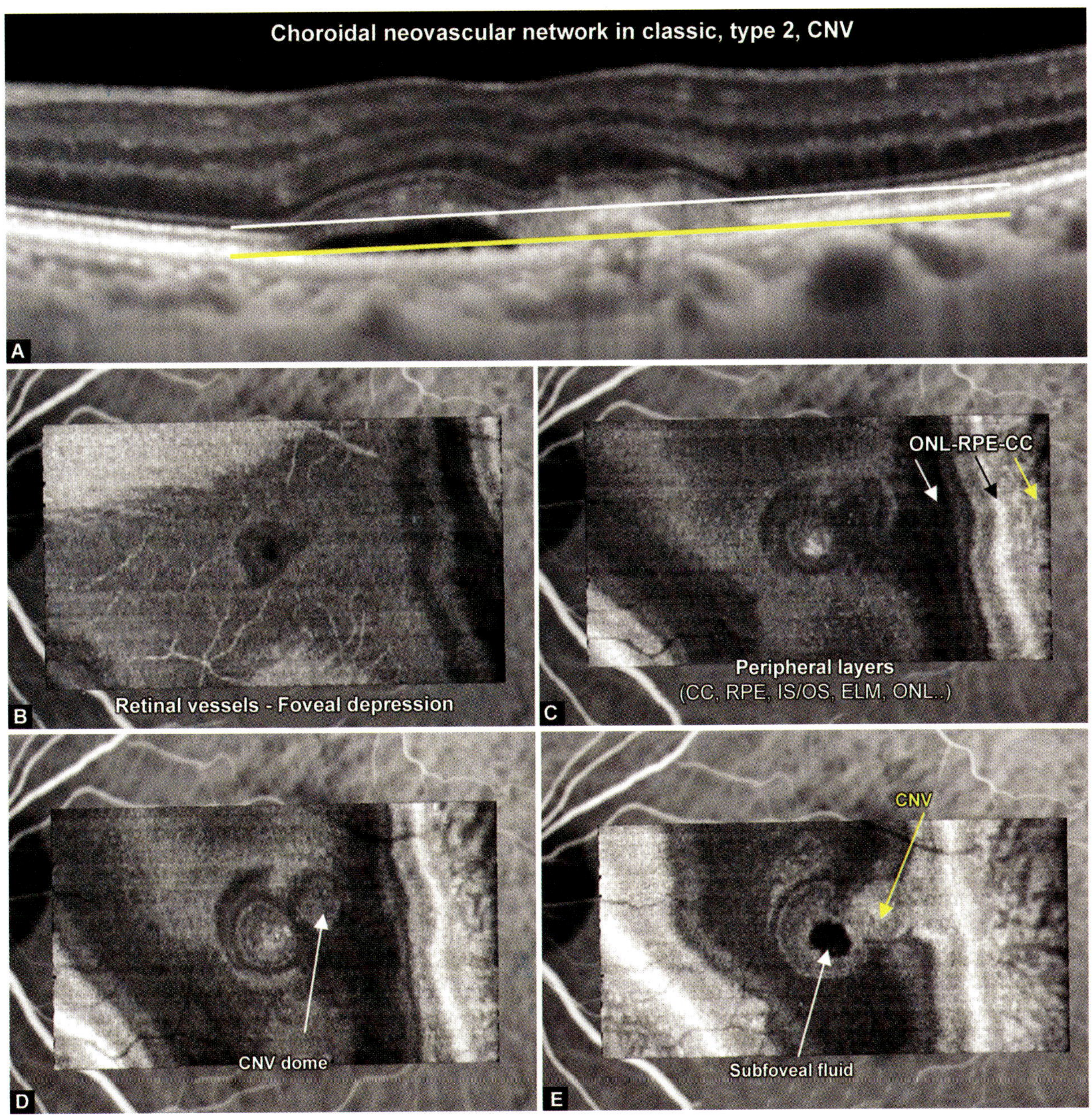

Figures 13A to E: Classic CNV, type 2 in AMD. Frozen images from the *en face* OCT video: Sections at the level of the foveal depression with the dome of juxtafoveal CNV
(Presented at *Gonin Club Meeting, Reykjavik*, 2012-06-21- G Coscas, F Coscas, G Querques, U De Benedetto, F Bandello, E Souied)[6-8]

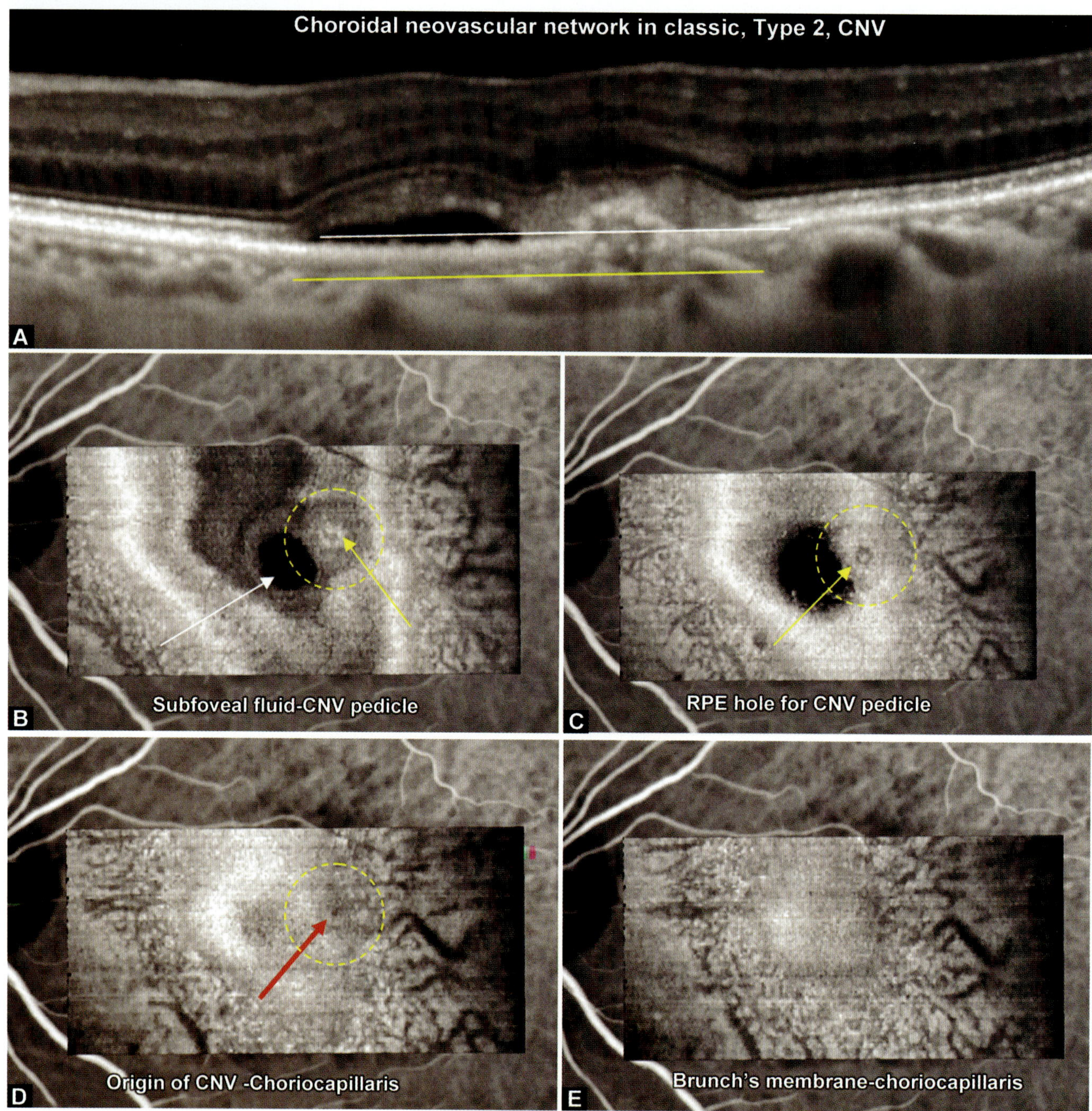

Figures 14A to E: Classic CNV, type 2 in AMD. Frozen images from the *en face* OCT video: Sections at the level of the CNV pedicle and hole in RPE, and origin CNV at the choriocapillaris

During the video and on the frozen images, it is possible to *recognize, the different elevated lesions* in the macular area:

Initially, the superficial layers (optic fibers) and the retinal vessels radiating toward the center and the foveal depression are visible.

Then, it becomes possible to analyze the different layers, (not only at the center but also at the periphery of the image) where are clearly distinguishable the choriocapillaris, the RPE, and the ONL.

Deeper, the dome of the CNV will appear which become progressively dense and hyperreflective with some subretinal fluid very close.

The precise analysis of the successive layers will allow a very specific image of the **CNV pedicle** and hole through the RPE layers and finally the origin of the CNV at the level of choriocapillaris **(Figures 14A to E)**.

The CNV are no more visible immediately behind the choriocapillaris.

6. Adult Onset Vitelliform Macular Dystrophy

Adult onset vitelliform macular dystrophy refers to a group of macular disorders with foveal macular accumulation of yellowish material, deeply at the level of the RPE layer and behind this layer, with highly variable clinical expression.

This *material* induces usually hypo-auto fluorescence and hypo-fluorescence on FA or ICGA with late or very late staining.

Usually there is *no fluid accumulation*. But during natural history, the material can progressively fragment with partial reabsorption, RPE atrophy and sub-RPE and even subretinal fluid accumulation (**Figures 15A to F**).

Diagnosis may become **very challenging**, as, moreover, in some rare cases, choroidal neovascularization may develop and be observed.

During the video and on the frozen images, it is possible to recognize, the different elevated lesions in the macular area: there is no changes in the inner retinal layers, retinal vessels and foveal depression, which is round and regular.

Progressively will appear the dome of material and the **material** itself which is moderately hyperreflective but not homogeneous and granular. The lesion is well delimited with hyper-reflective borders (RPE). Going deeper the material becomes more homogeneous and less reflective (**Figures 16A to F**).

At the level of RPE, the base of the lesion is irregular, hypo-reflective, suggesting partial atrophy of the RPE. At the reverse Bruch's membrane, choriocapillaris and choroid will appear normal.

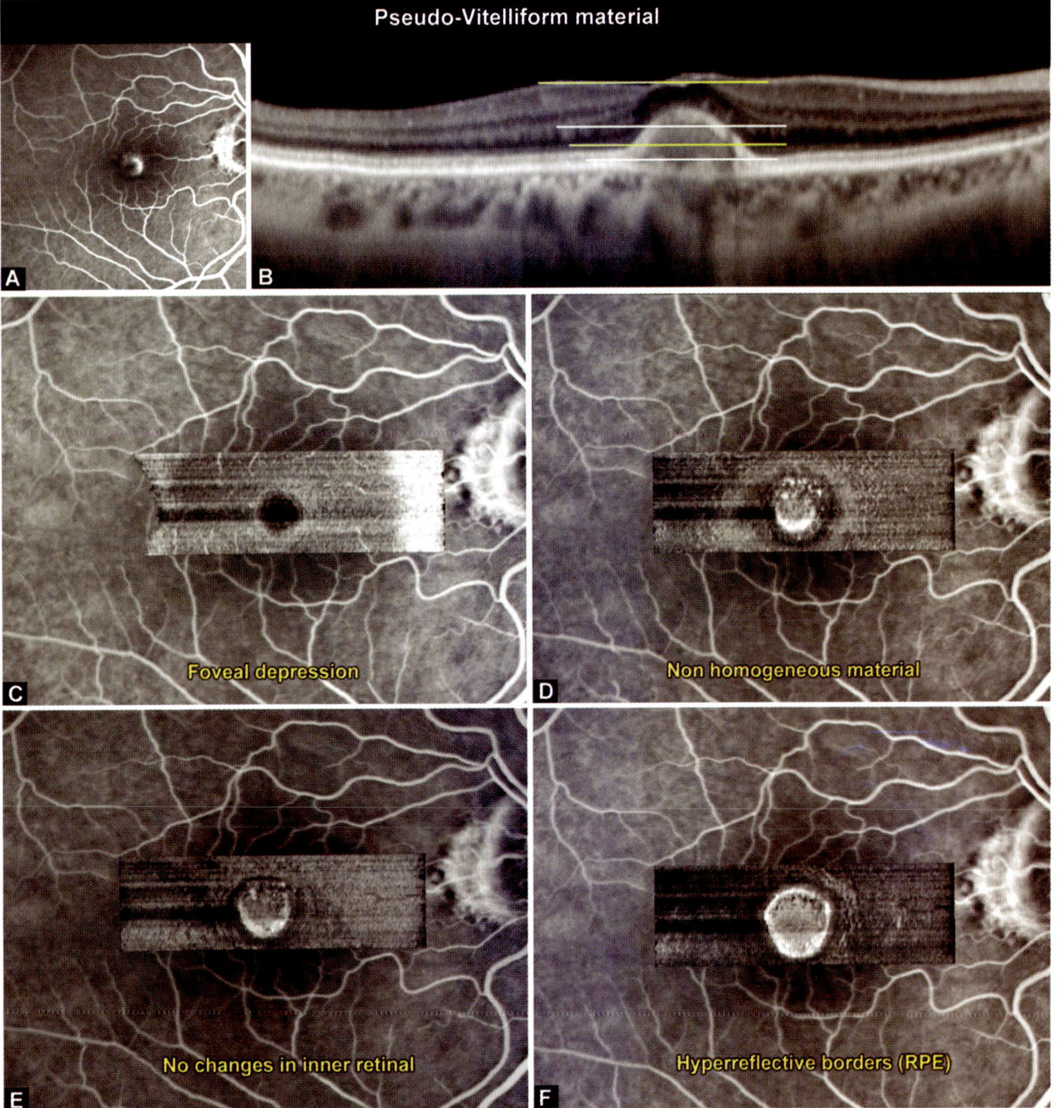

Figures 15A to E: Frozen images from the *en face* OCT Video (Pseudo-Vitelliform material): Sections at the level of the foveal depression and of the accumulated material

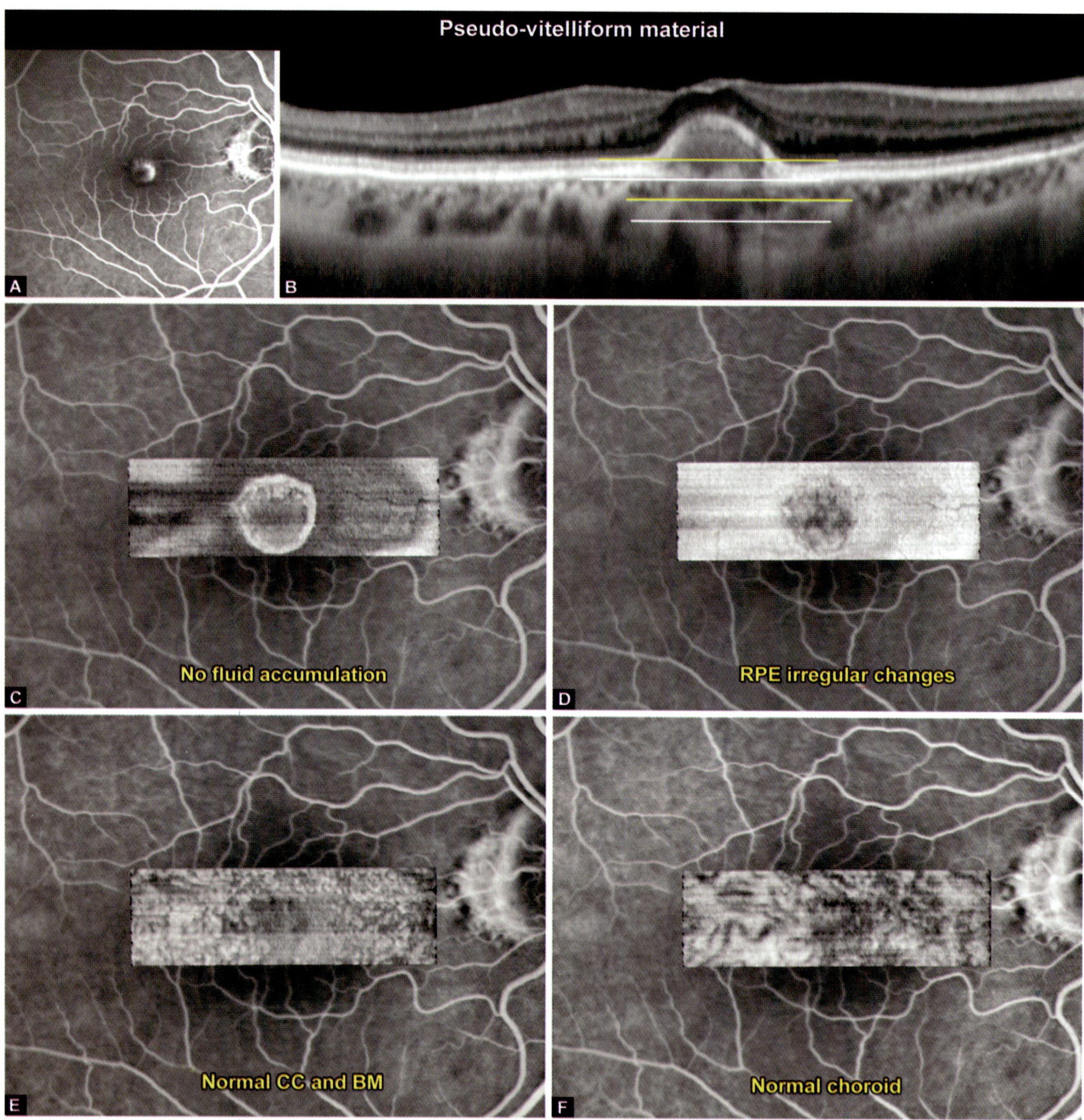

Figures 16A to F: Pseudo-Vitelliform material: Frozen images from the *en face* OCT video (sections at the level of the material, the RPE layer and the choriocapillaris)

7. Outer Retinal Tubulations

Outer retinal tubulations (or rosettes) have been recently identified in AMD (Zweifel, 2009). Initially visible like a roundish lesion in the outer retinal layers at the border of atrophic lesion, they have been also observed as multiple irregular cysts in front of fibrotic lesions.

It has been shown that they do not indicate persistence of active lesion but late irreversible degenerative changes, usually located at the level of ONL.

En face OCT examination has allowed recognizing that they are not roundish cysts but mainly of *tubular morphology* with more or less numerous ramifications. *En face* examination improved distinction between tubulations and any other cystoid serous cavities **(Figures 17A to F).**

In the successive images the tubulations become visible with *multiple ramifications* at different levels in front or inside the deep pre-epithelial fibrous tissue.[9]

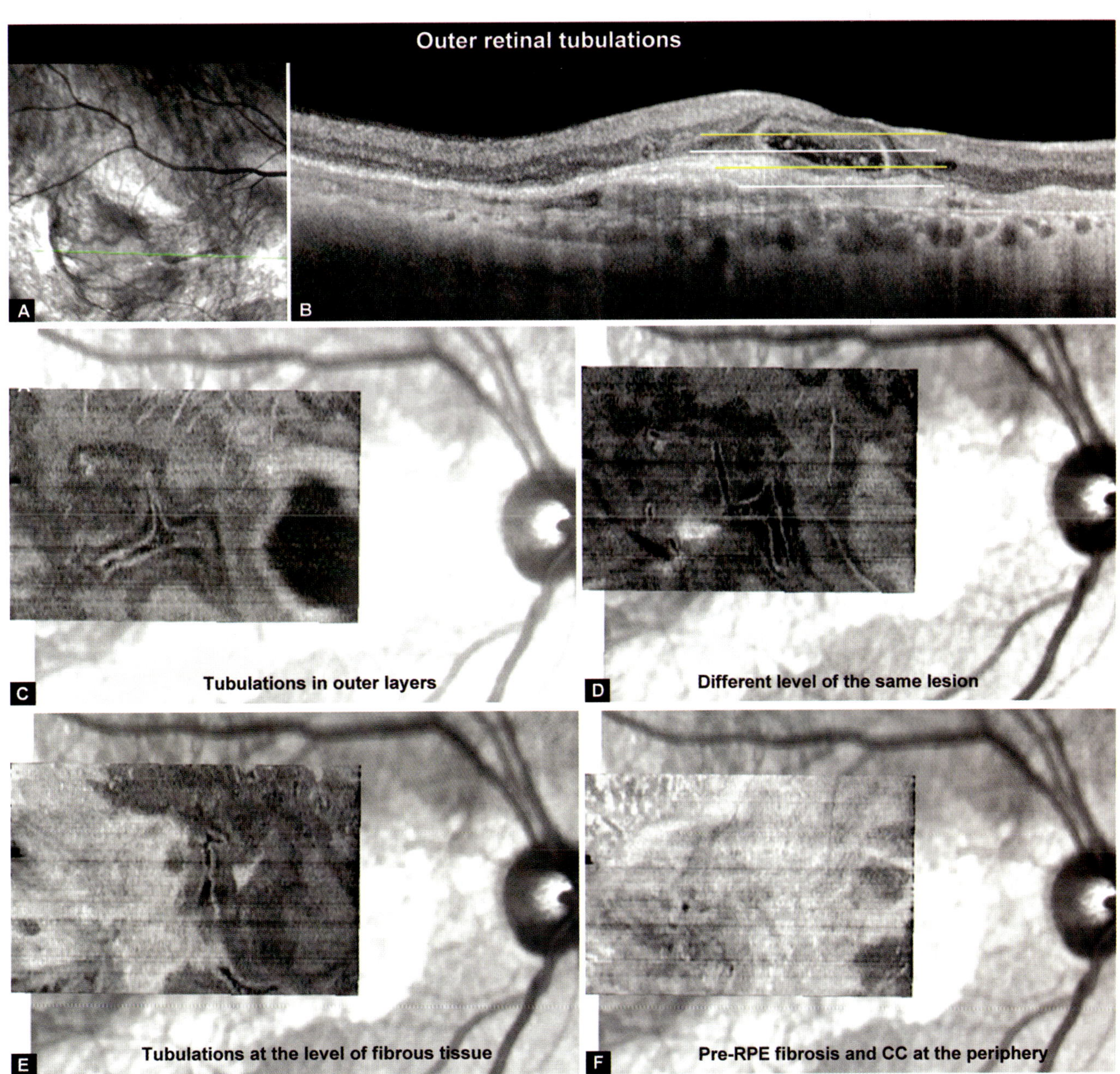

Figures 17A to F: Outer retinal tubulations or rosettes. Frozen images from the *en face* OCT video: Sections at different levels in front or inside the deep pre-epithelial fibrous tissue

8. Late and Cicatricial Lesions

Late and cicatricial lesions in the macular area will stain intensely with sometimes diffuse borders and severe symptoms. They are frequently elevated and could *masquerade* for still active lesions, as some vessels could be still perfused in ICG.

There is no sub-retinal fluid but some intraretinal cysts that make the diagnosis somewhat challenging.

En face OCT will show very precisely the lesion behind the RPE layer, hyper-reflective and dense and surrounded by well delimited hyper-reflective borders (RPE) (**Figures 18A to F**).

The analysis of the successively deeper images will show the posterior extension of the fibrotic lesion behind the RPE layer toward the choriocapillaris and superficial layers of the choroid.

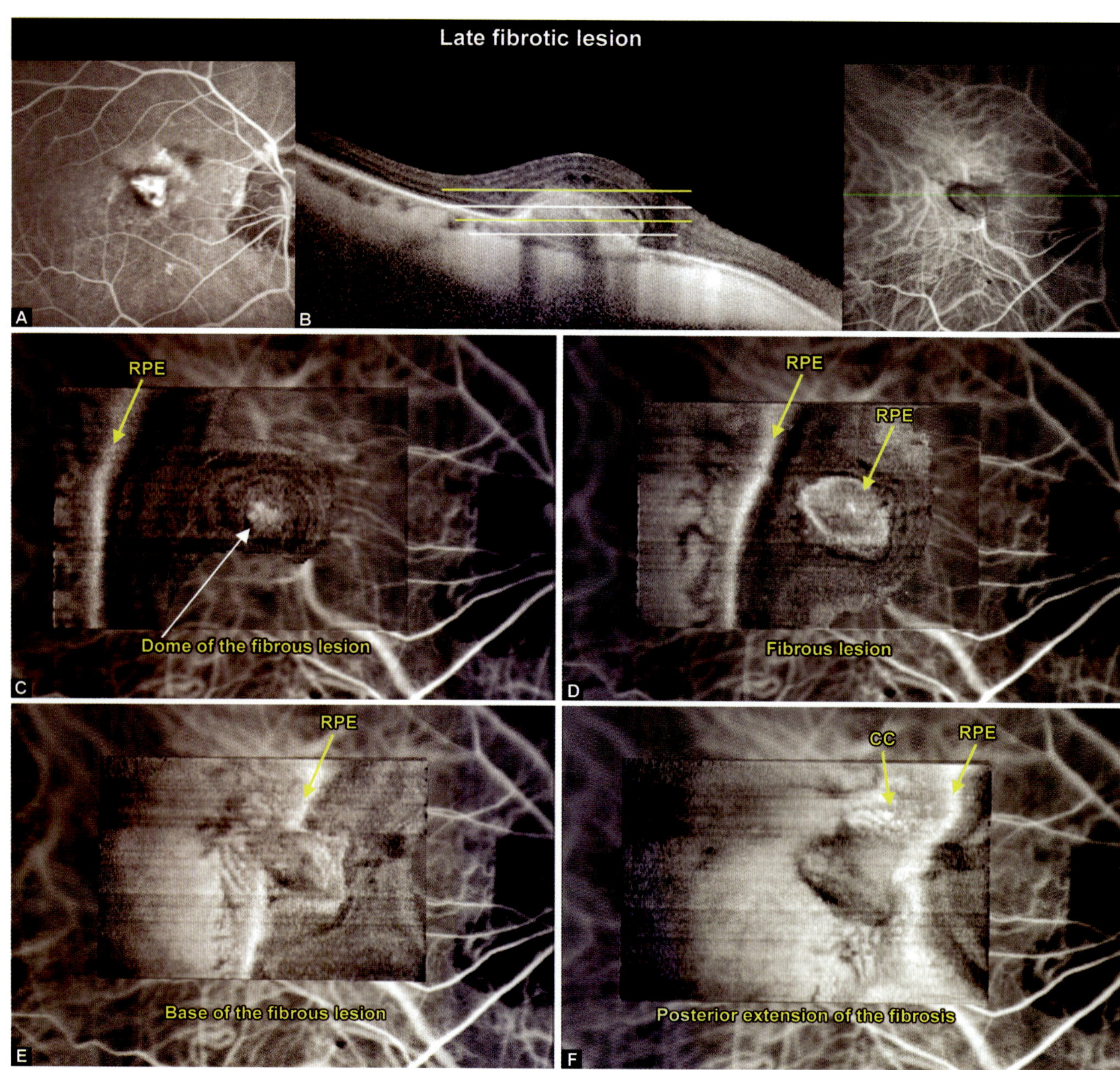

Figures 18A to F: Late fibrotic lesion: Frozen images from the *en face* OCT video: Sections at the level of the dome of the lesion, toward the choroid

Conclusion

Conventional SD-OCT provides mainly anterior-posterior sections that visualize essentially, the exudative and inflammatory reaction due to the neovascular network but also a pseudo histological section, allowing analysis of the different layers of the retina, RPE and choroid.

The more recent en face SD-OCT method of imaging simultaneously provides longitudinal images (B-scans) and transverse images (C-scans or frontal scans) of the macular region with very good pixel-to-pixel correspondence.

These *en face* images (C-scans) reconstructed from EDI-OCT B scans allow *segmentation* of subretinal and pre-retinal changes associated with many retinal diseases such as AMD in the various planes of the retina, choroid and CNV. Furthermore, interpretation of localized lesions *will take into account changes in adjacent structures and their interactions*.

In the future, this new OCT *en face* approach to retinal diseases will probably be useful for clinicians to be analysed and compared more accurately with the classic findings obtained with FA and ICG.

References

1. Coscas G, Coscas F, Vismara S, Zourdani A, Licalzi I. Optical coherence tomography in age-related macular degeneration. Springer Ed., Heidelberg, 2009, pp 384.
2. Spaide RF. Enhanced depth imaging optical coherence tomography of retinal pigment epithelial detachment in age-related macular degeneration. Am J Ophthalmol 2009;147:644-52.
3. Coscas F, Coscas G, Souied EH, Soubrane G. Optical Coherence Tomography identification of Occult Choroidal Neovascularization in age-related macular degeneration. Am J Ophthalmol 2007;144(4):592-99.
4. Lumbroso B, Savastano MC, Rispoli M, Balestrazzi A, Savastano A, Balestrazzi E. Morphologic differences, according to etiology, in pigment epithelial detachments by means of en face optical coherence tomography. Retina. 2011;31(3):553-8.
5. Coscas F, Coscas G, Querques G, Massamba N, Querques L, Bandello F, Souied EH. *En face* enhanced depth imaging OCT of fibrovascular PED. IOVS, 2012;53(7):4147-51.
6. Coscas G, Coscas F, Querques G, De Benedetto U, Bandello F, Souied E. *En face* Enhanced Depth Imaging Optical Coherence Tomography of Fibrovascular Pigment Epithelium Detachment. Presented at Macula Society meeting, Jerusalem, 2012-06-14.
7. Coscas G, Coscas F, De Benedetto U, Bandello F, Souied E. *En face* Enhanced Depth Imaging Optical Coherence Tomography of Polypoidal choroidal vasculopathy. Presented at Euretina Meeting, Milano, 2012-09-8.
8. Coscas G, Coscas F, Querques G, De Benedetto U, Bandello F, Souied E: *En face* Enhanced Depth Imaging Optical Coherence Tomography of Classic CNV, type 2 in AMD. Presented at Gonin Club Meeting, Reykjavik, 2012-06-21.
9. Wolff B, Matet A, Vasseur V, Sahel JA, Mauget-Faÿsse M. En Face OCT Imaging for the Diagnosis of Outer Retinal Tubulations in Age-Related Macular Degeneration.J Ophthalmol. 2012;2012:542417.

Other Types of Acquired Macular Degenerations

Fernando M Penha, Anderson Teixeira,
André Maia, Michel E Farah, Andre Romano

Introduction

Age related macular degeneration (AMD) is the major cause of blindness in elderly population and the main cause of acquired macular degeneration. In this chapter some cases of other types of acquired macular degenerations with interesting findings in the *en face* optical coherence tomography (OCT) imaging will be shown.

Dye Light Toxicity

Chromovitrectomy is a very common procedure in macular surgery in the past few years. Indocyanine green (ICG) was the first dye used for internal limiting membrane (ILM) staining, but it has been shown to be toxic to the retina and RPE.[1] Brilliant blue is now approved in Europe as a safe alternative to ICG with good ILM staining. Brilliant Peel (Fluoron, Geuder, Germany) is a ready-to-use product of 0.5 ml at a concentration of 0.125 mg/ml dye.[2] However, we have to be aware of the possibility of dye-light interaction which may induce retinal toxicity.[3] We present a case of cystic changes in the retina 10 days after the surgery with retinal atrophy and final visual acuity of 20/200 (**Figures 1A and B**). This patient underwent epiretinal membrane removal and internal limitant membrane peeling surgery with brilliant blue 0.125 mg/ml and a 420 nm irradiation using xenon light source, in a 20 minutes peeling maneuver. *En face* OCT imaging (C scan) of the retina surface showed the irregularity of the ILM on the peeled retina and also hyper-reflectivity due to outer retina changes.

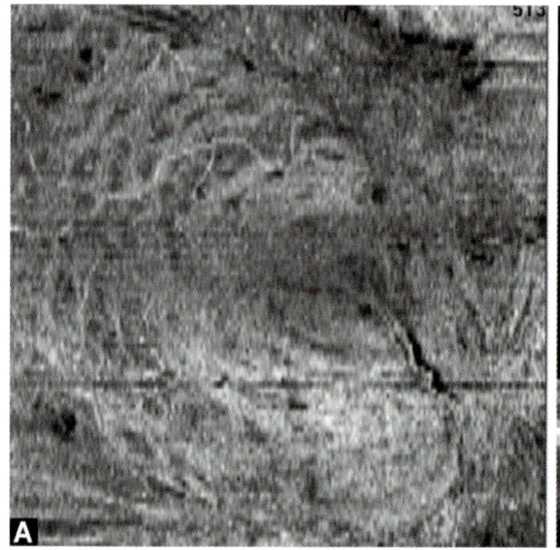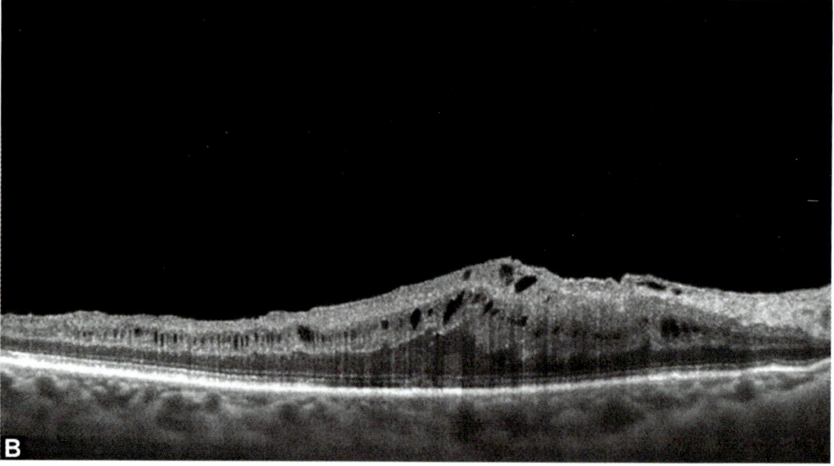

Figures 1A and B: A 54-year-old female underwent epiretinal membrane removal and internal limitant membrane peeling surgery with brilliant blue 0.125 mg/ml and a 420 nm irradiation using xenon light source, in a 20 minutes peeling maneuver. *En face* OCT imaging (C scan) of the retina surface showed the irregularity of the ILM on the peeled retina and also hyper-reflectivity due to outer retina changes. The B scan shows retinal edema and cystic changes with irregularities in the retinal surface

Vitelliform Macular Dystrophy

Vitelliform macular dystrophy (VMD) is a genetic disease that can cause central visual loss due to accumulation of lipofuscin and subsequent cell damage.[4] The classic form of the disease is called Best disease and it has an early onset, usually appears during childhood and the symptoms that may vary.[4] The adult onset form begins later in middle age and tends to cause relatively mild vision loss.[5] Not very commonly VMD can cause secondary choroidal neovascularization and vision loss.[5] We present a case of an adult onset vitelliform macular dystrophy in a 49-year-old female, with mild blurry central vision and 20/80 visual acuity. *En face* imaging of the retinal pigment epithelium (RPE) layer shows a hyporeflective ring secondary to retinal thinning in this area and a central dark spot that corresponds to the area of the vitelliform lesion (solid retinal pigmented epithelium elevation) in the center of the fovea (**Figures 2A and B**).

Macular Atrophy Related to Grid Laser Photocoagulation

Diabetic macular edema is the major cause of blindness in diabetic patients. The standard treatment was introduced after the Early Treatment Diabetic Retinopathy Study (ETDRS) showed that macular grid laser photocoagulation can improve or stabilize of best-corrected visual acuity in 17% of patients in 5 years.[6] More recently the DRCRnet group showed that pharmacotherapy with ranibizumab (Lucentis, Genentech, San Francisco, USA) can produce better results than laser.[7] The ETDRS showed that laser due to its scar can also produce reduction of visual field and visual acuity. We present a case with diabetic macular edema that was treated with modified macular grid laser photocoagulation that produced a severe retinal atrophy and pigment clumping on the RPE and consequent central vision loss. *En face* imaging shows a diffuse darkening of the scanned area and some spots of higher reflectivity related to pigment clumping (**Figures 3A and B**).

Solar Retinopathy

Solar retinopathy is an uncommon cause of macular atrophy and it is related to prolonged exposure to solar radiation or other bright light.[8] The outer retina is typical damaged due to a thermal and/or photochemical light injury.[8] This disease can occur after watching a solar eclipse, during religious rituals, after drug abuse typically during electronic parties. Patient's symptoms can be described as a small central dark spot or metamorphopsia and central vision loss in more severe cases.[8] After 6 months the visual acuity is usually in the range of 6/5 to 6/12, but frequently with a small central subjective scotoma. Visual acuity does not always recover and has reportedly remained as low as 3/60 with permanent retinal damage in the form of retinal holes and pseudo holes.[8] We report a case of solar retinopathy in a 47-year-old male patient with a history of excess solar light exposure and a chief complaint of a small central scotoma in both eyes. *En face* imaging shows a small central hyporeflective lesion caused by the absence of the IS/OS boundary in the foveal area leaving a bare RPE (**Figures 4A to D**).

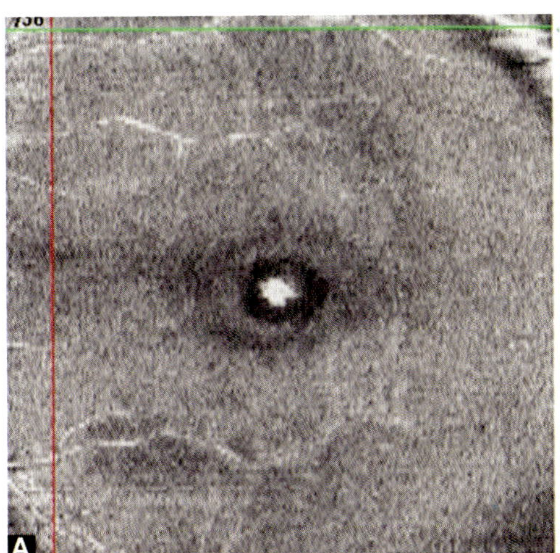
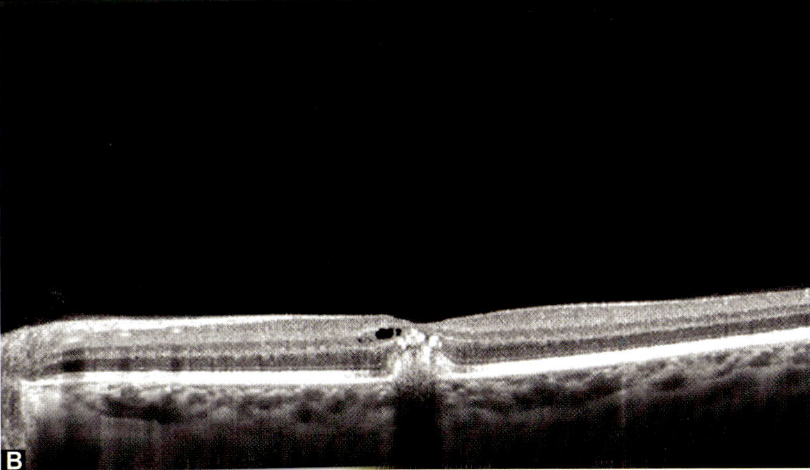

Figures 2A and B: A 49-year-old female with an adult onset vitelliform macular dystrophy, mild blurry central vision and 20/80 visual acuity. *En face* imaging of the RPE layer shows a hyporeflective ring secondary to retinal thinning in this area and a central dark spot that corresponds to the area of the vitelliform lesion (solid retinal pigmented epithelium elevation) in the center of the fovea. The B scan shows a retinal thinning and a vitelliform elevation of RPE over the fovea region

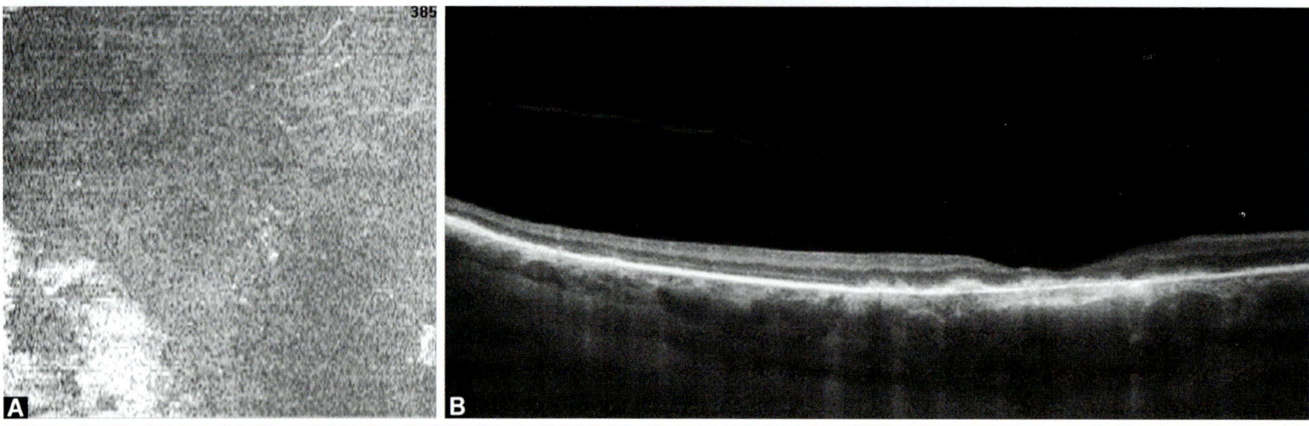

Figures 3A and B: A 40-year-old male, with diabetic macular edema that was treated with modified macular grid laser photocoagulation producing a severe retinal atrophy and pigment clumping on the RPE and consequent central vision loss. *En face* imaging shows a diffuse darkening of the scanned area and some spots of higher reflectivity related to pigment clumping

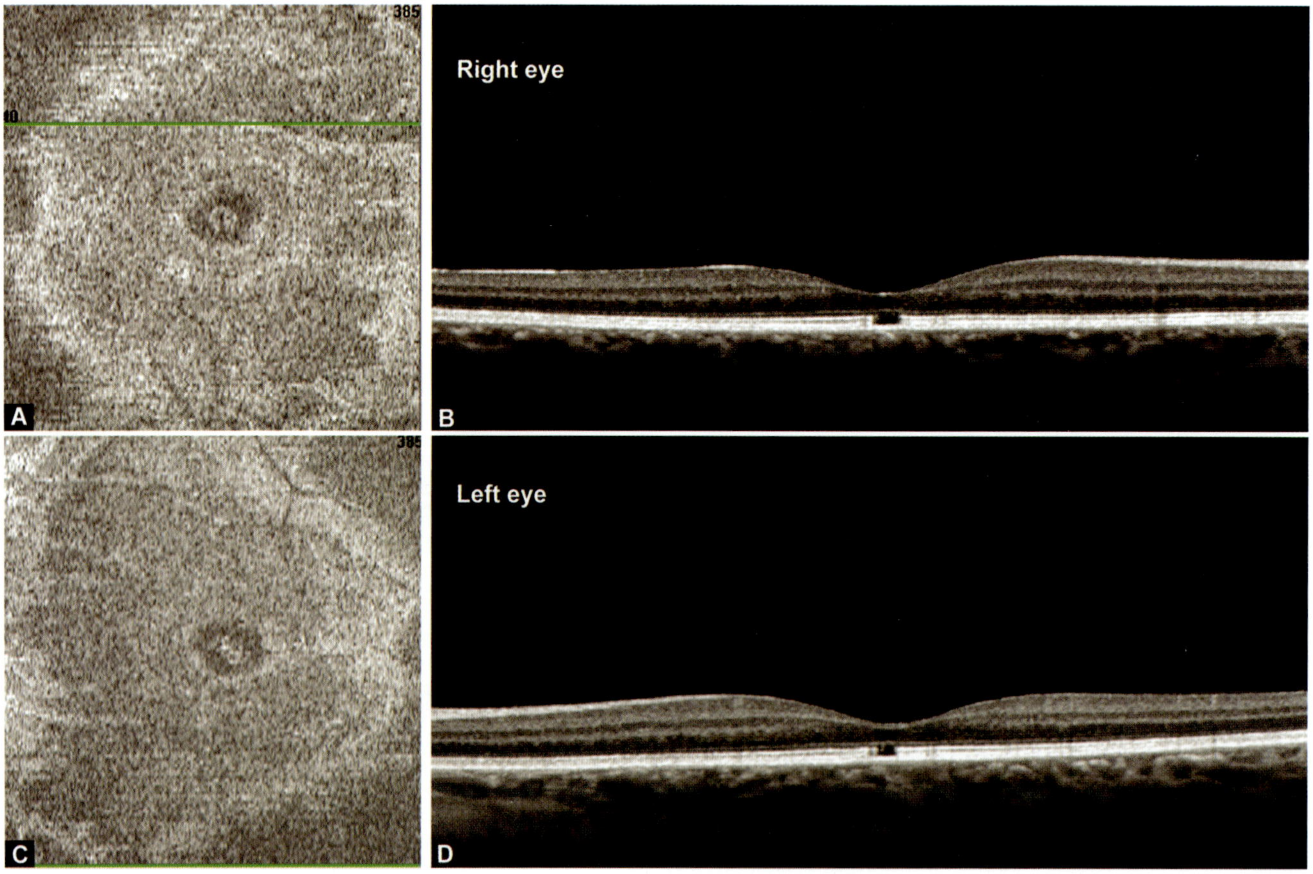

Figures 4A to D: A 47-year-old male with a history of excess solar light exposure and a chief complaint of a small central scotoma in both eyes. *En face* imaging shows a small central hyporeflective lesion caused by the absence of the IS/OS boundary in the foveal area leaving a bare RPE (B scan)

Inner Segment/Outer Segment Irregularity After Macular Hole Surgery

Full thickness macular hole is an idiopathic disease, mostly unilateral, more common in females over 50s which may lead to central vision loss or metamorphopsia.[9] The treatment is surgical with pars plana vitrectomy to relieve the anterior-posterior traction and ILM peeling to relief the tangential traction forces.[9] Patients usually recovers very well after the surgery and can achieve a visual acuity close to 20/30 even 20/20 in some cases. However, in some patients, despite a good anatomical outcome (macular hole closure) they could present a final visual acuity of 20/80 or 20/120. We present a case of a 79-year-old male that underwent pars plana vitrectomy and ILM peeling assisted with brilliant blue and after 2 months of the surgery had a final visual acuity of 20/20 with a visual vision discomfort. A discontinuity in the inner and outer photoreceptor segments (IS/OS) boundary that could explain the visual discomfort. *En face* imaging shows an irregularity in the retinal surface due to the ILM peeling and a central hyper-reflectivity due to the retinal atrophy (**Figures 5A to D**).

Central Areolar Choroidal Dystrophy

Central areolar dystrophy is a dominantly inherited macular dystrophy characterized by a bilateral, symmetrical, well-circumscribed loss of choroidal and retinal tissues.[10] Fluorescein angiography reveals normal choroidal filling with obvious hyperfluorescence in the areas of RPE atrophy.[10] A well-demarcated area of central loss evidences visual field defects.[10] We present a case of an 80-year-old white female with a chief complaint of central vision loss in the past 3 decades. In the *en face* OCT imaging it is possible to

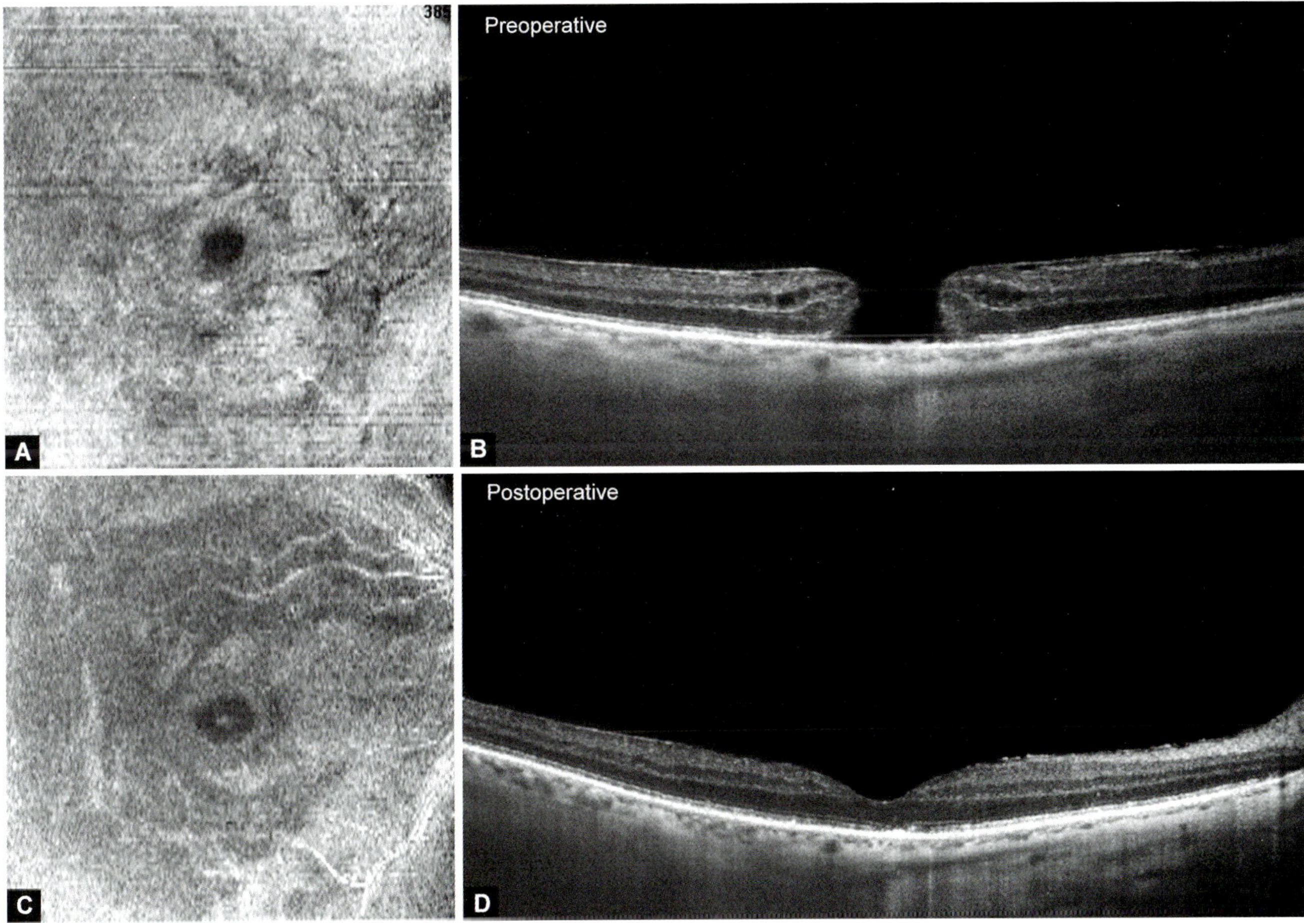

Figures 5A to D: A 79-year-old male that underwent pars plana vitrectomy and ILM peeling assisted with brilliant blue and after 2 months of the surgery the final visual acuity of 20/20 with a visual vision discomfort. A discontinuity in inner and outer photoreceptor segments (IS/OS) boundary that could explain the visual discomfort. *En face* imaging shows an irregularity in the retinal surface due to the ILM peeling and a central hyper-reflectivity due to the retinal atrophy

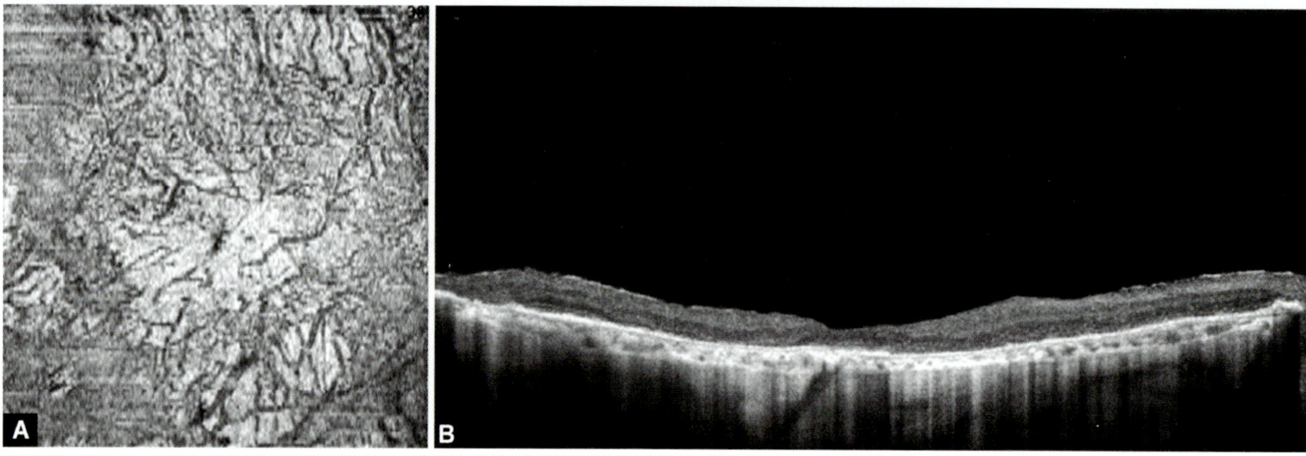

Figures 6A and B: An 80-year-old white female with a chief complaint of central vision loss in the past 3 decades. In the *en face* OCT imaging it is possible to appreciate a large area of retinal atrophy where the underlying choroidal vasculature can be observed and it correlates with the color fundus photography and SLO imaging. The B scan showed a severe retinal atrophy with a very substantial choroidal thinning

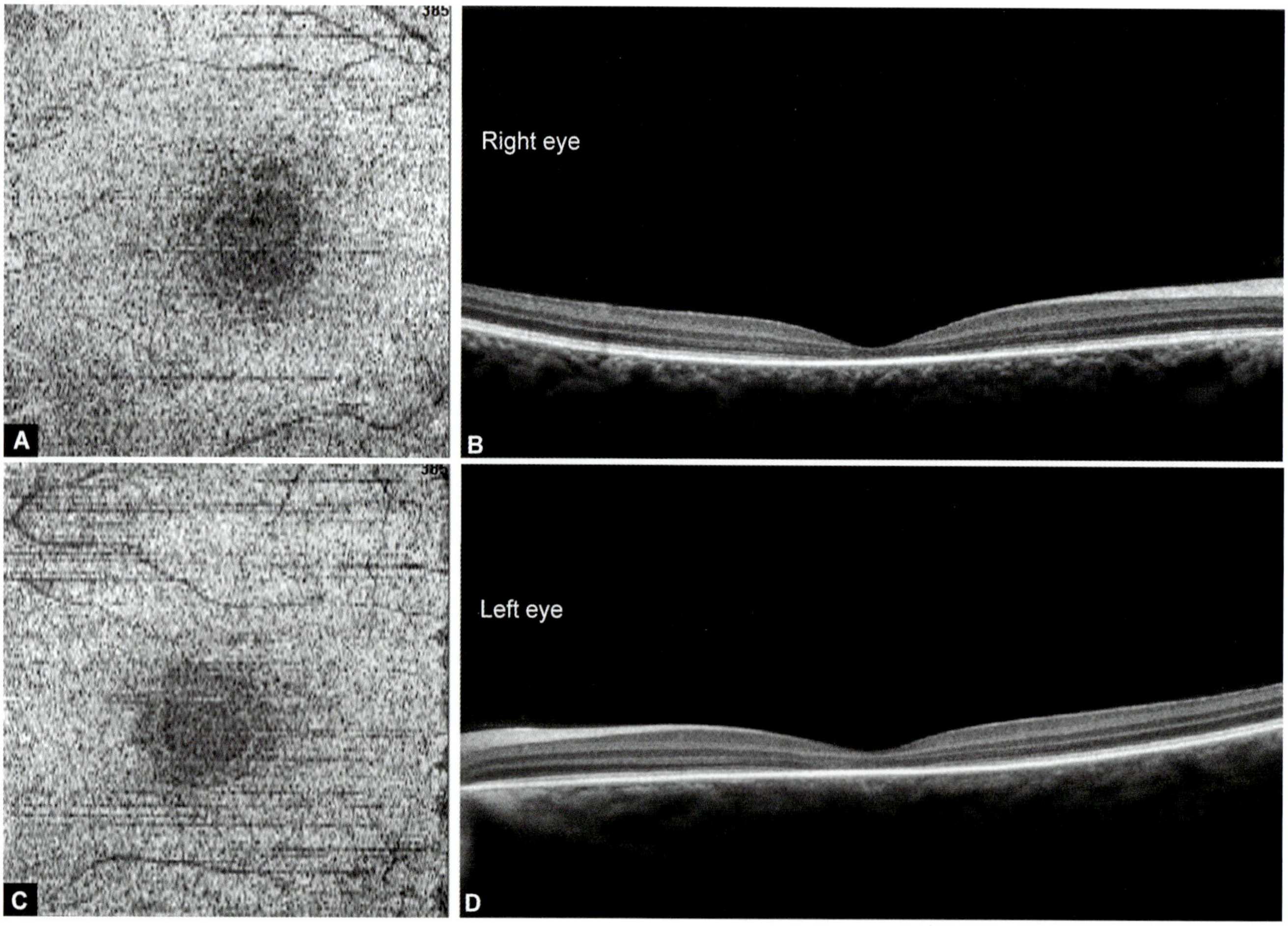

Figures 7A to D: The authors' present a case of a 19-year-old white female with a recent diagnosis of CRD. The B scan on the OCT showed a loss of IS/OS junctions. *En face* imaging shows a central hyporeflective lesion that corresponds to the area of cone loss

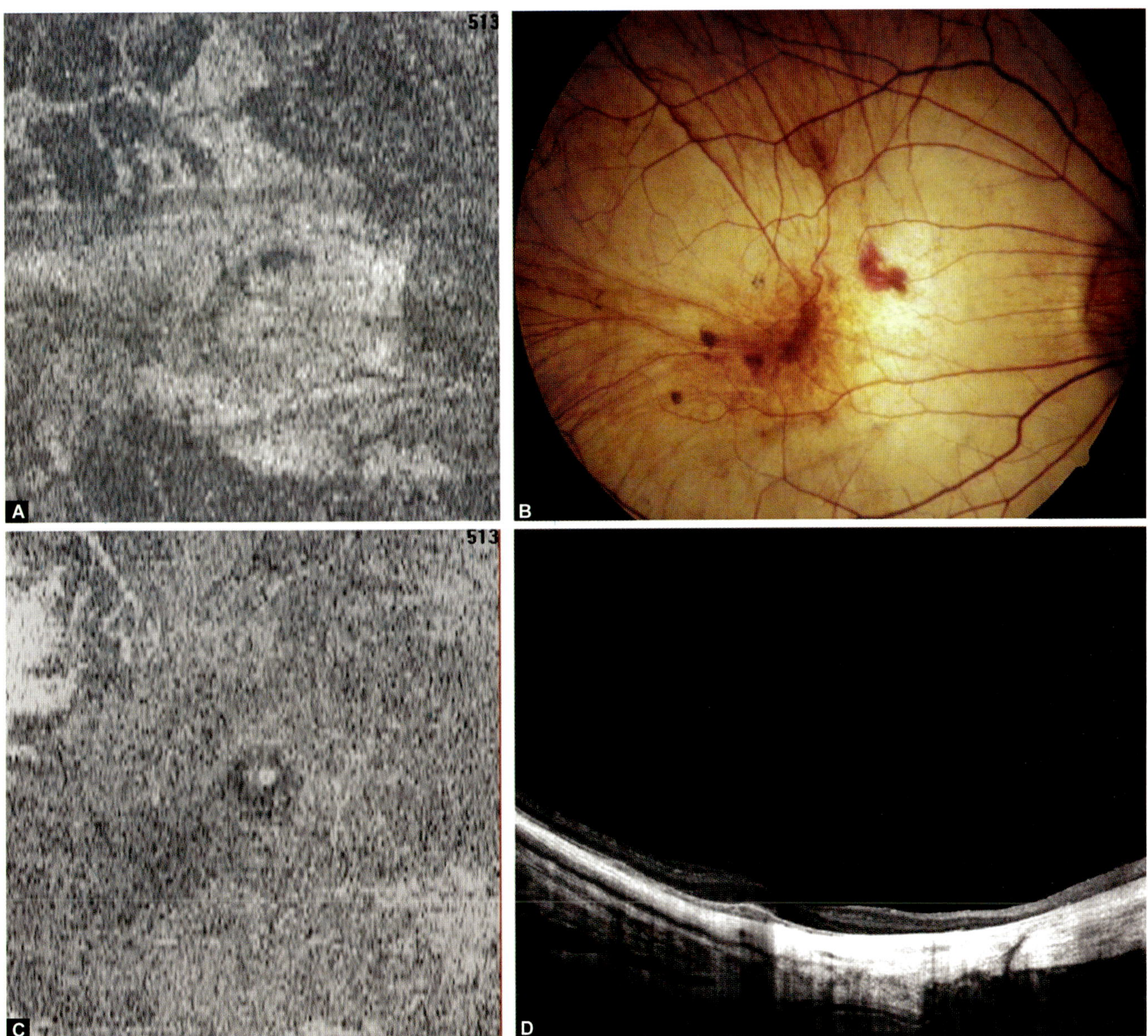

Figures 8A to D: A 35-year-old male underwent off-label treatment for retinitis pigmentosa in Cuba, Havana. The B scan revealed a severe retinal thinning and a high reflective tissue close to the sclera supposedly the fat tissue. *En face* image of that area showed some central hyper-reflective tissue possibly corresponding to the fat tissue under the sclera

appreciate a large area of retinal atrophy where the underlying choroidal vasculature can be observed and it correlates with the color fundus photography and systemic lupus erythematosus (SLO) imaging. The B scan showed a severe retinal atrophy with a very substantial choroidal thinning **(Figures 6A and B)**.

Cone-Rod Dystrophy

Cone-rod dystrophy (CRD) is an inherited progressive disease that causes deterioration of the cone and rod photoreceptor cells and often results in blindness.[11] It can be found as an autosomal dominant trait, but it is usually acquired as autosomal recessive.[11] Symptoms of CRD are seen as decreased visual acuity and color vision in the early stages followed by loss of peripheral vision.[11] The disease is similar to retinitis pigmentosa in this way, but there is no loss of night vision, the rate of rod and cone degeneration is equal, patterns of visual field loss are different, and the rate of rod electroretinogram (ERG) loss is significantly lower in CRD. We present a case of a 19-year-old white female with a recent diagnosis of CRD. The multifocal ERG showed a reduction of central cone response and the B scan on the OCT showed a loss of IS/OS junctions. *En face* imaging shows a central hyporeflective lesion that corresponds to the area of cone loss **(Figures 7A to D)**.

Retinitis Pigmentosa

Retinitis pigmentosa (RP) is an inherited, degenerative eye disease that can cause severe vision impairment and blindness.[12,13] Symptoms may vary such as: night blindness, visual field loss, changes in light-dark adjustment, blurry vision and severe visual loss in late stage of the diseases. Ocular findings in a typical case are bone spicules in the retinal mid-periphery, vascular thinning and optic disk pallor, but central changes may also occur in late stages. To date there is no treatment that has been proved to be effective to this genetic condition. Gene therapy,[13] retinal chip implant[12] and stem cell treatment are promising therapies that may give some hope to these patients. There is a controversial treatment for RP performed in Havana, Cuba, where a fat implant is placed intrascleral and it is postulate that patients can improve vision after this treatment. Here we present a case of a patient who went there for this alternative treatment, no improvement was observed. The B scan revealed a severe retinal thinning and a high reflective tissue close to the sclera supposedly the fat tissue. *En face* image of that area showed some central hyper-reflective tissue possibly corresponding to the fat tissue under the sclera **(Figures 8A to D)**.

References

1. Rodrigues EB, Costa EF, Penha FM, et al. The use of vital dyes in ocular surgery. Surv Ophthalmol. 2009;54(5):576-617.
2. Enaida H, Hisatomi T, Hata Y, et al. Brilliant blue G selectively stains the internal limiting membrane/brilliant blue G-assisted membrane peeling. Retina. 2006;26(6):631-6.
3. Malerbi FK, Maia M, Farah ME, et al. Subretinal brilliant blue G migration during internal limiting membrane peeling. Br J Ophthalmol. 2009;93(12):1687.
4. Boon CJ, Klevering BJ, Leroy BP, et al. The spectrum of ocular phenotypes caused by mutations in the BEST1 gene. Prog Retin Eye Res. 2009;28(3):187-205.
5. Dolz-Marco R, Gallego-Pinazo R, Díaz-Llopis M. Natural course of adult-onset foveomacular vitelliform dystrophy: a spectral-domain optical coherence tomography analysis. Am J Ophthalmol. 2012;153(2):389.
6. Early photocoagulation for diabetic retinopathy. ETDRS report number 9. Early Treatment Diabetic Retinopathy Study Research Group. Ophthalmology. 1991;98(5 Suppl):766-85.
7. Elman MJ, Bressler NM, Qin H, et al. Diabetic Retinopathy Clinical Research Network. Expanded 2-year follow-up of ranibizumab plus prompt or deferred laser or triamcinolone plus prompt laser for diabetic macular edema. Ophthalmology. 2011;118(4):609-14.
8. Yannuzzi LA, Fisher YL, Krueger A, et al. Solar retinopathy: a photobiological and geophysical analysis. Trans Am Ophthalmol Soc. 1987;85:120-58.
9. Bainbridge J, Herbert E, Gregor Z. Macular holes: vitreoretinal relationships and surgical approaches. Eye (Lond). 2008;22(10):1301-9.
10. Boon CJ, Klevering BJ, Cremers FP, et al. Central areolar choroidal dystrophy. Ophthalmology. 2009;116(4):771-82.
11. Kellner U, Kellner S. Clinical findings and diagnostics of cone dystrophy. Ophthalmologe. 2009;106(2):99-108.
12. Weiland JD, Cho AK, Humayun MS. Retinal prostheses: current clinical results and future needs. Ophthalmology. 2011;118(11):2227-37.
13. Bennett J. Gene therapy for retinitis pigmentosa. Curr Opin Mol Ther. 2000;2(4):420-5.

chapter 21

Torpedo Maculopathy

Salomon Y Cohen, Lise Dubois

Description and Pathogenesis

In 1992, Roseman and Gass[1] described the features of "hypopigmented nevus of the retinal pigment epithelium (RPE)", which was later called *torpedo maculopathy*.[2] In all cases, asymptomatic, torpedo-shaped defect in the RPE was observed in the temporal macular region with a pointed, torpedo-like tip directed toward the foveola. Diagnosis is based on the typical pattern of a unique lesion that corresponds to a nonpigmented RPE lesion within the temporal region of the macula, ranging from immediately underneath the foveola to 1 mm from the foveola and approximately 2–3 mm in horizontal diameter and 1 mm in vertical diameter.

This defect closely resembles solitary congenital hypertrophy of retinal pigment epithelium (CHRPE), but differs in its nonrandom macular location and pointed torpedo shape.[1-6] Indeed, solitary CHRPE is located most often in the equatorial or peripheral fundus, randomly in various quadrants, and rarely in the macula (1%).[3] Both CHRPE and torpedo maculopathy are presumed to be congenital RPE abnormalities, but its random distribution and rounded appearance is unlike torpedo maculopathy. In the few reported cases, there have been no systemic associations.

Shields and coworkers pointed out the notable differences observed in the temporal part of the lesion, with two alternative configurations that include a "frayed tail" or a rounded margin. They described the "frayed tail" as composed of either linear or dotted, hyperpigmentation or hypopigmentation. On the contrary, the rounded margin was smooth and composed of either linear, rounded, or no hyperpigmentation at the temporal margin. The etiology of torpedo maculopathy remains speculative but based on fetal anatomical findings, torpedo maculopathy could represent a persistent defect in the development of the RPE in the fetal temporal bulge.

Imagery of Torpedo Maculopathy

Fundus autofluorescence (FAF) was seldom reported with the lesion appearing as dark. There was a corresponding scotoma noted on Humphrey visual field.

There have been several reports of OCT findings in torpedo maculopathy. Golchet and coworkers reported two cases, in which an abnormal and thin RPE signal was observed in the area of a large cleft. In one patient, repeat OCT, 2 and 4 years later, showed no change. This pattern of cleft was observed in one of our patient (**Figures 1A to D**). On the contrary, Tsang and coworkers reported three cases in which OCT scans collected in this case series revealed general attenuation and disorganization within the inner and outer retinal layers in the area subtended by the lesion. There was a disruption of the RPE layer yielding a hyper-reflective band of tissues inducing a shadowing of the underlying choroid in the area of the lesion. This pattern also was observed in some cases (**Figures 2A to D**).

Report of Cases

Authors analyzed seven cases of torpedo maculopathy. Two main subtypes were observed in OCT. They report here an example of each subtype.

Case 1

Seventeen years old girl showed: (a) typical depigmented lesion of the fundus; (b) autofluorescence photograph showed the lesion as dark with some hyper-autofluorescent dots at its margins; (c) horizontal B scan of the OCT showed that RPE is totally absent, giving an image of cleft and (d) *en face* OCT image focused on the deep layers also showed the RPE as absent, giving a homogeneous dark image.

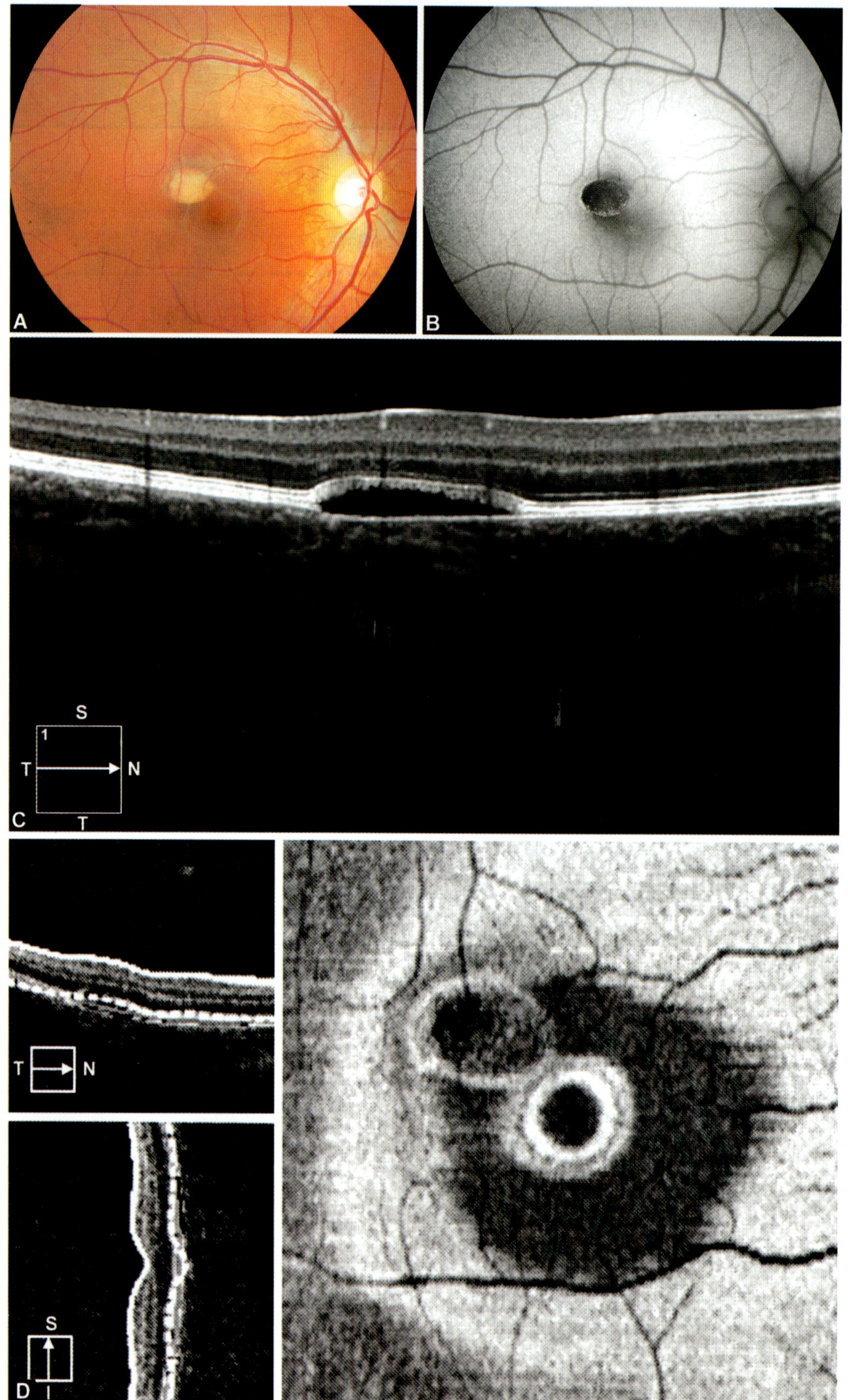

Figures 1A to D: (A) Typical torpedo maculopathy. (B) Autofluorescence photograph showed the lesion as dark with some hyper-autofluorescent dots at its margins. (C) Horizontal B scan of the OCT showed that RPE is totally absent, giving an image of cleft. (D) *En face* OCT image focused on the deep layers also showed the RPE as absent, giving a homogeneous dark image

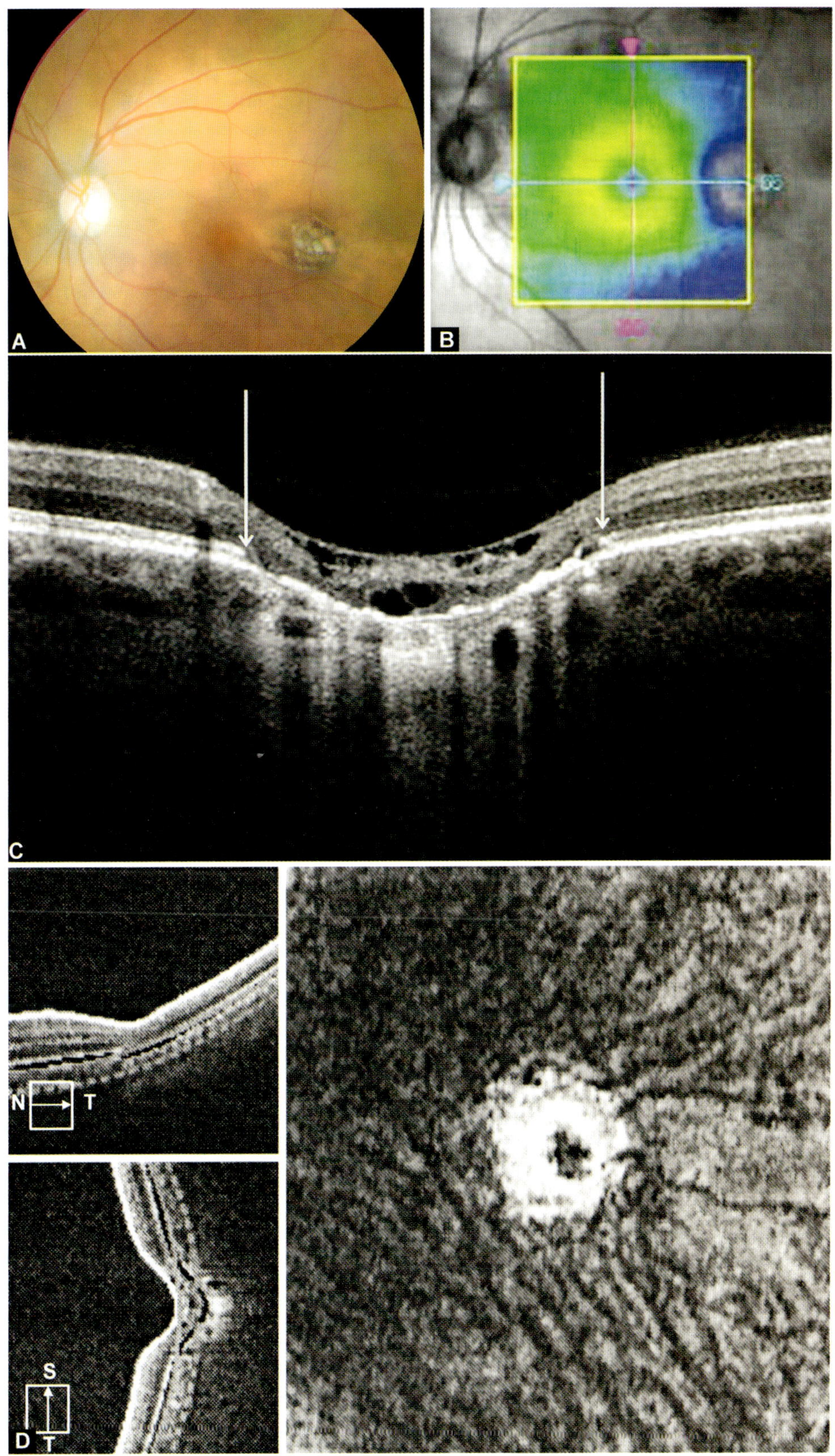

Figures 2A to D: (A) Partially pigmented torpedo maculopathy. (B) The retinal map of the OCT showed the lesion as a thinned area. (C) Magnification of the vertical scan of the OCT showed a disruption of the RPE layer, a disorganization of the retina, and an excavation of layers located below the RPE. (D) *En face* OCT image focused on the deep layers the lesion as whitish, inhomogeneous, contrasting with the adjacent choroid

Case 2

Forty-three years old woman showed: (a) partially pigmented torpedo lesion; (b) the retinal map of the OCT showed the lesion as a thinned area; (c) magnification of the vertical scan of the OCT showed a disruption of the RPE layer, a disorganization of the retina and an excavation of layers located below the RPE; (d) *en face* OCT image focused on the deep layers the lesion as whitish, nonhomogeneous, contrasting with the adjacent choroid.

Conclusion

Torpedo maculopathy still represents an imaging mystery. Some cases are characterized by focal absence of RPE giving a cleft in OCT imaging, while other cases are characterized by focal thinning of a present and hypoplastic RPE. OCT *en face* also showed images very different from one case to another. Torpedo maculopathy may correspond to a more or less complete defect in the development of the RPE, thus showing very variable imaging patterns among affected patients.

References

1. Roseman RL, Gass JD. Solitary hypopigmented nevus of the retinal pigment epithelium in the macula. Arch Ophthalmol. 1992;110:1358-9.
2. Daily MJ. Torpedo maculopathy or paramacular spot syndrome. New Dimensions in Retina Symposium. Chicago, 1993:11;7.
3. Shields CL, Guzman JM, Shapiro MJ, et al. Torpedo maculopathy at the site of the fetal "bulge." Arch Ophthalmol. 2010;128:499-501.
4. Richez F, Gueudry J, Brasseur G, et al. Bilateral torpedo maculopathy. J Fr Ophtalmol. 2010;33:296.
5. Tsang T, Messner LV, Pilon A, et al. Torpedo maculopathy: in vivo histology using optical coherence tomography. Optom Vis Sci. 2009;86:E1380-5.
6. Golchet PR, Jampol LM, Mathura JR Jr, et al. Torpedo maculopathy. Br J Ophthalmol. 2010;94:302-6.
7. Mahieu L, Mathis A. "Torpedo" maculopathy. J Fr Ophtalmol. 2003;26:533.
8. Rigotti M, Babighian S, Carcereri De Prati E, et al. Three cases of a rare congenital abnormality of the retinal pigment epithelium: torpedo maculopathy. Ophthalmologica. 2002;216:226-7.

chapter 22

En Face Optical Coherence Tomography in Retinal Dystrophies

Cinzia Mazzini, Andrea Sodi, Ugo Menchini

Introduction

In the last years the interest for retinal dystrophies has significantly grown because of the development of genetic diagnosis and the increased hopes for the availability of possible effective therapies.[1-3]

Anyway, the clinical evaluation of retinal dystrophies is often very difficult because in the most advanced stages some phenotypes may show similar features and overlap each other; moreover many patients present very poor visual acuity and severe visual field loss, preventing the chance to use visual function changes to monitor disease progression and its possible response to treatments.

Recently optical coherence tomography (OCT) technology allowed a safe, reliable and noninvasive method to analyze the details of retinal structure in retinal dystrophies.[4] Moreover, *en face* OCT approach[5] provided transversal scanning of the retina with a better visualization of the lateral extent of morphological abnormalities at the posterior pole. At present there is no detailed reports about the use of *en face* OCT in patients with retinal dystrophies; nevertheless this diagnostic approach may be helpful to disclose some peculiar clinical features of these disorders and to monitor their evolution with time.

Retinal dystrophies may be distinguished into retinal degenerations which primarily affect peripheral retina [i.e. retinitis pigmentosa (RP) and allied disorders, like choroidal dystrophies] or the macular area (a group of disorders more specifically named "macular dystrophies"); the most common macular dystrophies are Stargardt's disease (STGD), Best vitelliform maculopathy and juvenile retinoschisis.

Some *en face* OCT scans are reported in this chapter. All the images have been obtained by cirrus OCT (Carl Zeiss, Meditec) with the 512 × 128 macular cube acquisitions.

Retinitis Pigmentosa

Retinitis pigmentosa is characterized by progressive loss of photoreceptors; it usually primarily affects the rods with a later involvement of the cones.[6] Ophthalmoscopy shows a pale optic disk, attenuated retinal vessels, a diffuse RPE dystrophy with more or less numerous pigment clumping (**Figure 1A**). The macula is often spared until the last stages of the disease but in some cases peripheral retinal degeneration is associated with macular atrophic changes. In most of the cases the first symptom is night blindness, followed by the progressive loss in the peripheral visual field; in some cases the disease may progress to a very severe visual loss or even to blindness after several years. Electroretinographic response is typically abnormal.

In RP B scan OCT[7] often shows a normal laminar retinal architecture in the central retina around the macula with a progressive disruption or disappearance of the photoreceptors inner/outer segment junction (IS/OS line) in the more peripheral retinal areas (**Figure 1B**).

In this case *en face* OCT shows a central hyper-reflective island of survived outer retina surrounded by a hyporeflective ring of atrophic changes (**Figure 1C).**

Bietti Crystalline Dystrophy

This is a chorioretinal degeneration characterized by the presence of yellow-white glittering crystals scattered all over the eye fundus (**Figure 2A**). In most of the patients some crystalline deposits can be observed also in the corneal limbus. The symptoms include reduced visual acuity, poor night vision, abnormal retinal electrophysiology and visual field loss. Fluorescein angiography reveals diffused chorio-capillaris atrophy with residual islands of retinal structures (**Figure 2B**).[8]

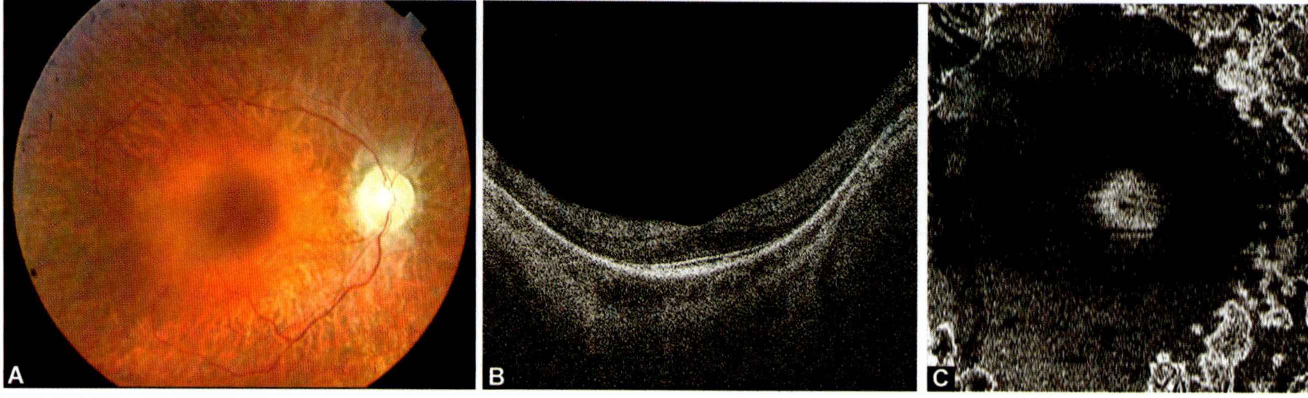

Figures 1A to C: Autosomal recessive retinitis pigmentosa. (A) Fundus picture: diffuse retinal dystrophy with small pigment clumping sparing the central retinal area; (B) B scan OCT: evident hyper-reflective layer in the macular area corresponding to the still surviving photoreceptors; (C) *En face* OCT (11 μ above RPE level): hyper-reflective island of survived outer retina surrounded by a hyporeflective ring of atrophic changes

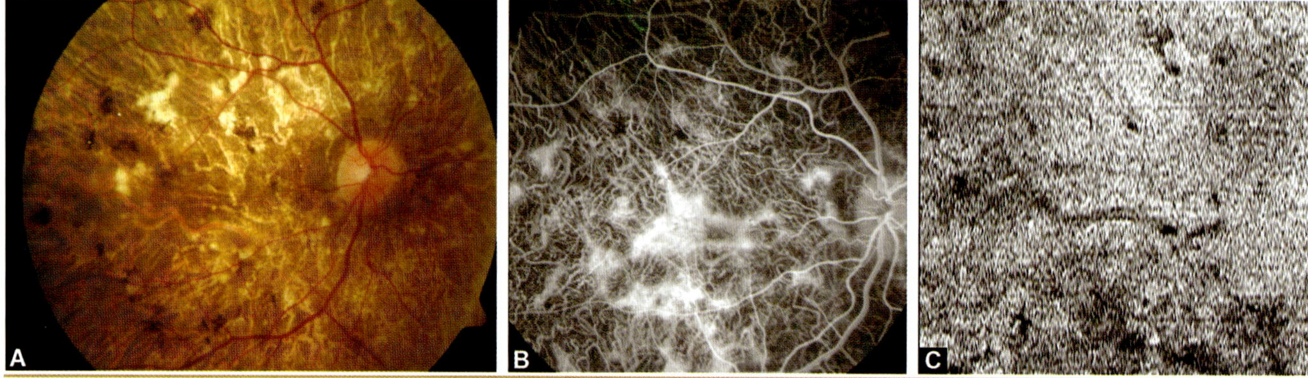

Figures 2A to C: Bietti's crystalline dystrophy. The patient carries a CYP4V2 mutation in heterozygosis on both alleles. (A) Fundus picture: diffuse chorioretinal degeneration with small glittering crystals scattered at the posterior pole and beyond the arcades; (B) Fluorescein angiography: diffused retinal and choriocapillaris atrophy with visualization of the deep choroidal circulation and island of survived retina; (C) *En face* OCT (at the RPE level): diffuse atrophic RPE changes with visualization of the underlying choroid; a few small hyper-reflective structures probably corresponding to the crystals can be appreciated

B scan OCT may show reduced retinal thickness, associated with some hyper-reflective spots at the level of the RPE,[9] while *en face* OCT presents diffused atrophic RPE changes with very small hyper-reflective structures probably corresponding to the crystals.

Stargardt Disease

Stargardt disease (STGD) is the most prevalent inherited juvenile macular dystrophy. Fundoscopy usually shows a macular atrophy, often associated with typical fish-tail white-yellowish spots spread at the posterior pole and sometimes at midperiphery (flecks) **(Figure 3A)**.[10,11] The disease is characterized by a diffuse accumulation of toxic metabolites (lipofuscins) at the level of the RPE with consequent impairment of the same RPE and photoreceptors atrophy.

Fluoroangiography shows very often a homogeneous dark aspect of choroid ("dark or silent choroid"), determined by the masking effect of lipofuscin storage in RPE on the underlying choroidal fluorescence. Electroretinogram (ERG) abnormalities can be recorded in patients with advanced stages of the disease.

In STGD B scan OCT usually shows foveal thinning, determined by the progressive photoreceptors loss and a significant disorganization or absence of IS/OS junction beneath the macula **(Figure 3B)**.[12] *En face* OCT at the level of RPE shows an irregular pattern at the posterior pole, with central photoreceptors atrophy **(Figure 3C)**.

In another case the flecks are located at the posterior pole and beyond the arcades **(Figure 4A)**; they are clearly visible in the fluorescein angiography **(Figure 4B)** and in most of the cases seem to be hyper-reflective at the *en face* OCT imaging **(Figure 4C)**.

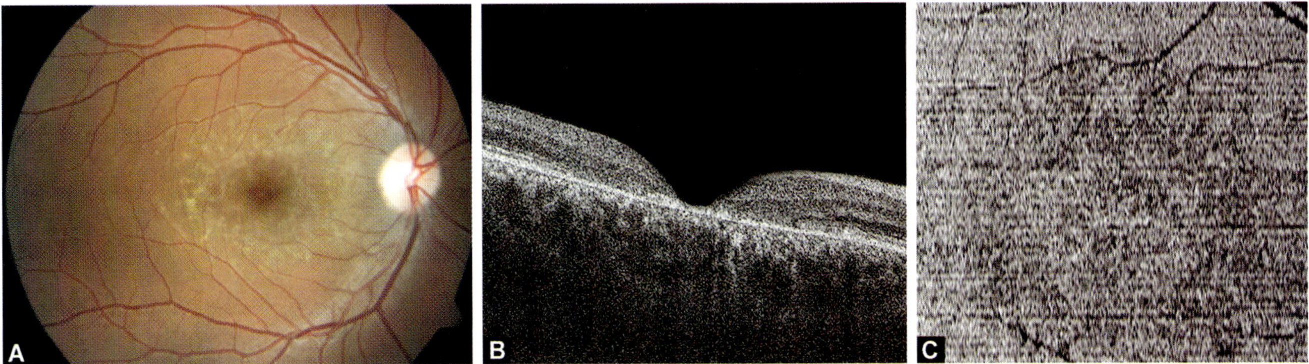

Figures 3A to C: Stargardt disease. The patient carries a complex allele with three ABCA4 mutations. (A) Fundus picture: macular atrophy surrounded by flecks at the posterior pole; (B) B scan OCT: reduced central retinal thickness and disappearance of the photoreceptors IS/OS junction at the posterior pole; (C) *En face* OCT (at the RPE level): irregular hyporeflective atrophic changes at the posterior pole

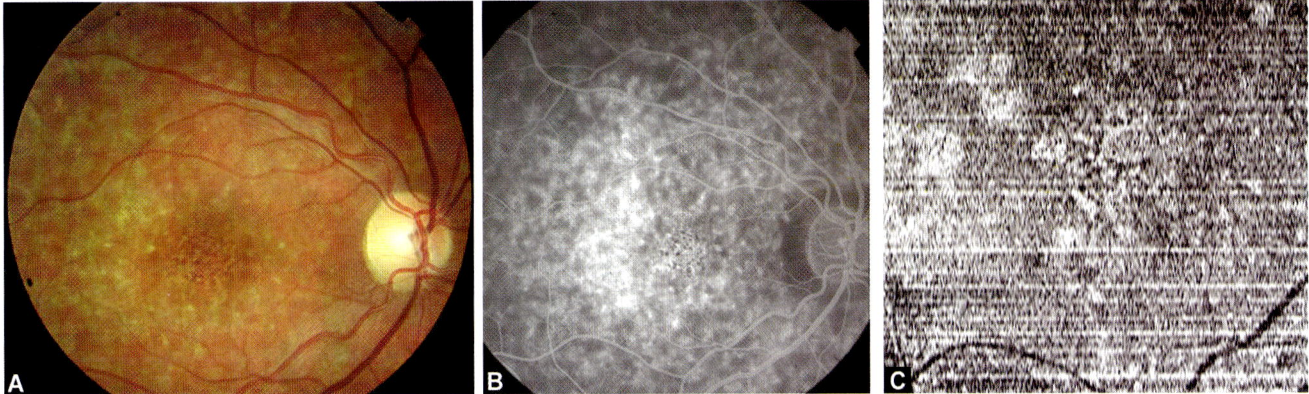

Figures 4A to C: Stargardt disease. The patient carries an ABCA4 mutation in heterozygosis in both alleles. (A) Fundus picture: macular atrophy with flecks at the posterior pole and beyond the arcades; (B) Fluorescein angiography: irregular fluorescence abnormalities at the posterior pole; flecks can be hyper- or hypo-fluorescent according to their stage of evolution toward atrophy; this patient does not show an evident dark choroid; (C) *En face* OCT (7µ above RPE level): hyper-reflective alterations in the central retina, probably corresponding to flecks and more generally to lipofuscins deposits

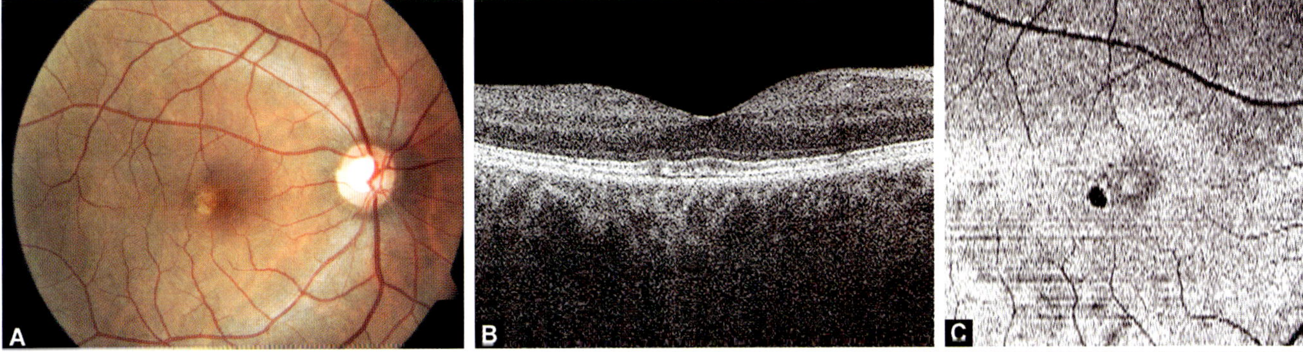

Figures 5A to C: Best vitelliform macular dystrophy. Previtelliform stage. The patient carries a single BEST1 mutation on one allele. His son carries the same mutation and shows a typical vitelliform disk. (A) Fundus picture: mild RPE paramacular atrophy; (B) B scan OCT: localized disorganization of the RPE layer; (C) *En face* OCT (9 µ above RPE level); hyporeflective paramacular spot corresponding to limited RPE atrophic changes

Best Vitelliform Macular Dystrophy

Best vitelliform macular dystrophy[13] is characterized by yellowish yolk-like lesion in the macula which over time progressively disintegrates with the development of macular atrophy or fibrosis. Like other macular dystrophies the disorder is associated with the accumulation of lipofuscin at the level of the RPE. During the course of the disease the macular lesions seem to progress through various stages: previtelliform (with a mild dystrophy of macular RPE) (**Figure 5A**), vitelliform, pseudohypopyon (with an accumulation of the vitelliform material in the lower part of the disk) (**Figure 5B**) vitelliruptive (with an irregular scattering of the vitelliform material within the disk), atrophic and cicatricial. EOG abnormalities can be recorded in all the patients, with very few exceptions.[14]

The vitelliform substance and the associated alterations of the RPE and of the photoreceptors are well imaged by B scan OCT imaging (**Figures 5C and 6A**).[15]

In the previtelliform stage *en face* OCT may detect the localized atrophy of the RPE at the posterior pole (**Figure 6B**) while in the pseudohypopyon stage (**Figure 6C**) the disk presents itself with a regular roundish shape and thickened hyper-reflective walls; the contents are not homogeneous with a deposit of the hyper-reflective vitelliform material in the lower part of the lesion.

Autosomal Recessive Bestrophinopathy

This peculiar phenotype has recently been described in association with biallelic BEST1 mutations.[16,17] It is characterized by irregular yellowish deposits at the posterior pole (**Figure 7A**), widespread RPE dystrophy, macular edema, EOG and ERG abnormalities. B scan OCT shows the macular intraretinal fluid (**Figure 7B**).

En face OCT at the RPE level offers a description of the hyper-reflective deposits located in the outer retina (**Figure 7C**) while more superficial scans describe the morphological features of the macular edema: it seems to correspond to a central larger cyst surrounded by smaller cavities. The borders of the whole lesion are thickened and hyper-reflective (**Figure 7D**).

Juvenile Retinoschisis

Its main clinical feature is a foveal schisis with a typical "star-like" or "spoke-like" appearance (**Figure 8A**) (occurring in almost all of the patients) and a peripheral retinoschisis (which is present in about half of the patients), usually in the inferotemporal retina.[18,19] Electronegative ERG response is frequently associated with the disease.

B scan OCT often shows cleavage of the retina at the level of the nerve fiber layer but retinal splitting in deeper layers has been described too (**Figure 8B**).[20]

En face OCT clearly images the morphology of the macular schisis, showing a central larger cavity with surrounding smaller cysts with an ordinate radial disposition. The wall of the macular lesion is thin and irregular (**Figure 8C**).

Pattern Dystrophies

These retinal dystrophies are characterized by pigment deposits arranged in a variety of patterns in the macular area (**Figure 9A**).[21] They are usually associated with mild central vision abnormalities and present a relatively good

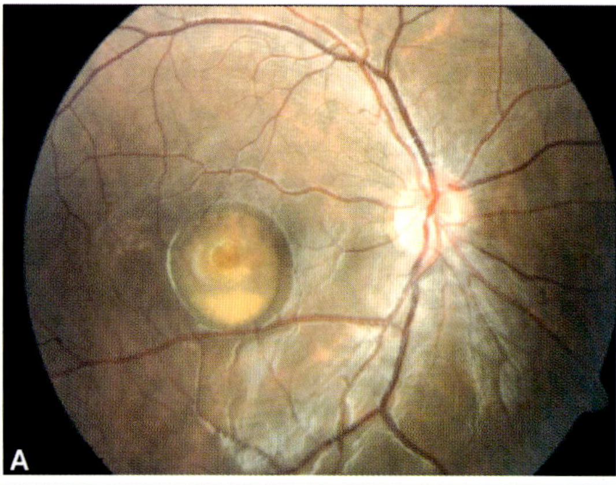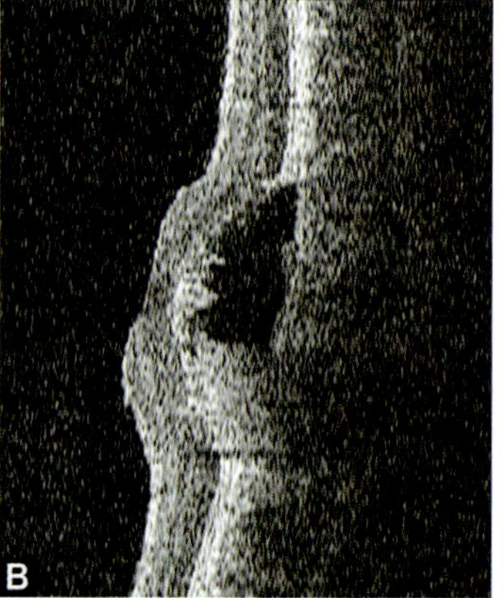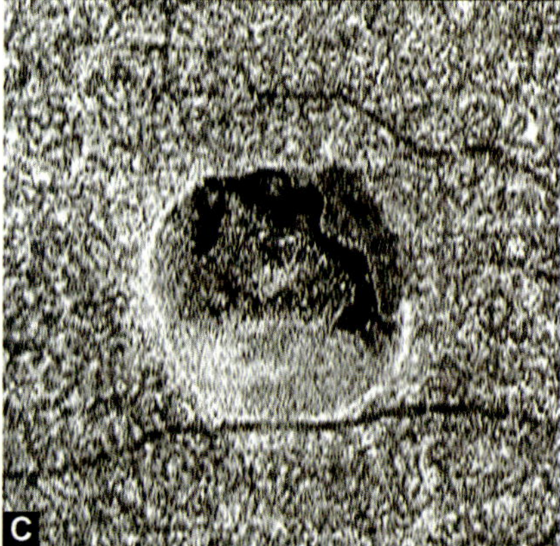

Figures 6A to C: Best vitelliform macular dystrophy. Pseudohypopion stage. The patient carries a single BEST1 mutation on one allele. (A) Fundus picture: vitelliform disk with accumulation of the vitelliform material in the lower part of the disk. (B) B scan OCT (vertical scan): Hyper-reflective vitelliform material located in the lower part of the disk while the superior part is optically empty. (C) *En face* OCT (at the RPE level): Roundish vitelliform disk with thickened hyperreflective walls; the contents are not homogeneous with deposit of the hyperreflective vitelliform material in the lower part of the lesion

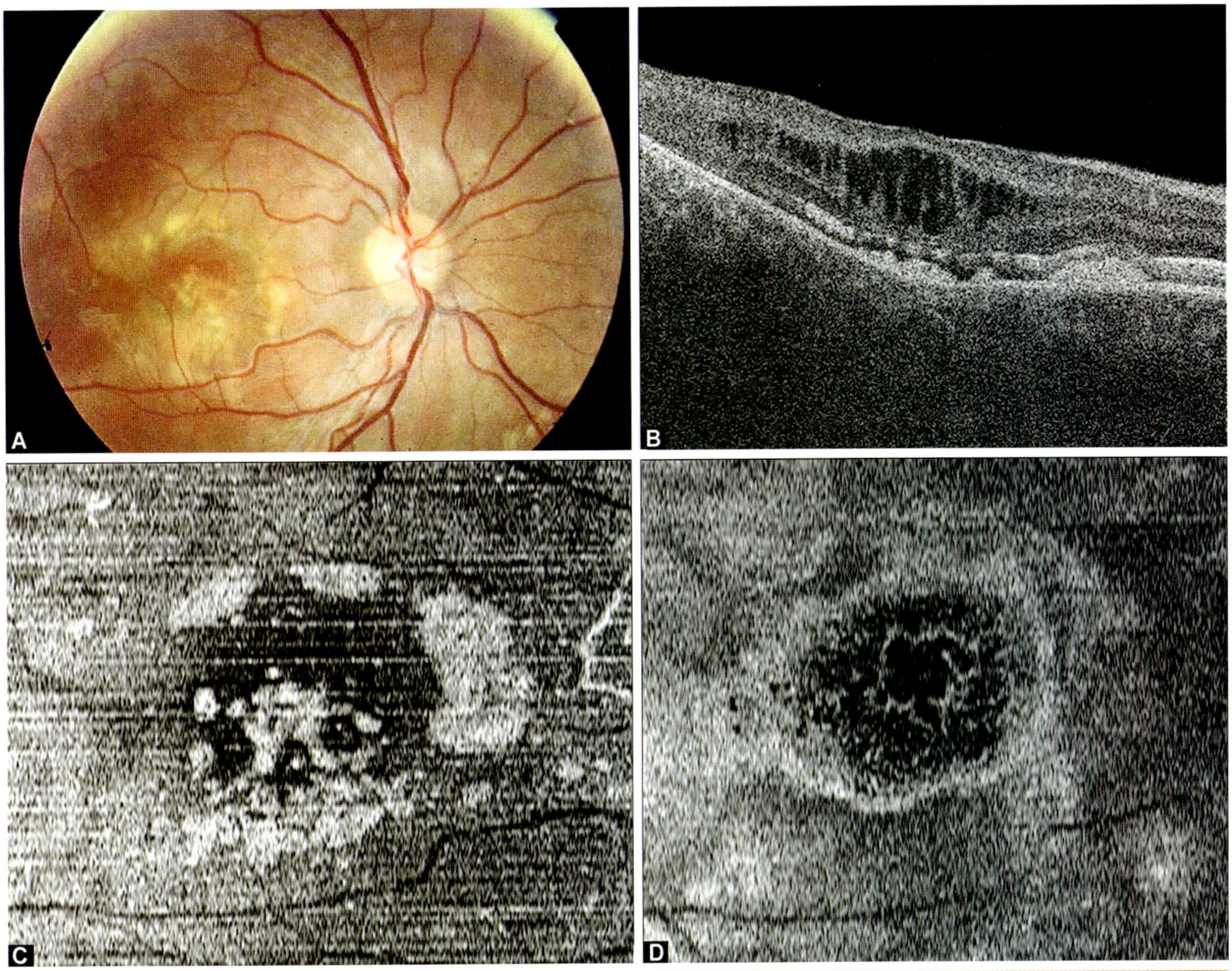

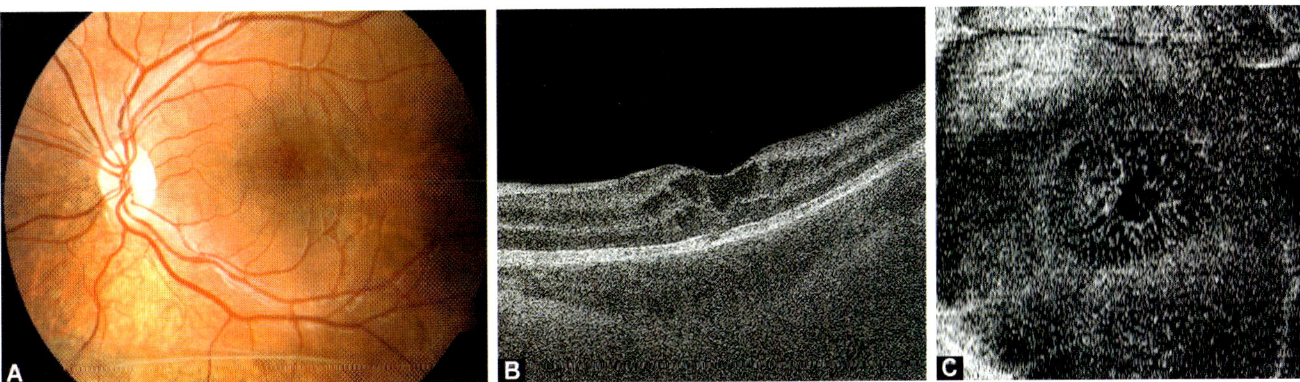

Figures 7A to D: Autosomal recessive bestrophinopathy. The patient carries a BEST1 mutation on both alleles in compound heterozygosis. (A) Fundus picture: diffused RPE dystrophy with yellowish deposits at the posterior pole, macular edema; (B) B scan OCT: in the macular area intraretinal optically empty cavities with localized thickening of the RPE layer; (C) *En face* OCT (3 µ above RPE level): hyper-reflective deposits regularly distributed at the posterior pole; (D) *En face* OCT (240 µ above RPE level): macular edema with a central cyst surrounded by smaller cavities; the borders of the whole lesion are thickened and hyper-reflective

Figures 8A to C: Juvenile retinoschisis. (A) Fundus picture: Macular cysts with radial distribution. (B) B scan OCT: Intraretinal splitting with optically empty cavities mostly located in the more superficial retinal layers. (C) *En face* OCT (191 µ above RPE level): Macular schisis with a central larger cavity surrounded by smaller cysts with an ordinate radial disposition; the wall of the macular lesion is thin and irregular

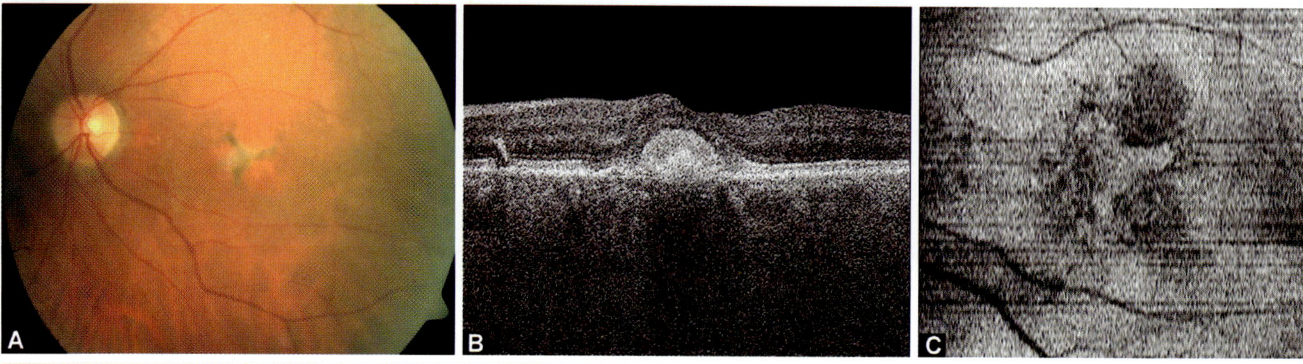

Figures 9A to C: Pattern dystrophy. (A) Fundus picture: macular RPE deposits distributed with a regular pattern (in this case with a triangular shape); (B) B scan OCT: localized dome-shaped thickening of the hyper-reflective RPE layer; (C) *En face* OCT (at the RPE level): at the posterior pole hyper-reflective deposist with an approximate triangular disposition

prognosis. B scan OCT often shows a localized dome-shaped thickening of the hyper-reflective RPE layer **(Figure 9B)** while *en face* OCT at the RPE level reveals the presence of hyper-reflective deposits with peculiar and apparently regular disposition **(Figure 9C)**.

En face OCT investigation of retinal dystrophies is presently taking its first steps. From now on, this diagnostic approach may provide some information about peculiar details of retinal architecture which cannot be imaged with other techniques; moreover it will probably represent a useful tool to monitor the natural history of inherited retinal degenerations and their response to possible innovative treatments.

References

1. Gass JDM. Heredodystrophic disorders affecting the pigment epithelium and retina. In: Strescopic Atlas of Macular Disease. Diagnosis and Treatment. St. Louis-London-Philadelphia-Sydney-Toronto: Mosby; 1997. pp. 303-435.
2. Puech B. Dystrophies maculaires hereditaires. In: Dufier JL, Kaplan J (Eds). Oeil et genetique. Societè Française d'Ophtalmologie, Paris: 2005. pp. 273-301.
3. Simonelli F, Sodi A. Distrofie Maculari Eredofamiliari. Fabiano, Canelli (AT), 2011.
4. Meunier I, Arndt C, Zanlonghi X, et al. Spectral-domain optical coherence tomography in hereditary retinal dystrophies. Intech, Rijeka-Shangai, 2012. pp. 147-70.
5. Van Velthoven MEJ, Verbraak FD, Yannuzzi LA, et al. Imaging the retina by *en face* optical coherence tomography. Retina. 2006;26:129-36.
6. Hartong DT, Berson EL, Dryia TP. Retinitis Pigmentosa. Lancet. 2006;368:1795-809.
7. Mitamura Y, Mitamura-Aizawa S, Nagasawa T, et al. Diagnostic imaging in patients with retinitis pigmentosa. J Med Invest. 2012;59:1-11.
8. Kaiser-Kupfer MI, Chan CC, Markello TC, et al. Clinical biochemical and pathologic correlations in Bietti's crystalline dystrophy. Am J Ophthalmol. 1994;118:569-82.
9. Pennesi ME, Weleber RG. High-resolution optical coherence tomography shows new aspects of Bietti crystalline retinopathy. Retina. 2010;30:531-2.
10. Noble KG, Carr RE. Stargardt's Disease and fundus flavimaculatus. Arch Ophthalmol. 1979;97:1281-5.
11. Passerini I, Sodi A, Giambene B, et al. Torricelli F. Novel mutations in of the ABCR gene in italian patients with Stargardt disease. Eye. 2010;24:158-64.
12. Ergun E, Hermann B, Wirtitsch M. Assessment of central visual function in Stargardt's disease/fundus flavimaculatus with ultrahigh-resolution optical coherence tomography. Invest Ophthalmol Vis Sci. 2005; 46:310-6.
13. Boon CJF, Klevering BJ, Leroy BP, et al. The spectrum of ocular phenotypes caused by mutations in the BEST1 gene. Progr Ret Eye Res. 2009;28:187-205.
14. Testa F, Rossi S, Passerini I, et al. A normal electro-oculography in a family affected by best disease with a novel spontaneous mutation of the BEST1 gene. Br J Ophthalmol. 2008;92(11):1467-70.
15. Querques G, Regenbogen M, Quijano C, et al. Definition optical coherence tomography features in vitelliform macular dystrophy. Am J Ophthalmol. 2008;146:501-7.
16. Burgess R, Millar ID, Leroy BP, et al. Biallelic mutation of BEST1 causes a distinct retinopathy in humans. Am J Hum Genet. 2008;82:19-31.
17. Sodi A, Menchini F, Manitto MP, et al. Ocular phenotypes associated with biallelic mutations in BEST1 in Italian patients. Mol Vis. 2011;17:3078-87.
18. Simonelli F, Cennamo G, Ziviello C, et al. Clinical features of X linked juvenile retinoschisis associated with new mutations in the XLRS1 gene in Italian families. Br J Ophthalmol. 2003;87:1130-4.
19. Sikkink SK, Biswas S, Parry NR, et al. X-linked retinoschisis: an update. J Med Genet. 2007;44:225-32.
20. Gregori NZ, Berrocal AM, Gregori G, et al. Macular spectral-domain optical coherence tomography in patients with X linked retinoschisis. Br J Ophthalmol. 2009;93: 373-8.
21. Marmor MF, Byers BE. Pattern dystrophy of the pigment epithelium. Am J Ophthalmol. 1977;84:32-44.

Section 6

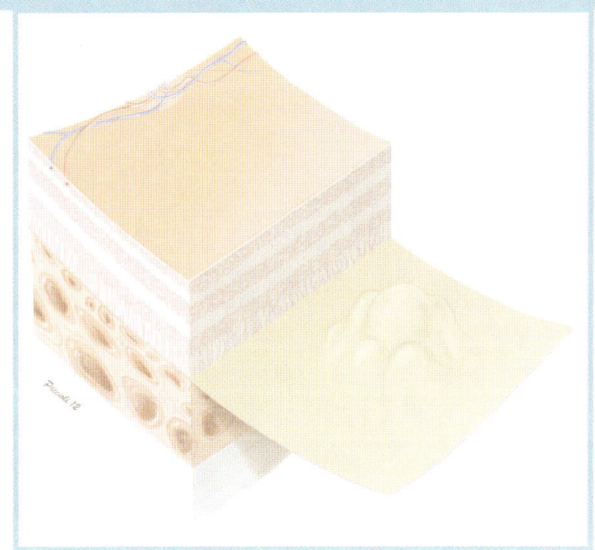

Retinal *En Face* Optical Coherence Tomography Examination: Other Macular Diseases

chapter 23

Central Serous Chorioretinopathy (By Means of Scans Adapted to RPE Concavity)

Luca Di Antonio, Leonardo Mastropasqua

Introduction

Central serous chorioretinopathy (CSC) is a common disease in young to middle aged adults characterized by an idiopathic serous detachment of the neuroepithelium secondary to one or more retinal pigment epithelium (RPE) leakage points as observed on fluorescein angiography (FA) **(Figures 1, 2 and 4)** and green indocyanine angiography (ICGA) **(Figures 3A to C)**.[1,2] Optical coherence tomography (OCT), specially spectral domain OCT (SD-OCT) provides important information on the structure and morphology of both neuroepithelium and PED in CSC and not surprisingly, a thickening of the choroid.[3] *En face* OCT, a noninvasive technique, produces images with high pixel to pixel correspondence to confocal fundus images.[4] CSC features have been described by means of an *en face* OCT in both longitudinal and transversal scan mode.[4]

First OCT instruments produced scans perfectly plane (C scan) to the pigmented epithelium concavity. The images thus acquired were interesting, but difficult to understand.[5]

New instruments recently introduced allows to perform *en face* scans fitting the pigmented epithelium concavity giving both interesting and well-understanding information in several macular diseases. In CSC *en face* OCT is able to detect the focal leak point seen in both FA and ICGA, size and location of serous detachment, presence of hyper-reflective dots, presence of thickened fibrinous fluid; presence, size, location and number of pigment epithelium detachment (PED) **(Figure 7)**.[4]

It allows showing the morphologic aspects of PED. PED shape is predominantly circular, inner silhouette is mostly smooth, contents are clear and wall aspects are frequently uniform in CSC **(Figures 6A and B)**.[6] *En face* OCT detects the irregularities of both photoreceptor outer segment and RPE surface previously seen by fundus autofluorescence, SD-OCT and *en face* OCT.[7-9] *En face* OCT highlights diffuse hyper-reectivity at the level of outer plexiform layer and outer nuclear layer suggesting that the presence of subretinal fluid results in alterations of intraretinal layers that are not directly adjacent to the subretinal fluid **(Figure 8)**.[10]

Recently it has been shown as an association between visual acuity and integrity of the inner and outer segment junction in patients with CSC.[11] Detection of intensity abnormalities in the inner and outer segment *en face* image is useful for monitoring the integrity of photoreceptor cells in the course of disease progression and therapeutic intervention **(Figures 5A and B)**.[12]

Moreover, *en face* OCT may confirm "polyp-like" dilations in polypoidal choroidal vasculopathy masquerading as CSC already described in ICGA **(Figures 9A to E)**.[13-16] *En face* OCT is able to give an instant overview of the whole macular area and provides new information not available with standard B scan **(Figures 10A and B)**.[4] It is to be in a position to detect structural and morphological changes of CSC before and after treatment (i.e. medical, photocoagulation and photodynamic therapies) **(Figures 10 to 14)**.

This improves and supports early diagnosis when use of contrast imaging technique is restricted (i.e. pregnancy, allergy) **(Figure 15)**. In short *en face* OCT is a good alternative in the diagnosis and follow-up of the patients with CSC and it can be considered a new breakthrough in retinal imaging.

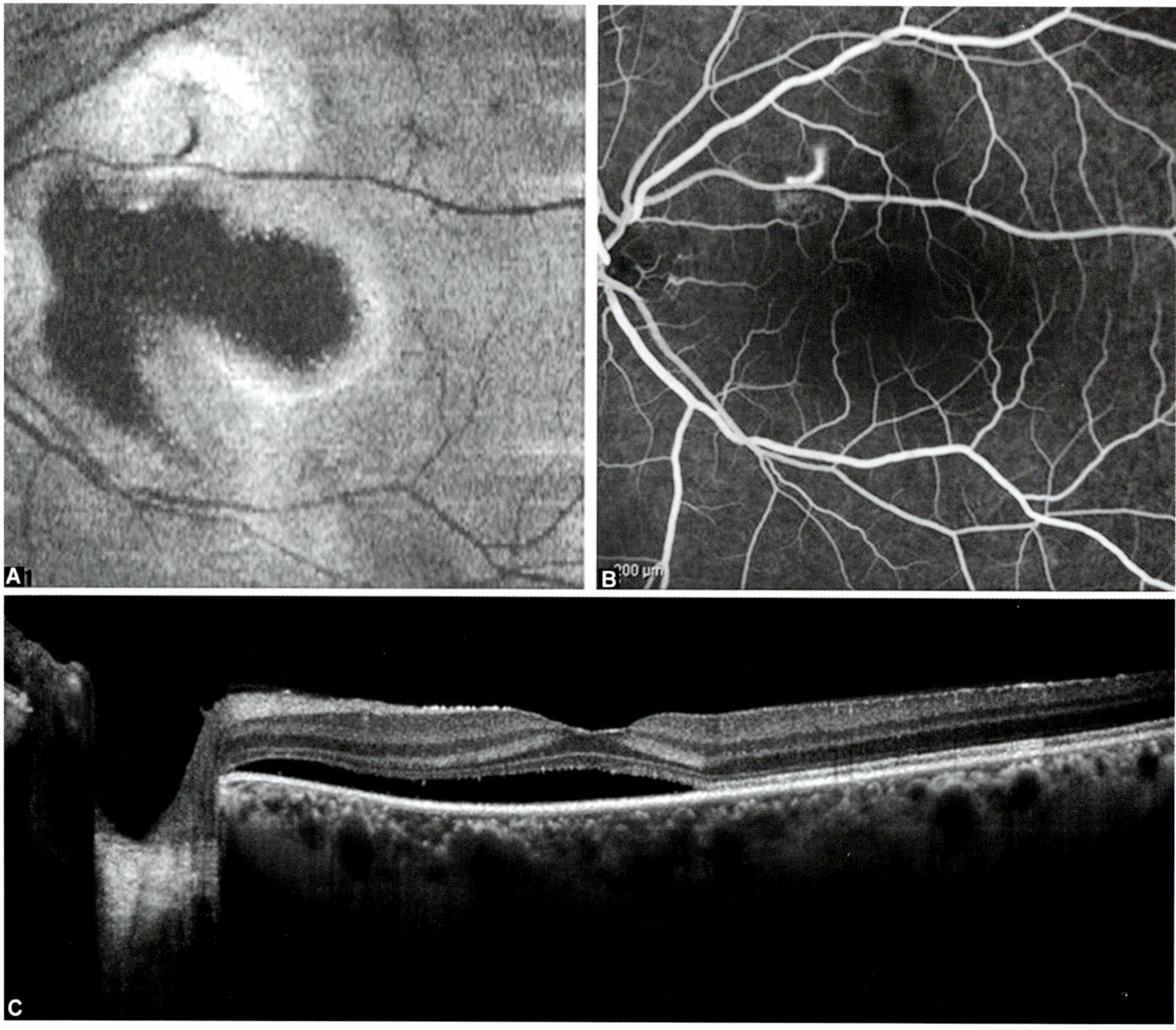

Figures 1A to C: Smokestack leak. (A) *En face* optical coherence tomography scan highlights a smokestack pattern corresponding to focal leak at the level of the retinal pigment epithelium seen in early frame of fluorescein angiography; (B) *En face* shows a hyporeflective area which corresponding to the serous detachment in the macular region. Note multiple highly reflective dot-like precipitates aligning the outer layer of the detached neurosensory retina; (C) The slightly elongated photoreceptor outer segments are seen below the serous neurosensory detachment in longitudinal scan. High reflectivity of Sattler's layer and a vessel dilation of Haller's layer are visible together with a thickened choroid

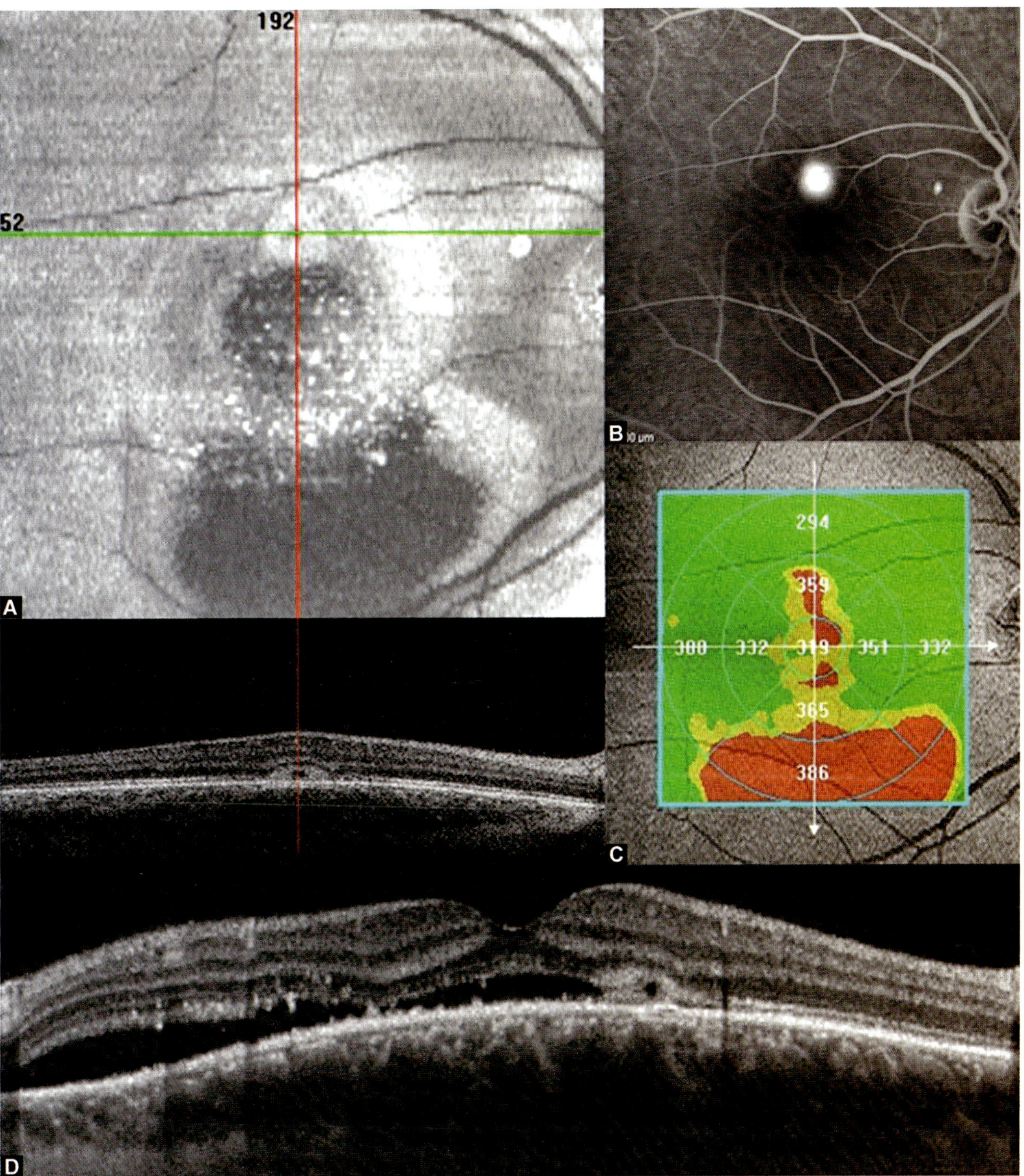

Figures 2A to D: Inkblot leak. (A) *En face* optical coherence tomography scan highlights an inkblot pattern corresponding to focal leak at the level of the retinal pigment epithelium seen in fluorescein angiography; (B) accompanied by a gravitating serous detachment in macular region and a small pigment epithelium detachment nasally to the fovea; (C) Full thickness macular map showing a retinal thickening; (D) The posterior surface of the detached retina became thin and granular at the macula, and fibrinous exudates around the leakage site are seen in both frontal (A) and longitudinal scan (D)

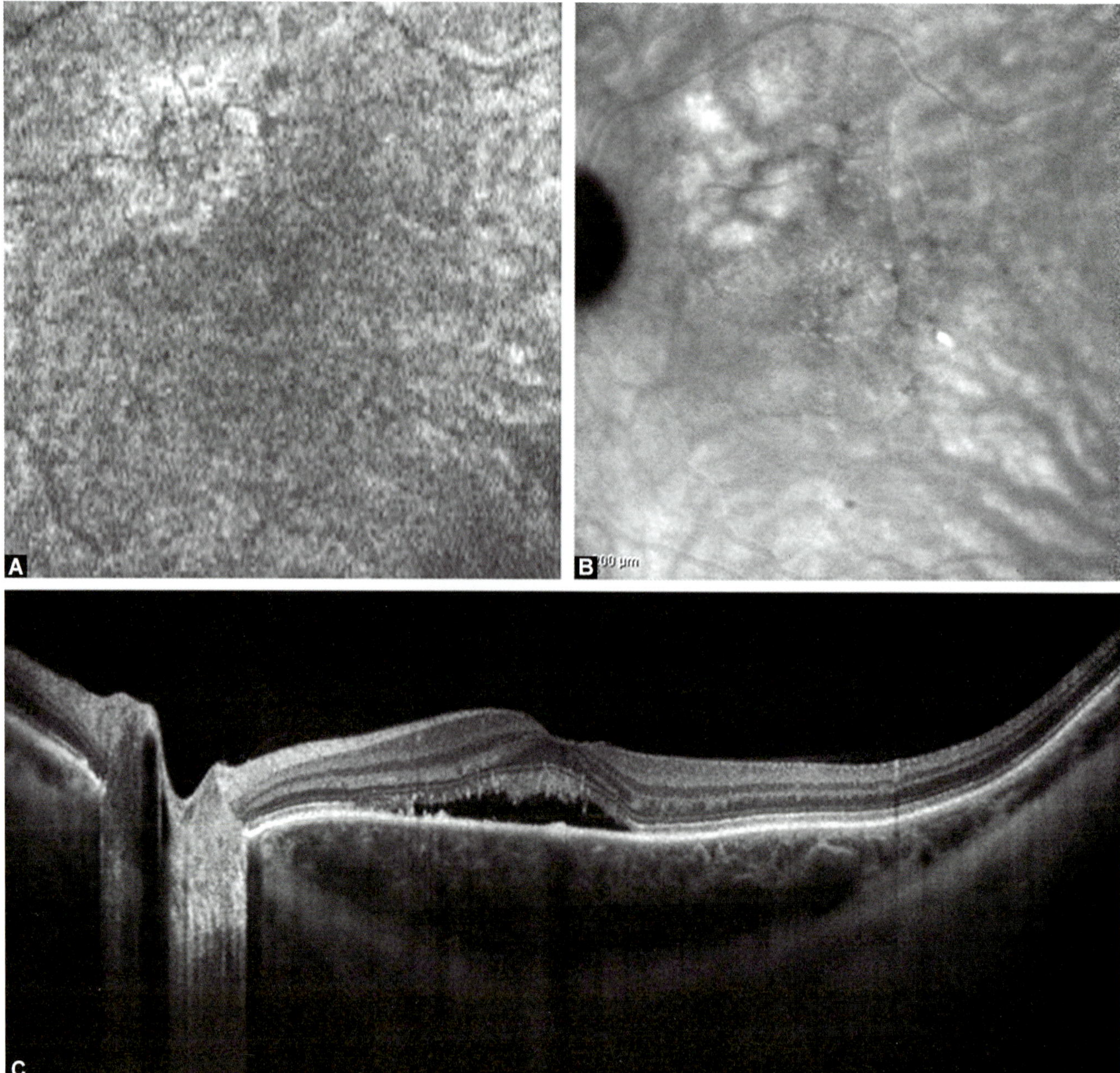

Figures 3A to C: Choroidal staining. (A) *En face* section is parallel to the pigmented epithelium and slices the choroid 83 µm below the epithelium; it shows a highly reflective area corresponding to hyper cyanescens island of inner choroidal vessels staining seen in late frame of indocyanine green angiography (B); (C) Thickening of the choroid, serous detachment and irregularities of both outer photoreceptor segment and retinal pigment epithelium are evident in longitudinal scan

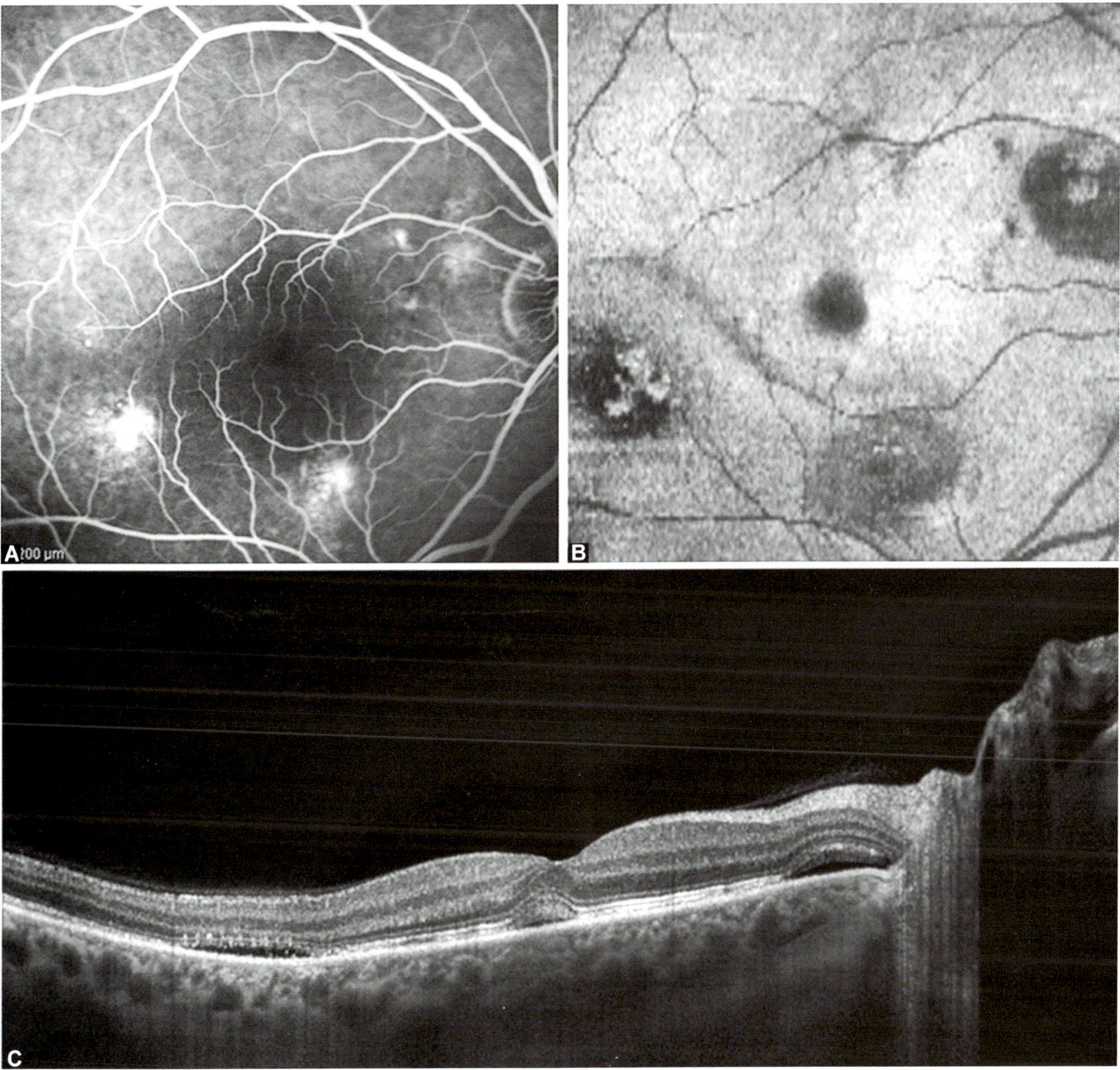

Figures 4A to C: Chronic central serous choroidopathy. (A) There may be focal or multifocal retinal pigment epithelium (RPE) leaks evident on both fluorescein angiography and (B) *En face* optical coherence tomography section; (C) There are multiple persistent and exudative detachments of the neurosensory retina resulting from a zonal or diffuse impermeability state of the RPE, resulting in fluid accumulation from the choroid through abnormal junctions of the RPE into the subretinal space

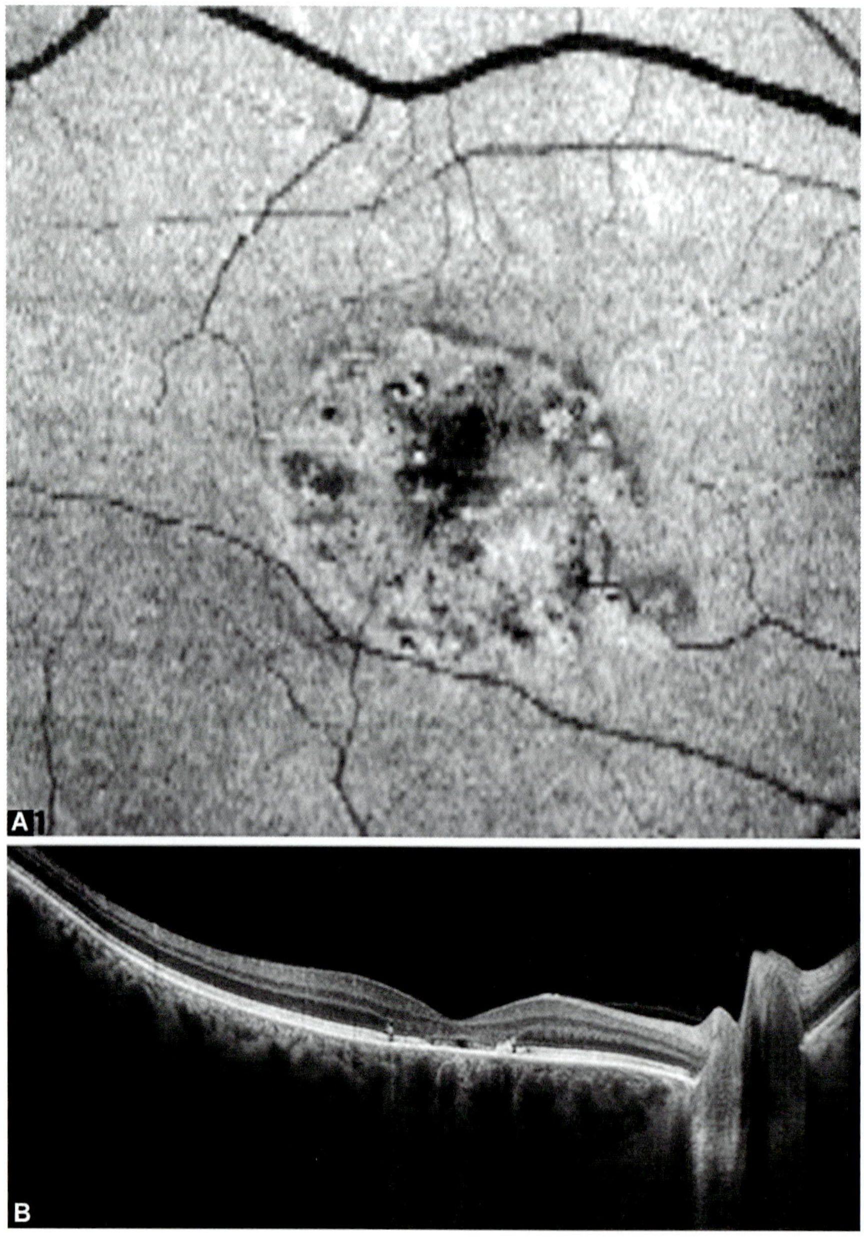

Figures 5A and B: Chronic central serous chorioretinopathy. (A) The inner and outer segment *en face* image displayed some regions of lower intensity resulting from decreased reflectance from the inner and outer segment junction associated to increased reflectance due to retinal pigment epithelium mottling. A circular area of moderate reflectance corresponding to a mark of prior neurosensory elevation; (B) Incomplete posterior vitreous detachment, preservation of external limiting membrane, discontinuity in the inner and outer segment junction, clumps and irregularities of RPE are present in longitudinal scan together with a thickened choroid

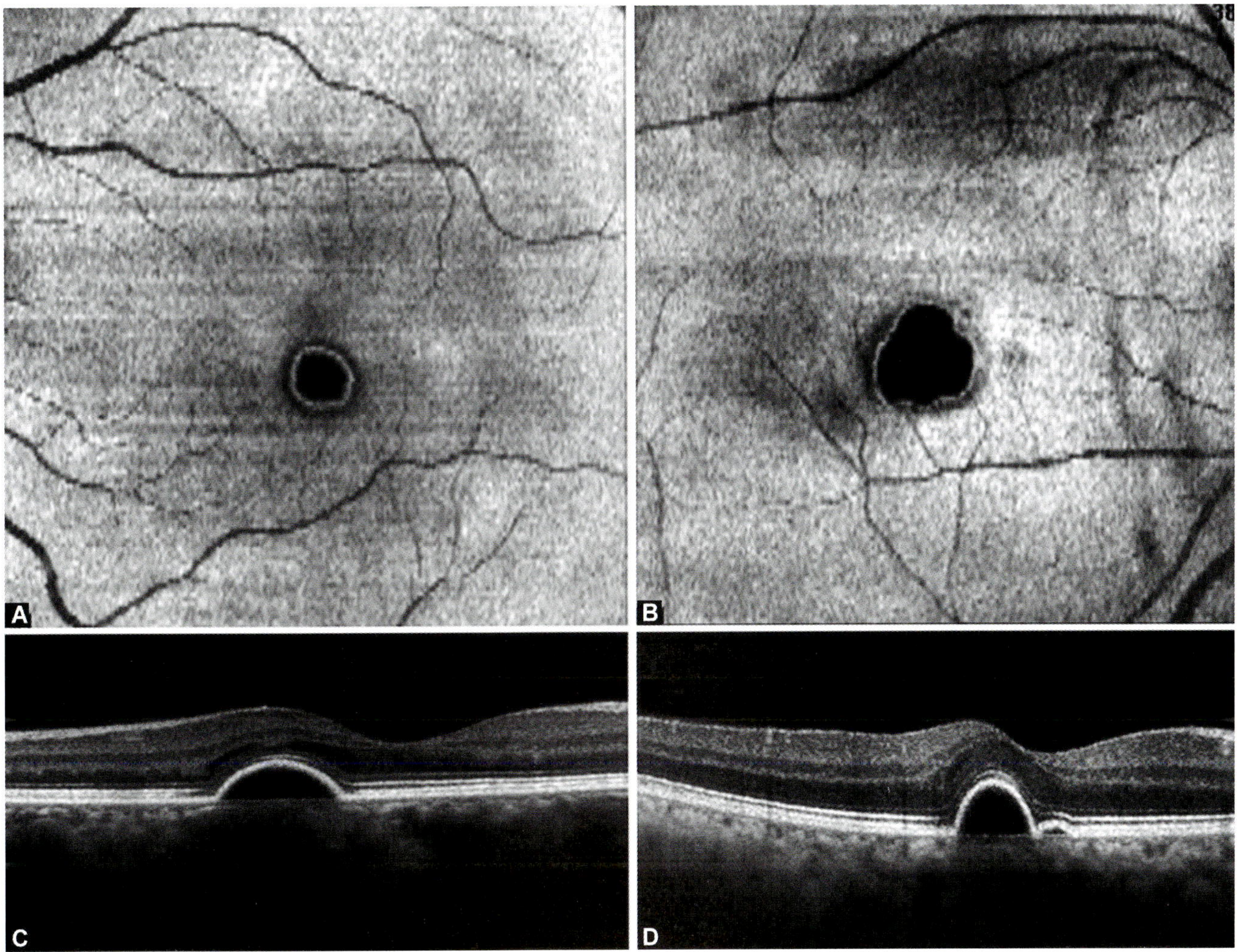

Figures 6A to D: Pigment epithelium detachment in central serous chorioretinopathy. (A and B) Pigment epithelium detachment (PED) shape is predominantly circular, inner silhouette is mostly smooth, contents are clear and wall aspects are frequently uniform; (C and D) PED appear to be optically empty, the uplift forms an angle greater than 45° with Bruch's membrane that appears clearly visible as a thin highly reflective line in longitudinal scan

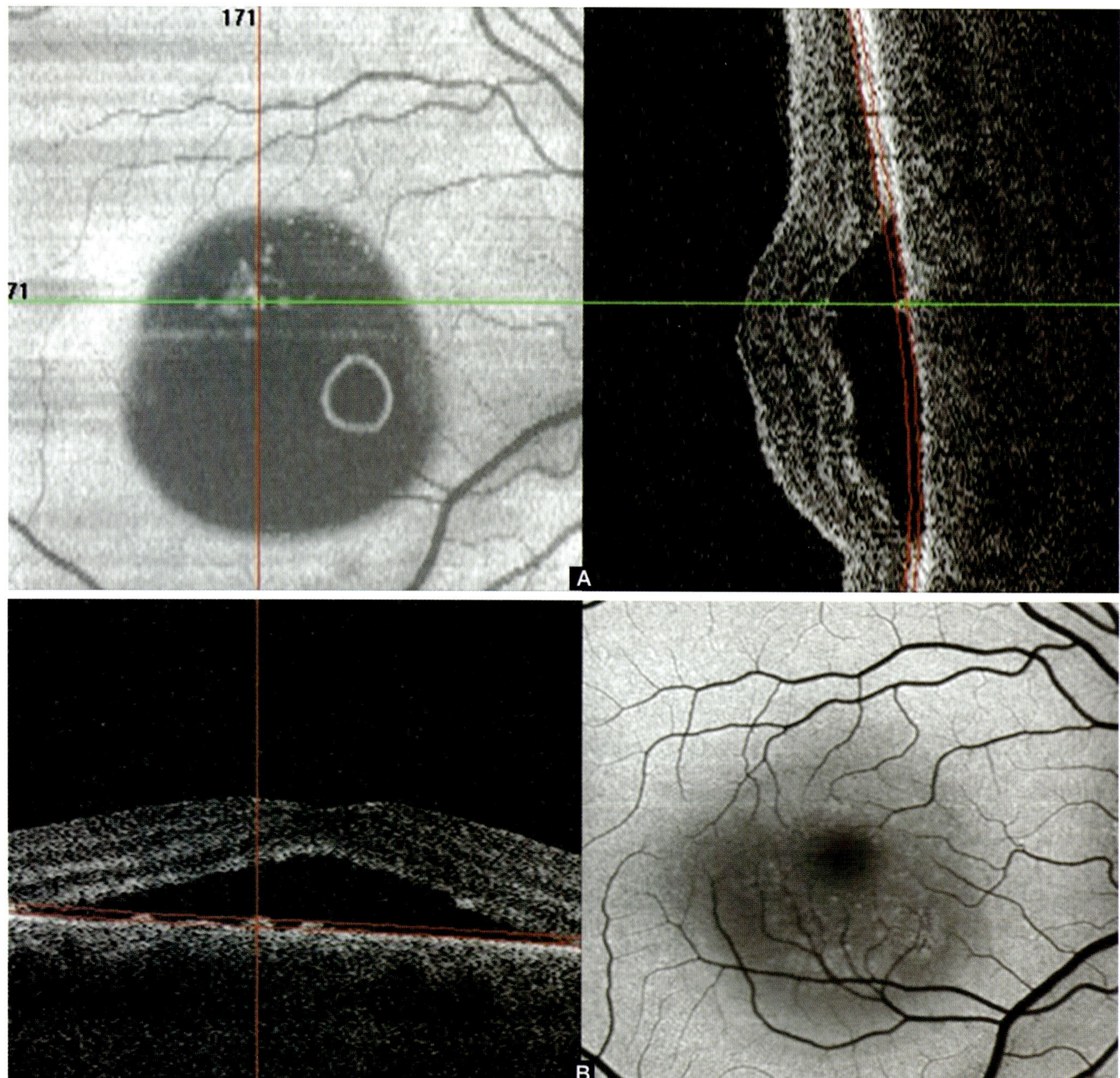

Figures 7A and B: Acute central serous chorioretinopathy. (A) *En face* optical coherence tomography section fits to the retinal pigment epithelium (RPE) concavity shows a serous detachment of neuroepithelium accompanied by a pigmented epithelium detachment; (B) The highly reflective dots exactly corresponding to the alterations of RPE surface easily, seen as hyper-autofluorescence points in fundus autofluorescence

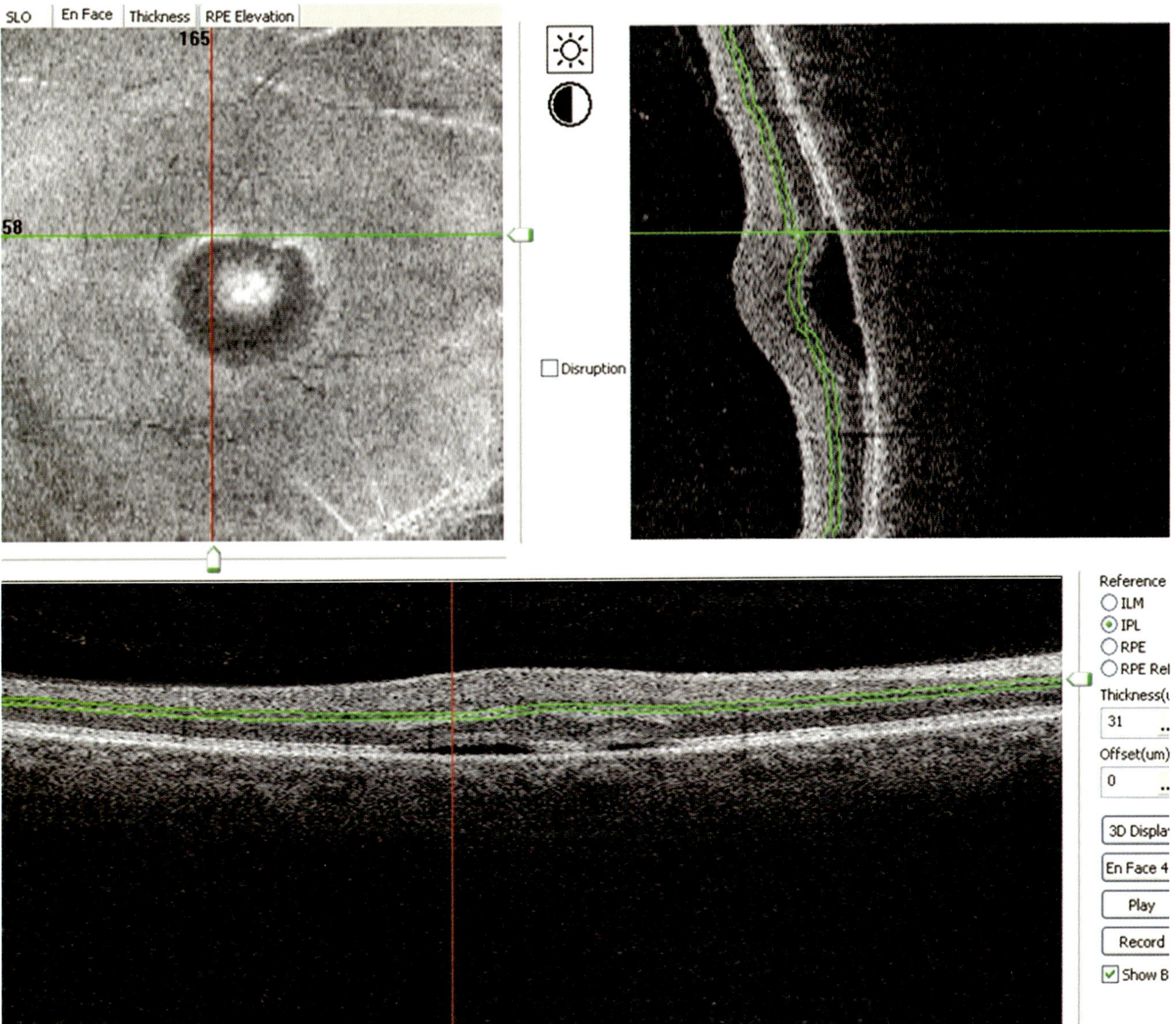

Figure 8: Hyper-reflective intraretinal layers. Ring of hyper-reflectivity of the outer plexiform layer and outer nuclear layer is more distinctive in regions marginal to subretinal fluid or at the edges of retinal bending

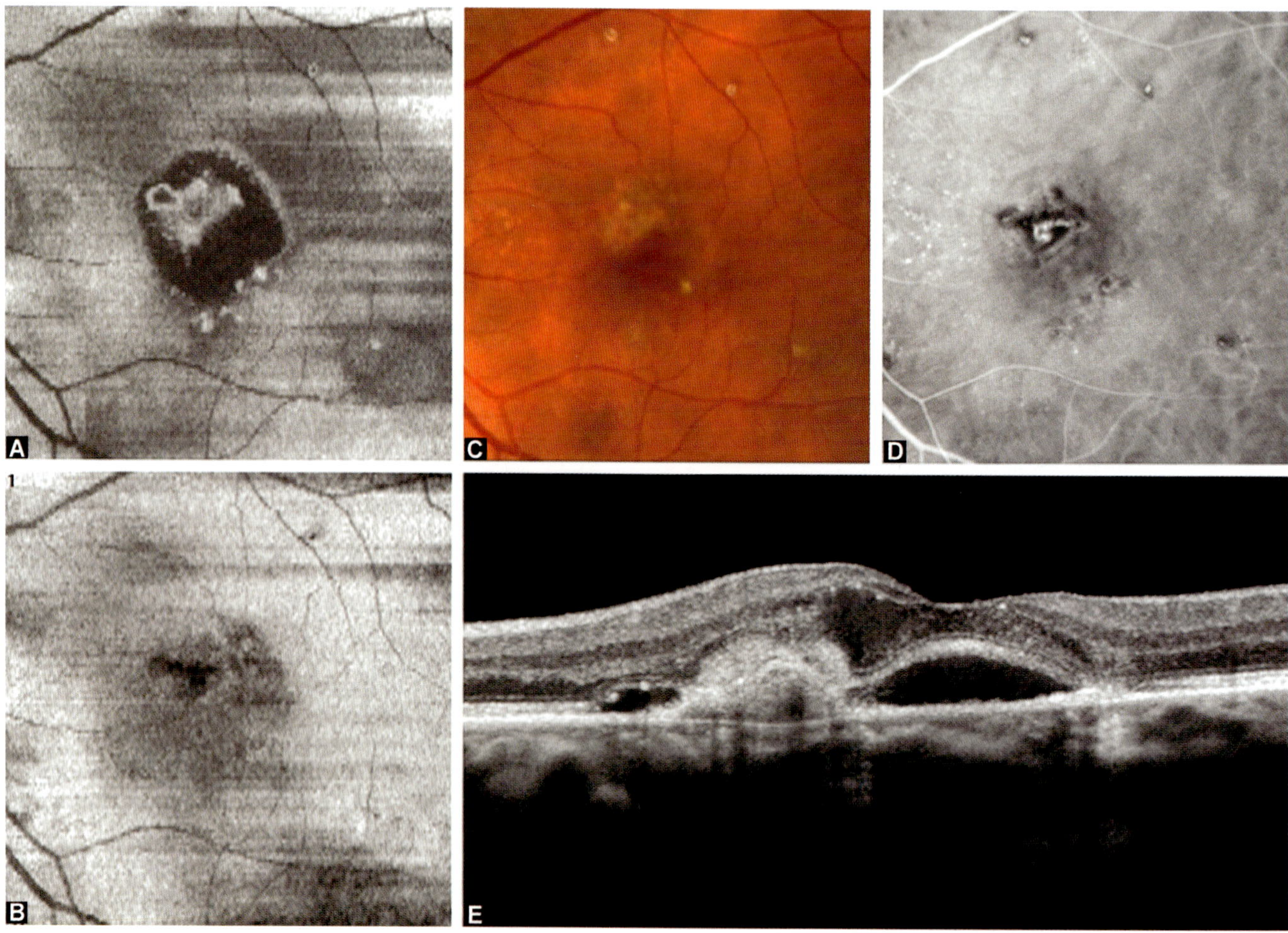

Figures 9A to E: Polypoidal choroidal vasculopathy masquerading as central serous chorioretinopathy in a patient with history of chronic decompensation of retinal pigment epithelium (RPE). (A) *En face* optical coherence tomography scan fits to RPE, shows a serous detachment associated with small pigment epithelium detachment. Note some highly reflective dots at the edge, inner and over the neurosensory detachment corresponding to both reddish-orange "polyp-like" and small cluster of numerous polypoidal choroidal dilations respectively seen in color photograph; (B) *En face* section beneath the RPE highlights a number of round protrusions of the RPE corresponding to the polypoidal lesions; (C and D) Indocyanine green angiogram; (E) Longitudinal sectional image reveals sharp protrusions of the RPE with moderate inner reflectivity, corresponding to the polypoidal lesions. These protrusions are accompanied by a slight elevation of the RPE that corresponds to the branching vascular network. Subretinal fluid, intraretinal pseudocystic cavity and intraretinal exudation are visible

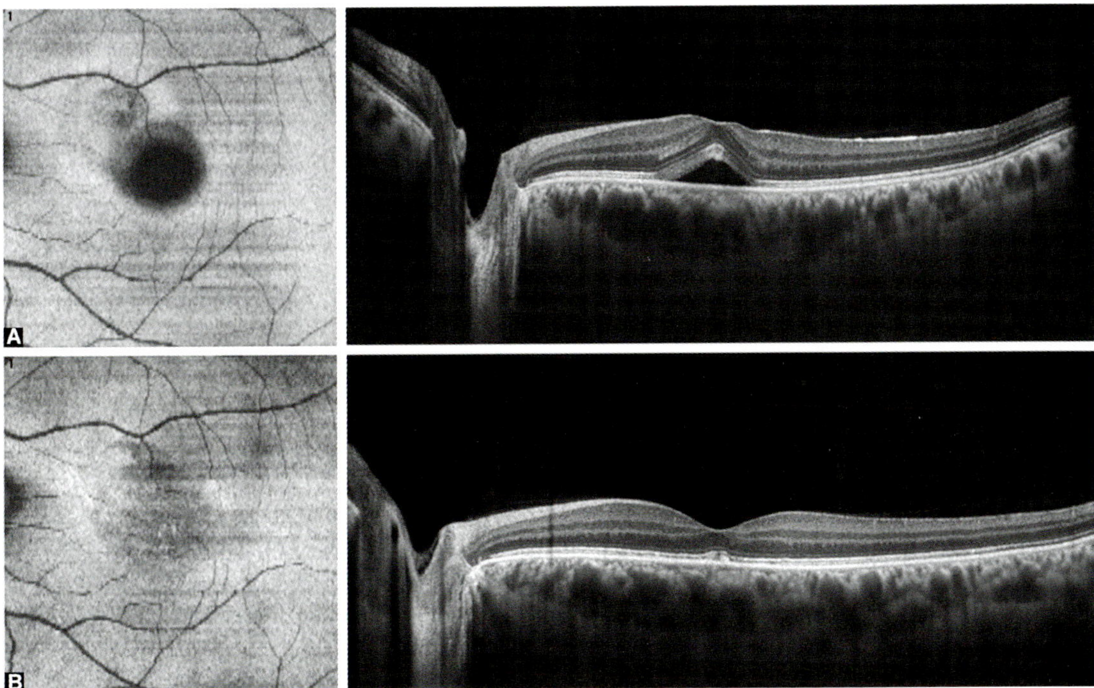

Figures 10A and B: Acute central serous chorioretinopathy. (A) *En face* optical coherence tomography in acute phase of disease shows a hyporeflective area due to serous detachment; (B) *En face* optical coherence tomography after carbonic anhydrase inhibitor therapy shows a complete resolution of serous detachment. In longitudinal scan the external limiting membrane and the inner/outer photoreceptor segment junction are preserved while pigmented epithelium highlights some irregularities. Thickened choroid is visible

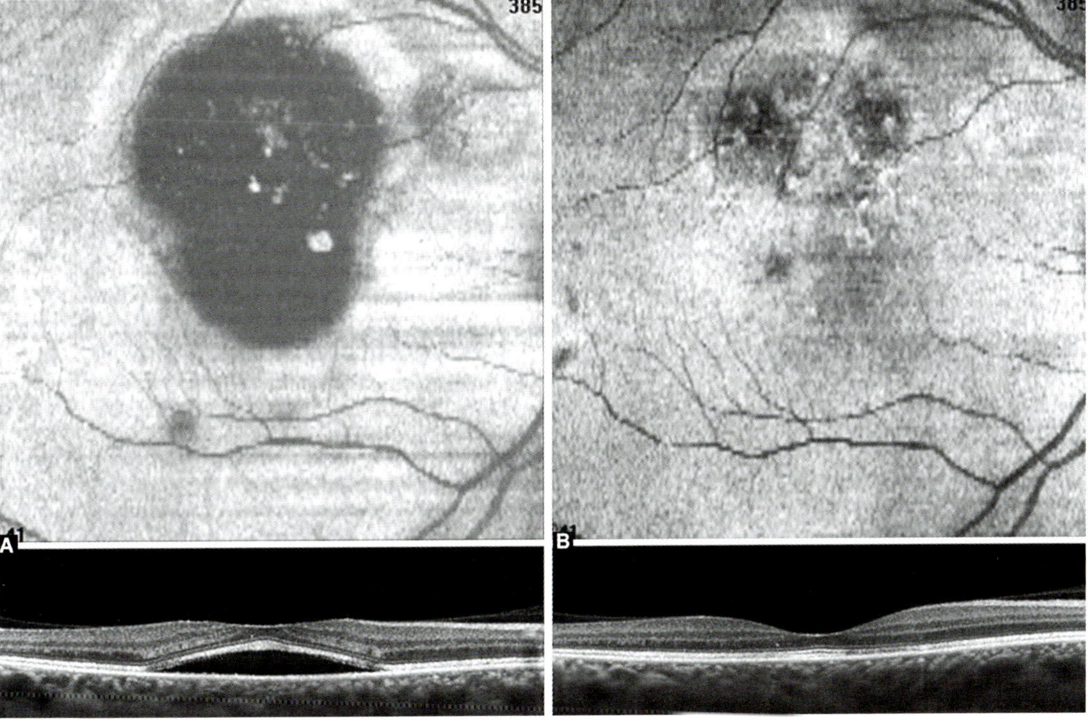

Figures 11A and B: Acute central serous chorioretinopathy. (A) *En face* optical coherence tomography in acute phase of disease shows a hyporeflective area due to serous detachment; (B) *En face* optical coherence tomography scan after angiotensin-converting-enzyme inhibitor therapy shows a resolution of serous detachment associated with irregularities at level of the retinal pigment epithelium

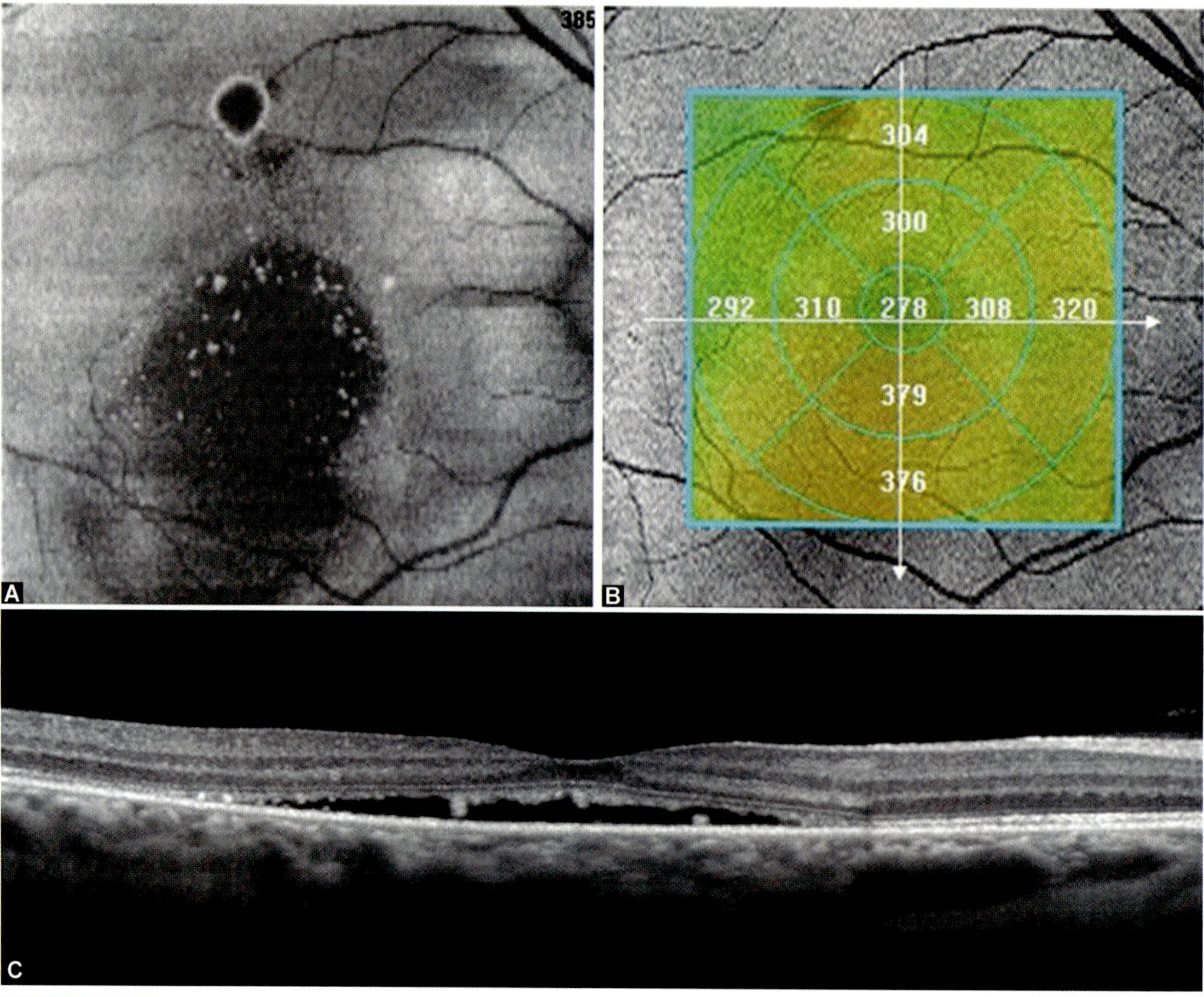

Figures 12A to C: Central serous chorioretinopathy before photocoagulation treatment. (A) Three-dimensional reference scan shows an area of hyporeflectivity due to neuroepithelium detachment in the macular area, associated with highly reflective dots due in part to elongated photoreceptor outer segment and in part to the retinal pigment epithelium (RPE) villosities alterations. RPE detachment appears as a highly reflective ring over the vascular arcades; (B) The full thickness macular map shows an increase of mean central retinal thickness; (C) Longitudinal scan shows shallow serous neuroepithelium detachment. The photoreceptor outer segment appears irregular and elongated probably due to cone disk distress and rod engorgement. Pigmented epithelial villosity alterations are visible

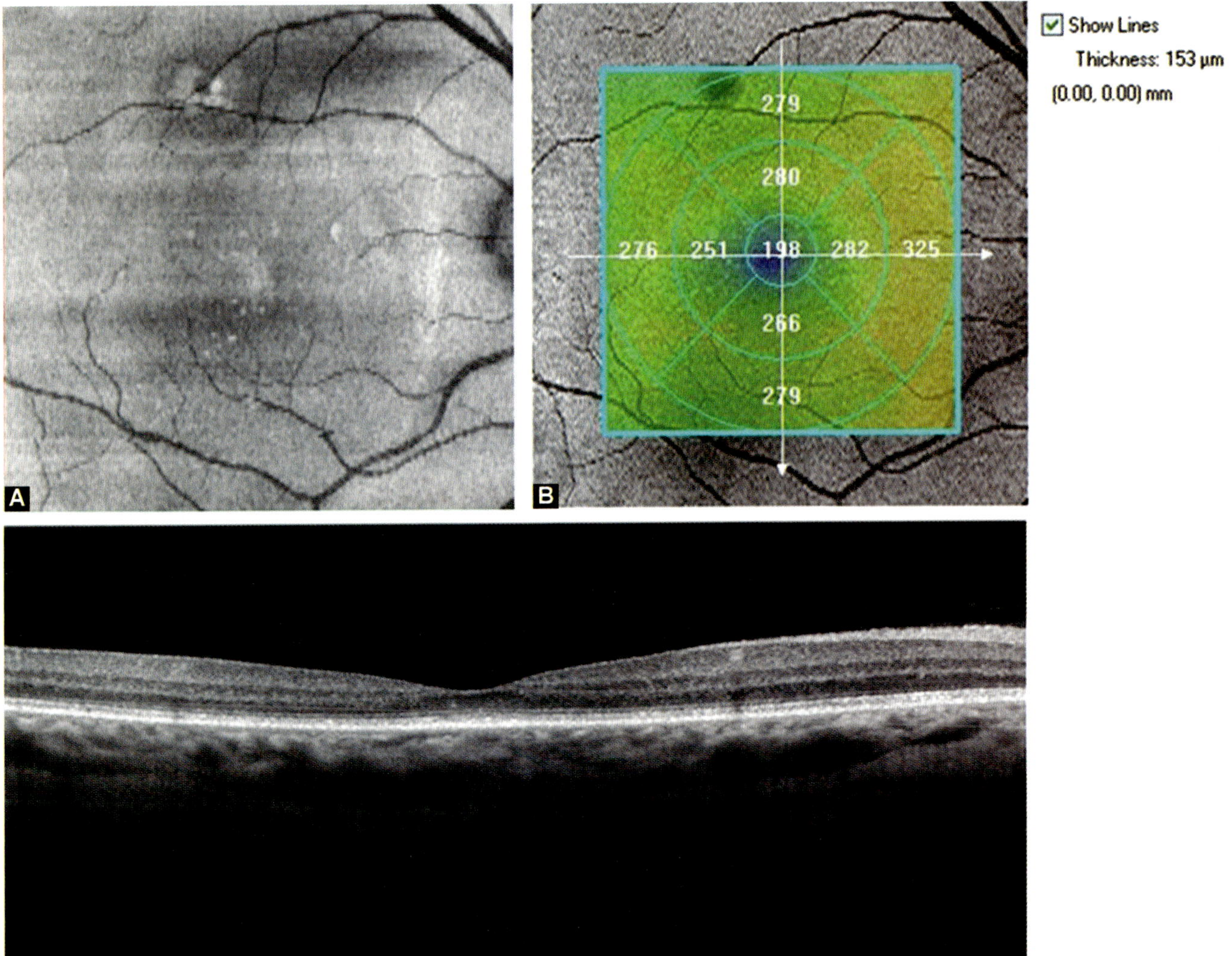

Figures 13A to C: Central serous chorioretinopathy 4 weeks after photocoagulation. (A) *En face* optical coherence tomography shows a resolution of both neuroepithelium and pigment epithelium detachments with a reduction of most of highly reflective dots; (B) The full thickness macular map shows a decrease of mean central retinal thickness; (C) Longitudinal scan shows a normal profile of retina with some highly reflective dots due to retinal pigment epithelium irregularities

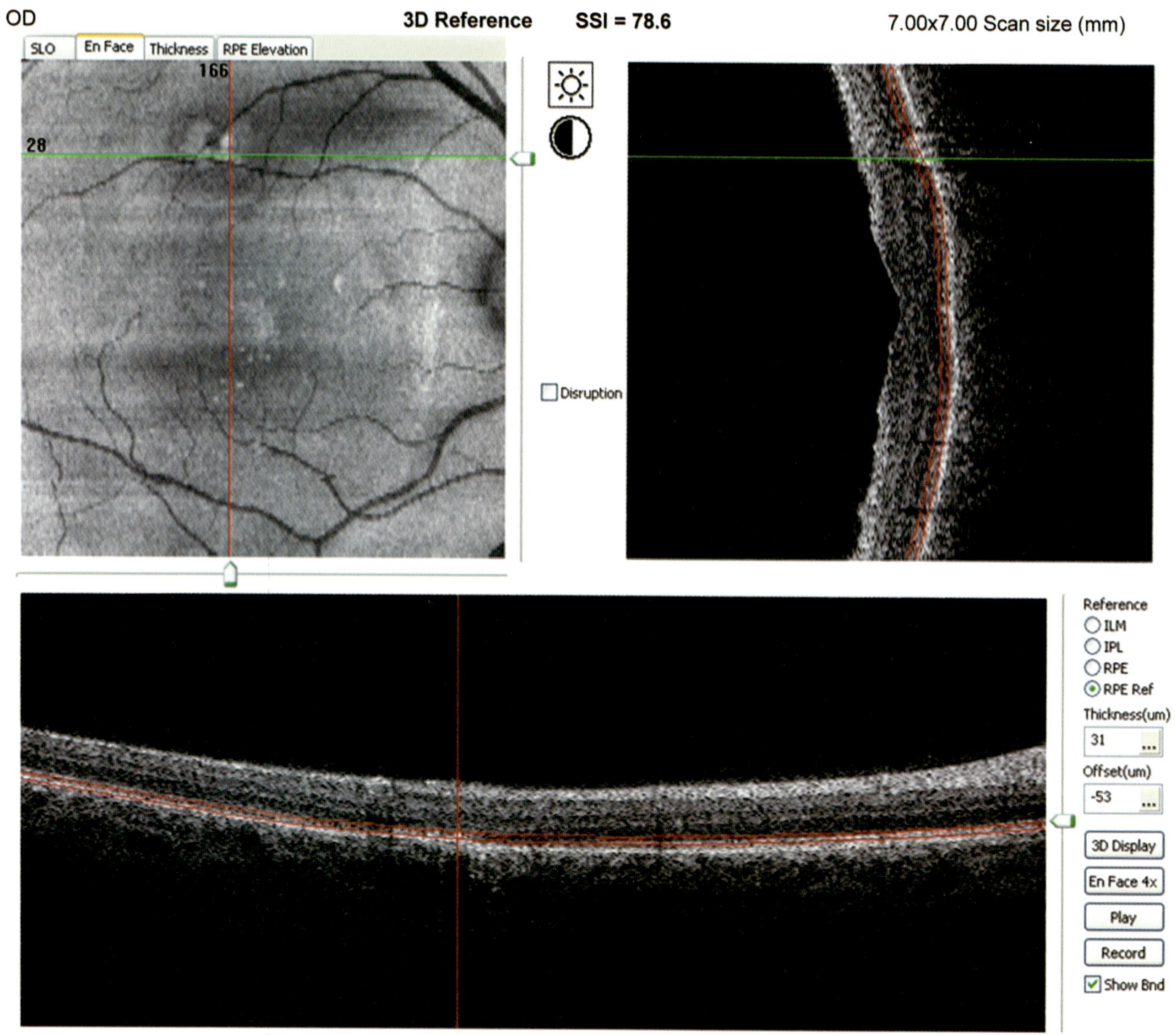

Figure 14: Laser photocoagulation scarring. *En face* optical coherence tomography section fits to the concave shape of retinal pigment epithelium shows some highly reflective points due to laser lesions limited to outer retina, especially retinal pigment epithelium and photoreceptor layer in correspondence of the focal leak point previously treated by photocoagulation

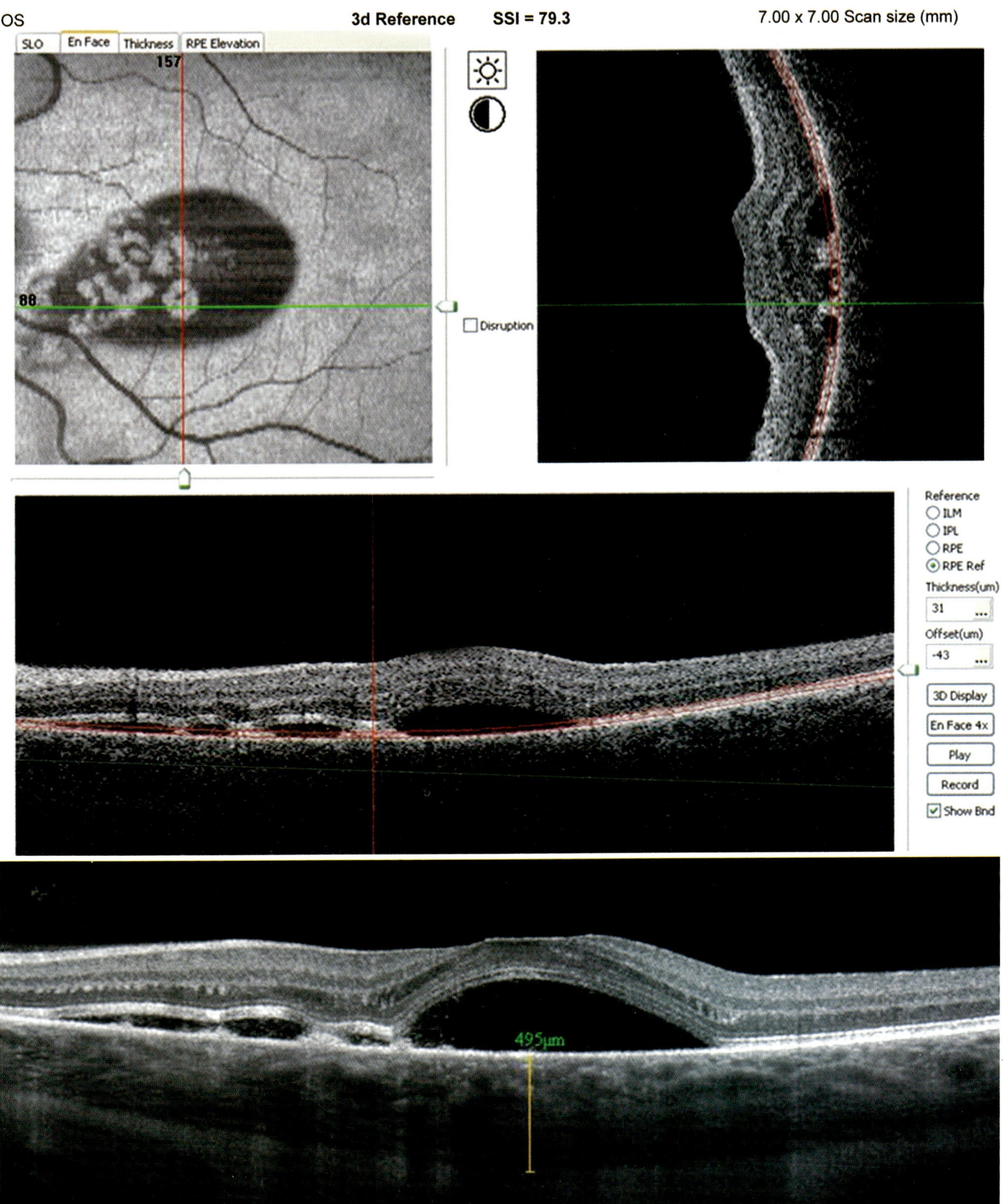

Figure 15: Acute central serous chorioretinopathy in pregnancy. *En face* section depicts a large serous detachment with hyper-reflective spots due to fibrinous exudates typically of acute central serous chorioretinopathy during pregnancy. Longitudinal scan shows high reflectivity of outer plexiform layer, outer nuclear layer, and dome-shaped macular detachment containing several tiny dots of moderate reflectance associated with fibrinous exudates between serous detachment and retinal pigment epithelium. Note thickened choroid

References

1. Gass JD. Pathogenesis of disciform detachment of the neuroepithelium. Am J Ophthalmol. 1967;63:Suppl: 1-139.
2. Guyer DR, Yannuzzi LA, Slakter JS, et al. Digital Indocyanine green videoangiography of central serous chorioretinopathy. Arch Ophthalmol. 1994;112:1057-62.
3. Imamura Y, Fujiwara T, Margolis R, et al. Enhanced depth imaging optical coherence tomography of the choroid in central serous chorioretinopathy. Retina 2009;29:1469-73.
4. van Velthoven ME, Verbraak FD, Garcia PM, et al. Evaluation of central serous retinopathy with *en face* optical coherence tomography. Br J Ophthalmol. 2005;89: 1483-8.
5. Lumbroso B, Rispoli M. Retinal Oct: Analysis and interpretation method. Publisher Optovue Inc. 2010.
6. Lumbroso B, Savastano MC, Rispoli M, et al. Morphologic differences, according to etiology, in pigment epithelial detachments by means of *en face* optical coherence tomography. Retina. 2011;31:553-8.
7. Matsumoto H, Kishi S, Sato T, et al. Fundus autouorescence of elongated photoreceptor outer segments in central serous chorioretinopathy. Am J Ophthalmol. 2011;151: 617-23.
8. Fujimoto H, Gomi F, Wakabayashi T, et al. Morphologic changes in acute central serous chorioretinopathy evaluated by fourier-domain optical coherence tomography. Ophthalmology. 2008;115:1494-500.
9. Hirami Y, Tsujikawa A, Sasahara M, et al. Alterations of retinal pigment epithelium in central serous chorioretinopathy. Clin Experimental Ophthalmol. 2007;35:225-30.
10. Ahlers C, Geitzenauer W, Stock G. Alterations of intraretinal layers in acute central serous chorioretinopathy. Acta Ophthalmol. 2009;87:511-6.
11. Piccolino FC, de la Longrais RR, Ravera G, et al. The foveal photoreceptor layer and visual acuity loss in central serous chorioretinopathy. Am J Ophthalmol. 2005;139(1):87-99.
12. Wanek J, Zelkha R, Lim JI, et al. Feasibility of a method for *en face* imaging of photoreceptor cell integrity. Am J Ophthalmol. 2011;152(5):807-14.
13. Yannuzzi LA, Freund KB, Goldbaum M, et al. Polypoidal choroidal vasculopathy masquerading as central serous chorioretinopathy. Ophthalmology. 2000;107:767-77.
14. Rosen RB, Hathaway M, Rogers J, et al. Multidimensional *en face* OCT imaging of the retina. Opt Express. 2009; 17(5):4112-33.
15. Saito M, Iida T, Nagayama D. Cross-sectional and *en face* optical coherence tomographic features of polypoidal choroidal vasculopathy. Retina. 2008;28(3):459-64.
16. Kameda T, Tsujikawa A, Otani A, et al. Polypoidal choroidal vasculopathy examined with *en face* optical coherence tomography. Clin Experiment Ophthalmol. 2007;35(7): 596-601.

chapter 24

Optical Coherence Tomography *En Face* in Central Serous Chorioretinopathy

Mathieu Lehmann, Benjamin Wolff, Vivien Vasseur, Nadine Manasseh, Virginie Martinet, José Alain Sahel, Martine Mauget-Faÿsse

Introduction

Central serous chorioretinopathy (CSC) is a common and idiopathic clinical disease that affects mostly young to middle aged men. Currently, the etiology of this disease still remains unclear and numerous hypotheses have been suggested. The retinal pigment epithelium (RPE) and choroidal vessels are involved and various anatomical and functional changes affecting these important structures have been described. Patients with CSC develop a serous retinal detachment (SRD), always associated to a more or less depictable serous retinal pigment epithelium detachment (PED). The leakage areas are clearly seen during fluorescein angiography (FA), showing focal leak(s) at the level of the RPE and gradually expanding into the shape of a smokestack or an inkblot pattern. Indocyanine green angiogram (ICGA) shows the presence of dilation and hyperpermeability of the choroidal vessels (Table 1). Generally, retinal detachments resulting from acute CSC resolve spontaneously within a few months[1] and the patient's visual acuity (VA) returns to normal, without any treatment. Nevertheless, some patients will develop chronic and widespread RPE decompensation with progressive retinal cystoid degeneration.

Optical coherence tomography (OCT) is a complementary diagnostic tool that provides useful visualization of changes in foveal structures, such as outer segment protruding, PED, subretinal or intraretinal fluid and choroidal thickening.

In acute forms, B scan OCT usually shows bulges protruding from the RPE layer[2] under an optically empty space (i.e. SRD). The retinal thickness of the detached retina is relatively preserved. Enhanced depth imaging (EDI) combined with OCT demonstrates an important thickening of the choroid (generally more than 500 µ).

In chronic forms, B scan OCT shows additional progressive RPE atrophy areas sometimes associated with cystoid retinal cavities (Table 2).

A new automated image reconstruction method based on spectral domain OCT (SD-OCT) imaging called *en face* OCT, combining OCT and confocal ophthalmoscopy, provides additional information about retinal and especially choroidal abnormalities in CSC.

The following description of *en face* OCT in CSC was obtained with an SD-OCT (Spectralis® Heidelberg Engineering, Heidelberg, Germany).

Table 1: Central serous chorioretinopathy angiogram

	Early stage	Intermediate stage	Late stage
Fluorescein angiography	Leaking point(s)	Leakage of the dye (smoke stack or inblot pattern) Retinal pigment epithelium alterations	Pooling of the dye into the SRD Retinal cyst staining (in cystoid macular degenerations)
Indocyanine green angiography	Focal ischemia Dilation of the choroidal vessels	Dilation of the choroidal vessels Retinal pigment epithelium alterations	Hyperpermeability of the choroidal vessels Retinal pigment epithelium area staining

Table 2: Optical coherence tomography B scan

Acute central serous chorioretinopathy	Serous retinal detachment	Pigment epithelium detachment (bulges protruding from the retinal pigment epithelium)	Choroidal thickening
Chronic central serous chorioretinopathy	Cystoid cavities and cystoid macular degeneration, inconstant serous retinal detachment	Retinal pigment epithelium alterations with inner segment/outer segment alterations	Choroidal thickening

Description of Retinal Changes

Serous retinal detachment observed with *en face* OCT **(Figures 1 and 2)** appears like a hyporeflective area surrounded with concentric circles of retinal layers [from the photoreceptor inner segment/outer segment junction (IS-OS) to the internal limiting membrane][3,4] whereas FA only shows a progressive staining. Inside the SRD, small hyper-reflective deposits can be seen.

When analyzing the C scan sections, deeper to the choroid, it is possible to observe the highly hyper-reflective RPE layer. Small uprisings at the level of the RPE layer are frequently noticed. During active phases, small PED and RPE hyperplasia are often located where the leaking points are observed in FA **(Figures 3A to F)**. The shape of the PED appears predominantly circular,[5] with a mostly "smooth inner silhouette", clear contents and frequently uniform appearance of the reflective wall. This particular feature with

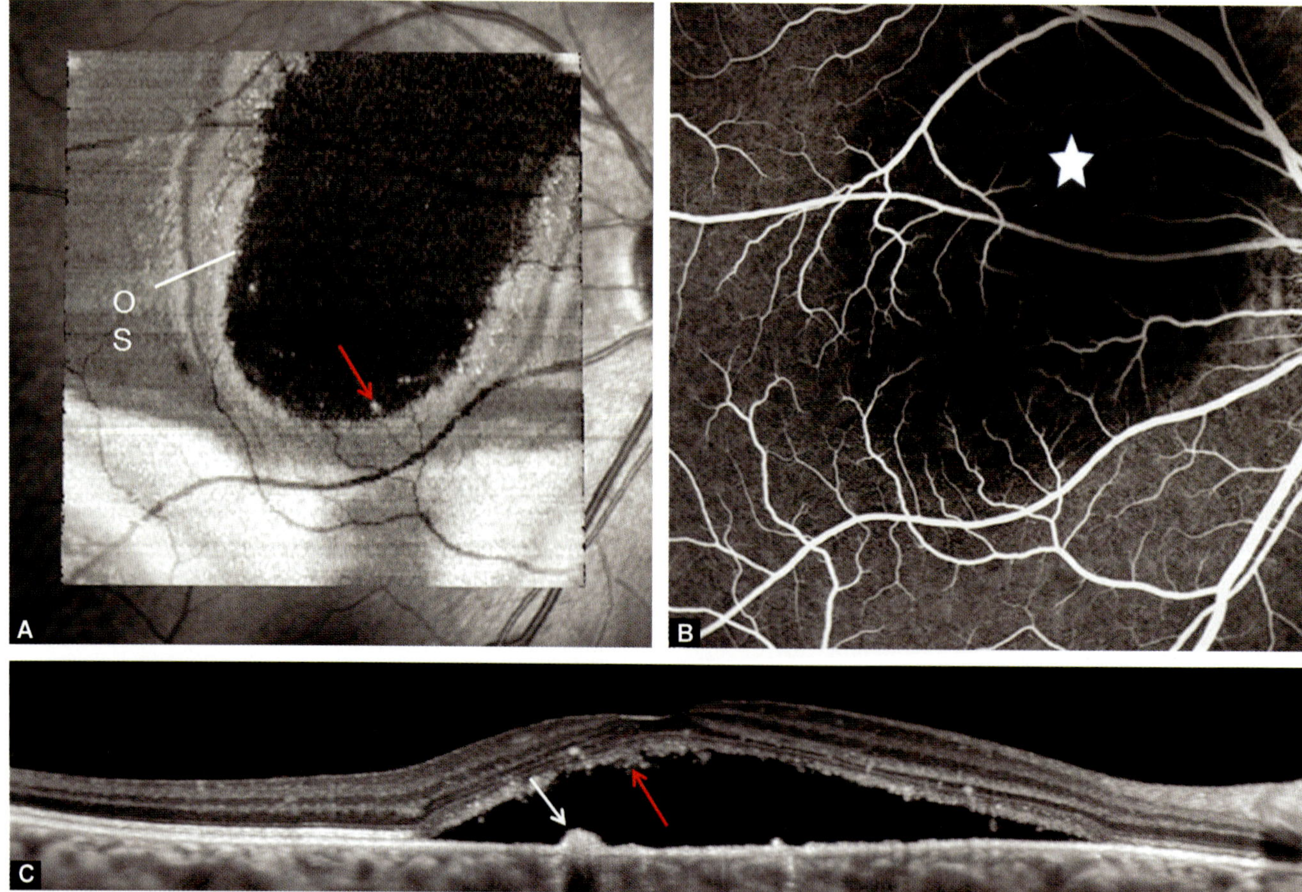

Figures 1A to C: Serous detachment of the neurosensory retina. (A) *En face* optical coherence tomography showing a regular hyporeflective retinal detachment surrounded by the outer segment of the photoreceptor with hyper-reflective deposits inside (red arrow). Note that the retinal vessel can be seen inside the detachment thanks to their shadow posterior cone; (B) Early stage of fluorescein angiography showing a wide mask effect (white star); (C) B scan showing neurosensory retinal detachment, small pigment epithelium detachment (white arrow), and hyper-reflective deposits on the outer side of the retinal detachment (red arrow)

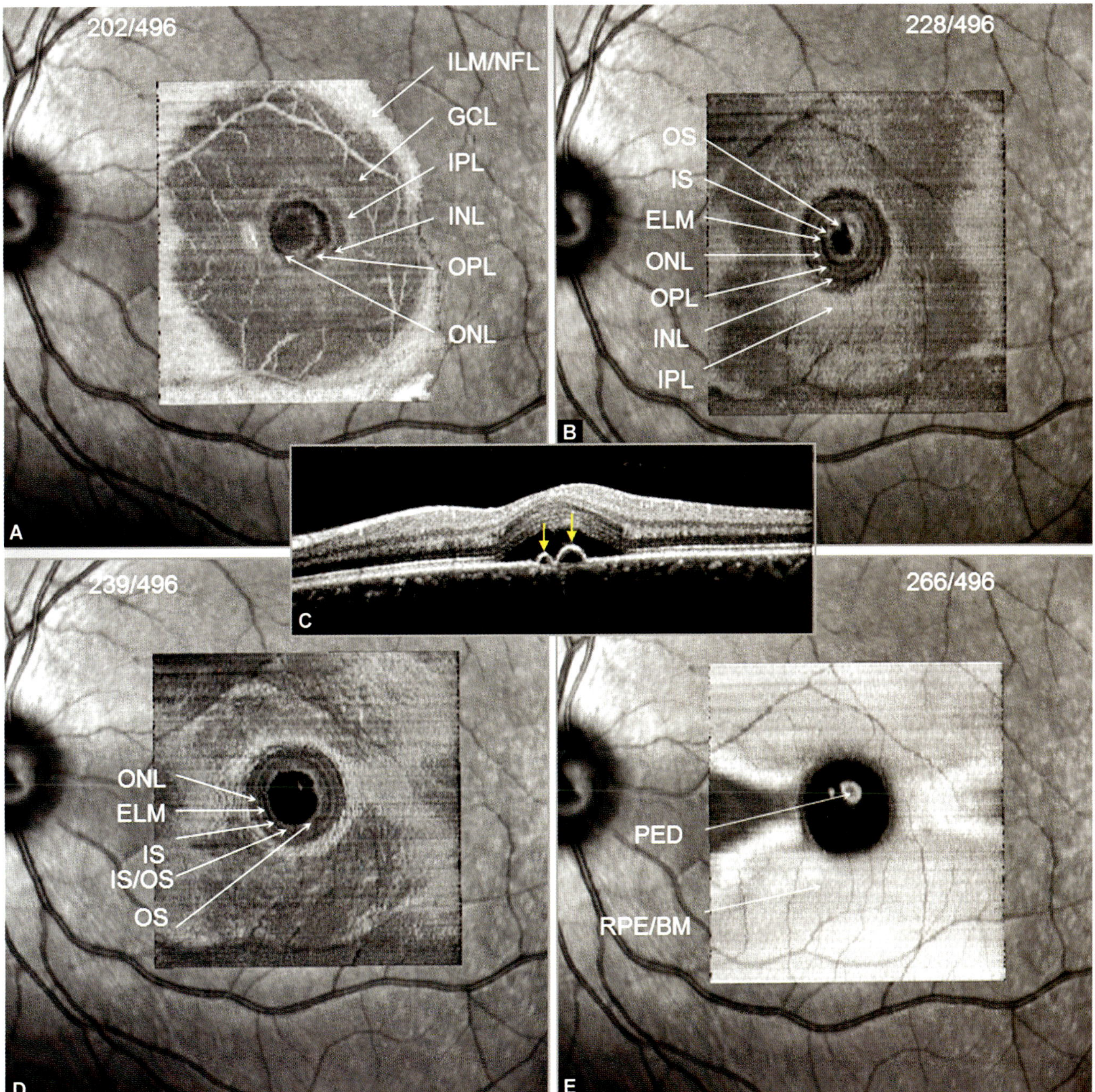

Figures 2A to E: (A, B and D) Serous detachment of the neurosensory retina in the foveolar area with visualization of concentric circles of retinal layers. (C) B scan OCT: 2 small uprisings at the level of the RPE layer (yellow arrows). (E) *En face* OCT deep in the SRD showing a small PED
(ILM/NFL: Internal limiting membrane/nerve ber layer; ELM: External limiting membrane; GCL: Ganglion cell layer; INL: Inner nuclear layer; IPL: Inner plexiform layer; IS: Photoreceptor inner segment layer; IS/OS: Photoreceptor inner and outer segment junction; ONL: Outer nuclear layer; OPL: Outer plexiform layer; OS: Photoreceptor outer segment layer; RPE/BM: Retinal pigment epithelium/Bruch's membrane)

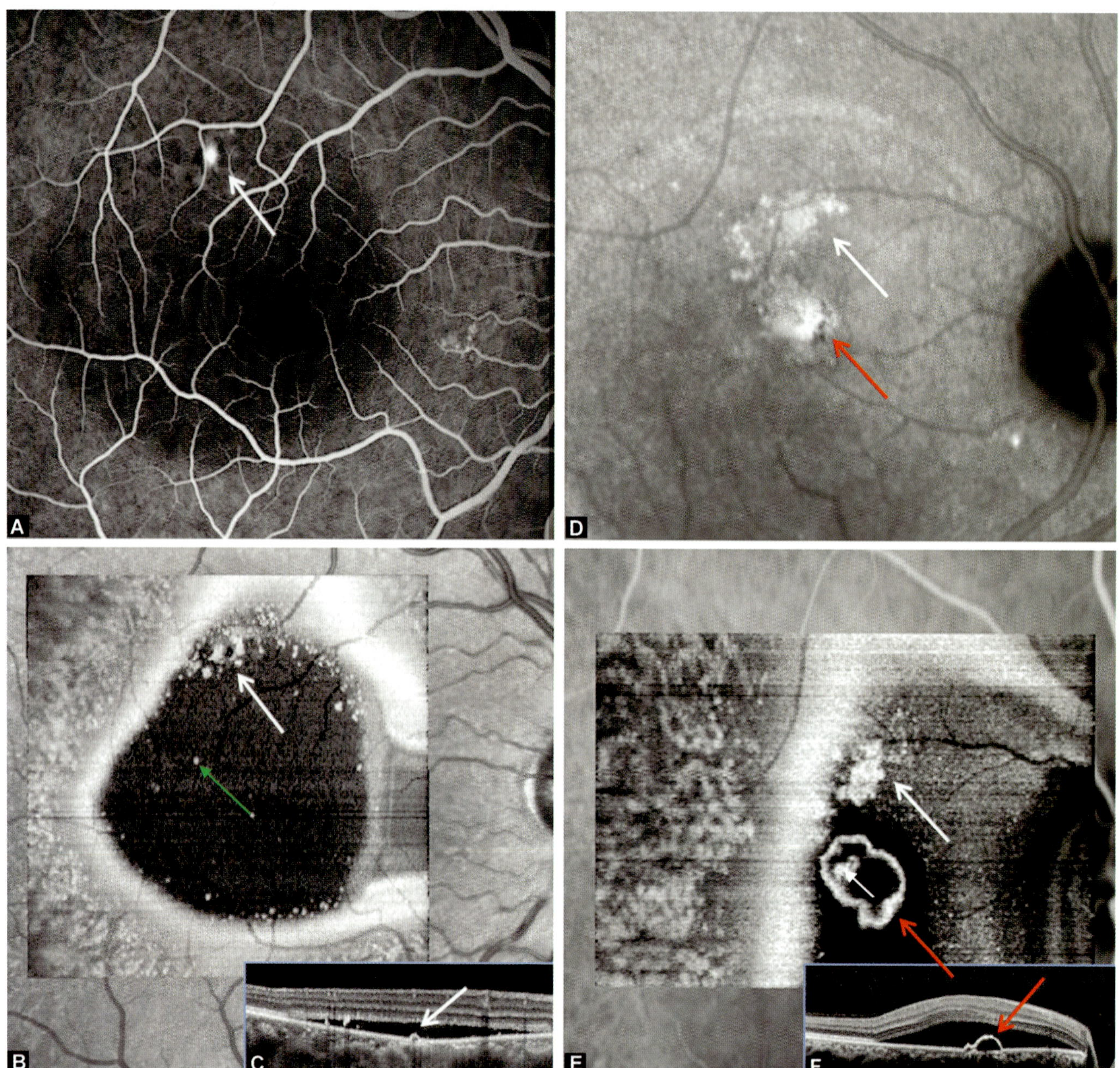

Figures 3A to F: Serous retinal detachment with focal leak and RPE alterations. (A) Intermediate stage on fluorescein angiography showing the focal leak on an acute and active central serous chorioretinopathy; (B) *En face* optical coherence tomography (OCT) into the retinal detachment. The white arrow shows the small pigment epithelium detachment (PED) where the fluid leaks and hyper-reflective deposits inside the serous retinal detachment (green arrow); (C) B scan, of the same small PED inside the neurosensory retinal detachment; (D) Late indocyanine green angiography stages of the right eye of another patient. The red arrow points to the small PED without any leakage. The white arrows depict some retinal pigment epithelium (RPE) hyperplasia with late hyperfluorescence; (E) *En face* OCT confirms the round PED with a regular outline and clear contents; (F) The same finding can be seen with the classic B scan with very little information on the RPE hyperplastic changes

en face OCT differentiates them from PEDs in age-related macular degeneration, which usually have an irregular wall aspect. Sometimes hyper-reflective lesions, corresponding to RPE hyperplasia, can be described above the RPE layer.

In chronic forms, cystoid cavities and cystoid macular degenerations[6,7] are perfectly shown with *en face* OCT images **(Figure 4A)**. It reveals a "moth-eaten" aspect of the outer retina. Both B scans and C scans show multiple hyporeflective cysts inside the outer retina, and through the whole retina in the foveolar area due to intraretinal exudation and cystoid changes. This appearance can only be seen with chronic evolution of CSC. *En face* OCT, in this case, allows us to estimate the area of retina affected by such degeneration **(Figures 4B and C) (Table 3)**.

Description of Choroidal Changes

En face OCT always shows choroidal dilatation of the vascular network,[8] irrespective of whether the disease is active (acute, chronic or recurrent) or quiescent and this observation is true even when ICGA could not show the same dilation **(Figures 5A to E)**.[9,10] With *en face* imaging, unlike the retinal vessels that appear hyper-reflective, the choroidal vessels are hyporeflective, probably because of their thin inner surface lacking of pericytes.

Sometimes, above the choroidal dilatation, choroidal cavities can be observed defined as hyporeflective cysts, without any outline and just below the choriocapillary layer. They may correspond to ischemic lesions **(Figures 6A to E)**.

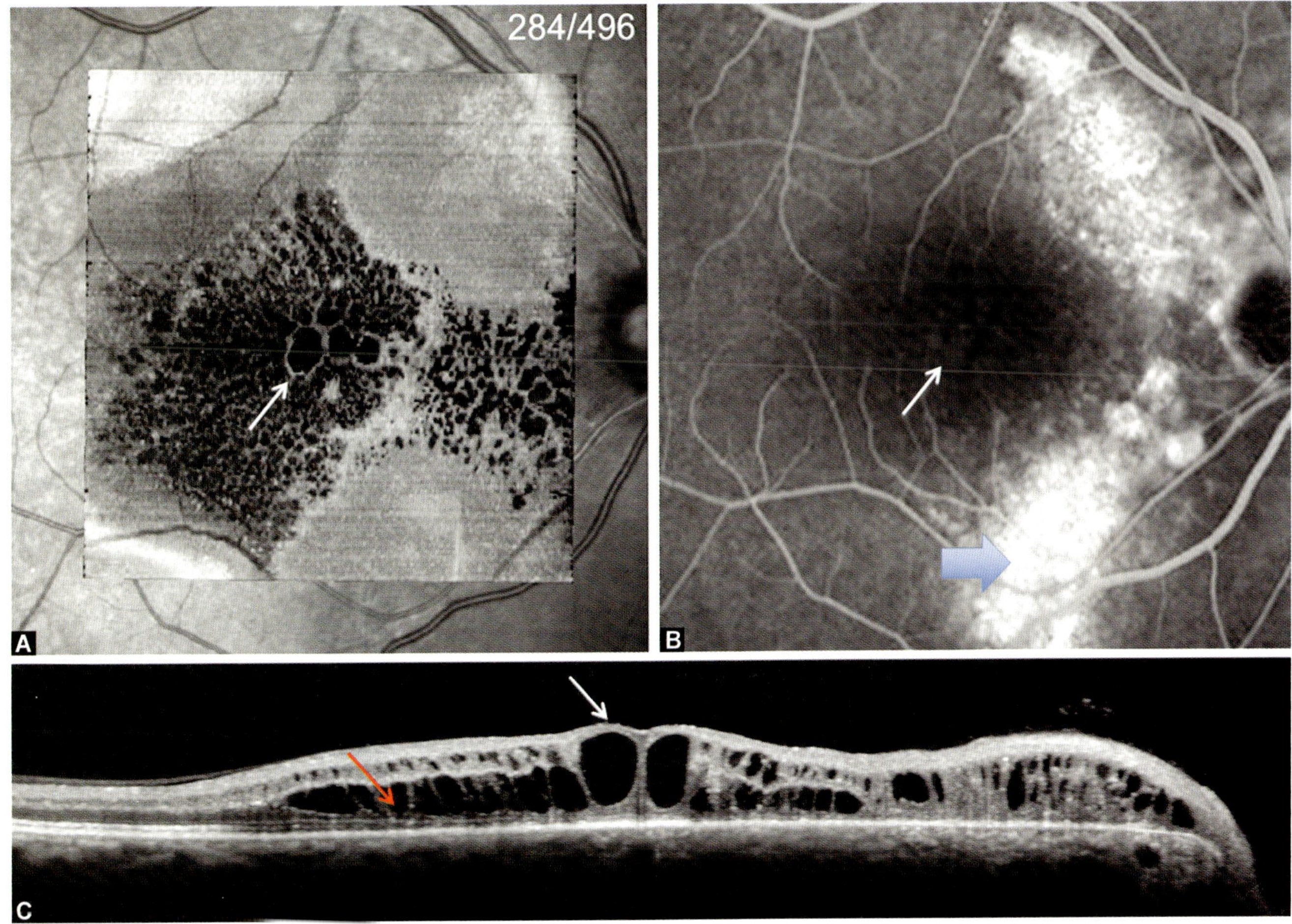

Figures 4A to C: Macular cystoid edema. (A) *En face* optical coherence tomography: central cystoid degeneration (white arrow) with a moth-eaten appearance of the surrounding outer retina; (B) Intermediate stage of fluorescein angiography with staining of the retinal cysts like a flower petal. Blue arrow: Large areas of retinal pigment epithelium alteration with a window defect due to chronic central serous chorioretinopathy; (C) B scan: cystoid macular edema (white arrow) and outer retinal cyst (red arrow). No retinal detachment

Table 3: Optical coherence tomography C scan combined with enhanced depth imaging

		Retinal changes	Choroidal changes
Acute central serous chorioretinopathy	Serous retinal detachment (hyporeflective area) surrounded with concentric circles of retinal layers	Retinal pigment epithelium layer (highly hyper-reflective) Circular pigment epithelium detachment (smooth inner silhouette, clear contents, uniform wall appearance)	Choroidal dilation of the vascular network
	Small hyper-reflective deposits inside	Retinal pigment epithelium hyperplasia above the retinal pigment epithelium layer (hyper-reflective lesions)	
Chronic central serous chorioretinopathy	Hyper-reflective deposits inside inconstant retinal detachment	Moth-eaten aspect of the outer retina with hyporeflective cysts (macular cystoid degeneration)	Choroidal dilatation of the vascular network Choroidal cavitations (hyporeflective cysts)
	Circular chronic pigment epithelium detachment		Hyper-reflective points inside the choriocapillary layer

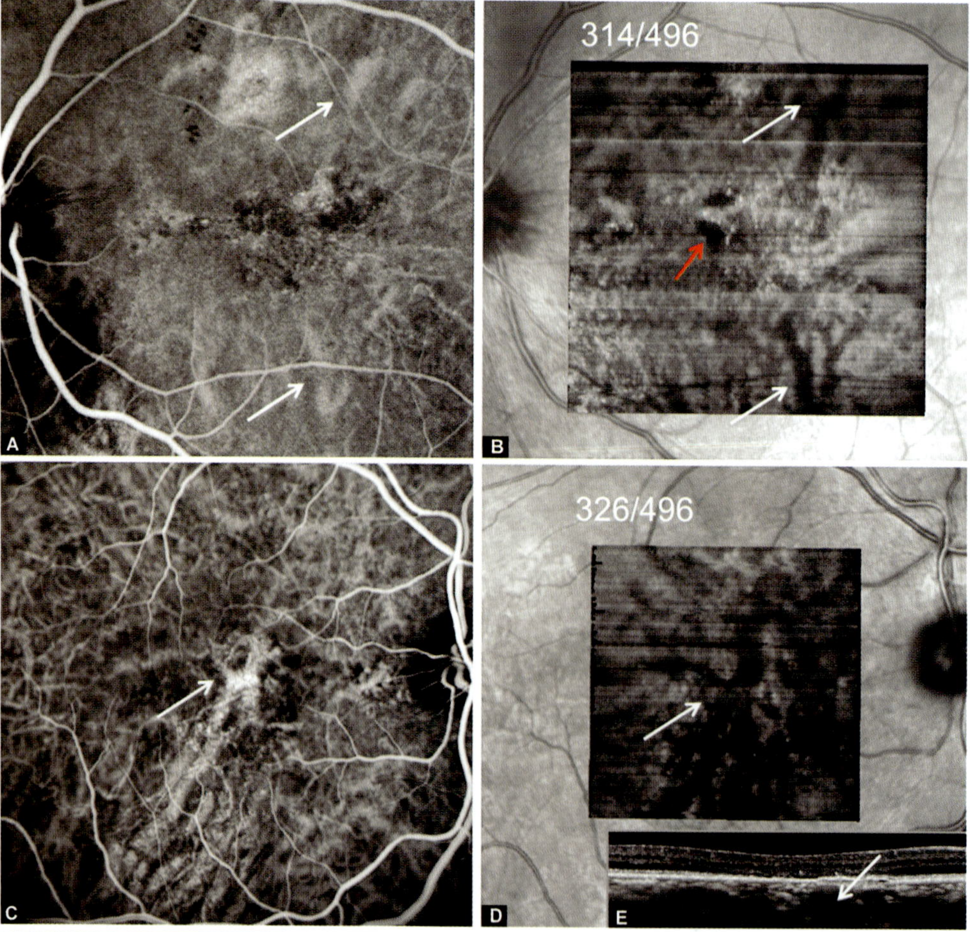

Figures 5A to E: Standard indocyanine green angiography (ICGA) in early stage compared with *en face* optical coherence tomography (OCT). (A) Early stage of ICGA: dilation of the choroidal network is hardly visible in the early and late stages of ICGA (white arrow); (B) However, *en face* OCT clearly depicts these vascular dilations in the choroid beneath the area of retinal pigment epithelium alterations and choroidal decompensation. Shadow of a small pigment epithelium detachment (red arrow); (C and D) ICGA and *en face* OCT images of these choroidal dilations in the foveal area; (E) B scan showing dilation of the choroidal vessels (white arrow)

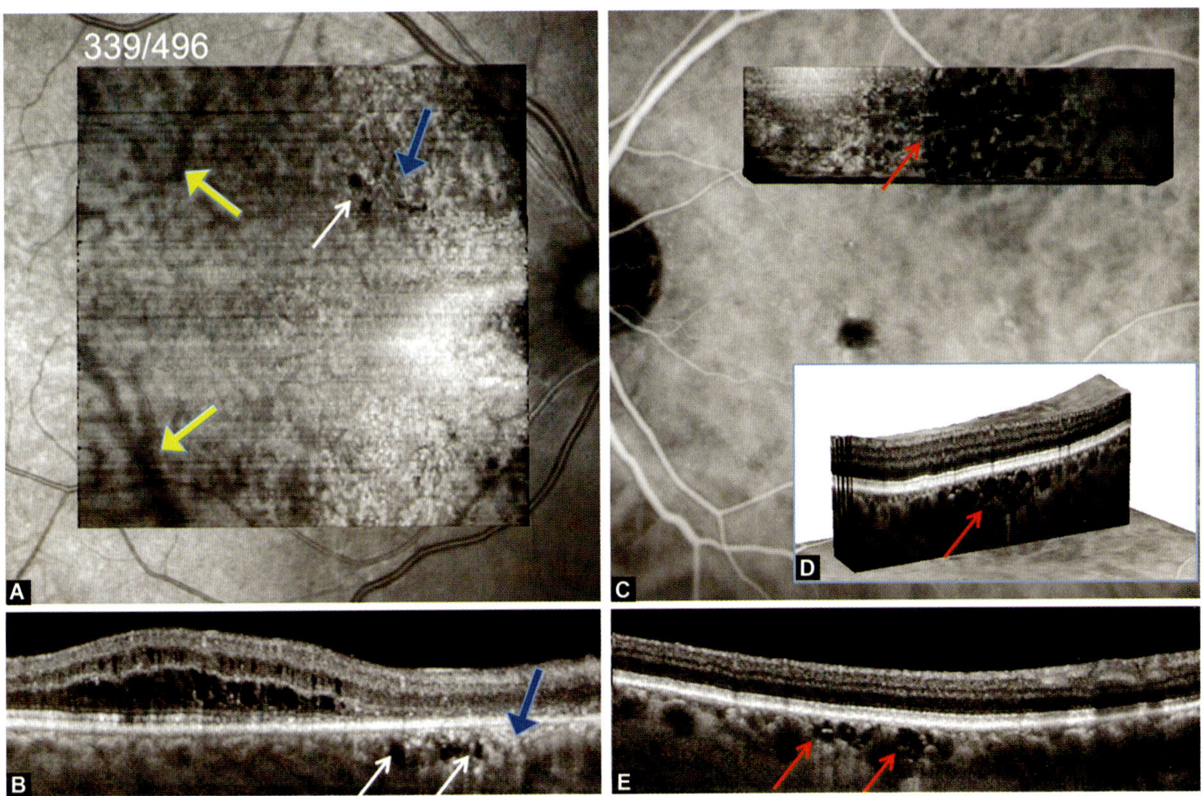

Figures 6A to E: Choroidal cavitations. (A) *En face* optical coherence tomography shows few choroidal cavitations (white arrow) beneath the choriocapillaris layer, as hyporeflective spots without any outline. The yellow arrows confirm the choroidal dilations in chronic central serous chorioretinopathy; (B) B scan through the cavitations (white arrows). The blue arrow shows alterations of the choriocapillaris layers with hyper-reflective points; (C) *En face* imaging of the choroidal cavitations (red arrow); (D) Three-dimensional reconstructions and (E) B scans shows hyporeflective cysts (darker than choroidal vessels)

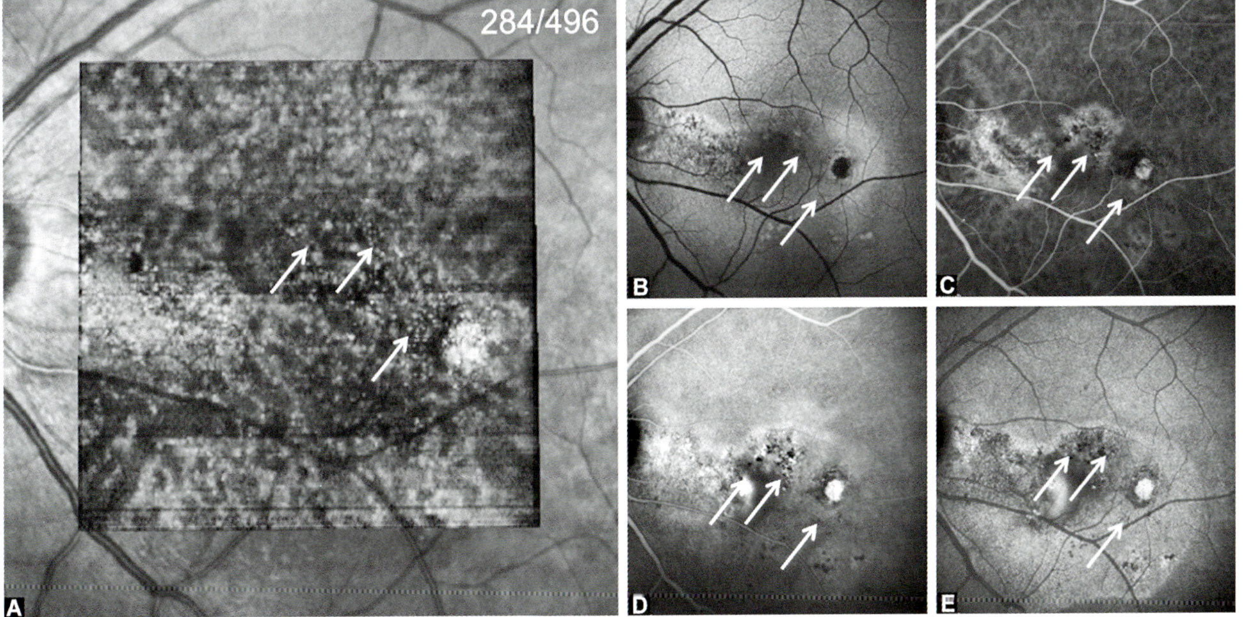

Figures 7A to E: Hyper-reflective pin points in the choriocapillaris layer. (A) *En face* optical coherence tomography: multiple hyper-reflective points inside the choriocapillaris layer in the area of choroidal hyper-permeability. The patient has an active recurrent central serous chorioretinopathy; (B) Autofluorescence; (C to E) Showing the early, intermediate and late stages of indocyanine green angiography of the same patient. White arrows depict the location of chronic lesions

Many patients have hyper-reflective points inside the choriocapillary layer with C scan analysis. These hyper-reflective points (or pinpoints) were focal or diffuse, located inside the granular aspect of the choriocapillary layer and observed under the area of the SRD **(Figures 7A to E)**. This is a novel observation and their presence might reveal disease activity since quiescent CSC did not show any hyper-reflective points **(Table 3)**.

Conclusion

En face SD-OCT combined with EDI is an easy, reproducible, noninvasive and effective technique to better understand retinal and choroidal modifications during the evolution of CSC. Currently, the choroid is a very poorly described tissue, but this new technique should be used as an essential examination in the future and might replace other examinations for the diagnosis, follow-up and treatment of CSC.

References

1. Gass JD. Pathogenesis of disciform detachment of the neuroepithelium, II: Idiopathic central serous choroidopathy. Am J Ophthalmol. 1967;63:587-615.
2. Montero JA, Ruiz-Moreno JM. Optical coherence tomography characterisation of idiopathic central serous chorioretinopathy. Br J Ophthalmol. 2005;89(5):562-4.
3. Ojima Y, Hangai M, Sasahara M, et al. Three-dimensional imaging of the foveal photoreceptor layer in central serous chorioretinopathy using high-speed optical coherence tomography. Ophthalmology. 2007;114:2197-207.
4. van Velthoven ME, Verbraak FD, Garcia PM, et al. Evaluation of central serous retinopathy with *en face* optical coherence tomography. Br J Ophthalmol. 2005;89:1483-8.
5. Lumbroso B, Savastano MC, Rispoli M, et al. Morphologic differences according to etiology, in pigment epithelial detachments by means of *en face* optical coherence tomography. Retina. 2011;31:553-8.
6. Piccolino FC, De La Longrais RR, Manea M, et al. Posterior cystoid retinal degeneration in central serous chorioretinopathy. Retina. 2008;28:1008-12.
7. Iida T, Yannuzzi LA, Spaide RF, et al. Cystoid macular degeneration in chronic central serous chorioretinopathy. Retina. 2003;23:1-7; quiz 137-8.
8. Iida T, Kishi S, Hagimura N, et al. Persistent and bilateral choroidal vascular abnormalities in central serous chorioretinopathy. Retina. 1999;19:508-12.
9. Fujimoto H, Gomi F, Wakabayashi T, et al. Morphologic changes in acute central serous chorioretinopathy evaluated by fourier-domain optical coherence tomography. Ophthalmology. 2008;115:1494-500.
10. Hirami Y, Tsujikawa A, Sasahara M, et al. Alterations of retinal pigment epithelium in central serous chorioretinopathy. Clin Experiment Ophthalmol. 2007;35:225-30.

chapter 25

En Face Optical Coherence Tomography in Idiopathic Macular Telangiectasia

Martine Mauget-Faÿsse, Benjamin Wolff, Chrysanthi Basdekidou, Alexandre Matet, Vivien Vasseur, Michel Paques, José-Alain Sahel

Introduction

Macular telangiectasia (MacTel), a retinal disease in which the hallmark is retinal parafoveolar or temporal-foveolar telangiectasia with aneurysmal dilations affecting venous, arterial and capillary vessels, was originally described in 1968 by Gass.[1,2] In 1993, Gass and Blodi classified this condition into five clinical stages according to disease development.[3] Yannuzzi, in 2006, published a simplified classification of this entity with only two distinct types: MacTel type 1 (aneurysmal telangiectasia) and MacTel type 2 (perifoveal telangiectasia).[4]

New clinical signs of MacTel, particularly of MacTel type 2, have been found using novel imaging techniques, such as fundus autofluorescence,[5] macular pigment optical density scanning,[6-8] confocal blue reflectance,[9] and more recently, polarization-sensitive optical coherence tomography (OCT)[10] and adaptive optics scanning laser ophtalmoscopy.[11]

The following description of *en face* OCT idiopathic macular telangiectasia was obtained with a spectral domain OCT (SD-OCT, Spectralis® Heidelberg Engineering, Heidelberg, Germany).

High-definition *en face* images depict retinal vessels through the other retinal structures as hyper-reflective curved tubes even without dye utilization while the "shadows" of the retinal vessels are identical but seen in deeper layers as hyporeflective curved tubes. On SD-OCT B scan and C scan, dense tissues, such as retinal vessels or melanin-containing structures produce a screen creating a shadow on the deeper layers. This important problem will probably be eliminated with the use of new devices, such as polarization-sensitive OCT and adaptive optics scanning laser ophthalmoscopy (**Figures 1A to C**).

Currently, without adequate software, it is difficult to follow the complete anatomical path of the vessels although segments can be analyzed and abnormalities identified.

En Face Imaging Patterns of the Normal Retinal Vasculature

In normal retina outside the fovea, three interconnected capillary layers[12,13] can be found (**Figures 2A to D**): a first layer in the ganglion cell layer in continuity with arterioles; a second layer at the outer plexiform layer/inner nuclear layer interface and a third layer in the external plexiform layer (**Table 1**). These layers are interconnected by orthogonal microvessels. Capillaries are identified as a dense network of thin, curved and interconnected hyper-reflective tubules in the posterior pole except in the central foveal area. In the foveolar zone, there are no capillaries. Perifoveolar capillaries are very dense close to the foveolar zone, leaving an avascular region of 400–500 microns in diameter. The diameter of the foveal avascular zone is closely correlated to the depth of the foveal pit (**Figure 3**).[14]

En Face Imaging in MacTel

The characteristics of MacTel type 1 and type 2 as observed through different diagnostic tests are summarized in **Tables 2 to 5**.

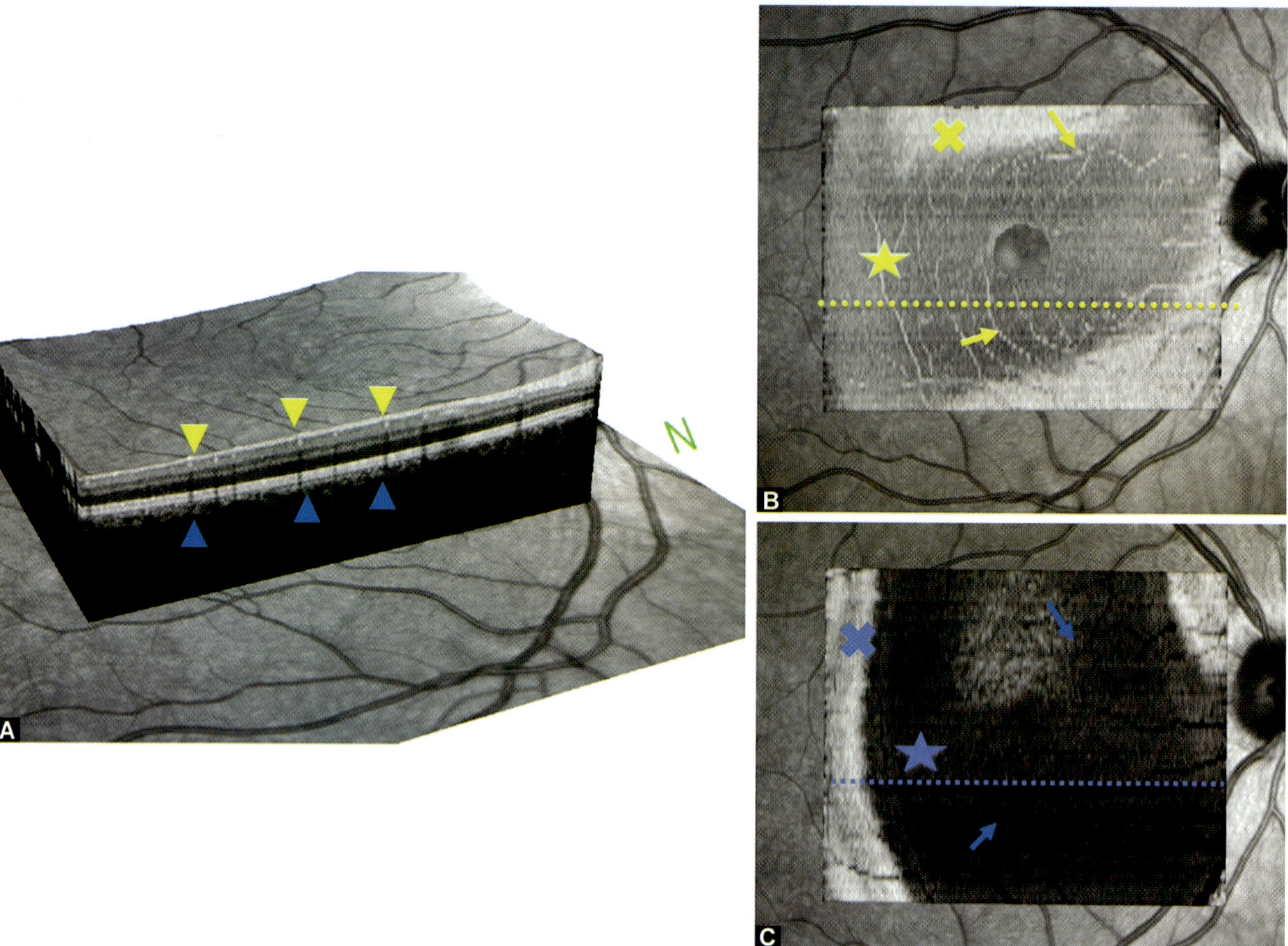

Figures 1A to C: B scan and *en face* (C scan) optical coherence tomography (OCT) imaging of normal retinal vessels with their shadows. (A) Three-dimensional imaging: the hyper-reflective spots (yellow arrow head) represent a section of secondary retinal arteries and veins. Underneath these small hyper-reflective spots and perpendicular to the photoreceptor line, hyporeflective thin lines (blue arrow head) are visible corresponding to the shadow of each hyper-reflective retinal secondary vessels; (B) *En face* OCT scan into the ganglion cell layer (yellow star): the hyper-reflective secondary retinal arteries and veins (yellow arrows) are visualized as hyper-reflective vessel segments; the hyper-reflective layer corresponds to the inner plexiform layer (yellow cross); (C) *En face* OCT scan into the outer nuclear layer (blue star): the hyporeflective secondary retinal vessel segments are the shadow of these vessels (blue arrows); the hyper-reflective layer here corresponds to the inner segment/outer segment junction (blue cross)

Table 1: Anatomical location of the normal retinal vessels revealed through an *en face* optical coherence tomography C scan

Intraretinal vessels location	Ganglion cell layer	Outer plexiform layer/Inner nuclear layer interface	External plexiform layer	Photoreceptor layer
Secondary arteria and vein	Presence	Absence	Absence	Absence
Three capillary layers (Second and third interconnected)	First capillary layer Presence	Second capillary layer Presence	Third capillary layer Presence	Absence

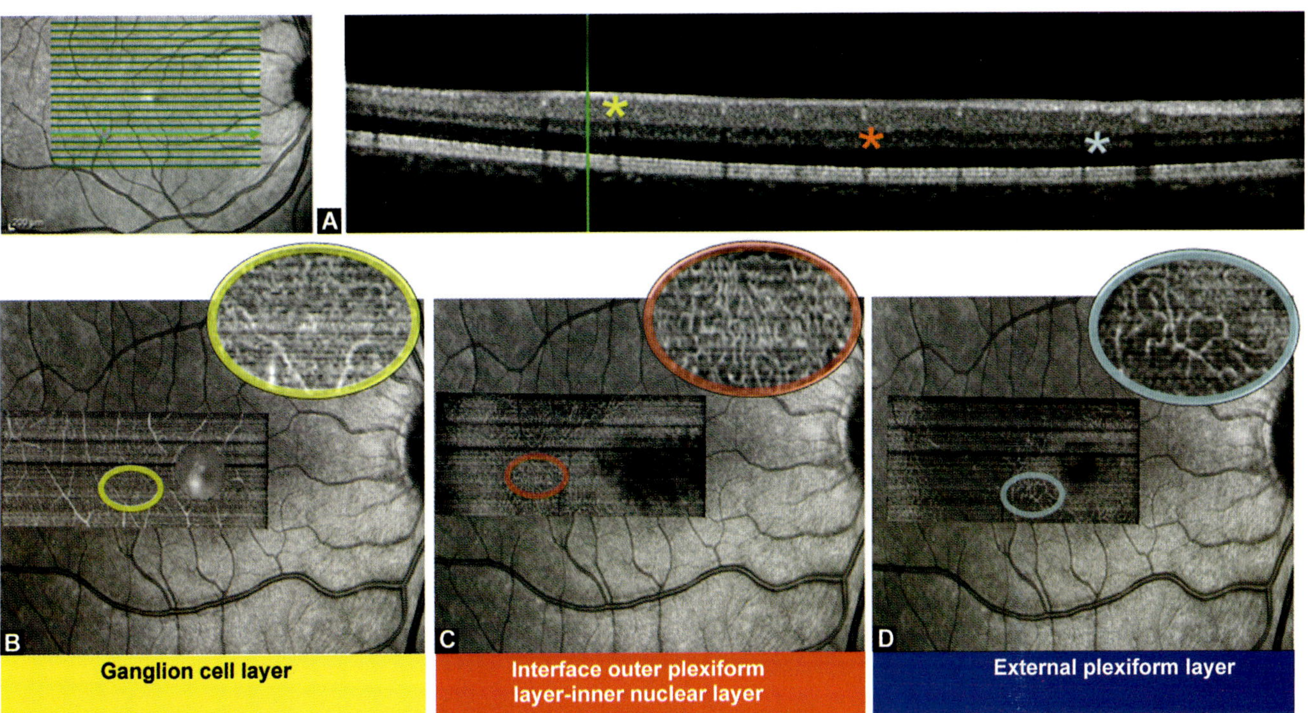

Figures 2A to D: B scan and *en face* imaging, with magnification, of the three capillary layers in the normal retina. (A) Spectral domain OCT B scan allows identification of anatomical layers of the neurosensory retina. By comparison with *en face* imaging, the tiny hyper-reflective round or oval spots located in three different depths correspond to the normal retinal capillaries; (B to D) *En face* optical coherence tomography (OCT) scan: the retinal capillaries can be seen, without dye, as hyper-reflective tiny interconnected network tubules in three different levels—the ganglion cell layer (yellow star), the interface outer plexiform layer—inner nuclear layer (red star) and the external plexiform layer (blue star)

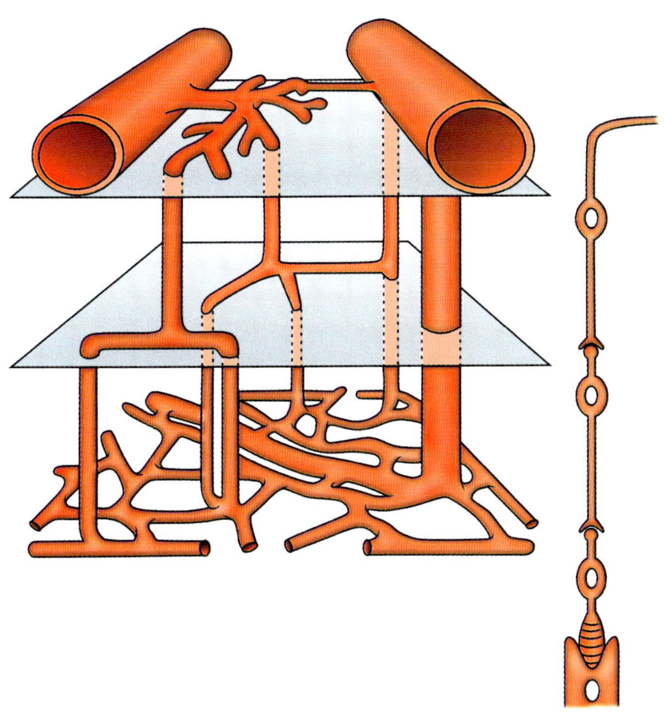

Figure 3: Structural and hemodynamic analysis of the mouse retinal microcirculation. Schematic representation of the microvessels array between an arteriovenous couple. The arteriole is in the top left of the image, the venule in the top right. The mouse retina has the same three layers of capillaries as in the human retina (*Source*: Paques M, Tadayoni R, Sercombe R, et al. Structural and hemodynamic analysis of the mouse retinal microcirculation. Invest Ophthalmol Vis Sci. 2003;44(11):4960-7)

Table 2: Clinical signs of macular telangiectasia type 1 and type 2[15-25]

Type of macular telangiectasia	Clinical signs		
MacTel type 1	Male	Unilateral	Decrease vision
MacTel type 2	No sex differences	Bilateral small telangiectasia	Scotomas and decrease vision

Table 3: Fundus macular telangiectasia

MacTel type 1	Capillary, venular and arteriolar aneurysms of the superficial and deep retinal vessels		Lipid deposition+++ Macular thickening ± Hemorrhages - No pigment proliferation - No crystalline deposit - No CNV		Sometimes: focal vascular change in the mid-periphery	
MacTel type 2	Telangiectasia not well visible Loss of retinal transparency	Cystic appearance to the fovea	Crystalline deposits	Squared angle vein or artery within 1 disk diameter of the foveola	Frequent retinal-retinal anastomosis and CNV	RPE hyperplasia Intraretinal pigment migration

Table 4: Characteristics of macular telangiectasia as observed through fluorescein angiography

	Early phase fluorescein angiography		Intermediate phase fluorescein angiography		Late phase fluorescein angiography	
MacTel type 1	Perifoveolar capillary, venular and arteriolar aneurysms		Sometimes minimal retinal ischemic areas		Leakage into the retina and cystoid macular edema	
MacTel type 2	Visualization of telangiectasia	Squared angle vein or artery	Frequent retinal-retinal anastomosis	Possible leakage from choroidal neovascularization	Some leakage	Mask effect by retinal pigment epithelium hyperplasia

Table 5: Characteristics of macular telangiectasia as observed through optical coherence tomography B scan

MacTel type 1	Macular thickening with focal exudative cystic change			Inconstant shallow serous retinal detachment			Visualization of intraretinal microangiopathy in superficial and deep circulations with aneurysms	
MacTel type 2	Small hyper-reflective spots in all the retinal layers	Inner and outer retinal cystic changes	Bright hyper-reflective material at the ganglion cell fiber level	Focal decrease in retinal thickness	Loss at the level of inner segment/ outer segment junction, thinning of the outer nuclear layer	Plexiform layer wrinkles	Hyper-reflective materials with a shadow cone behind it	Hyper-reflectivity at the level of choroidal neovascularization

Table 6: Characteristics of macular telangiectasia as observed through optical coherence tomography C scan

MacTel type 1	Hyporeflective intraretinal cystoid spaces	Hyper-reflective areas of lipid deposition	Hyporeflective areas as the shadow of lipid deposition	Slightly dilated retinal hyper-reflective tubules with telangiectasic aspect	Hyper-reflective round, oval or coma spots			
MacTel type 2	Hyper-reflective slightly dilated and scarsed tubules with telangiectasia aspect	Hypo-reflective cysts	Bright hyper-reflective dots at the ganglion cell fiber level	Hyper-reflective walls of the squared angle vein or artery	Intraretinal and subretinal anastomosis visualization	Retinal pigment epithelium hyper-reflectivity with hypo-reflective shadow underneath	Small hyporeflective defects at hyper-reflective retinal pigment epithelium/ inner segment/ outer segment junction layer	Hyper-reflective intraretinal neovascularization

MacTel Type 1: Aneurysmal Telangiectasia[4]

MacTel type 1 pathological patterns revealed with *en face* OCT C scans indicate (**Table 6**):

- Cystoid hyporeflective intraretinal cystoid spaces with hyper-reflective areas of lipid deposition (**Figures 4A to E**)
- Slightly dilated retinal hyper-reflective tubules with telangiectatic appearance (**Figures 5A to D**)
- Hyper-reflective round, oval or comma-shaped spots as visualization of the aneurysmal dilations (**Figures 6A to D**).

MacTel Type 2: Perifoveal Telangiectasia[16-24]

MacTel type 2 abnormalities revealed with *en face* OCT C scans indicate (**Table 6**):

- Crystalline deposits[24] (**Figures 7A to H**)
- Intraretinal capillary location and shape[25] (**Figures 8A and B**)
- Loss of the anastomotic perifoveal network[26] (**Figure 9**)
- Better visualization of retinal vessels and telangiectasia than on fluorescein angiography (**Figures 10A to D**)
- Visualization of intraretinal cysts[27] (**Figures 11A and B**)
- Extent and location of intraretinal neovascularization (**Figures 12A to E**) and hyperplastic pigment plaques (**Figures 13A to H**)
- Outer plexiform layer folding toward the outer retinal layers[28] (**Figures 14A and B**)
- Hyper-reflective spots in the outer retina and photoreceptor loss[29-31] (**Figures 15A to E**)
- Choroidal cavities (**Figures 16A and B**).

Conclusion

Spectral domain OCT and particularly *en face* OCT technology allows the imaging of anatomic elements by way of their specific reflectivity. However, there will always be a posterior shadow cone behind the hyper-reflective structures. This may lead to difficulties and pitfalls when interpreting *en face* OCT imaging. Considering all these elements, *en face* imaging in idiopathic macular telangiectasia facilitates new understanding of the nature and effect of these vascular abnormalities on the macula.

En face OCT is a very useful technique in the visualization of the real extent of the intraretinal anomalies related to idiopathic macular telangiectasia type 2A compared with fluorescein angiography. It allows for more stable image analysis of the capillary network and the cysts' depth and extent within the retina. It should therefore be considered as an indispensable complementary examination in the early diagnosis and follow-up of macular telangiectatic lesions.

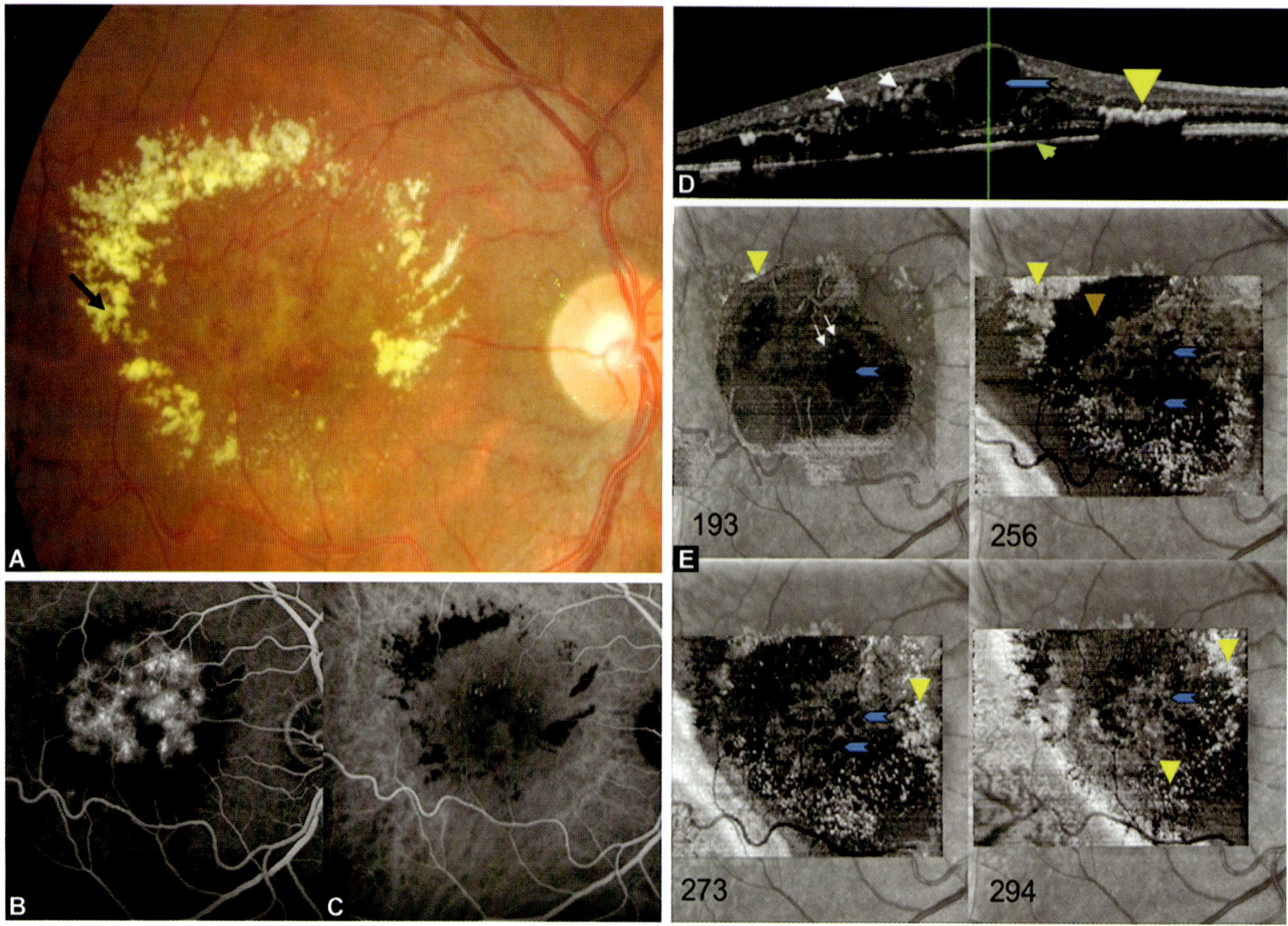

Figures 4A to E: Macular telangiectasia type 1 in a 52-year-old male with progressive decrease in vision in the right eye. (A) Fundus color photograph shows lipid exudates (black arrow). Capillary, venular and arteriolar vessels dilations are visible in the posterior pole; (B) Fluorescein angiogram shows parafoveolar capillary dilations in the early phase and progressive leakage into the retina with cystoid macular edema in the late phase; (C) Indocyanine green angiogram clearly depicts the central aneurysms; (D) B scan spectral domain optical coherence tomography shows macular thickening with focal exudative cystic changes (blue arrowhead) and hyper-reflective lipid deposits (yellow arrowhead) with a shallow serous retinal detachment (green arrow) and vascular aneurysms (white small arrows); (E) *En face* optical coherence tomography imaging at different depths—depth 193: visualization of the cystoid hyporeflective central large cyst (blue arrowhead) and vascular abnormalities (small white arrows), depths 256, 273 and 294: visualization of the highly hyper-reflective lipid deposits (yellow arrowheads) mixed with the shadow of the above accumulation of lipid exudates (brown arrowhead). Small hyporeflective areas represent cystoid spaces (blue arrowhead)

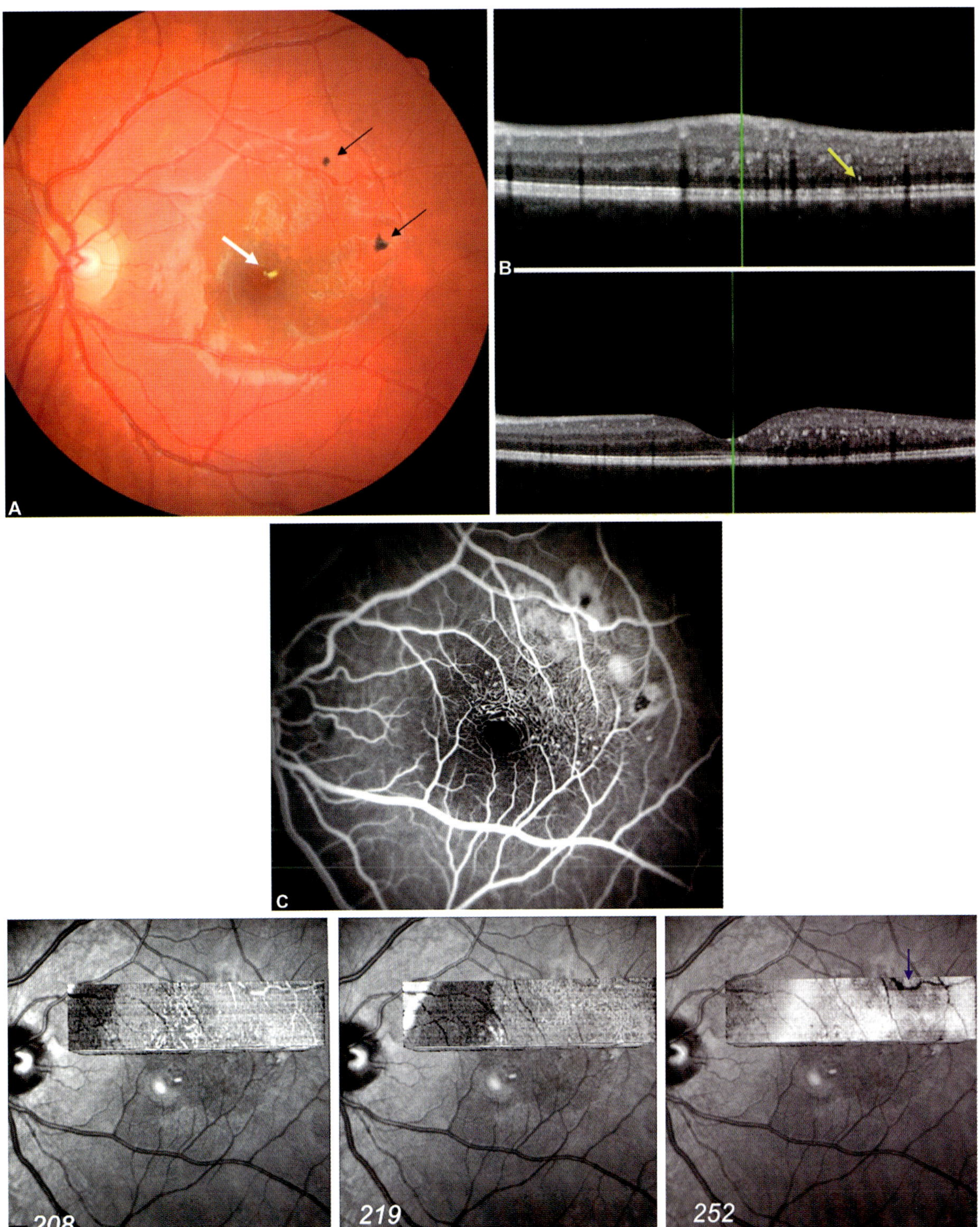

Figures 5A to D: Macular telangiectasia type 1 in a 12-year-old male with 20/20 vision in the left eye which had undergone laser photocoagulation 2 years ago. (A) Fundus color photograph: residual paracentral lipid exudates (white arrow) and laser photocoagulation scars (black arrow); (B) B scan spectral domain optical coherence tomography: abnormal increase in the number and diameter of intraretinal hyper-reflective round or ovoid small spots. Note also the presence of these spots as far as the outer limiting membrane (yellow arrow); (C) Fluorescein angiogram: Abnormal vascular and capillary network with macular telangiectasia and laser scars; (D) *En face* C scan optical coherence tomography at different depths, without dye, showing the slightly dilated intraretinal hyper-reflective capillaries with the telangiectasia (depth 219). In depth 252, the tiny hyporeflective spots correspond to the shadows of the telangiectasia. Note the black shadow of the temporal secondary artery with telangiectasia (blue arrow)

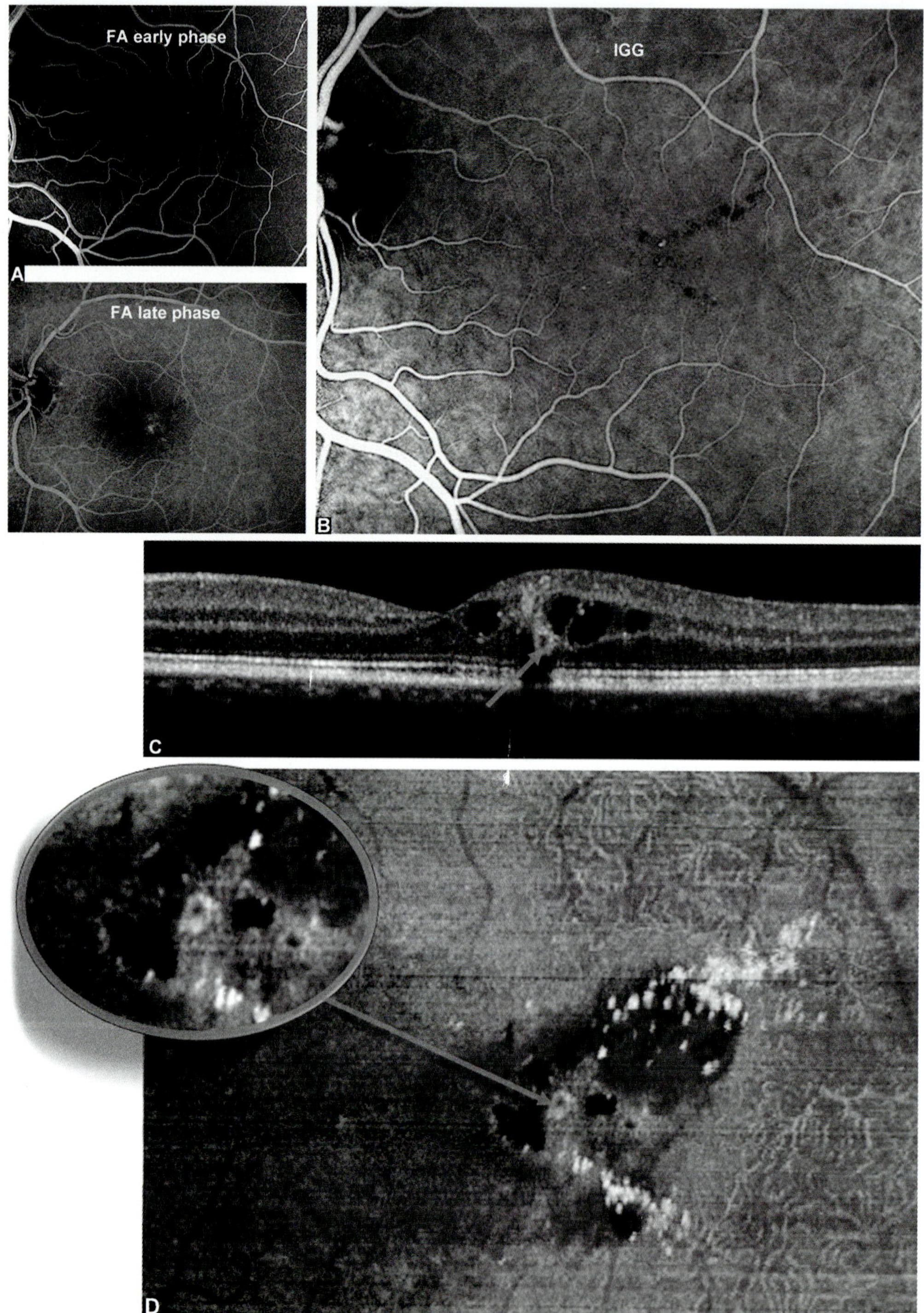

Figures 6A to D: Macular telangiectasia type 1 in a 46-year-old male with unilateral decrease in vision. Fundus examination reveals unilateral venular and arteriolar aneurysms with macular thickening and lipid deposition. (A) Angiograms confirm the diagnosis of aneurysmal telangiectasia with visualization of parafoveal capillary dilations on fluorescein in the early phases and leakage in the late phases; (B) On indocyanine green angiography, the telangiectasias are even better depicted[32] as well as the hyporeflective mask effect of lipid deposition. (C) B scan optical coherence tomography: visualization of an aneurysm in the outer plexiform layer associated with focal texudative cystic changes in the inner nuclear layer and slight thickening of the macula. Also, increase in the number and diameter of intraretinal hyper-reflective spots corresponding to an abnormal vascular network; (D) *En face* optical coherence tomography: surrounding dilated capillaries in the outer plexiform layer are clearly visible. A large aneurysm is located at the level of this retinal layer and is surrounded by irregular hyporeflective cavities of cystoid macular edema. The hyper-reflective white dots represent lipid deposits. The secondary retinal vessel shadow is clearly visible

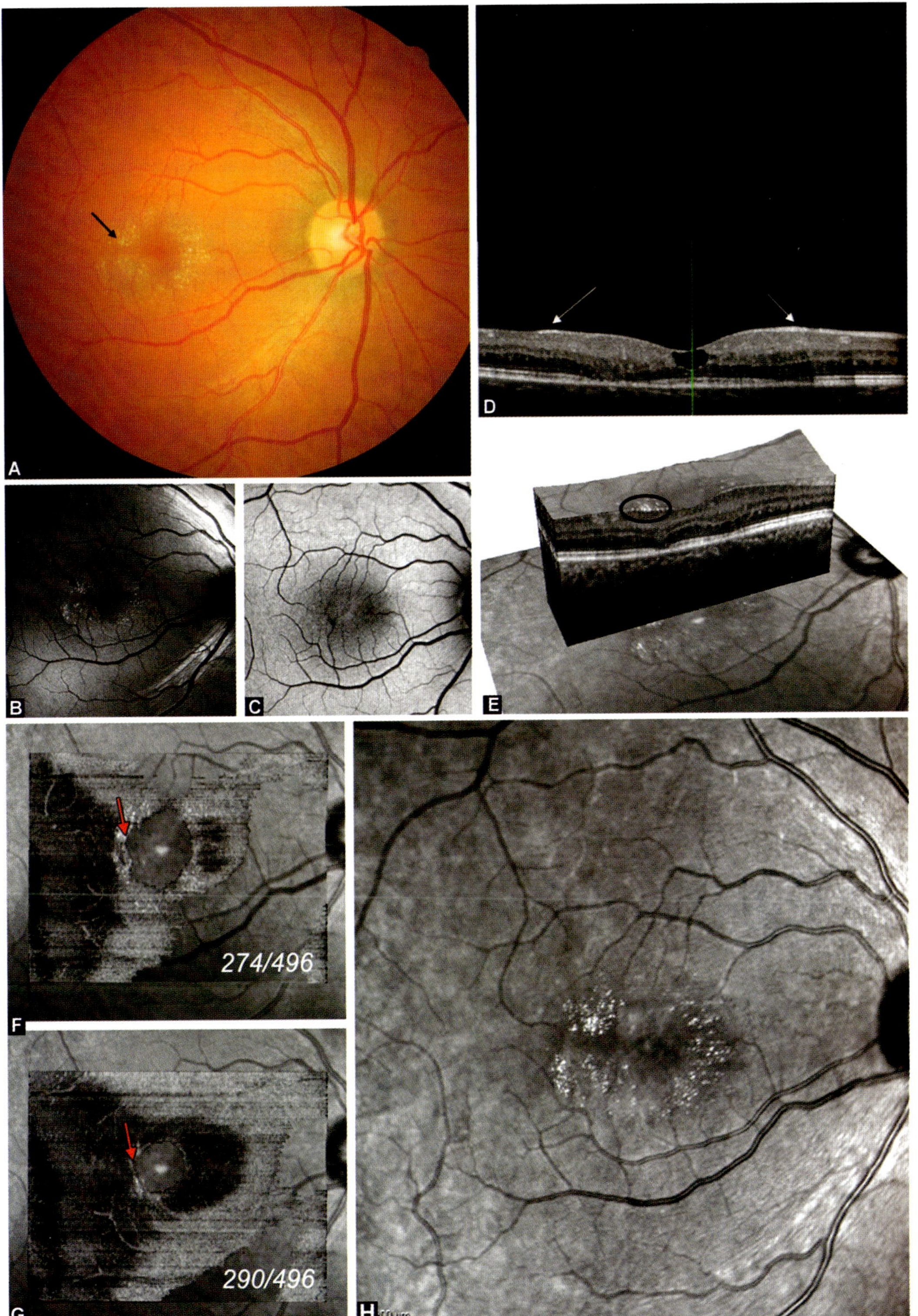

Figures 7A to H: Macular telangiectasia type 2 in a 62-year-old male with visual acuity of 20/32. (A) Color fundus photography revealed the presence of yellowish dot-like crystalline deposits in the perifoveal area (B) seen as hyper-reflective dots on red free; (C) and presenting hypoautofluorescence on autofluorescence image, (D) The optical coherence tomography (OCT) B scan reveals the presence of hyper-reflective crystalline deposits lying mostly within the superficial retinal layers. They are better visualized on three-dimensional image reconstruction (E). (F) On *en face* OCT the crystalline deposits are visualized as areas of high hyper-reflectivity in the nerve fiber layer; (G) Here, they are arranged along the nerve fiber within an annular area centered on the fovea (red arrow) and are better visualized than with infra-red imaging (H)

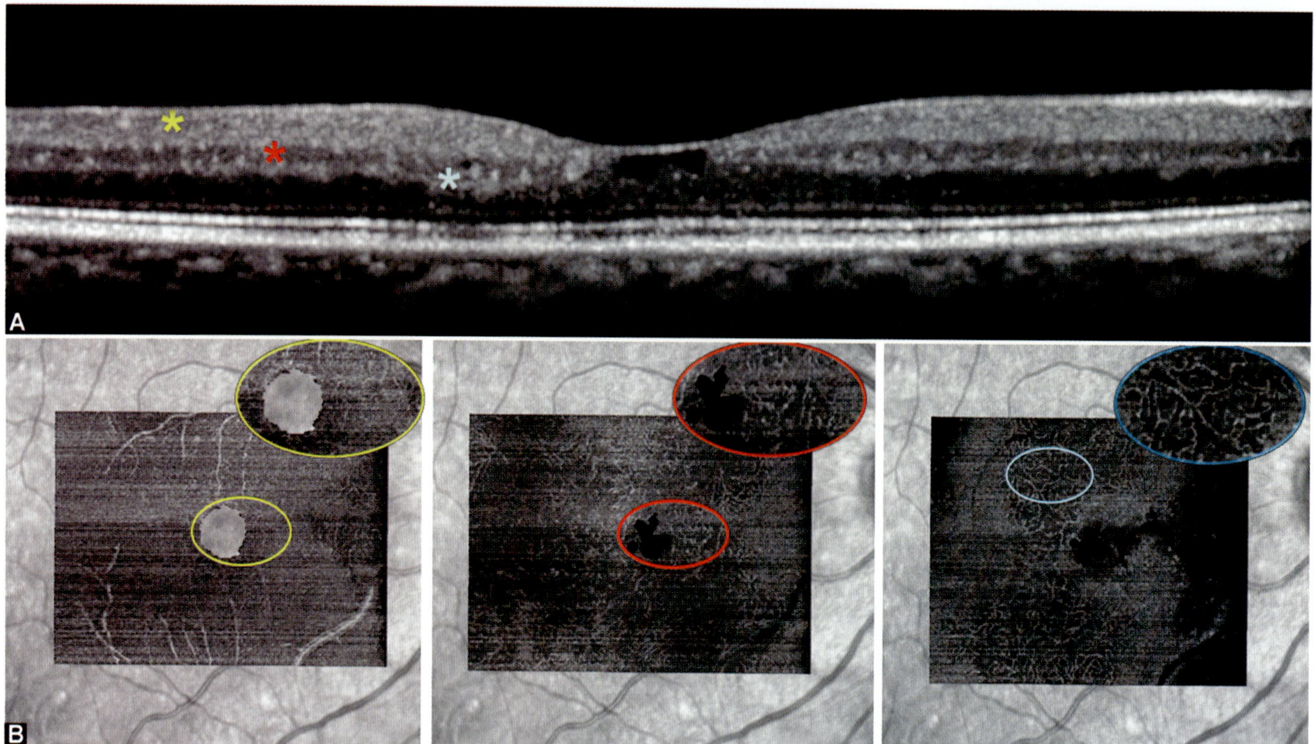

Figures 8A and B: A 64-year-old male with MacTel type 2 and decreased vision in the right eye. (A) Spectral domain optical coherence tomography (OCT) B scan shows a central inner retinal cavity. Numerous hyper-reflective tiny spots of different diameters are visible. The outer plexiform layer appears swollen in some places with a thinning of the facing outer nuclear layer; (B) *En face* OCT C scan shows capillaries with telangiectasia as hyper-reflective interconnected tubules almost similar in shape to normal eyes, whilst they seem slightly dilated and sparse. They are seen very deep in the retina, in the outer nuclear layer, as already published by Gass
(*Source*: Gass JD. Stereoscopic Atlas of Macular diseases: Diagnosis and Treatment. 4th edition. St Louis: CV Mosby; 1997. pp. 502-13)

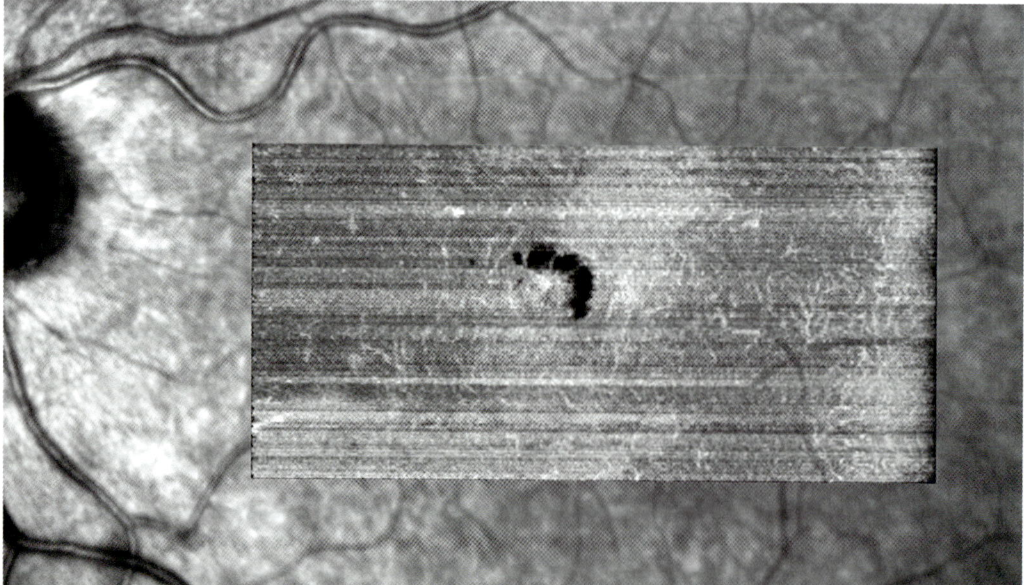

Figure 9: Anastomotic perifoveal network in MacTel type 2 patients. Capillaries differ in comparison with normal eyes: with a three well-defined layers are no more and the capillary network invades the foveolar zone with a partial loss of the anastomotic perifoveal network as already described by Mansour
(*Source*: Mansour AM, Schachat A. Foveal avascular zone in idiopathic juxtafoveolar telangiectasia. Ophthlamologica. 1993;207:9-12)

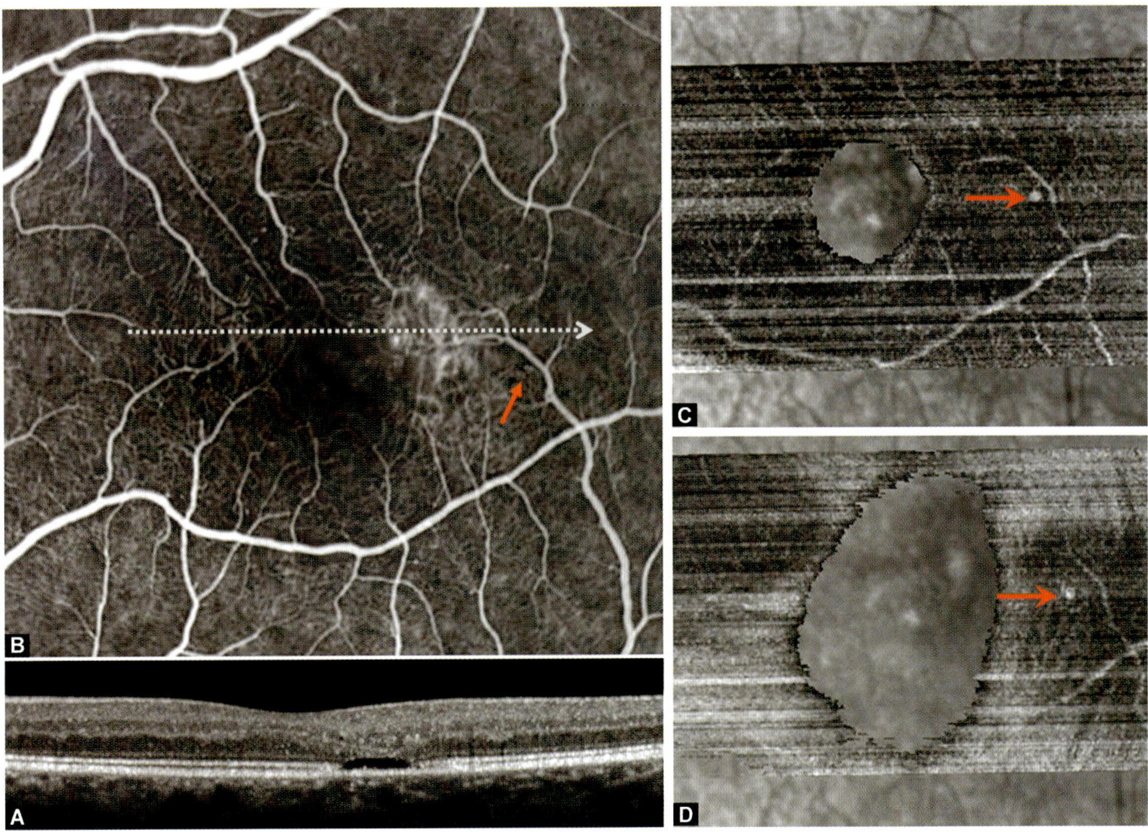

Figures 10A to D: (A) Spectral domain optical coherence tomography B scans. There is partial loss of the highly reflective junction of inner and outer photoreceptor segments (IS/OS junction). Above this photoreceptor damage, the outer nuclear layer is absent and is replaced with a moderately hyper-reflective tissue with small hyper and hyporeflective spots; (B) Fluorescein angiogram: telangiectasias are visualized in the temporal part of the fovea; (C and D) *En face* C scan at 2 different cuts; (C) In the inner nuclear layer and (D) in the outer plexiform-inner nuclear interface layer: telangiectasis are even more visible than on fluorescein angiography, without use of the dye in different cuts (red arrow)

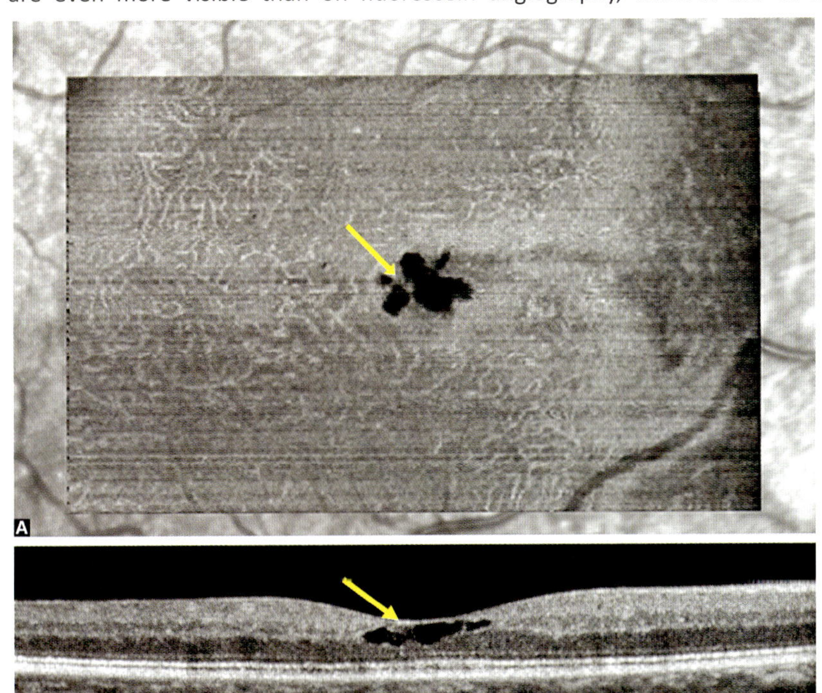

Figures 11A and B: Intraretinal cysts are inner lamellar cysts bordered anteriorly by the inner limiting membrane. They are seen on *en face* (A) and spectral domain OCT B scan (B) as hyporeflective areas, with well defined borders, in the fovea

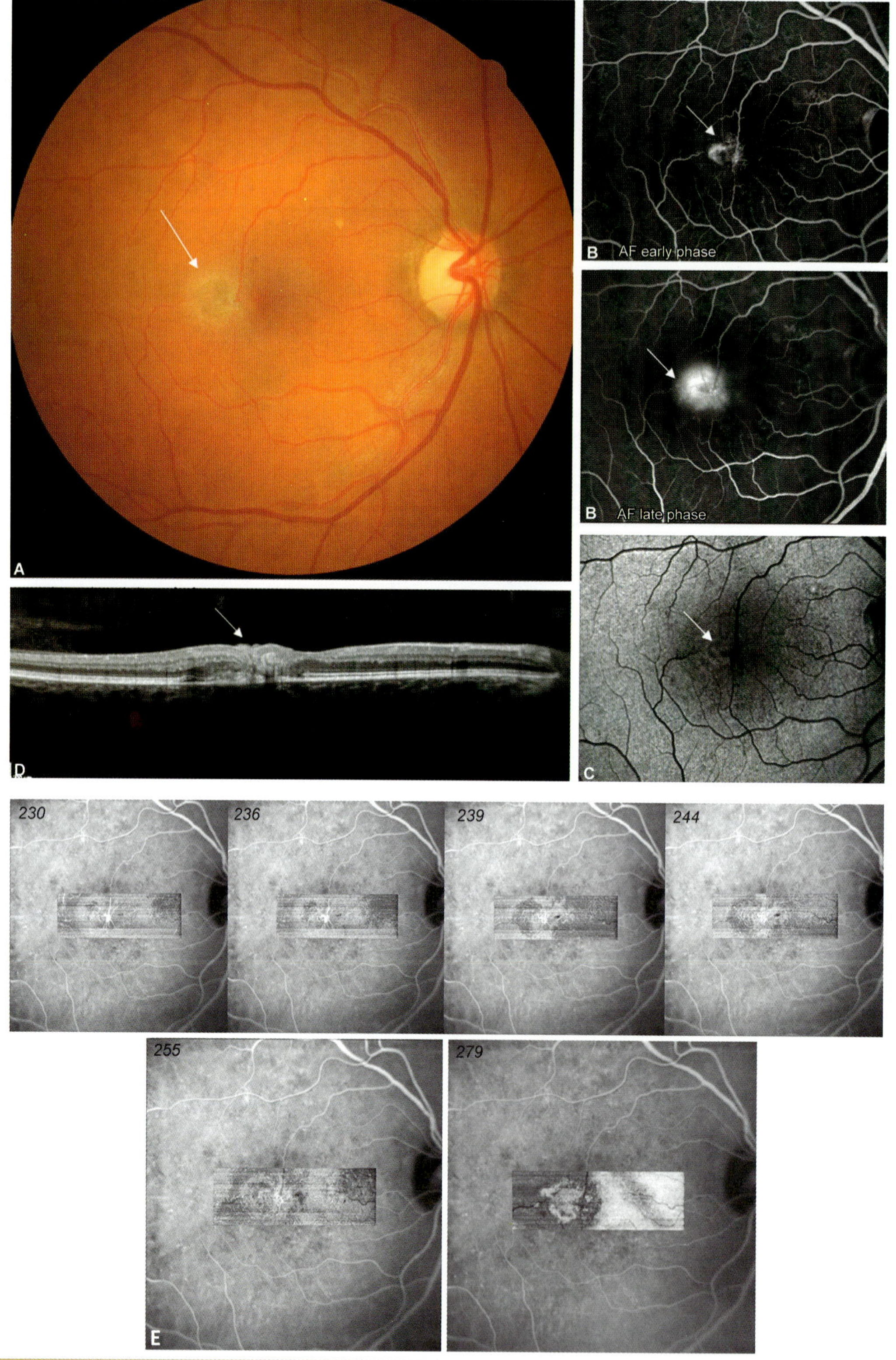

Figures 12A to E: A 66-year-old female with sudden decrease of vision and metamorphopsia in the right eye. Retinal-retinal anastomosis and neovascularization are frequent in MacTel patients. (A) Color fundus photograph; (B) Fluorescein angiography and (C) autofluorescence imaging: shows retinal-retinal anastomosis with a temporo-foveolar subretinal neovascularization; (D) Optical coherence tomography (OCT) B scan at the level of the anastomosis: shows hyper-reflective structures inside the retina with slight retinal thickening; (E) *En face* OCT scans at different depths: shows the retinal capillaries spreading into the foveolar zone. There is a retinal-retinal anastomosis communicating with the subretinal neovascularization. The neovascular tissue appears in depth 279 as a moderately hyper-reflective plaque

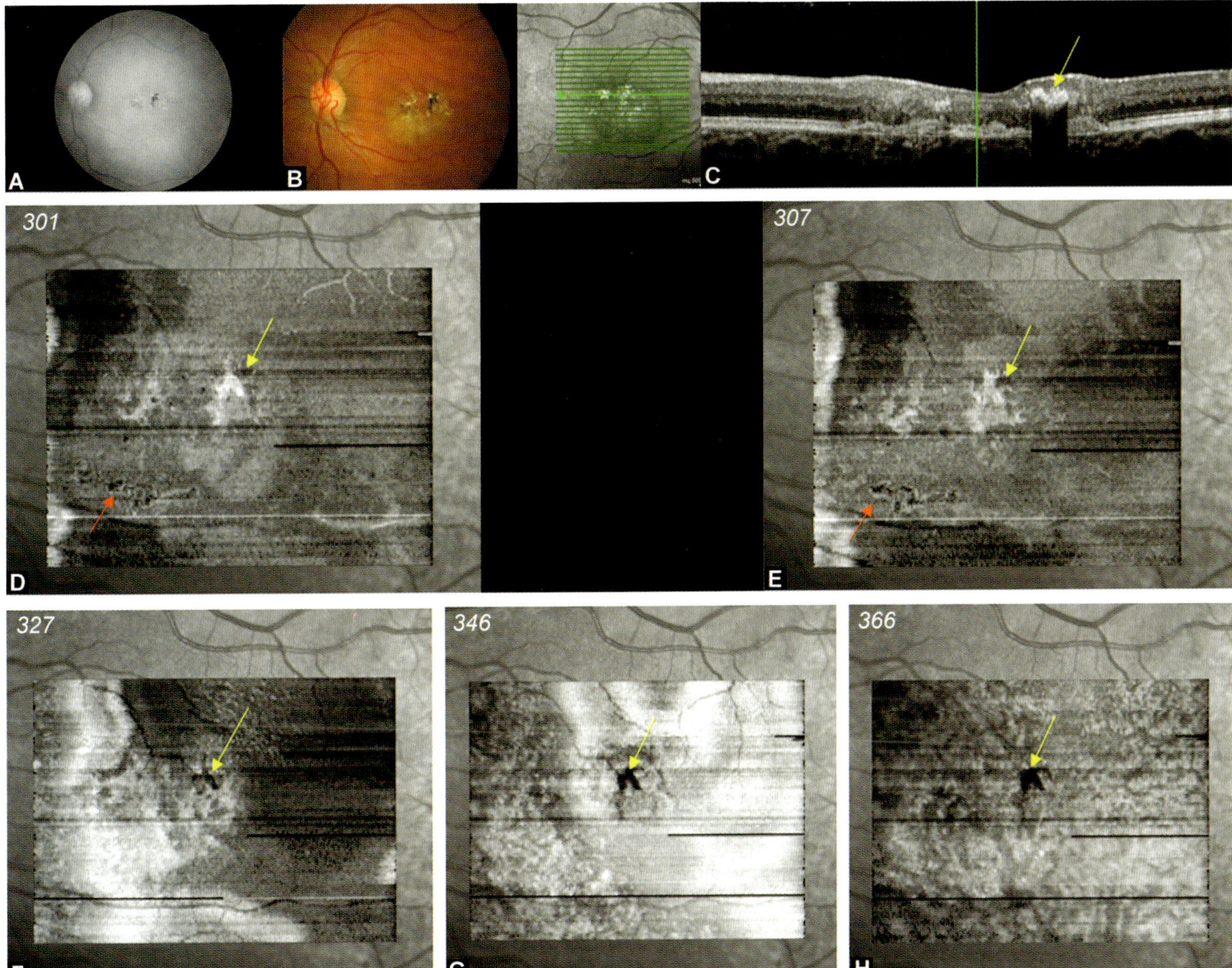

Figures 13A to H: (A) Red filter; (B) Color fundus photograph of a 66-year-old female left eye with progressive vision loss due to MacTel type 2. (C) Spectral domain optical coherence tomography (OCT) B scan shows an intraretinal hyper-reflective plaque temporal to the fovea with an intense shadow effect (yellow arrows). (D to H) *En face* OCT scan: the hyperplastic pigment plaques appear as hyper-reflective irregularly shaped areas with a shadow cone underneath. This cone shadow is visible until the choroidal layers (depth 366). In scans 301 and 307, outer retinal tubulations are visible (red arrows)

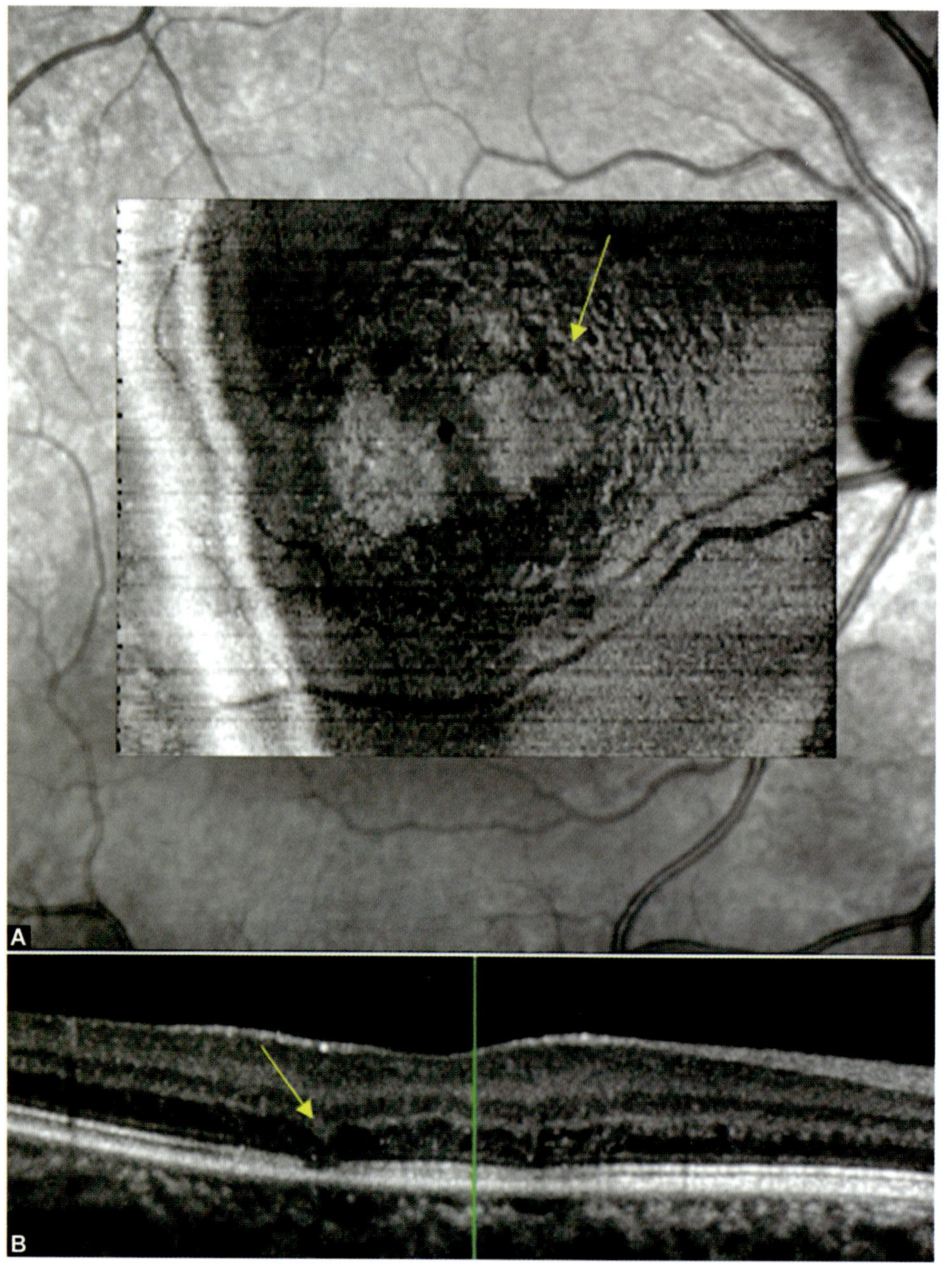

Figures 14A and B: Outer plexiform layer. (A) Spectral domain optical coherence tomography B scan shows sites of diffuse hyper-reflective haze located in the outer retinal layer (yellow arrows). This haze is almost always adjacent to areas with intraretinal cyst or disruption of the inner segment/outer segment junction. The outer plexiform layer has a wrinkled appearance and is often folded towards the outer retinal layers as seen here; (B) *En face* C scan cutting at the level of the outer plexiform layer, this layer appears wavy in all cases (yellow arrows)
(*Source*: Gillies MC, Zhu M, Chew E, et al. Familial asymptomatic macular telangiectasia type 2. Ophthalmology. 2009;116: 2422-9)

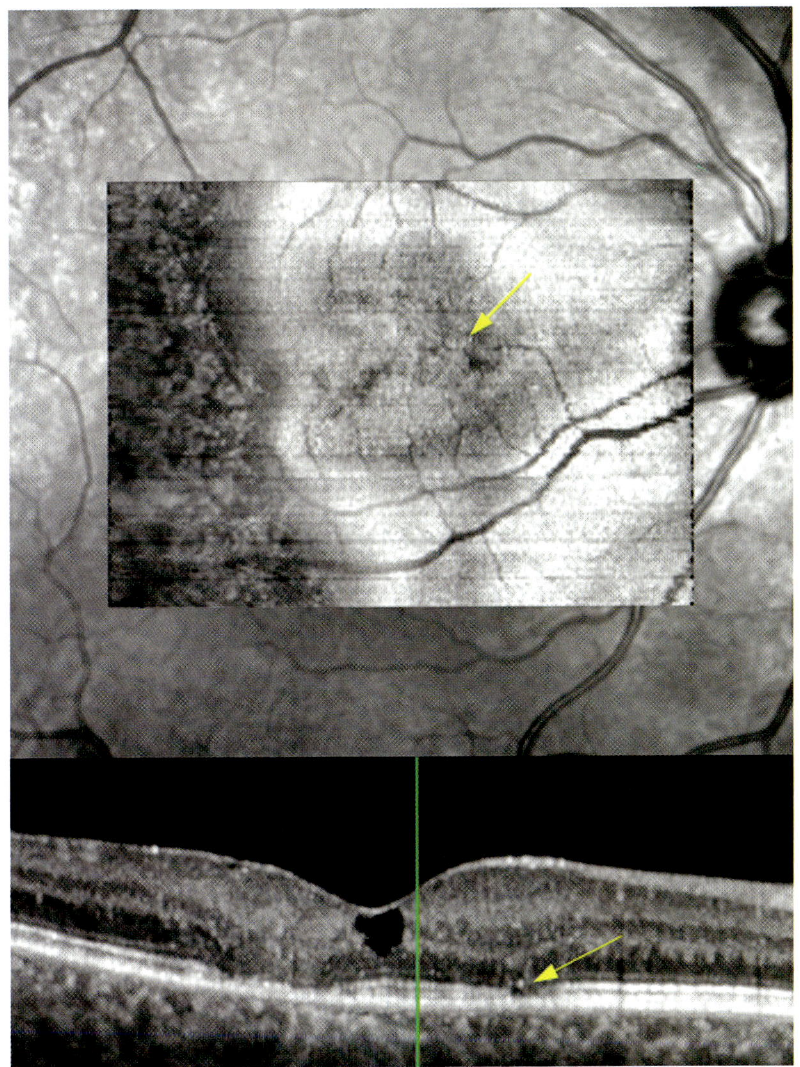

Figure 15A

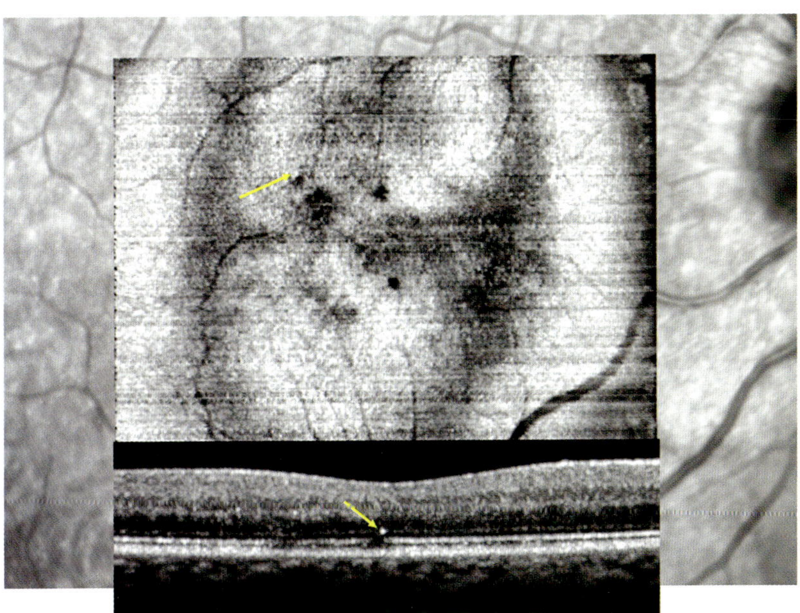

Figure 15B

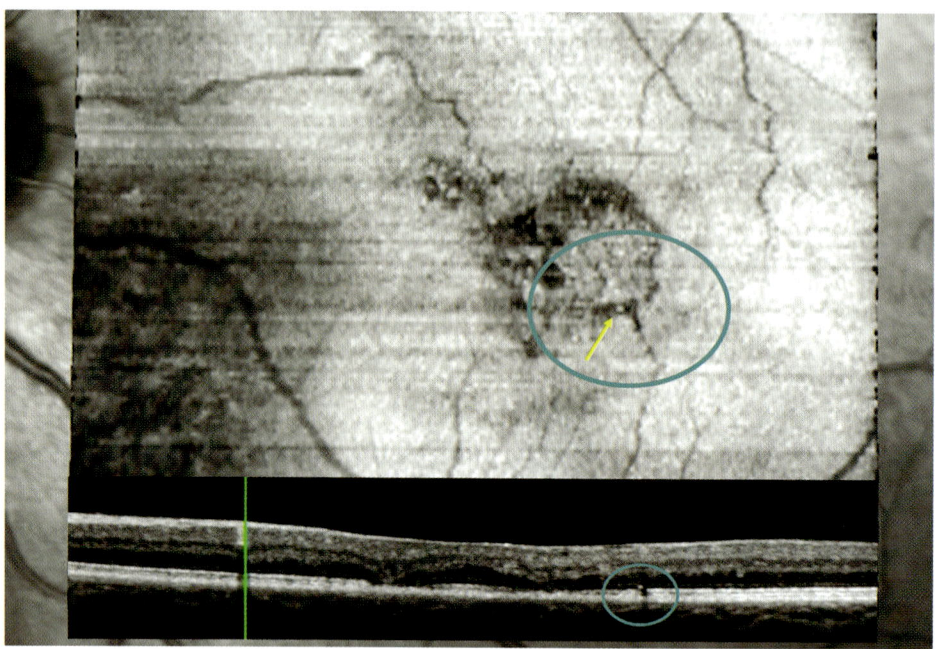

Figure 15C

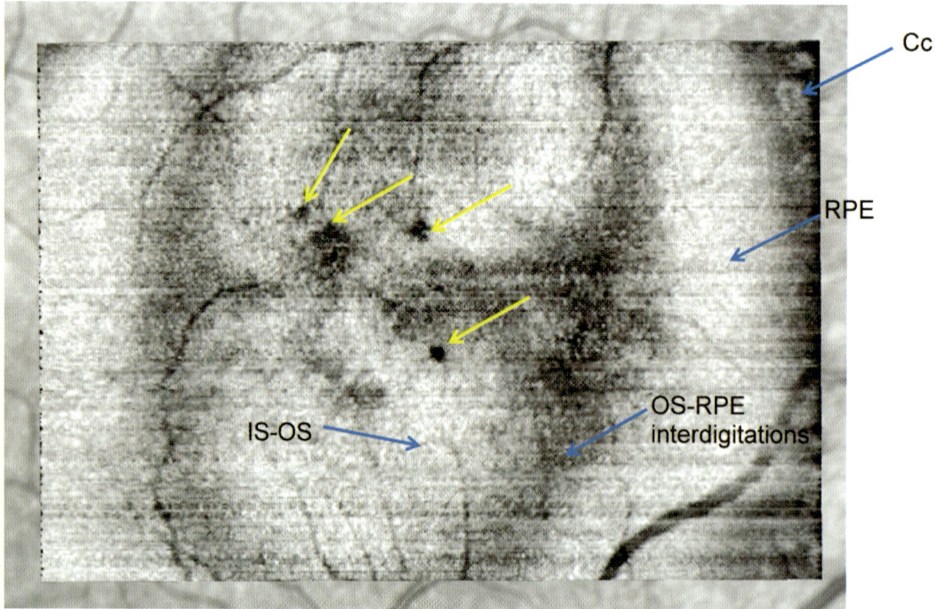

Figure 15D

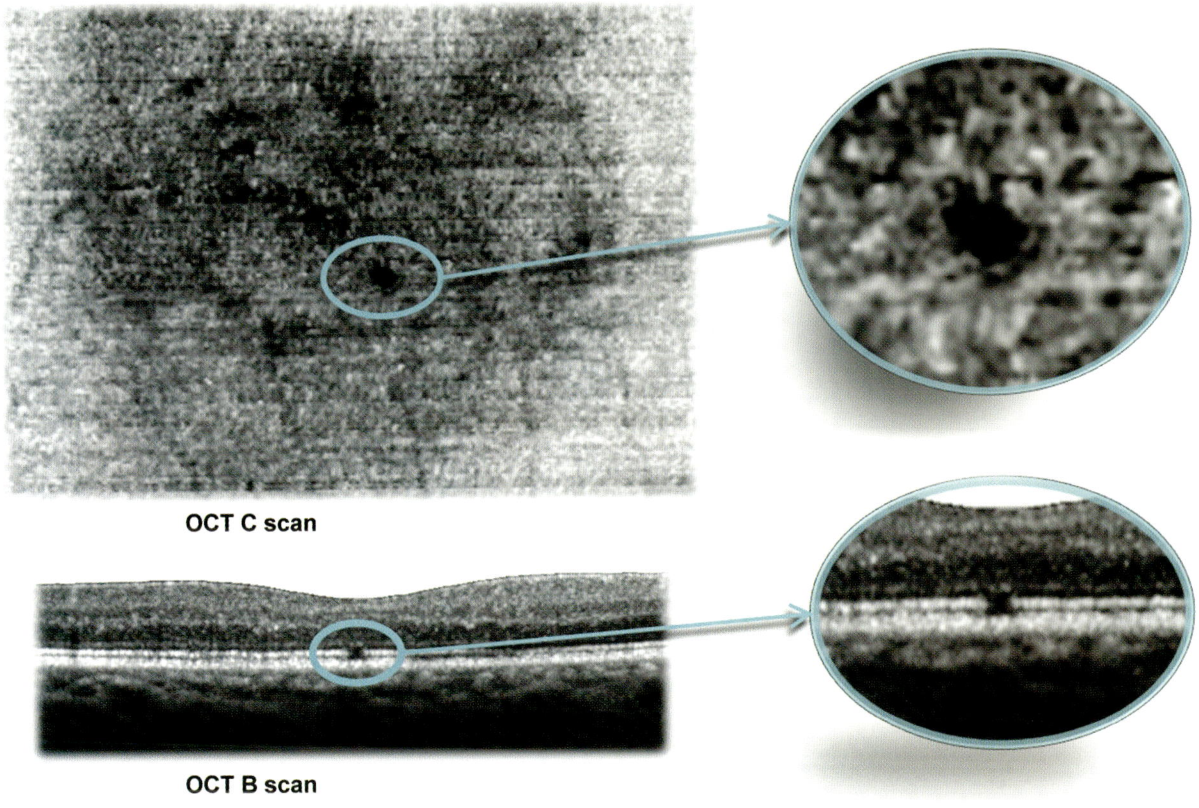

Figure 15E

Figures 15A to E: Photoreceptor loss observed with spectral domain optical coherence tomography (OCT) B scans and *en face* OCT in MacTel patients type 2. (A) Hyper-reflective bright spots are seen at the level of the outer nuclear layer or the outer limiting membrane (yellow arrow). The photoreceptor loss always appears at the level of the inner segment/ outer segment (IS/OS) border and outer segment-retinal pigment epithelium (RPE) interdigitation as hyporeflective areas; (B) Bright hyper-reflective spots were seen in case of photoreceptor loss, very close to the disruption of the IS/OS border and outer segment-RPE interdigitation and in the vicinity of intraretinal cystoid spaces (yellow arrow); (C) The hyper-reflective spots could correspond to degenerating Müller cells, accumulation of extravasated material from incompetent capillaries, visualization of capillary walls or pigment migration (yellow arrow); (D) *En face* OCT gives a more general appearance of disease damage than B scan images, showing hypo-reflective areas corresponding to photoreceptor loss (yellow arrows); (E) SD-OCT scan and *en face* OCT with magnification of an IS/OS defect (inside the oval blue)

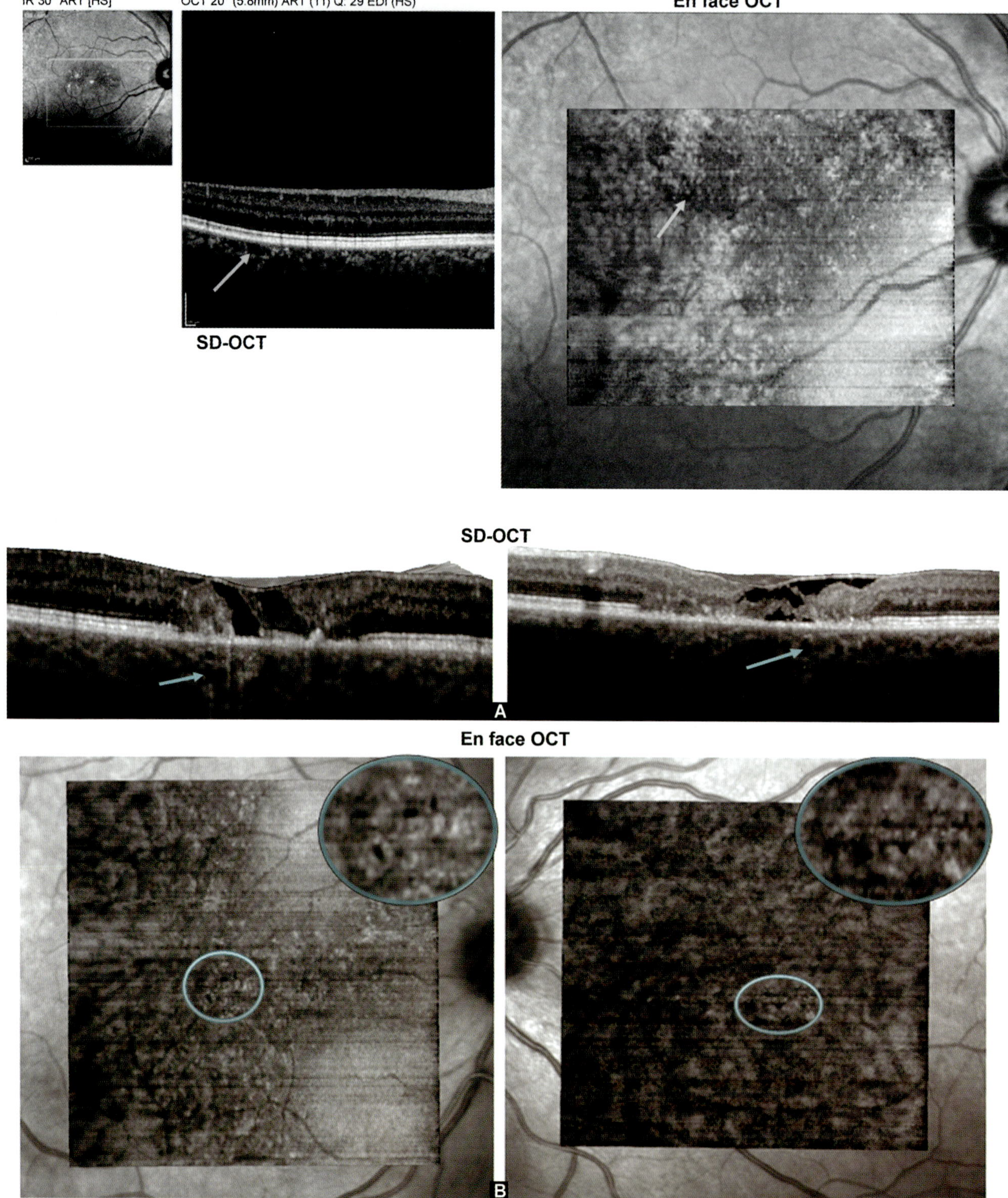

Figures 16A and B: Choroidal cavities in MacTel patients type 2. (A) EDI-OCT B scan: cavities are seen in the choroidal layer as small hyporeflective cysts (blue arrow). (B) *En face* EDI C scan: the cavities are seen as small hyporeflective areas in the foveolar or juxtafoveolar areas. They have to be differentiated from hyperplastic pigment plaque shadows

References

1. Gass JD. A fluorescein angiographic study of macular dysfunction secondary to retinal vascular disease. V. Retinal telangiectasis. Arch Ophthalmol.1968;80:592-605.
2. Gass JD, Oyakawa RT. Idiopathic juxtafoveolar retinal telangiectasis. Arch Ophthalmol. 1982;100(5):769-80.
3. Gass JD, Blodi BA. Idiopathic juxtafoveolar retinal telangiectasis. Update of classification and follow-up study. Ophthalmology. 1993;100(10):1536-46.
4. Yannuzzi LA, Bardal AM, Freund KB, et al. Idiopathic macular telangiectasia. Arch Ophthalmol. 2006;124(4): 450-60.
5. Wong WT, Forooghian F, Majumdar Z, et al. Fundus autofluorescence in type 2 idiopathic macular telangiectasia: correlation with optical coherence tomography and microperimetry. Am J Ophthalmol. 2009;148:573-83.
6. Charbel Issa P, van der Veen RL, Stijfs A, et al. Quantification of reduced macular pigment optical density in the central retina in macular telangiectasia type 2. Exp Eye Res. 2009;89:25-31.
7. Helb HM, Charbel Issa P, van der Veen RL, et al. Abnormal macular pigment distribution in type 2 idiopathic macular telangiectasia. Retina. 2008;28:808-16.
8. Zeimer MB, Padge B, Heimes B, et al. Idiopathic macular telangiectasia type 2: distribution of macular pigment and functional investigations. Retina. 2010;30(4):586-95.
9. Charbel Issa P, Berendschot TT, Staurenghi G, et al. Confocal blue reflectance imaging in type 2 idiopathic macular telangiectasia. Invest Ophthalmol Vis Sci. 2008;49:1172-7.
10. Schütze C, Ahlers C, Pircher M, et al. Morphologic characteristics of idiopathic juxtafoveal telangiectasia using spectral-domain and polarization-sensitive optical coherence tomography. Retina. 2012;32:256-64.
11. Ooto S, Hangai M, Takayama K, et al. High-resolution photoreceptor imaging in idiopathic macular telangiectasia type 2 using adaptive optics scanning laser ophthalmoscopy. Invest Ophthalmol Vis Sci. 2011;52(8): 5541-50.
12. Constantin J, Pournaras, et al. Pathologies vasculaires oculaires. Société Française d'Ophtalmologie. Elsevier Masson SAS: 2008. pp 33-5.
13. Paques M, Tadayoni R, Sercombe R, et al. Structural and hemodynamic analysis of the mouse retinal microcirculation. Invest Ophthalmol Vis Sci. 2003;44(11):4960-7.
14. Tick S, Rossant F, Ghorbel I, et al. Foveal shape and structure in a normal population. Invest Ophthalmol Vis Sci. 2011;29;52(8):5105-10.
15. Gaudric A, Ducos de Lahitte G, Cohen SY, et al. Optical coherence tomography in group 2A idiopathic juxtafoveolar retinal telangiectasis. Arch Ophthalmol. 2006;124:1410-9.
16. Paunescu LA, Ko TH, Duker JS, et al. Idiopathic juxtafoveal retinal telangiectasis: new findings by ultrahigh-resolution optical coherence tomography. Ophthalmology. 2006; 113:48-57.
17. Cohen SM, Cohen ML, El-Jabali F, et al. Optical coherence tomography findings in nonproliferative group 2a idiopathic juxtafoveal retinal telangiectasis. Retina. 2007;27:59-66.
18. Barthelmes D, Gillies MC, Sutter FK. Quantitative OCT analysis of idiopathic perifoveal telangiectasia. Invest Ophthalmol Vis Sci. 2008;49:2156-62.
19. Charbel Issa P, Holz FG, Scholl HP. Findings in fluorescein angiography and optical coherence tomography after intravitreal bevacizumab in type 2 idiopathic macular telangiectasia. Ophthalmology. 2007;114:1736-42.
20. Surguch V, Gamulescu MA, Gabel VP. Optical coherence tomography findings in idiopathic juxtafoveal retinal telangiectasis. Graefes Arch Clin Exp Ophthalmol. 2007;245(6):783-8.
21. Albini TA, Benz MS, Coffee RE, et al. Optical coherence tomography of idiopathic juxtafoveolar telangiectasia. Ophthalmic Surg Lasers Imaging. 2006;(2):120-8.
22. Gillies MC, Zhu M, Chew E, et al. Familial asymptomatic macular telangiectasia type 2. Ophthalmology. 2009;116: 2422-9.
23. Koizumi H, Iida T, Maruko I. Morphologic features of group 2A idiopathic juxtafoveolar retinal telangiectasis in three-dimensional optical coherence tomography. Am J Ophthalmol. 2006;142:340-3.
24. Sallo FB, Leung I, Chung M, et al. Retinal crystals in type 2 idiopathic macular telangiectasia. Ophthalmology. 2011;118:2461-7.
25. Gass JD, Stereoscopic Atlas of Macular diseases: Diagnosis and Treatment. 4th edition. St Louis: CV Mosby; 1997. pp. 502-13.
26. Mansour AM, Schachat A. Foveal avascular zone in idiopathic juxtafoveolar telangiectasia. Ophthlamologica. 1993;207:9-12.
27. Charbel Issa P, Scholl HP, Gaudric A, et al. Macular full-thickness and lamellar holes in association with type 2 idiopathic macular telangiectasia. Eye (Lond). 2009;23(2): 435-41.
28. Bottoni F, Eandi CM, Pedenovi S, et al. Integrated clinical evaluation of Type 2A idiopathic juxtafoveolar retinal telangiectasis. Retina. 2010;30(2):317-26.
29. Baumüller S, Charbel Issa PC, Scholl HP, et al. Outer retinal hyper-reflective spots on spectral-domain optical coherence tomography in macular telangiectasia type 2. Ophthalmology. 2010:117;2162-8.
30. Bolz M, Schmidt-Erfurth U, Deak G, et al. Optical coherence tomographic hyper-reflective foci: a morphologic sign of lipid extravasation in diabetic macular edema. Ophthlamology. 2009;116:914-20.
31. Ahlers C, Götzinger E, Pircher M, et al. Imaging of the retinal pigment epithelium in age-related macular degeneration using polarization-sensitive optical coherence tomography. Invest Ophthalmol Vis Sci. 2010;51:2149-57.
32. Bourhis A, Girmens JF, Boni S, Pecha F, Favard C, Sahel JA, Paques M. Imaging of macroaneurysms occurring during retinal vein occlusion and diabetic retinopathy by indocyanine green angiography and high resolution optical coherence tomography. Graefes Arch Clin Exp Ophthalmol. 2010;248(2):161-6.

Section 7

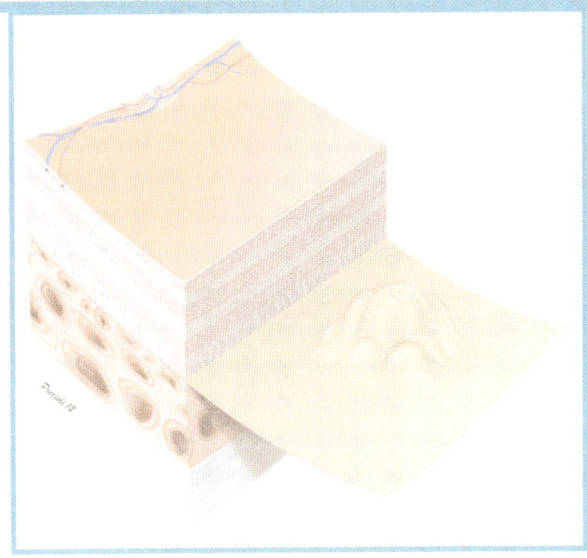

Retinal *En Face* Optical Coherence Tomography Examination: Vascular Diseases and Infections

chapter 26

Retinal Venous Occlusion

Min Wang, Gezhi Xu

Introduction

Retinal vein occlusion is the obstruction of the retinal venous system by thrombus formation, external compression, or disease of the vein wall. Engorgement and dilatation of the retinal veins with secondary intraretinal hemorrhages and intraretinal edema, retinal ischemia, retinal exudates and macular edema are the main features of the disease. Many of these features can be visualized on an *en face* optical coherence tomography (OCT).

Case 1

A 57-year-old man with the diagnosis of central retinal vein occlusion (CRVO) underwent OCT. At the inner plexiform layer (IPL) level of *en face* OCT, cystoid macular edema (CME) showed as meshwork changes at the macular area **(Figure 1)**. These meshwork lesions correspond to the structural changes of CME on OCT scan across the fovea **(Figure 2)** and they can not be visualized on color fundus photo **(Figure 3)**.

Case 2

A 40-year-old man was diagnosed with CRVO in his left eye **(Figure 4)**. *En face* OCT at the level of internal limiting membrane (ILM) and IPL demonstrates a large area of scattered high and low reflectivity patches that represent the intraretinal hemorrhages and exudates **(Figure 5)**. On retinal pigment epithelium (RPE) level, the shadows of the patches are still visible. Horizontal and vertical OCT scans confirmed the intraretinal hemorrhages and exudates **(Figure 6)**.

Case 3

A 40-year-old woman was diagnosed with CRVO **(Figure 7)**. Spoke-like changes represent the epiretinal membrane

(ERM) and the central dark area represents the CME at the level of ILM of *en face* OCT. The distribution of cystoid edema is identified better at the level of IPL. At the level of RPE and RPE reference, the shadows of ERM and CME are aware of **(Figure 8)**. The cross-line OCT scan indicates typical and severe CME **(Figure 9)**.

Case 4

A 56-year-old woman was diagnosed with branch retinal vein occlusion (BRVO) in her right eye **(Figure 10)**. On *en face* OCT, intraretinal hemorrhages were displayed both at the levels of ILM and IPL superior and temporal to the fovea featuring as irregular high and low reflectivity patches **(Figures 11 and 12)**. The shadows of intraretinal hemorrhages can be observed at the level of RPE. The patches of intraretinal hemorrhages on *en face* OCT correspond to the OCT vertical scan that is drawn across the upper hemorrhage area **(Figure 12)**. OCT horizontal line scan also indicates the intraretinal hemorrhage **(Figure 13)**.

Case 5

A 44-year-old woman had the diagnosis of BRVO in her right eye. The following lesions were detected at the ILM level of the *en face* OCT: CME (red arrow), intraretinal exudates (arrowhead) and the edge of hemorrhage (blue arrow) above the fovea **(Figure 14)**. CME and exudates do not display clearly on fundus photo **(Figure 15)**, but OCT revealed these lesions on horizontal and vertical scans **(Figure 16)**. There were some artifacts on RPE level of *en face* OCT due to minor eye movement. The shadow of the hemorrhage was recognized at RPE reference level.

Case 6

A 40-year-old woman had the diagnosis of BRVO **(Figure 17)**.

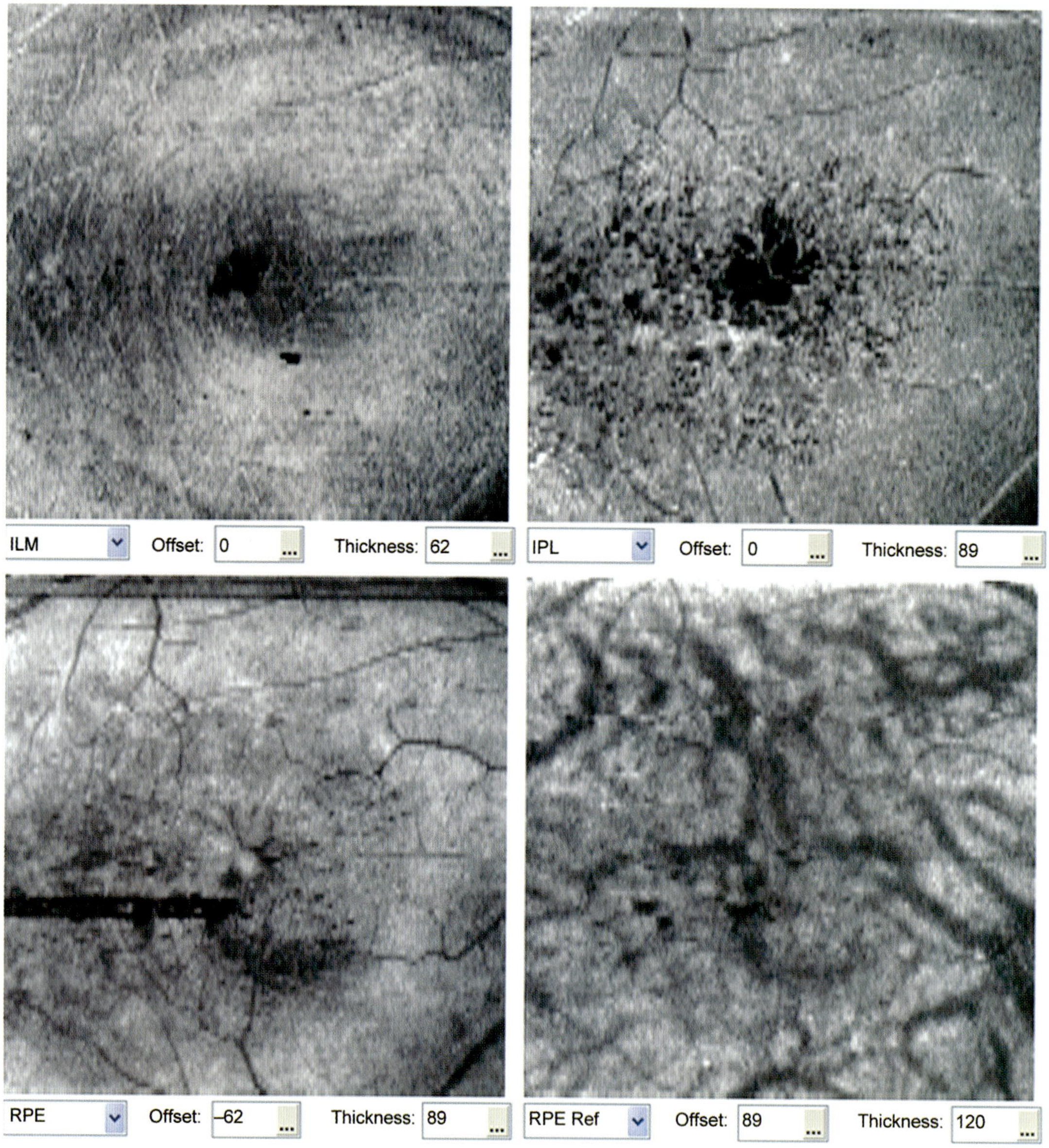

ILM   Offset: 0   Thickness: 62   IPL   Offset: 0   Thickness: 89

RPE   Offset: −62   Thickness: 89   RPE Ref   Offset: 89   Thickness: 120

Figure 1: *En face* OCT showing cystoid macular edema as meshwork changes at IPL level

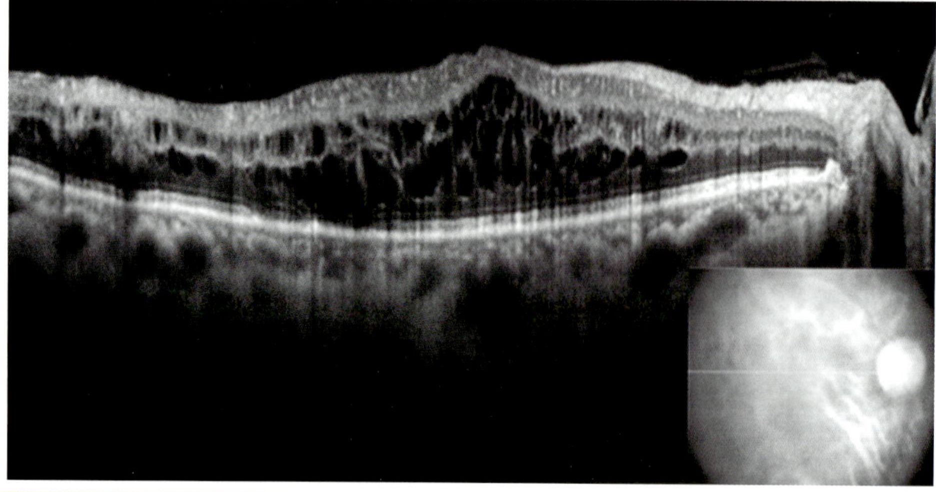

Figure 2: OCT line scan demonstrating cystoid macular edema

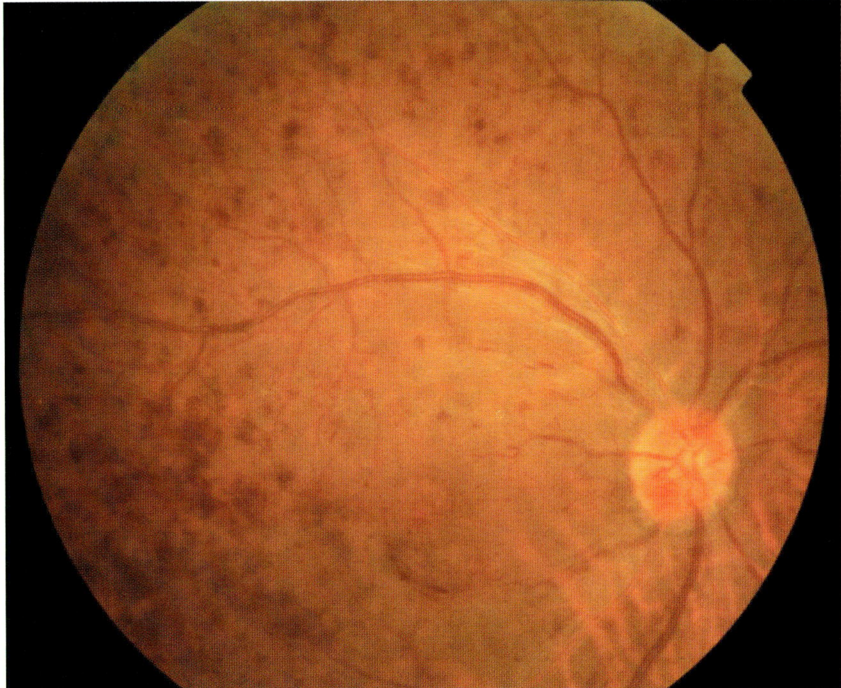

Figure 3: A 57-year-old man diagnosed with central retinal vein occlusion in his right eye

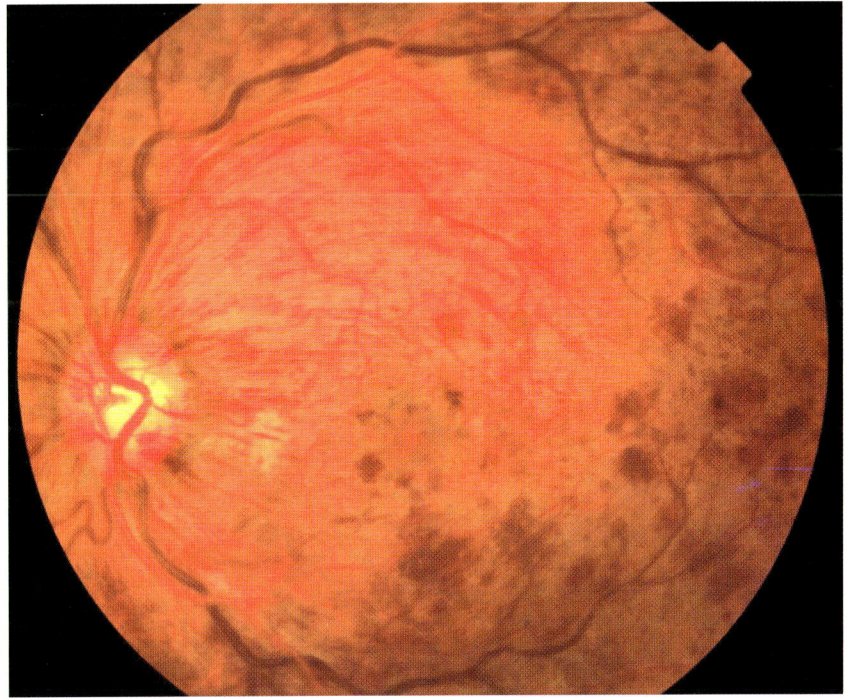

Figure 4: A 40-year-old man suffering from central retinal vein occlusion in his right eye

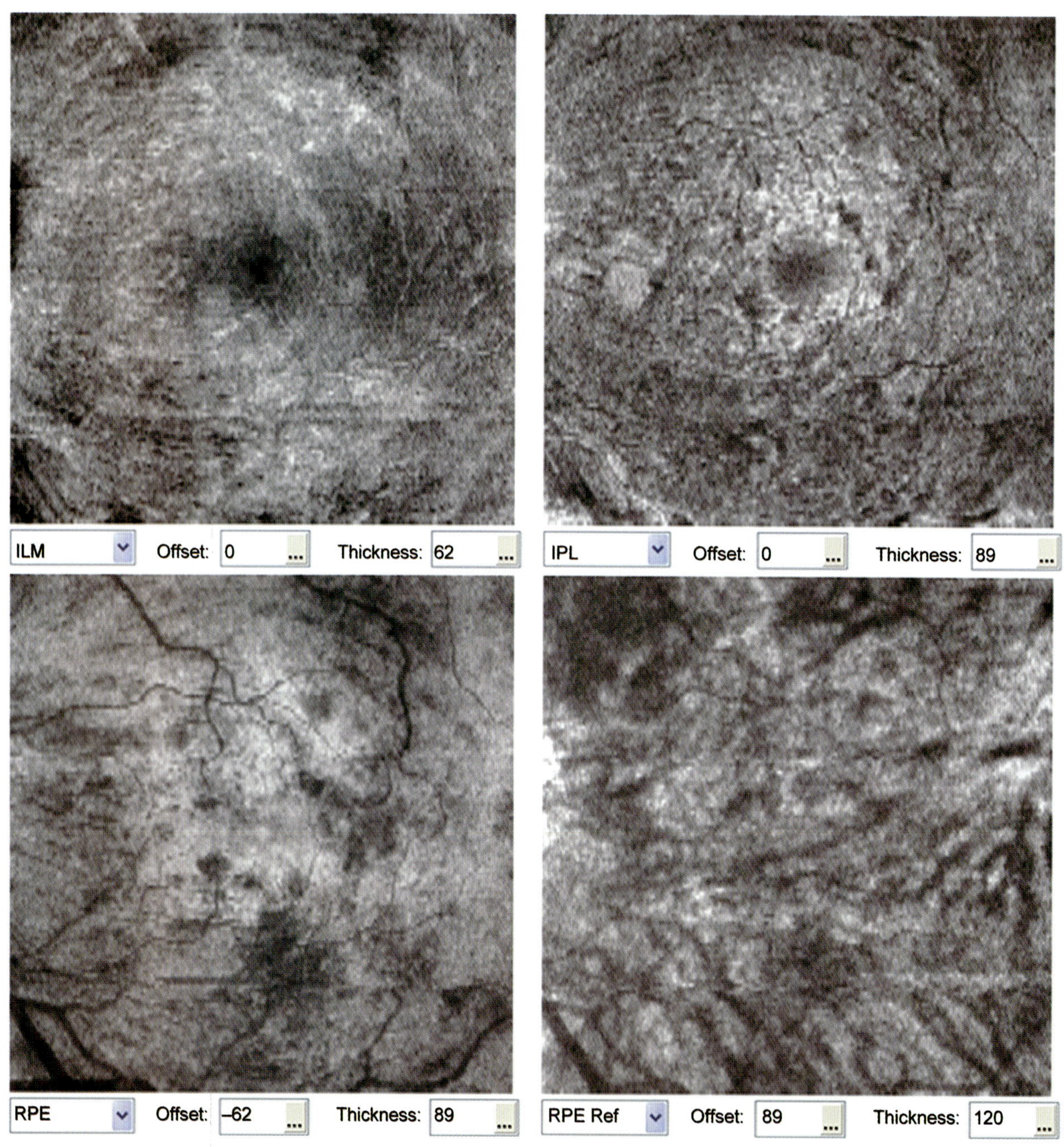

Figure 5: *En face* OCT showing high and low reflectivity patches representing intraretinal hemorrhage and exudates at ILM and IPL levels

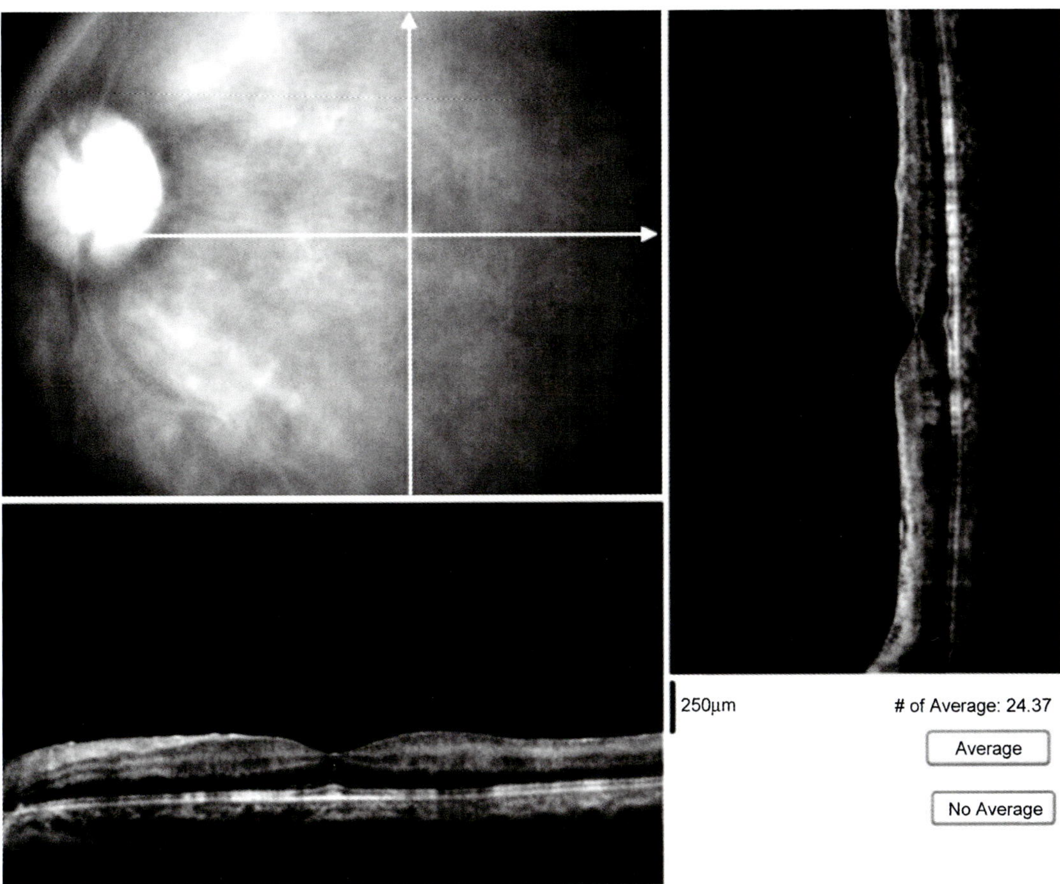

Figure 6: Horizontal and vertical OCT line scan showing intraretinal hemorrhage and exudates

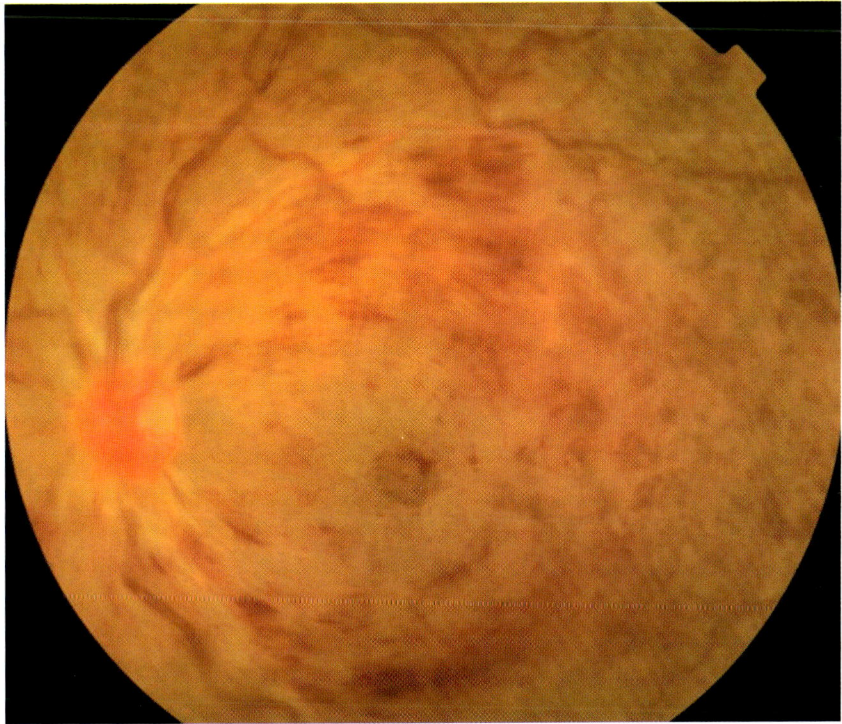

Figure 7: A 40-year-old woman diagnosed to be suffering from central retinal vein occlusion

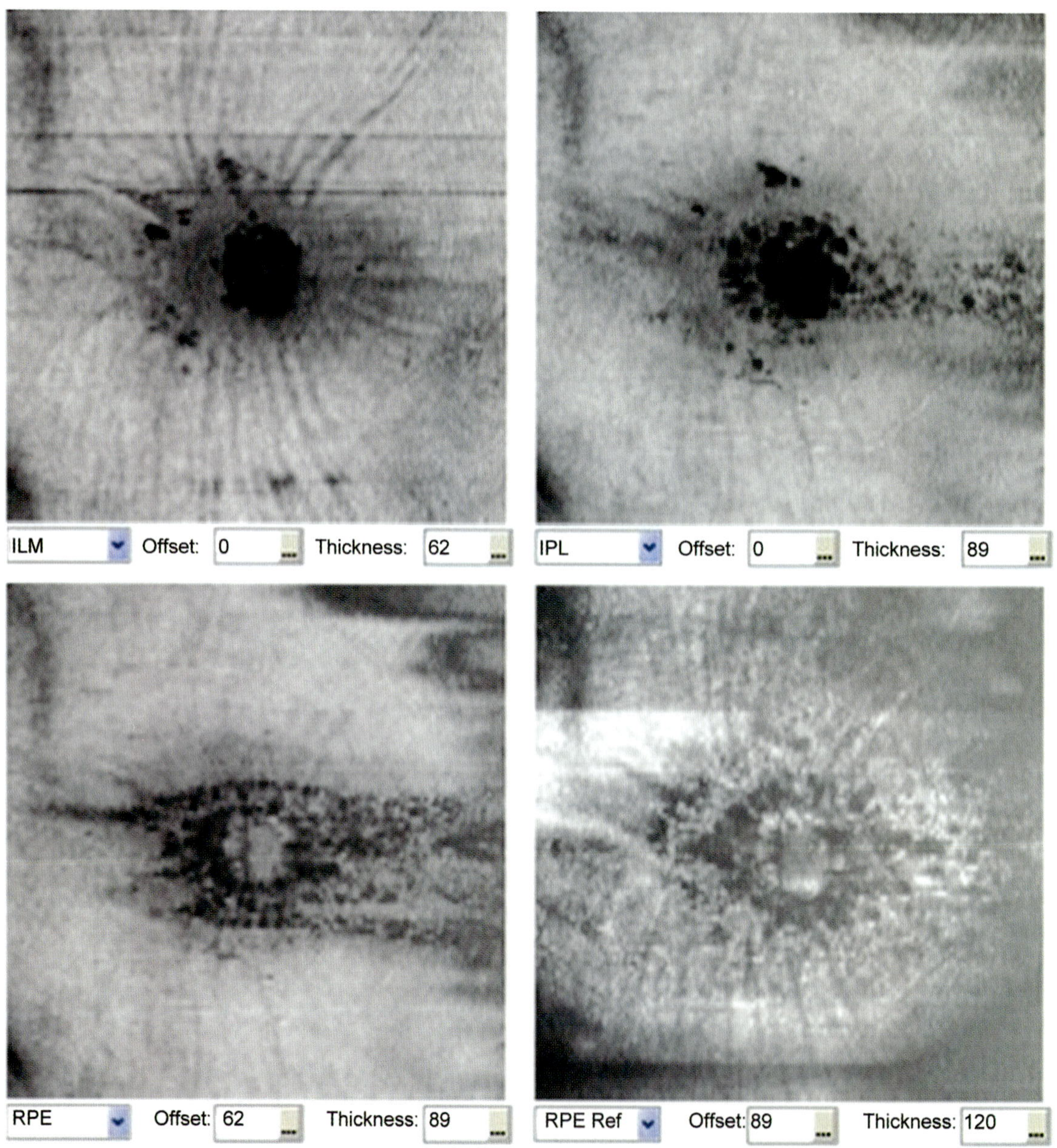

Figure 8: *En face* OCT showing ERM as spoke-like changes at ILM level and cystoid macular edema demonstrating at IPL level

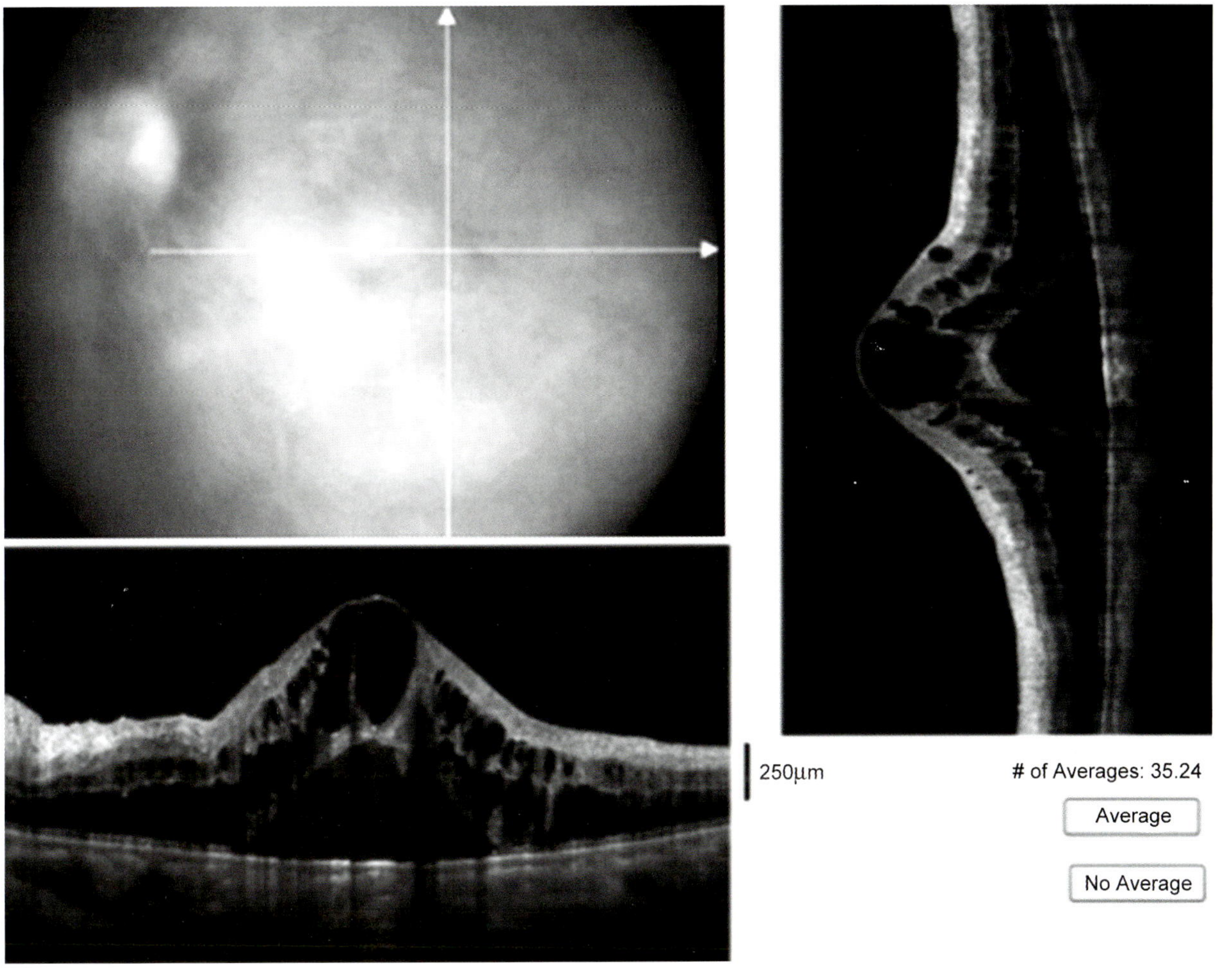

Figure 9: Horizontal and vertical OCT line scan showing cystoid macular edema

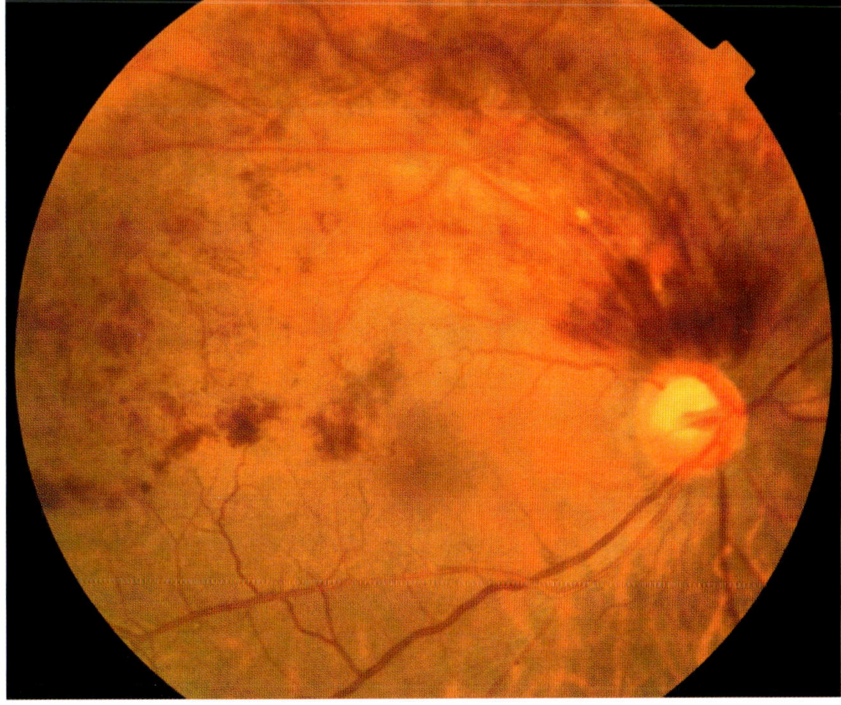

Figure 10: A 56-year-old woman suffering from branched retinal venous occlusion in the right eye

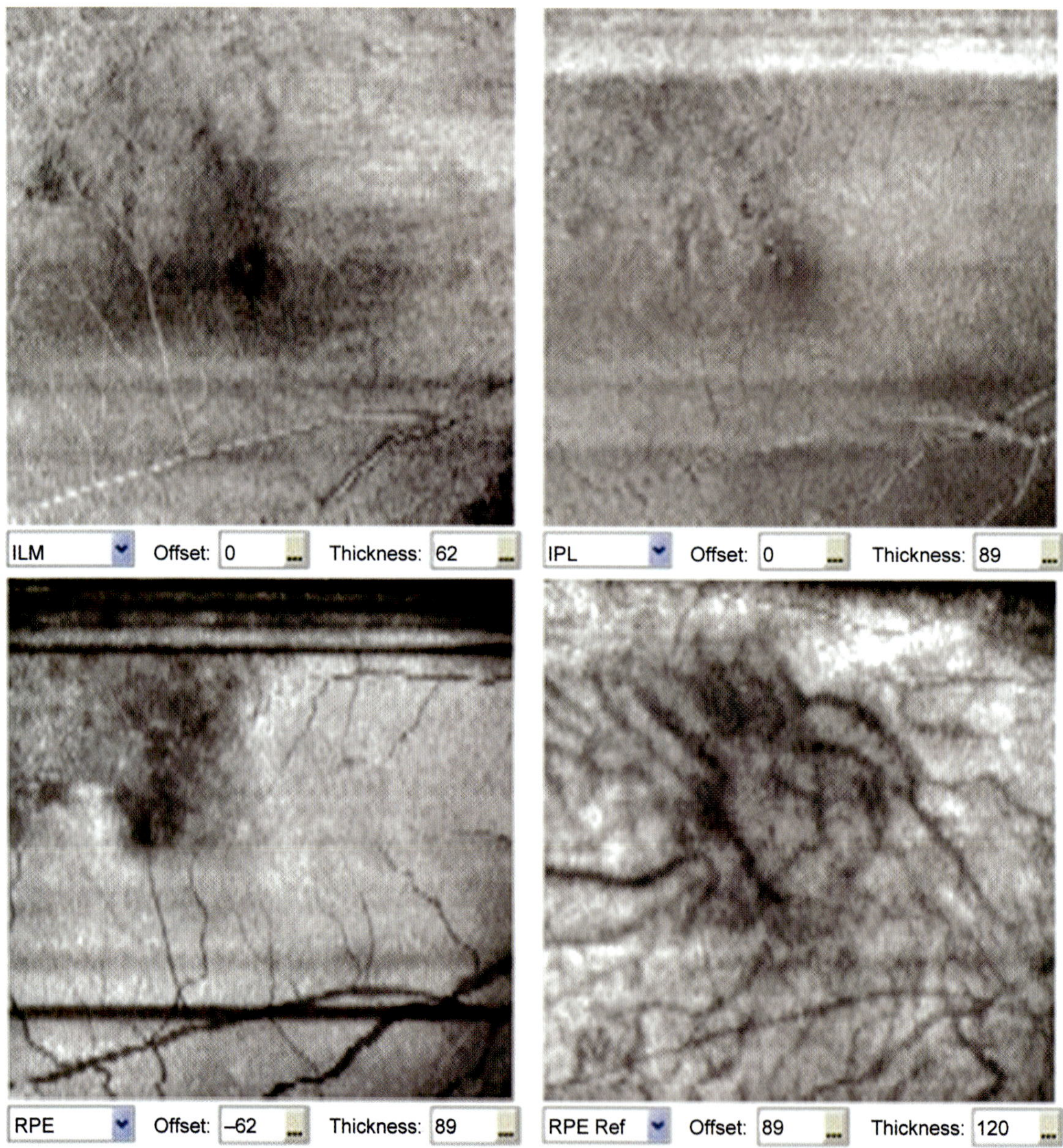

Figure 11: *En face* OCT showing intraretinal hemorrhage as irregular high and low reflectivity patches at ILM and IPL level superior-temporal to the fovea

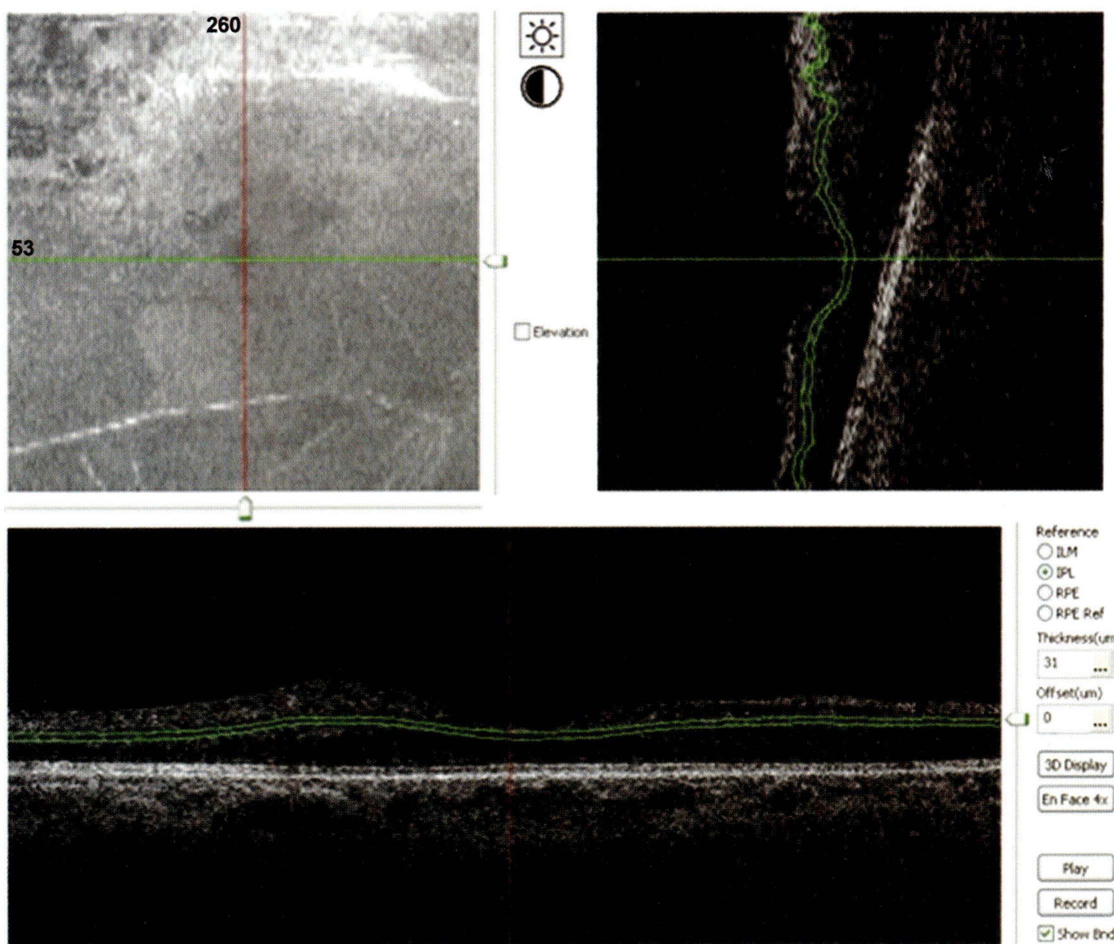

Figure 12: Superior-temporal patches on *en face* OCT corresponding to the upper hemorrhage area across vertical OCT scan

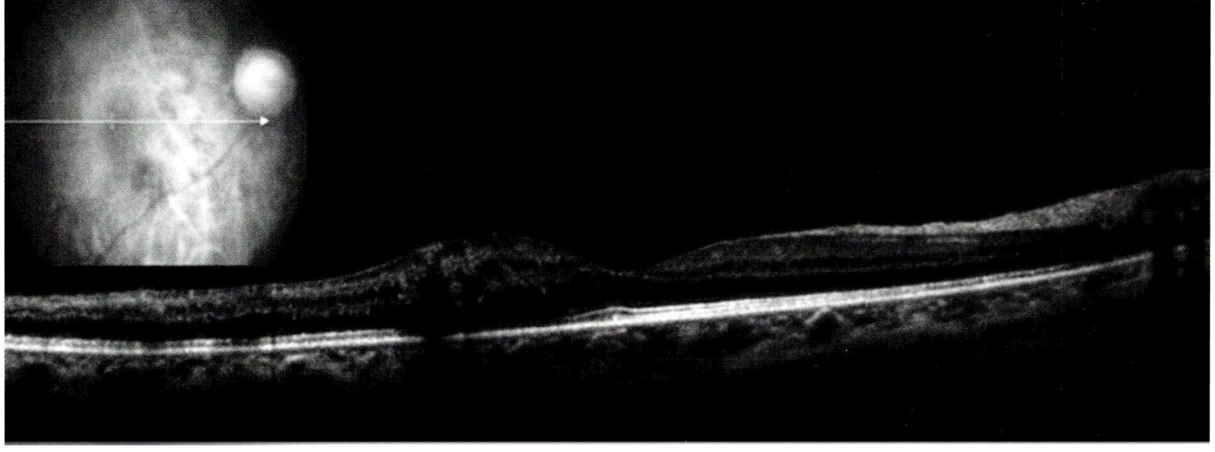

Figure 13: OCT line scan showing intraretinal hemorrhage

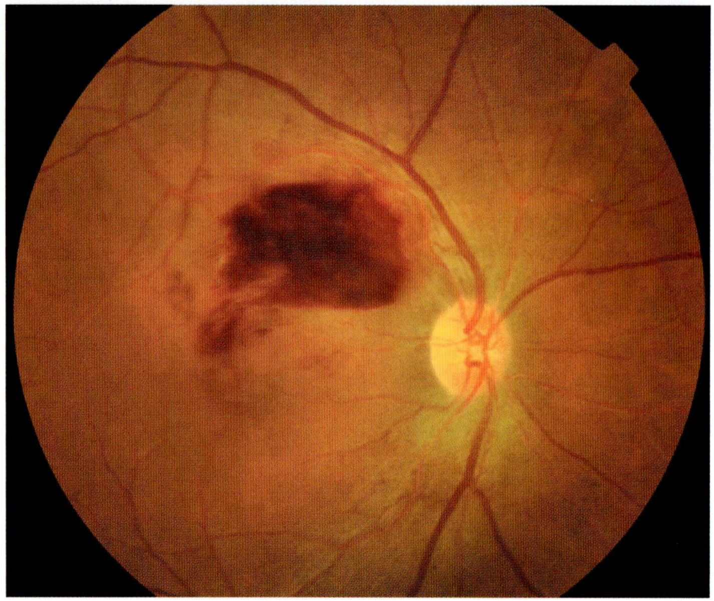

Figure 14: A 44-year-old woman suffering from branched retinal venous occlusion in the right eye

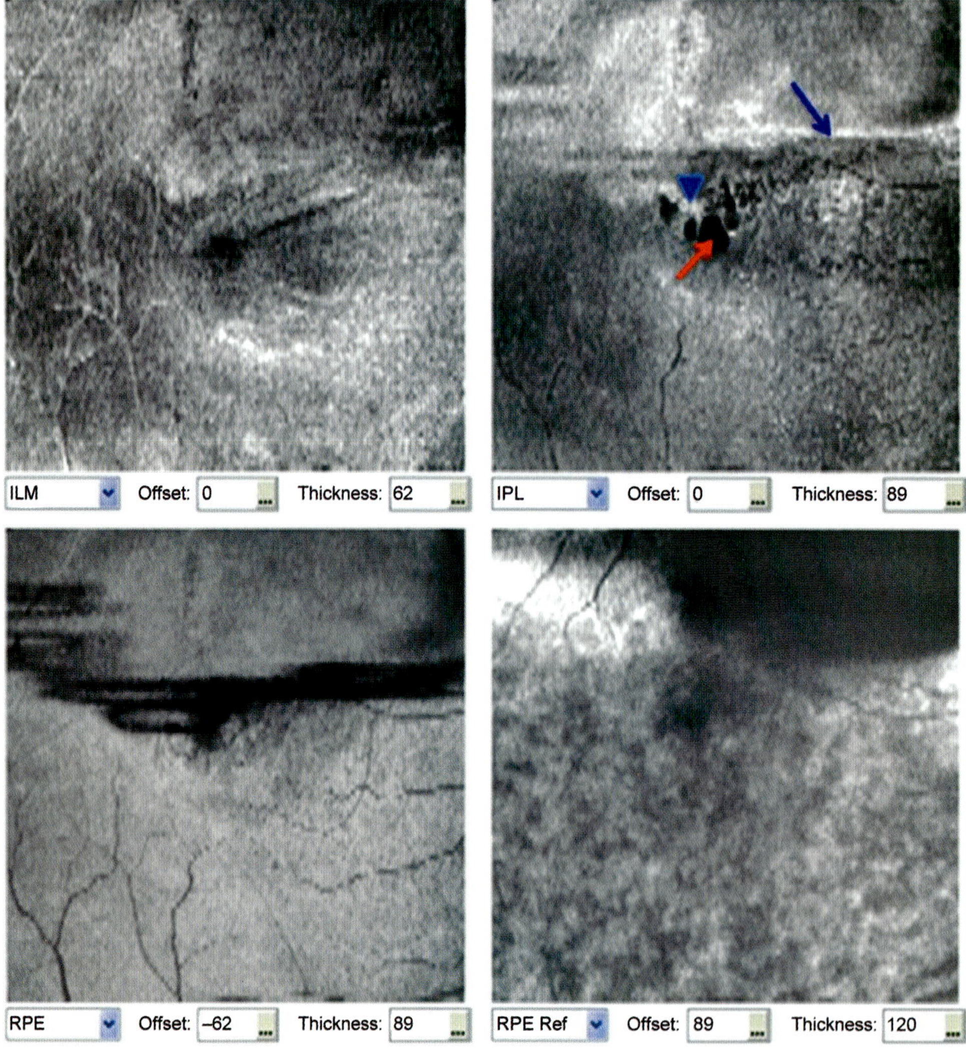

Figure 15: *En face* OCT showing cystoid macular edema (red arrow), intraretinal exudates (arrowhead) and the edge of hemorrhage (blue arrow)

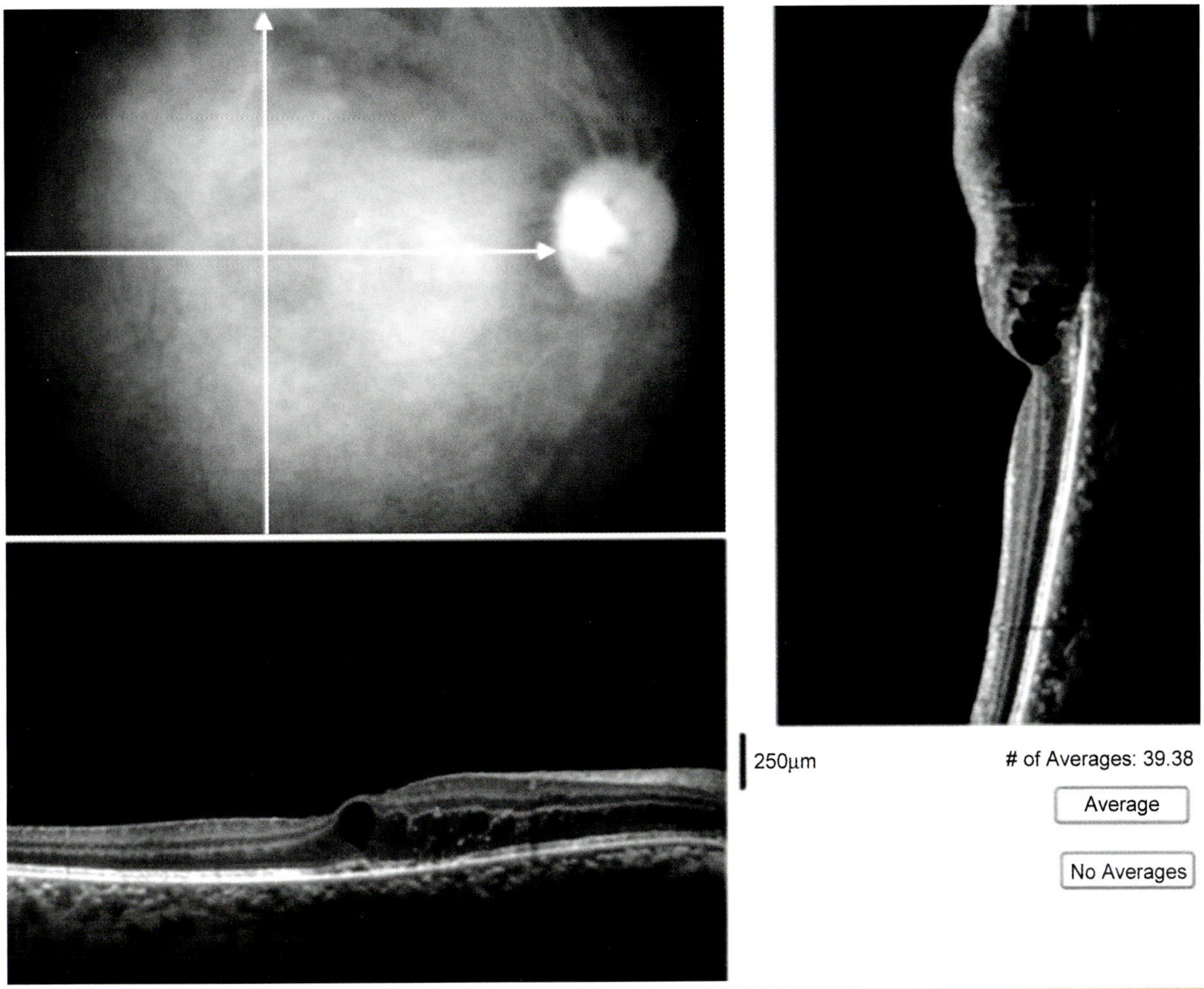

Figure 16: OCT showing cystoid macular edema and hemorrhage

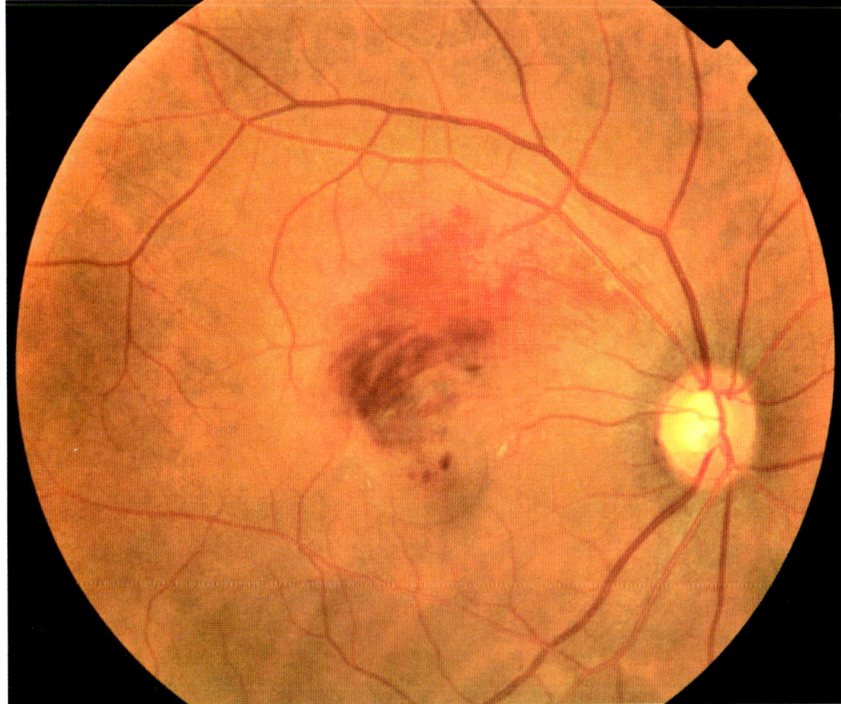

Figure 17: A 40-year-old woman suffering from branched retinal venous occlusion

En face OCT demonstrates CME (red arrow), exudates (blue arrow) and intraretinal hemorrhage at the level of IPL **(Figure 18)**. The ranges of the serous detachment of neuroretina with fluid accumulation and intraretinal hemorrhage were observed on the RPE level **(Figure 19)**. There is an artifact at the RPE level due to minor eye shifting. OCT scans confirm all the above characteristics **(Figure 20)**.

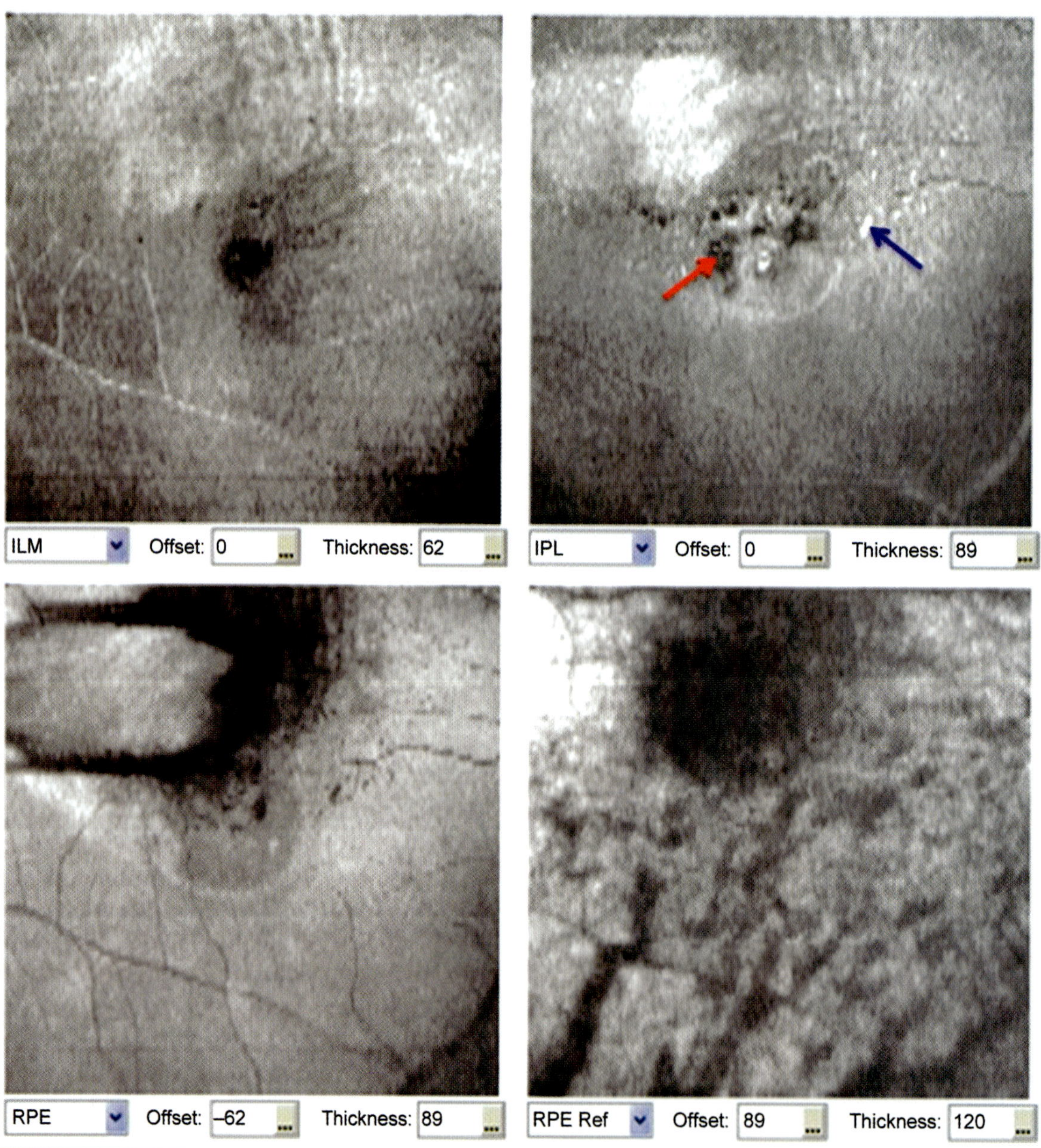

Figure 18: *En face* OCT demonstrating cystoid macular edema (red arrow), exudates (blue arrow) and hemorrhage at IPL level

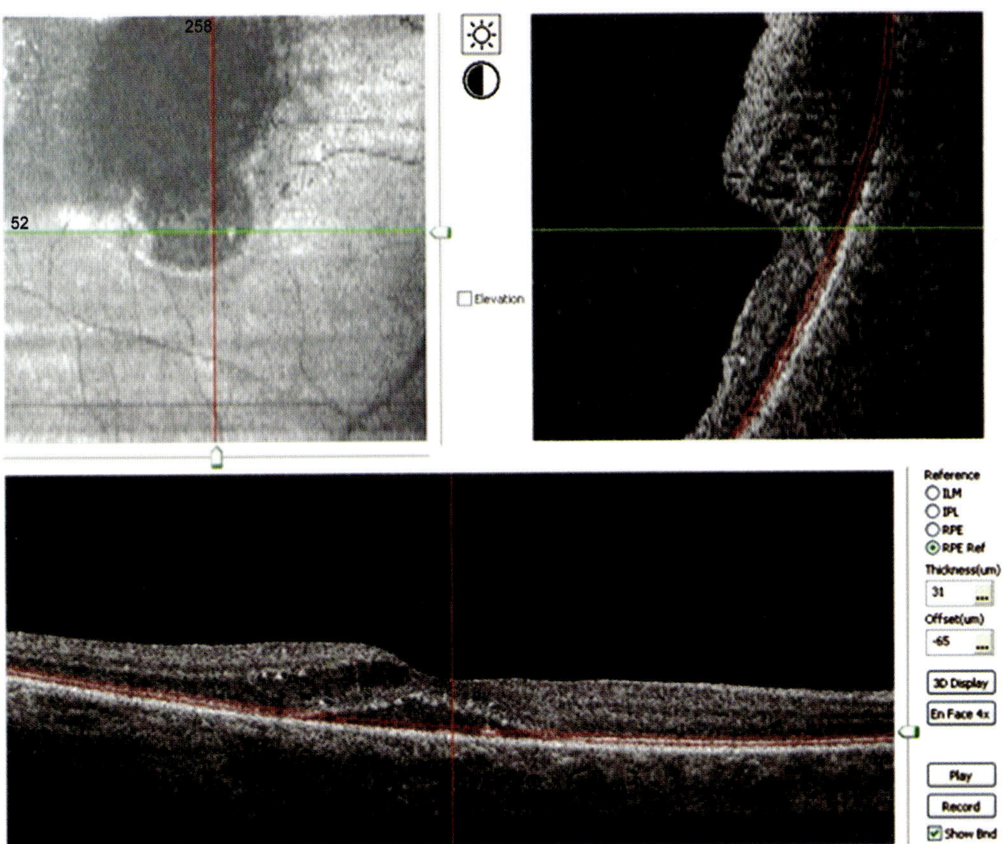

Figure 19: *En face* OCT showing the range of the serous detachment of neuroretina with fluid accumulation and intraretinal hemorrhage at RPE level

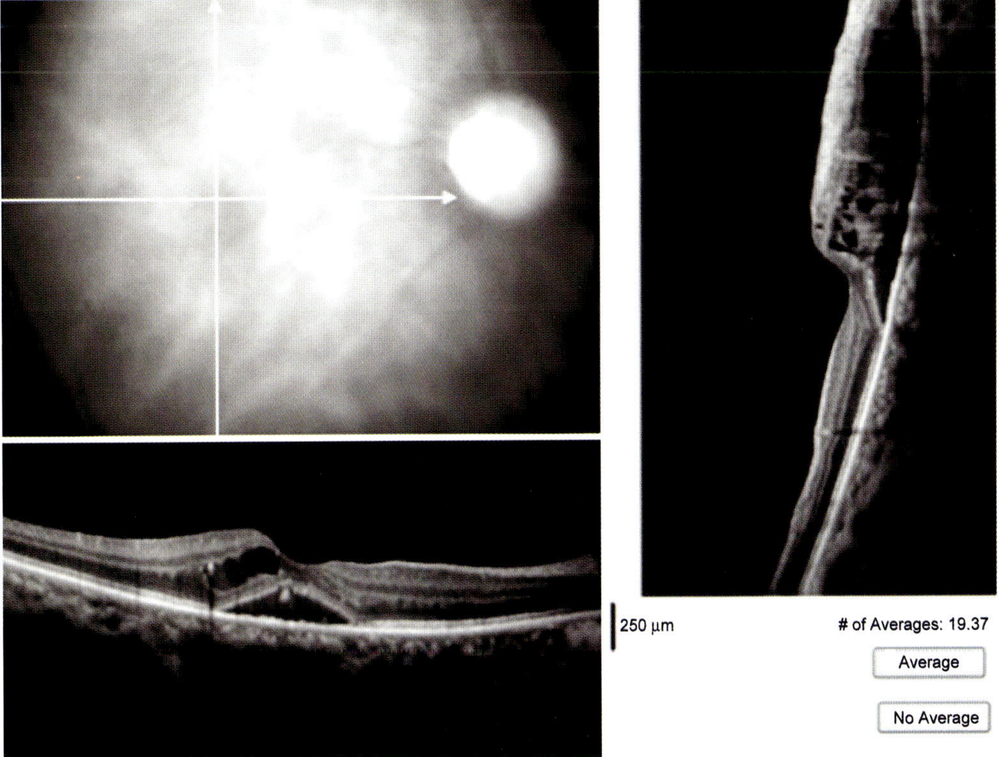

Figure 20: OCT scan showing cystoid macular edema, serous neuroretinal detachment, intraretinal hemorrhage and exudates

chapter 27

Diabetic Maculopathy and *En Face* Optical Coherence Tomography

Lucia Pelosini, John Marshall

Introduction

Diabetic macular oedema (DME) represents a significant cause of visual loss occurring in 27% of patients within 9 years of onset of diabetes.[1]

The Early Treatment Diabetic Retinopathy Study (ETDRS) demonstrated that over a 3-year period focal laser treatment reduced the risk of moderate visual loss by 50% compared with controls.[2] By contrast, diffuse DME involving the center of the macula was associated with higher risk of permanent visual loss and limited functional improvement following grid laser.[3]

Definition of Macular Edema

Macular edema is a nonspecific sign of ocular disease caused by abnormal accumulation of fluid in the retina secondary to a variety of conditions and leading to loss of vision.[4,5] The term "cystoid macular edema" refers to the accumulation of fluid in multiple cyst-like compartments, resembling a cyst but having no enclosing capsule. Investigation of DME with scanning electron microscopy (ESM) and optical coherence tomography (OCT) *en face* demonstrate how "cystoid" represents a misnomer and how fluid fills a continuous space within the compact retinal architecture.

Light microscopy of DME (**Figure 1**) shows round cavities separated by vertical strands of tissue connecting the outer retina to the inner retinal layers. OCT B scan provides a similar picture (**Figure 1,** inset) with low-signal cavities separated by high-signal vertical structures, suggesting the presence of fluid-filled cavities. By contrast, SEM (**Figure 2**) shows a 3D image with vertical tissue columns surrounded by a continuous fluid-filled space and connecting the outer retina to the inner retina. Similarly, OCT *en face* shows a

continuous space interrupted by high signal elements representing the cross section of tissue columns and connecting the inner to the outer retina (**Figure 3**).

This chapter will describe the application of OCT *en face* to identify predictors of visual function and will discuss the following aspects of DME:
1. Fluid dynamics in DME: Sources of fluid and fluid location within the retinal architecture.
2. Observation of DME with OCT imaging: Quantitative and qualitative approaches in the evaluation of fluid.
3. Quantitative analysis of tissue integrity in DME with OCT *en face* and predictors of visual function.

Fluid Dynamics in DME: Sources of Fluid and Fluid Location in the Retina

DME is caused by an imbalance of fluid transport across the retina.[4,5] Fluid transport always involves a two-ways system, an inflow and an outflow or drainage. According to Starling, tissue edema develops when the rate of capillary filtration exceeds the rate of fluid removal from the perivascular interstitium.[6] Therefore, failure of one or both mechanisms may lead to abnormal fluid accumulation.

The retinal circulation is a watertight system and is formed by two main vascular plexuses: the inner retinal plexus and the outer retinal plexus. There are two blood retinal barrier (BRB) systems to prevent fluid access to the retina. The inner BRB is formed by a continuous layer of endothelial cells and tight cell junctions whereas the outer BRB is formed by the retinal pigment epithelium (RPE) and intercellular junction complexes with RPE cells pumping the fluid into the choriocapillaris.[7,8] DME may either result from excessive leakage of retinal capillaries or from loss of pumping capacity of the RPE. In DME, the former mechanism is thought to be the causal agent.[4,5]

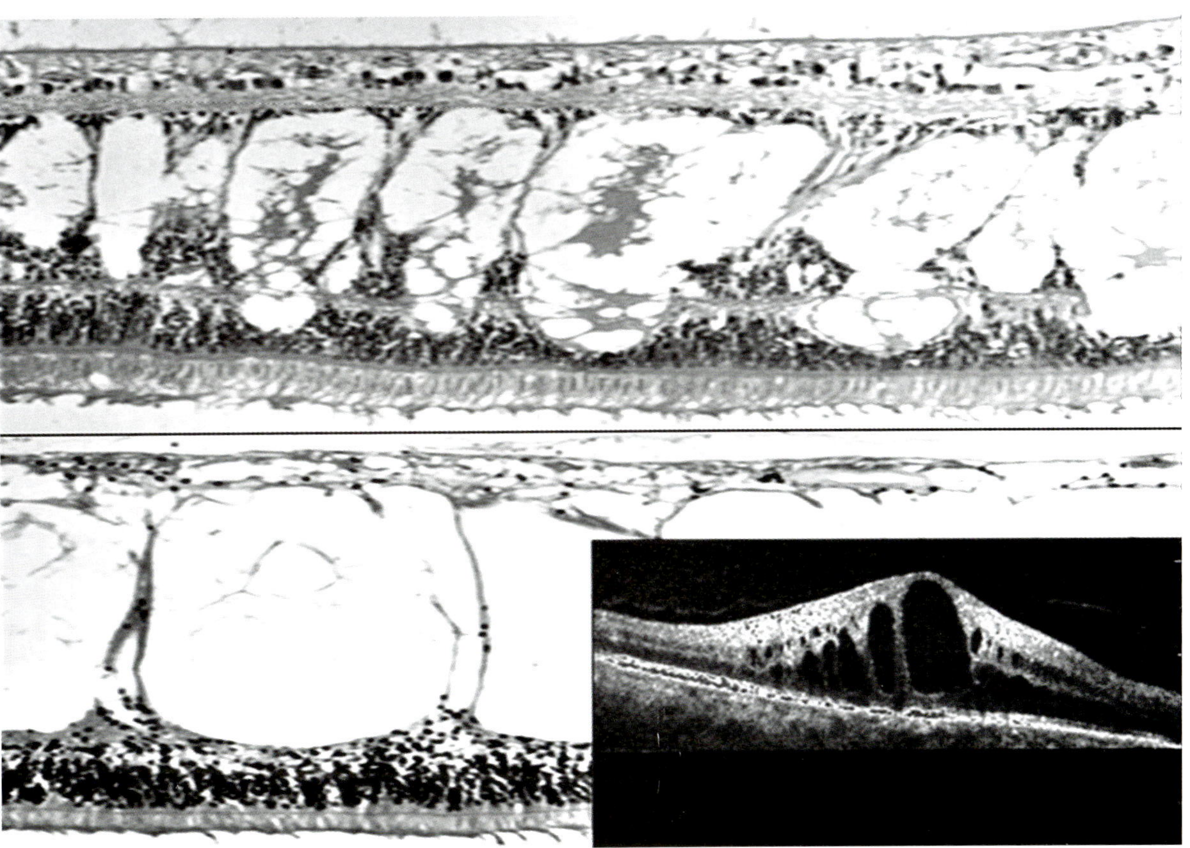

Figure 1: Similarity between light microscopy and OCT B scan of DME (*Courtesy* of Prof J Marshall)

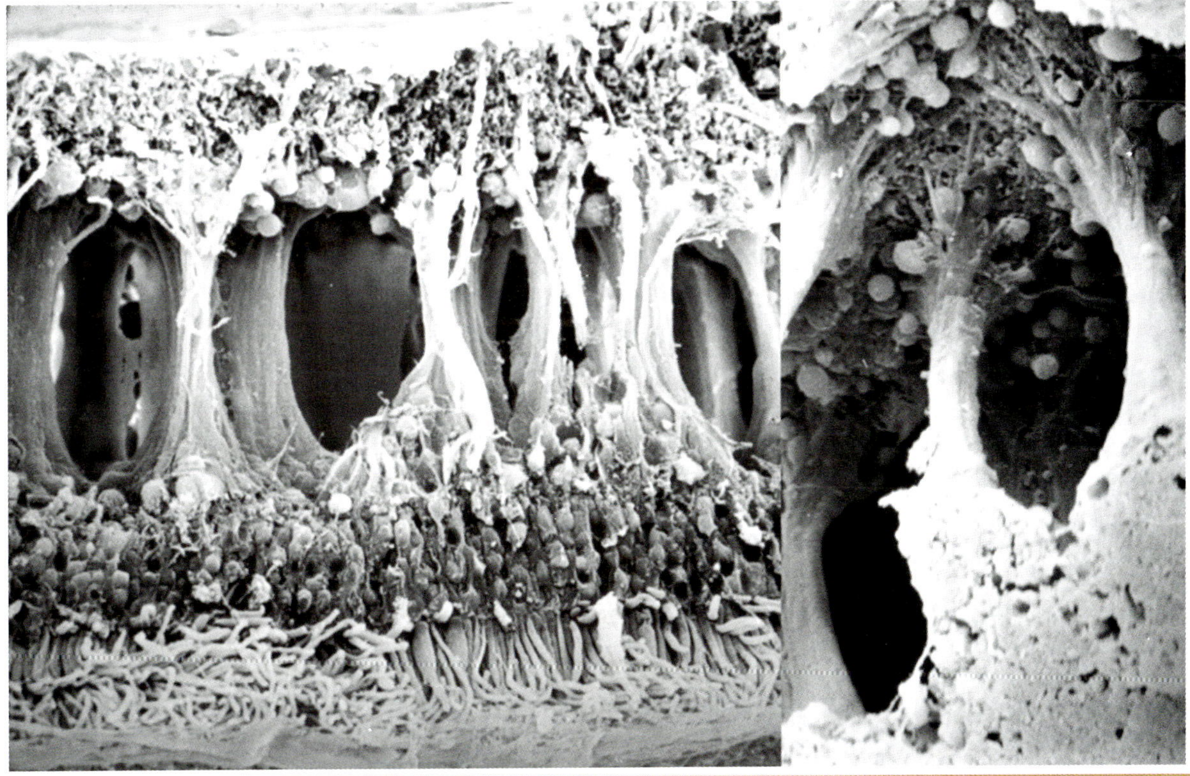

Figure 2: SEM image of DME (*Courtesy* of Prof J Marshall)

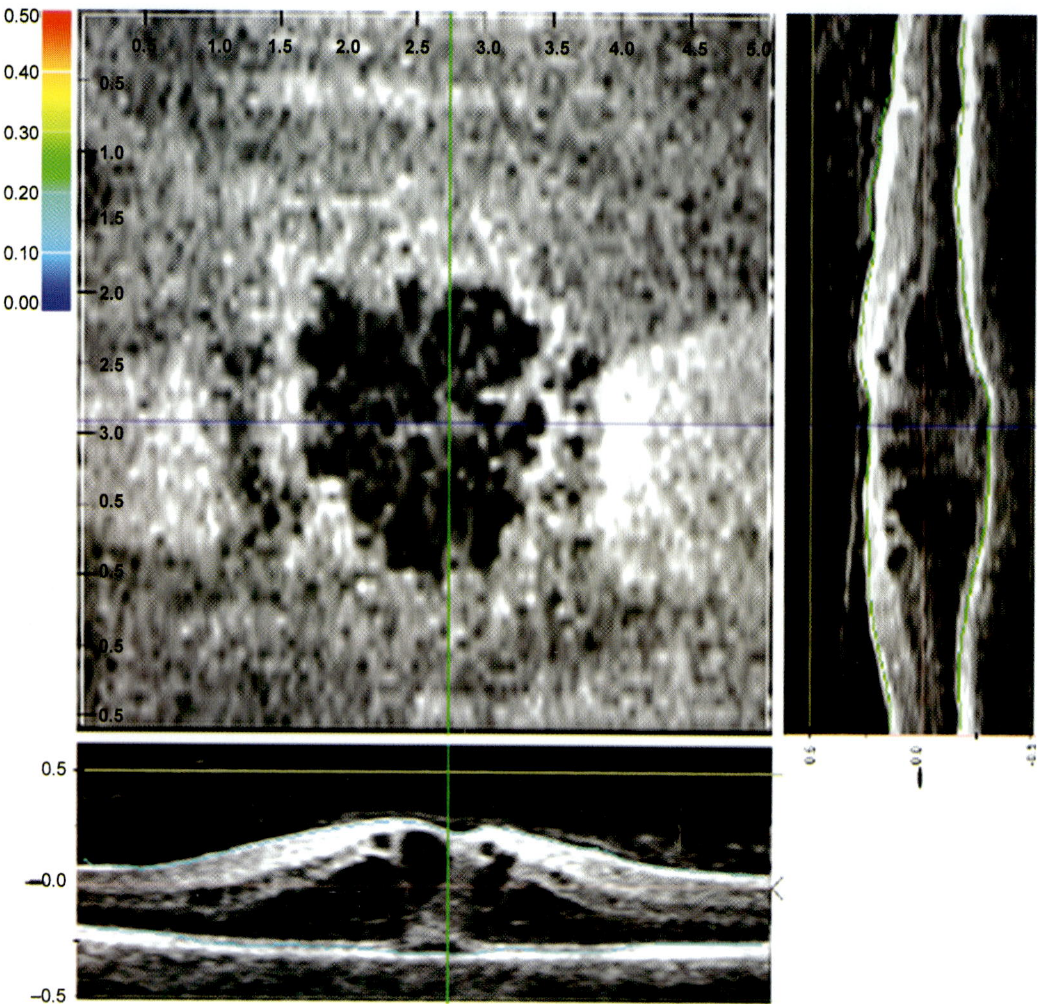

Figure 3: OCT *en face* of DME shows a continuous fluid space interrupted by cross-sections of vertical elements connecting the outer to the inner retina

Microscopic Location of Fluid

There is a long standing debate in the literature about microscopic location of fluid in respect to cellular components of the retina. The Fine-Brucker theory of progressive intracellular fluid accumulation was attributing the majority of cytological changes to Müller cells, given their role in the biochemical balance of the retina and ionic transport.[9] Gass et al postulated an alternative theory suggesting a predominant extracellular location of fluid, giving rise to cellular displacement and compression.[10] Gass demonstrated an expansion of the extracellular space in the inner nuclear and outer plexiform layer with no evidence of Müller cells degeneration on electron microscopy.

Macroscopic Fluid Location in Relation to Retinal Layers

The retina is a high density tissue with high resistance to deformation and minimal extracellular space. The first effect of fluid accumulation within the retina is represented by displacement of retinal components and overall increase in retinal volume. Fluid accumulation in the retina is determined by the presence of high resistance permeability barriers and separation planes in the retina.

Antcliff et al demonstrated the presence of two high resistance barriers in the retina—the inner plexiform layer (IPL) and the outer plexiform layer (OPL).[11] Hence, fluid would accumulate either between the barriers or outside the barriers, at the level of the inner nuclear layer (INL), outer nuclear layer (ONL) and Henle's fiber layer (HFL) **(Figure 4)**. The HFL represents a site of low resistance to separation where fluid may easily displace the fibers and create a vertical space along the z plane **(Figures 5 and 6)**.

The presence of retinal planes with low resistance to separation would explain how fluid accumulates in horizontal spaces **(Figure 7)**. Pre-retinal hemorrhages occur behind the posterior hyaloid membrane or in the nerve fiber layer (NFL),

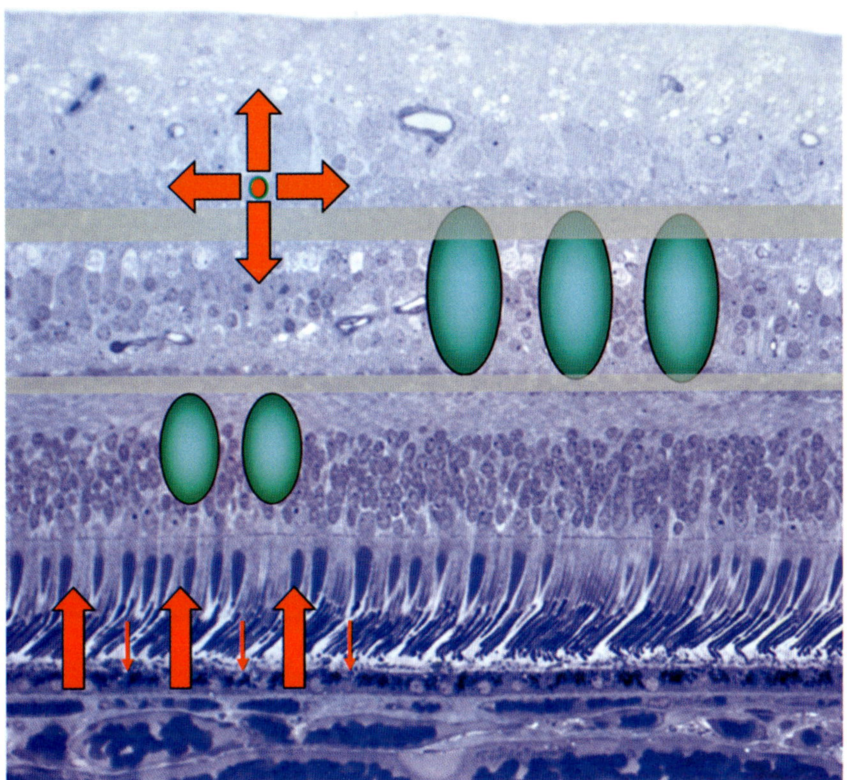

Figure 4: High resistance permeability barriers (thick gray band=IPL; thin gray band=OPL) in the retina and location of fluid

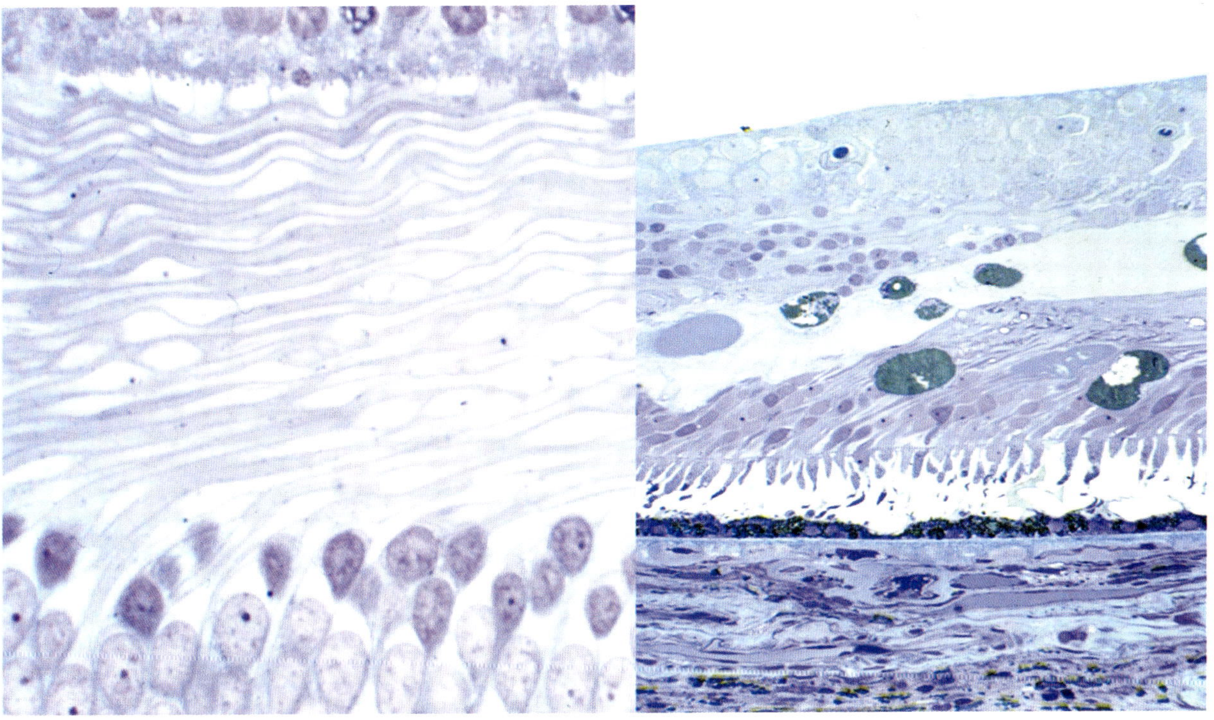

Figure 5: Light microscopy image showing the oblique pathway of the fibers in the Henle's layer of the fovea (*Courtesy of Prof J Marshall*). The foveola has an area of 0.07 mm^2; it contains approximately 2,500 cone cells and is formed by the cone outer segment, inner segment and the cone inner connecting fibers, forming the Henle's fiber layer

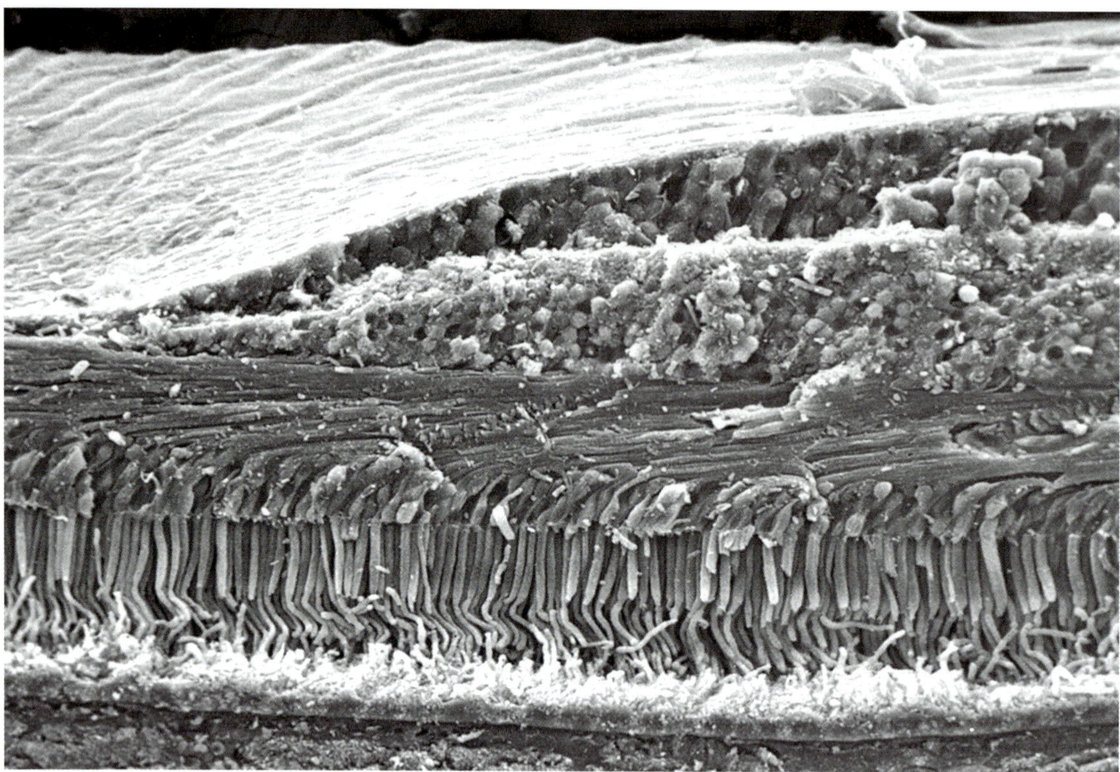

Figure 6: Scanning electron microscopy image of the human retina showing the photoreceptors and the Henle's layer with tightly packed cone inner connecting fibers (*Courtesy* of Prof J Marshall)

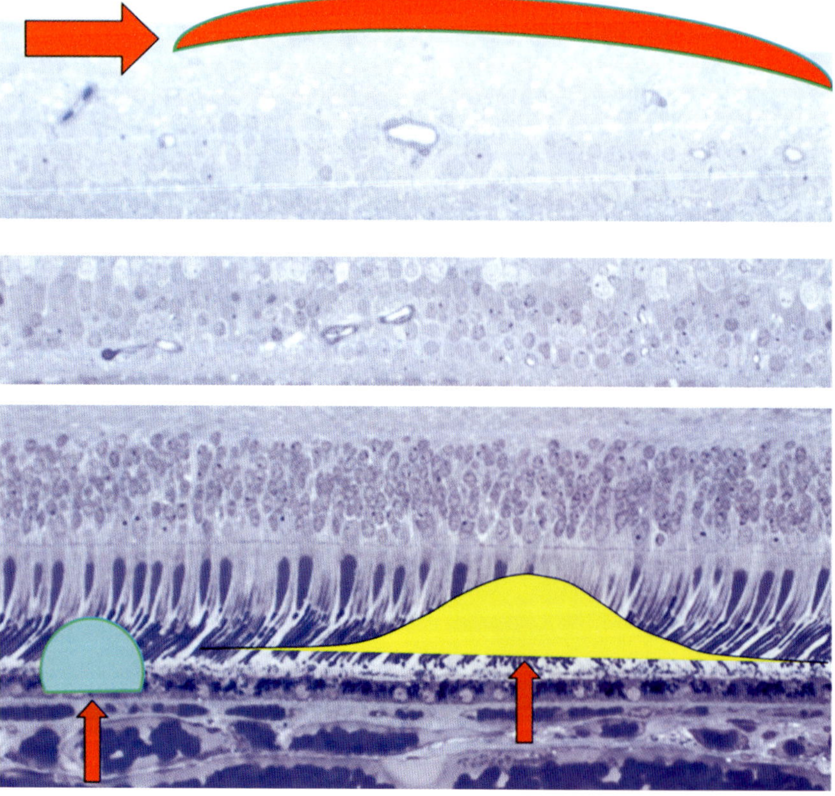

Figure 7: Horizontal separation planes of the retina: pre-retinal hemorrhages (red), CSR (yellow), PED (blue)

central serous retinopathy (CSR) consists of fluid accumulated between the photoreceptors and RPE, pigment epithelium detachments (PED) occur when fluid accumulates under the RPE.

From observation of OCT scans it appears that there are four preferential sites of fluid accumulation:
1. Fluid in the INL causes stretching and compression of the IPL and the OPL **(Figure 8)**.
2. Fluid at the level of HFL and ONL causes stretching and compression of the IPL and OPL and the outer limiting membrane (OLM) **(Figure 9)**.
3. Fluid between the photoreceptor layer (PL) and the RPE causes a serous detachment of the retina with stretching and compression of the photoreceptors and disconnection of the photoreceptor outer segment from the RPE cells. Example of CSR is shown in **Figure 10**.

4. Fluid under the RPE produces a detachment of the RPE with distortions of the PL and the RPE layer. Example of PED is shown in **Figure 11**.

Observation of DME with OCT Imaging: Quantitative and Qualitative Approaches in the Evaluation of Fluid

Quantitative Approaches for the Evaluation of Fluid

Previous studies of DME have investigated the relationship between central macular thickness (CMT) and VA in the attempt of identifying an OCT parameter that could be used as surrogate of visual function **(Figure 12)**. At present, OCT measurement of CMT represents the accepted standard despite its weak correlation with VA (R^2 values ranging from 0.08 to 0.54).[12]

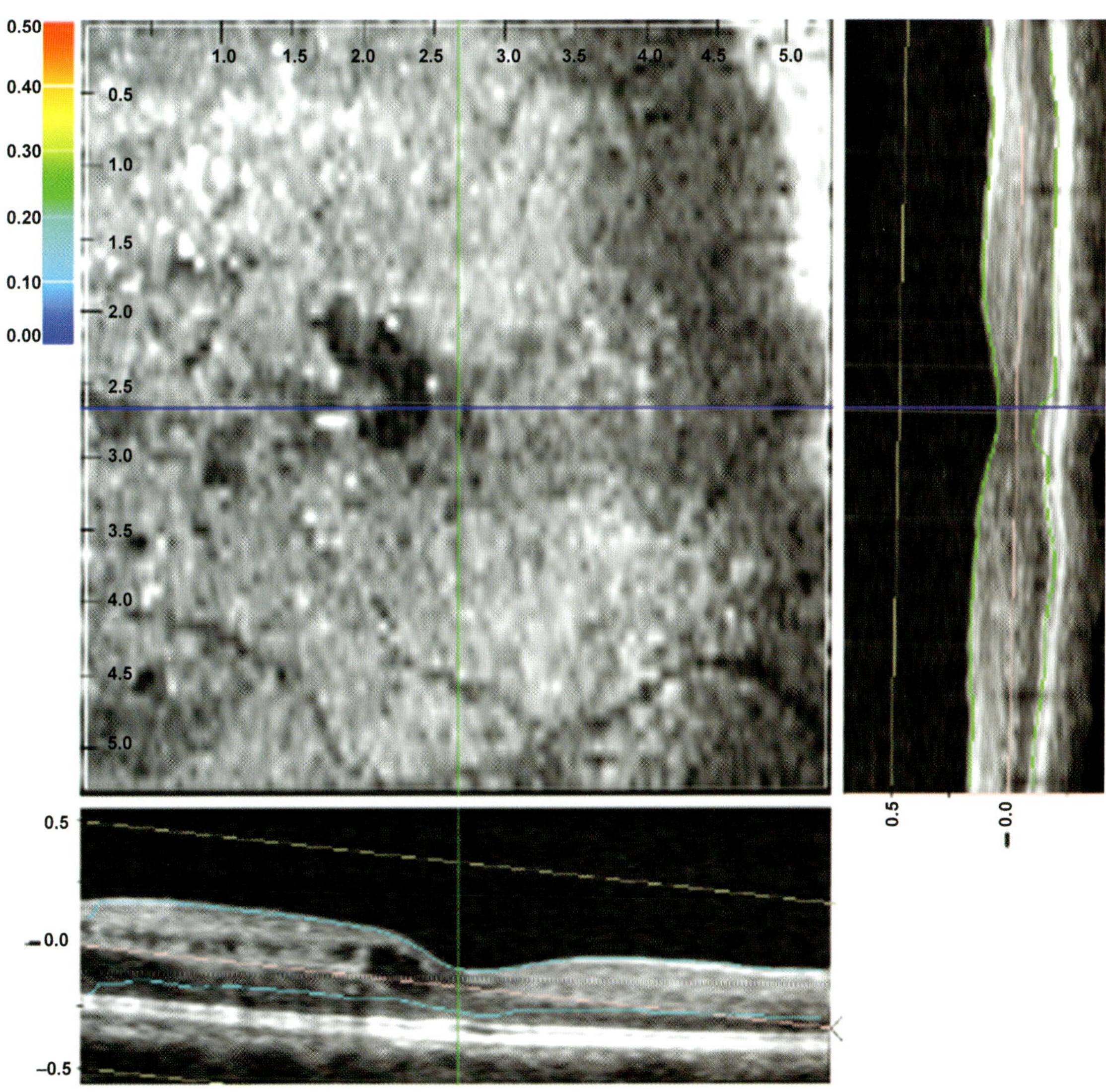

Figure 8: Fluid in the INL

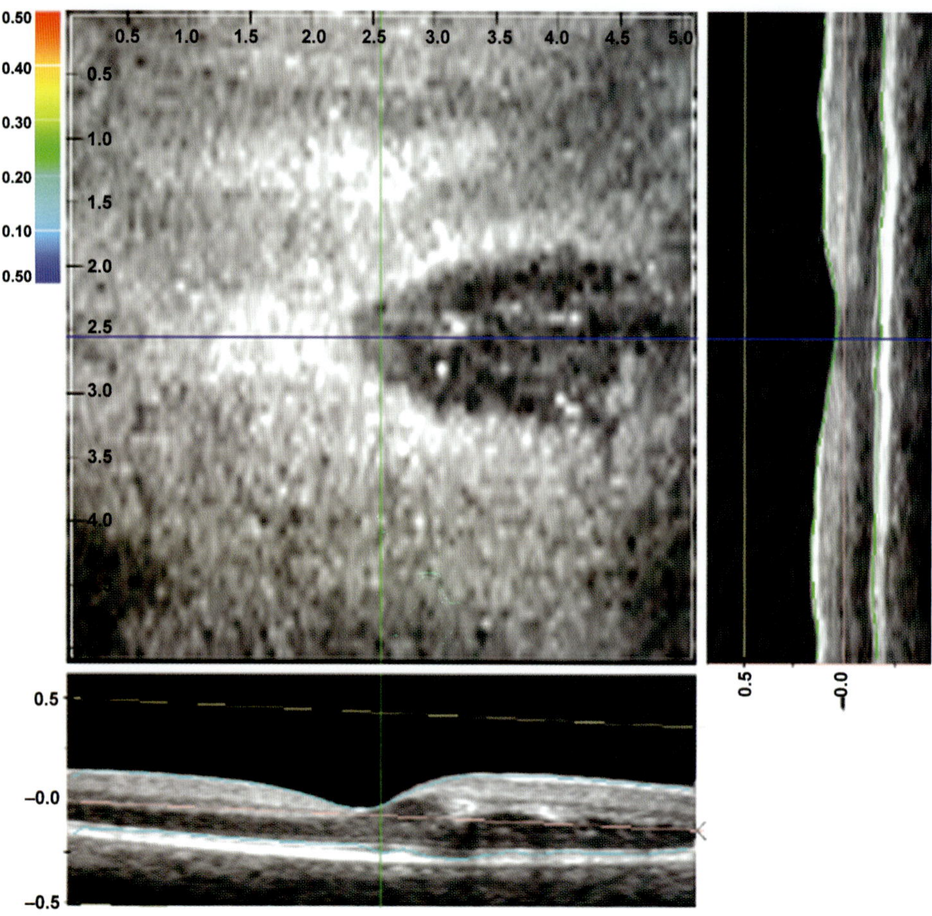

Figure 9: Fluid in the HFL and ONL

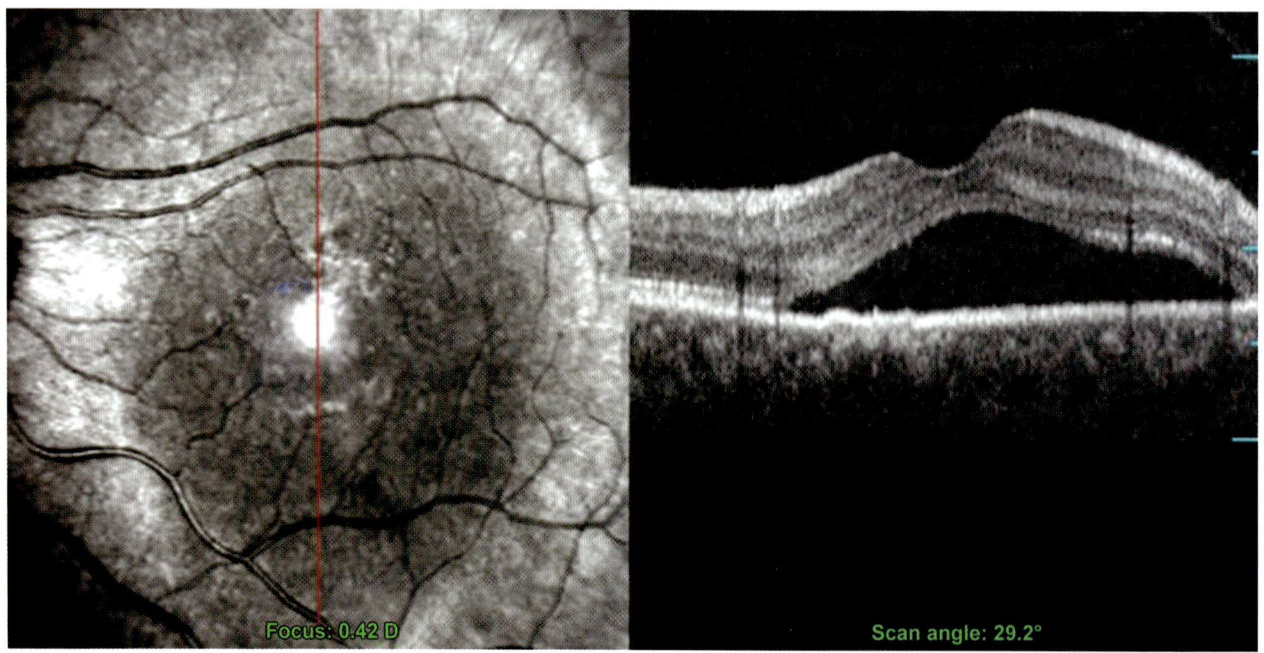

Figure 10: Central serous retinopathy

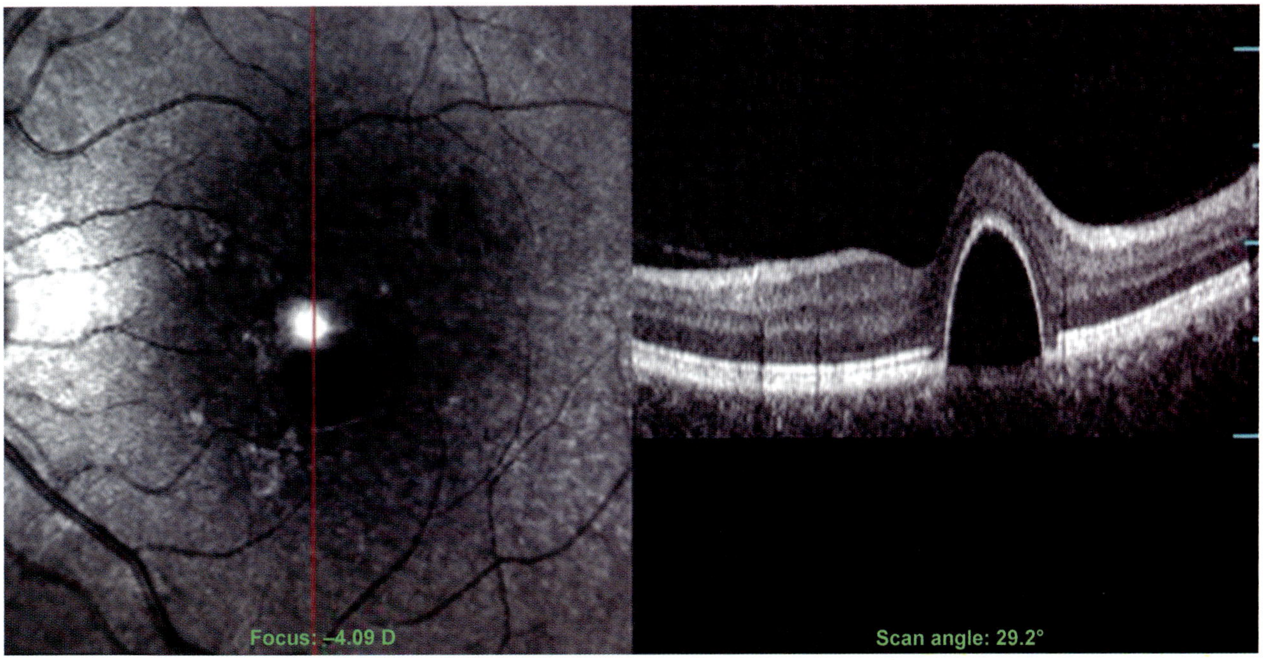

Figure 11: Pigment epithelium detachment

Among other studies, the measurement of the height of cysts,[13] the area and number of cysts[14] and the number of thickened subfields[15] has demonstrated higher correlation with VA, compared to CMT. However, measuring specific retinal dimensions is time consuming and has demonstrated low repeatability. In conclusion, apart from research settings, these alternative parameters have not found a clinical application.

Qualitative Approaches for the Evaluation of Fluid

Qualitative investigations of DME have correlated OCT patterns of fluid distribution with four main angiographic patterns: petalloid (**Figure 13**), honeycomb (**Figure 14**), diffuse DME (**Figure 15**) and serous retinal detachment.[16] Although there is a correlation between angiographic and OCT patterns, no studies have identified how this correlation may help clinical management. In conclusion, the description of patterns does not appear to discriminate between patients likely to benefit from the treatment and patients unlikely to respond.

Overall, the majority of image analysis investigations described so far looked at the volume of fluid and its effect on overall retinal dimensions. Retinal neurones are displaced, compressed, stretched and finally damaged as a consequence of fluid accumulation. The evaluation of tissue integrity in DME may provide a stronger predictor of VA. The next experiment illustrates a quantitative image analysis method for the evaluation of residual tissue in DME.

Quantitative Evaluation of Bipolar Integrity with OCT *En Face*

The three neurones responsible for visual function (photoreceptors, bipolar and ganglion cells) are located at three different levels of the retina and may be differently affected by accumulation of fluid (**Figure 16**). The retinal glia forms a rigid framework and holds together the remaining cells.

In DME the vertical structures connecting the IPL with the OPL consist of columns of Müller's fibers together with the axonal elements of bipolar cells.[17-19] The bipolar cells are the sole communication pathway between photoreceptors and ganglion cell, therefore any loss of connectivity between these cells will compromise visual function. Progressive fluid accumulation produces stretching and distortion of the bipolar axons and it may lead to permanent damage with effect on visual function.

In **Figure 17**, we illustrate two cases of DME with similar CMT (538 and 522 microns, respectively). The Log MAR visual acuity (Log MAR VA) was 0.3 and 1.0, in patients A and B respectively. The two cases had different volume of residual tissue forming the columnar structures between the OPL and the IPL. The first case showed considerable amount of residual inter-plexiform connections and a preserved architecture of the inner retina. By contrast, the second case showed extensive loss of connections with advanced thinning of the inner retinal layers.

Given the fundamental role of bipolar axons in visual transmission, a method was developed for quantitative

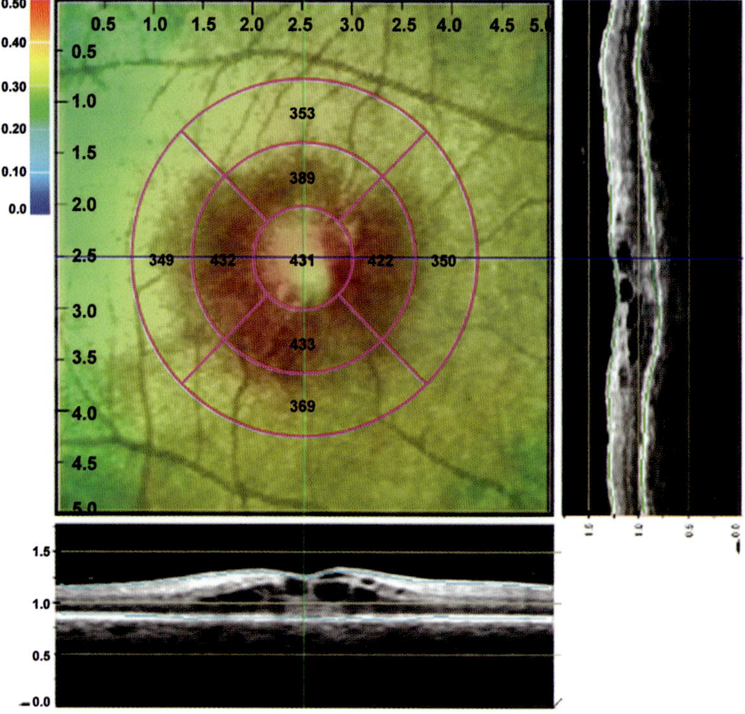

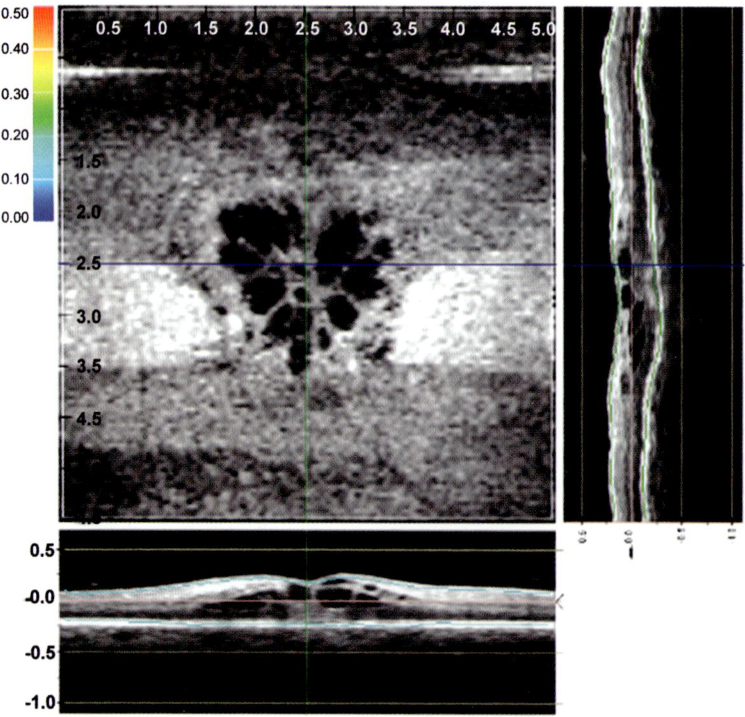

Figure 12: Topography map showing CMT measured on the z plane (top image); OCT *en face* showing the extent and distribution of fluid along the x-y plane (lower image)

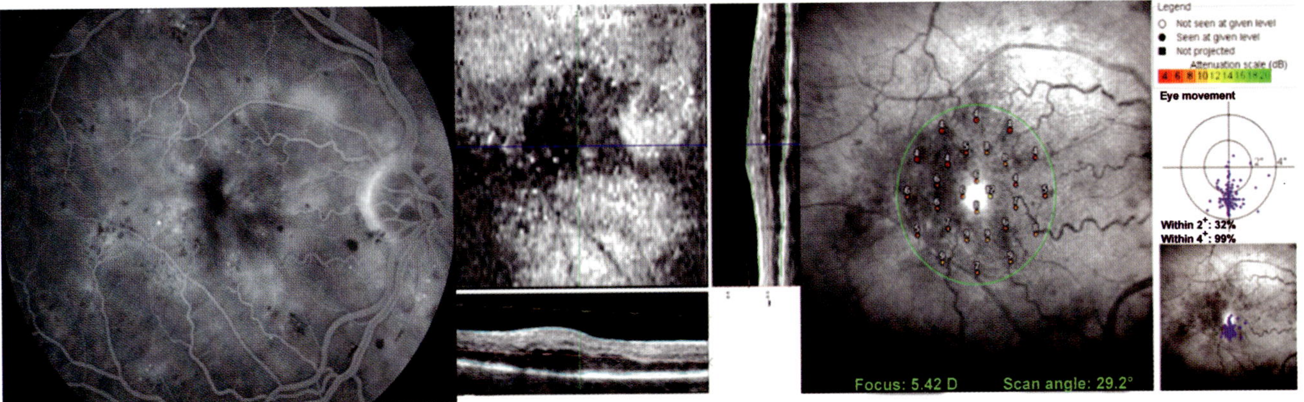

Figure 13: Fluorescein angiogram, OCT *en face* and microperimetry of DME with petalloid pattern (fluid in the OPL): showing vascular leakage, morphology and photoreceptor function

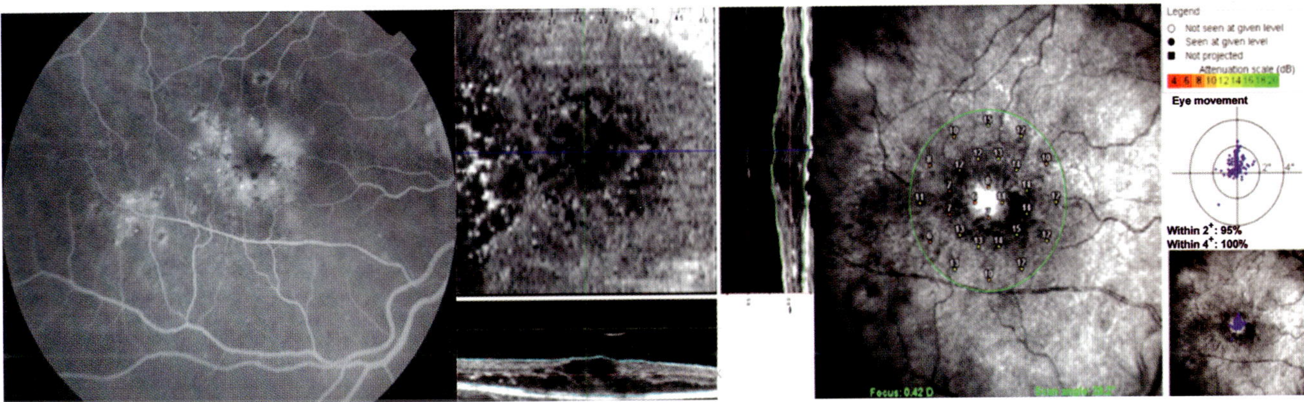

Figure 14: Fluorescein angiogram, OCT *en face* and microperimetry of DME with honeycomb pattern (fluid in OPL and INL)

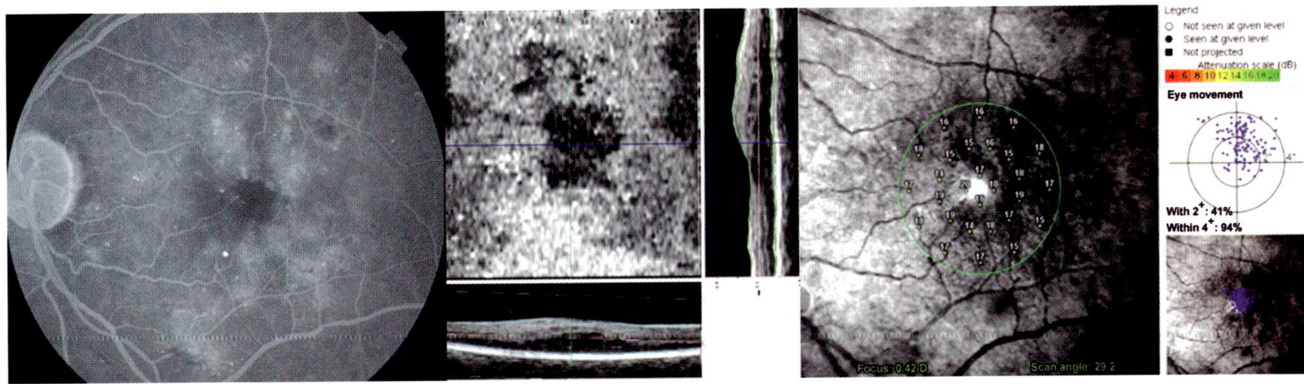

Figure 15: Fluorescein angiogram, OCT *en face* and microperimetry of DME with diffuse pattern

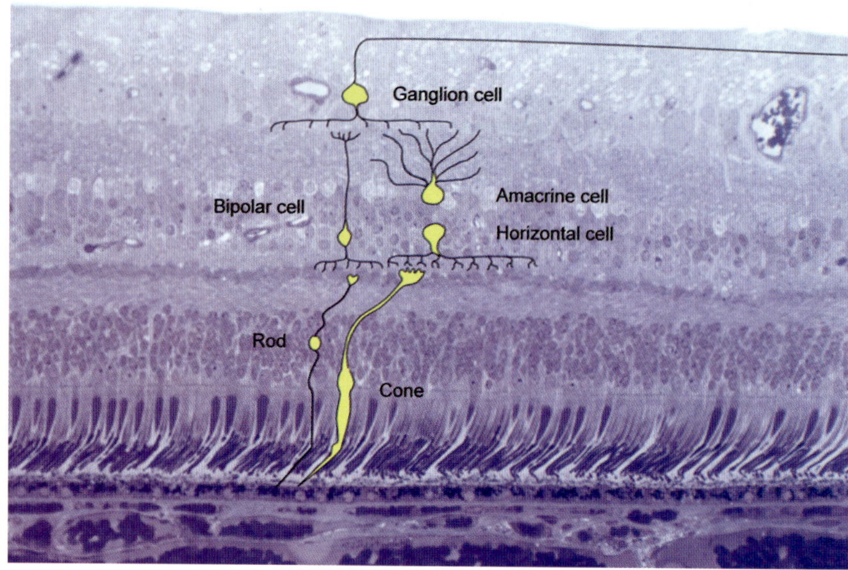

Figure 16: Light microscopy image of normal human retina and schematic representation of retinal neurones (*Courtesy* of Prof J Marshall)

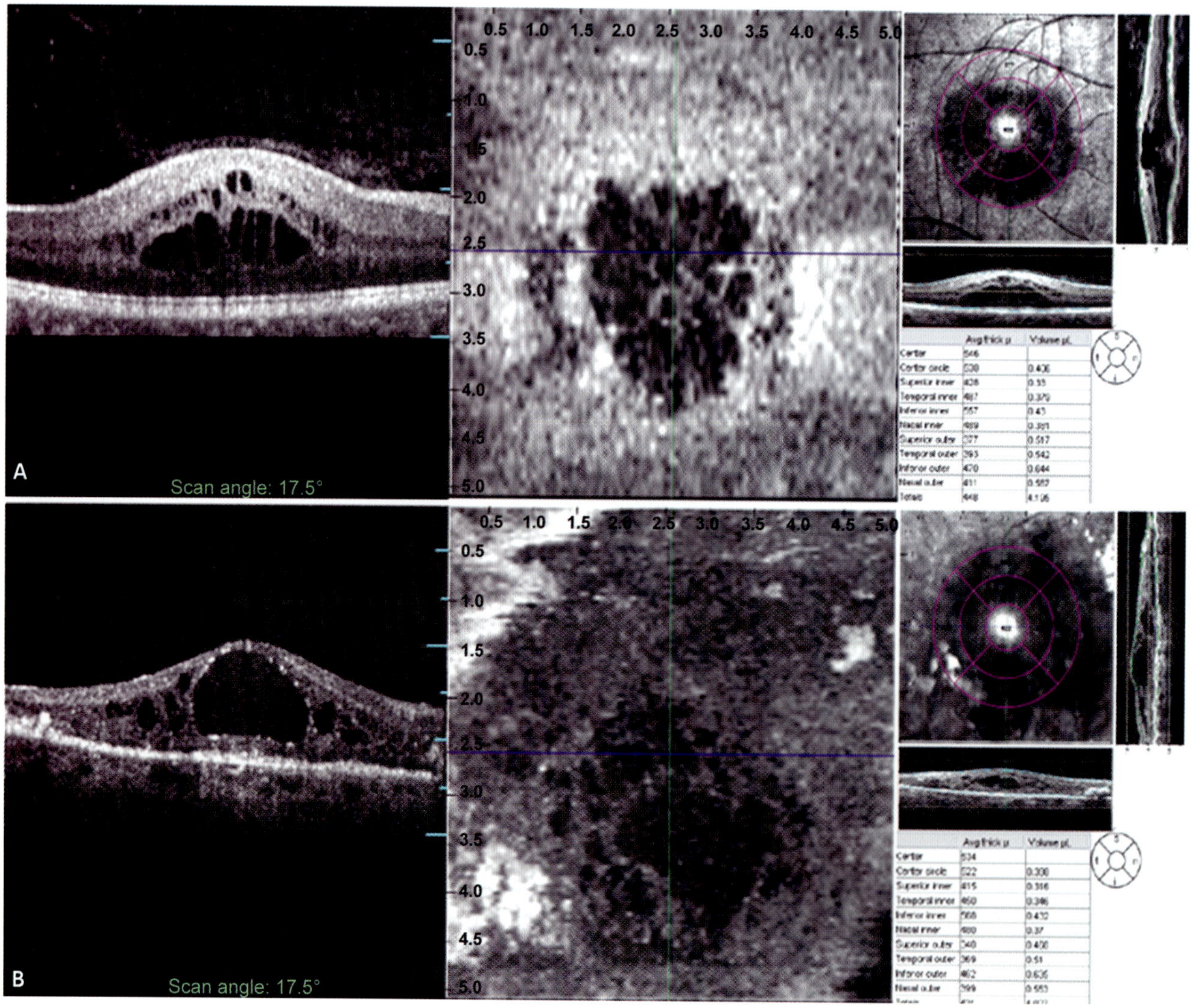

Figure 17: Two cases of DME with different amount of tissue integrity

evaluation of tissue integrity in DME.[20] Raster scans of the macula, OCT *en face* and 3D topographies were recorded using the Opko OCT/SLO. (Opko Health, Inc. Miami, USA). OCT *en face* scans were obtained by selecting the mid-point between the ganglion cell layer and the innermost aspect of the OPL, in most cases to mid depth of the cysts.

An image analysis system was created to extract the residual volume of tissue passing between the two plexiform layers, the number of vertical elements, their diameter and eccentricity from the fovea, in function of VA. Data were collected from a series of concentric rings of 500 µm, 1000 µm, 1500 µm, 2000 µm, 2500 µm radii respectively **(Figure 18)**.

The images were segmented by compressing the grayscale **(Figure 19)** such that tissue became white and edema black.[21] The number of white pixels within each ring was counted and the number of pixels of spared tissue within each annulus was converted to area in mm².

Best corrected Log MAR VA was correlated with retinal tissue integrity evaluated as number of pixels of tissue at increasing eccentricities from the fovea.[20] A linear regression model was developed to assess if the amount of glia and bipolar cells could be used to predict visual acuity. This

study demonstrated a strong correlation between Log MAR VA and the volume of tissue passing between the two plexiform layers in the central retina as determined by OCT *en face* in DME.[20] The volume of retinal tissue between the plexiform layers in ring 1 and 2 (up to 1000 µ from the foveal center) predicted 80% of visual acuity. By contrast, central macular thickness within the central 1000 µ predicted only 14% of visual acuity. The correlation between tissue integrity and VA appeared to fall progressively for rings 3, 4 and 5 **(Figure 20)**.

Furthermore, from the linear regression model, it appears that a minimum of 50% of preserved retinal tissue within ring 1 is necessary in order to maintain a visual acuity of 0.4 LogMAR or better, whereas at least 70% of the retinal tissue within ring 2 is necessary to achieve 0.4 Log MAR VA or better. While there was still reasonable correlation within ring 3, presumably due to signals derived from photoreceptors at the extreme edges of the fovea, correlation was lost within rings 4 and 5.

This experiment showed a strong correlation between retinal tissue integrity in DME assessed with OCT *en face* and Log MAR VA.[20] It will be of interest to apply the current analysis to future trials designed to modulate DME. The

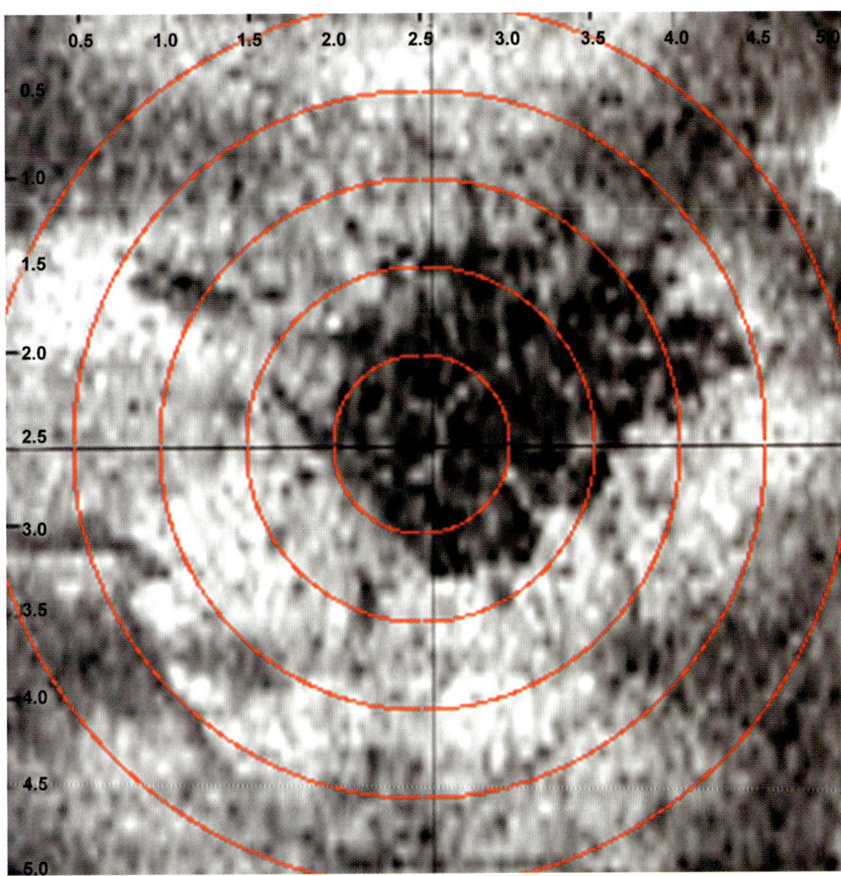

Figure 18: Example of OCT *en face* with overlay of five concentric rings (500 µm, 1000 µm, 1500 µm, 2000 µm, 2500 µm radii) for analysis of tissue integrity at increasing eccentricity from the fovea

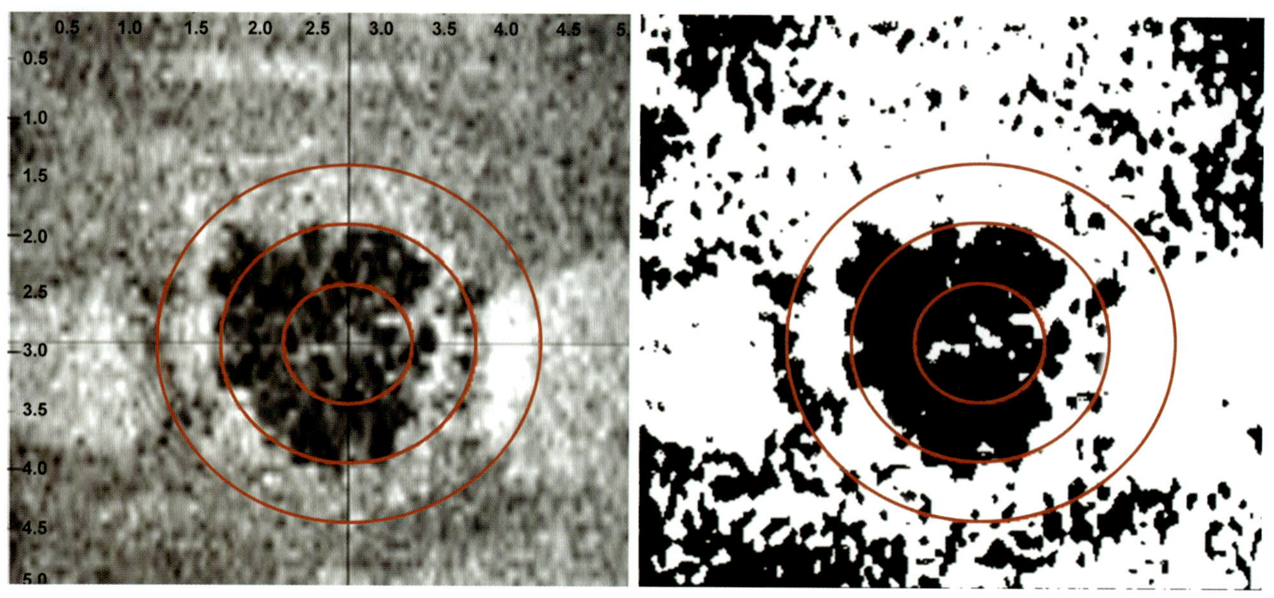

Figure 19: Example of OCT *en face* in grayscale (left) and segmented (right) image with white pixels representing tissue, black pixels representing fluid

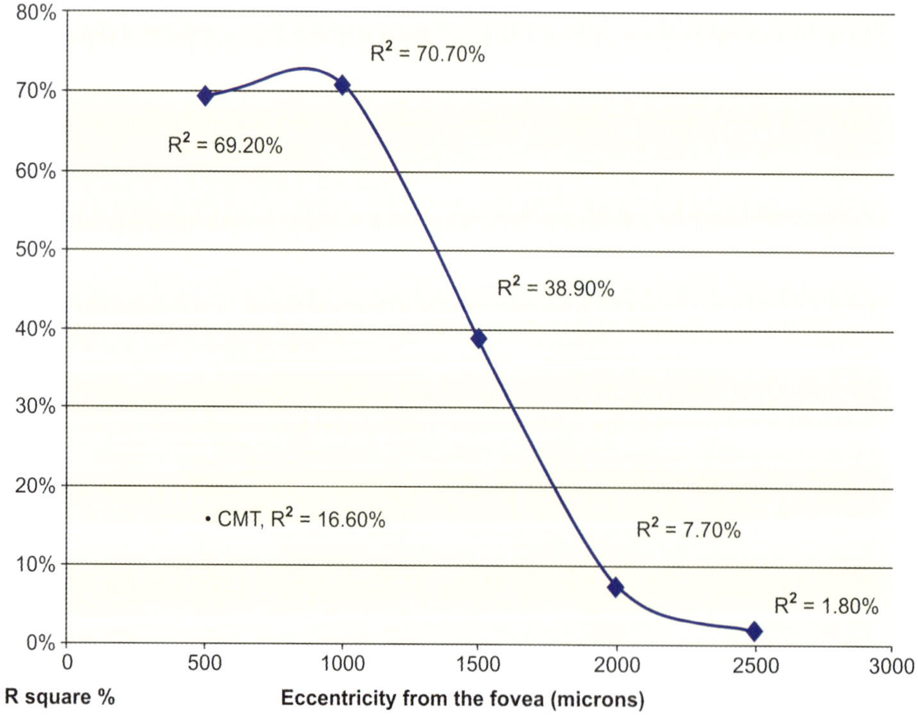

Figure 20: Diagram illustrating the relationship between tissue integrity and Log MAR VA ($R^2\%$ on y axis) at 500, 1000, 1500, 2000, 2500 microns from the fovea (x axis)

ability to determine the potential visual outcome for patients prior to the commencement of any treatment trial will be highly beneficial in that it will allow exclusion of those individuals who could not benefit from intervention.

Summary

OCT *en face* represents an essential tool for the diagnosis, description and prognostic evaluation of DME. The advantages of imaging DME with OCT *en face* versus OCT B scan include:

- OCT *en face* produces images of the x-y plane of the retina across a square area of 5.5 mm by 5.5 mm
- OCT *en face* provides information on the extent and distribution of fluid and exudates across the whole macular region and can be used as a guide during focal/grid laser treatment
- OCT *en face* images can be analysed quantitatively to obtain an estimation of residual connectivity in the inter-plexiform layer of the retina and prognostic evaluation of visual function
- OCT *en face* can be correlated with fluorescein angiography and microperimetry in order to combine morphological information with vascular perfusion and photoreceptor function.

References

1. Progression of retinopathy with intensive versus conventional treatment in the Diabetes Control and Complications Trial. Diabetes Control and Complications Trial Research Group. Ophthalmology. 1995;102(4): 647-61.
2. Early Treatment Diabetic Retinopathy Study Research Group. Photocoagulation for diabetic macular edema: Early Treatment Diabetic Retinopathy Study report number 4. Int Ophthalmol Clin. 1987;27:265-72.
3. Lee CM, Olk RJ. Modified grid laser photocoagulation for diffuse diabetic macular edema: long term visual results. Ophthalmology. 1991;98:1594-1602.
4. Tso MOM. Pathology of cystoid macular edema. Ophthalmology. 1982;89:902-15.
5. Wolter JR. The histopathology of cystoid macular edema. Albrecht Von Graefes Arch Klin Exp Ophthalmol. 1981;216: 85-101.
6. Starling EH. On absorptions of fluids from the connective tissue spaces. J Physiol (London) 1896;19:312.
7. Hogan MJ, Alvarado JA, Weddell JE. Histology of the Human Eye: An Atlas and Textbook. WB Saunders, Philadelphia, 1971.
8. Cunha-Vaz JG, Travassos A. Breakdown of the blood-retinal barriers and cystoid macular oedema. Surv Ophthalmol. 1984;28:485-92.
9. Fine BS, Brucker AJ. Macular edema and cystoid macular edema. Am J Ophthalmology. 1981;92:466-81.
10. Gass JD, Anderson DR, Davis EB. A clinical, fluorescein angiographic and electron microscopic correlation of cystoid macular edema. Am J Ophthalmol. 1985;100:82-86.
11. Antcliff RJ, Hussain AA, Marshall J. Hydraulic conductivity of fixed retinal tissue after sequential excimer laser ablation: barriers limiting fluid distribution and implications for cystoid macular edema. Arch Ophthalmol. 2001;119:539-44.
12. Diabetic Retinopathy Clinical Research Network. Relationship between optical coherence tomography measured central retinal thickness and visual acuity in diabetic macular oedema. Ophthalmology. 2007;114:525-36.
13. Antcliff RJ, Stanford MR, Chauhan DS, et al. Comparison between optical coherence tomography and fundus fluorescein angiography for the detection of cystoid macular edema in patients with uveitis. Ophthalmology. 2000;107:593-9.
14. Arend O, Wolf S, Harris A, Reim M. The relationship of macular microcirculation to visual acuity in diabetic patients. Arch Ophthalmol. 1995;113:610-4.
15. Browning DJ, Glassman AR, Aiello LP, et al. Diabetic retinopathy clinical research network. Optical coherence tomography measurements and analysis methods in optical coherence tomography studies of diabetic macular edema. Ophthalmology. 2008;115(8):1366-71.
16. Yeung L, Lima VC, Garcia P, et al. Correlation between spectral domain optical coherence tomography findings and fluorescein angiography patterns in diabetic macular edema. Ophthalmology. 2009;116(6):1158-67.
17. Yamada E. Some structural features of the fovea centralis in the human retina. Arch Ophthalmol 1969;82:151-9.
18. Gass JDM. Muller cell cone, an overlooked part of the anatomy of the fovea centralis. Arch Ophthalmol 1999;117:821-3.
19. Marshall J. The effects of ultraviolet radiation and blue light on the eye. In Marshall J. The susceptible visual apparatus. London, Macmillan. 1991:54-66.
20. Pelosini L, Hull C, Boyce JF, et al. Optical coherence tomography may be used to predict visual acuity in patients with macular oedema. Invest Ophthalmol Vis Sci. 2011;52(5):2741-8.
21. Barman SA, Hollick EJ, Boyce JF, et al. Quantification of posterior capsular opacification in digital images after cataract surgery. Invest Ophthalmol Vis Sci. 2000;41(12): 3882-92.

chapter 28

En Face OCT Morphologic Changes in Diabetic Maculopathy

Bruno Lumbroso, Marco Rispoli

En Face OCT Images Adapted to the Cup-shaped Retina in the Study of Diabetic Macular Edema

En face optical coherence tomography (OCT) images, adapted to the cup-shaped retina are an improvement on plane scans for clinical and research. purposes. Instead of making a flat section, the *en face* scan may be generated following a natural surface contour.

OCT scans adapted to the normal concavity of the retinal pigment epithelium (RPE) or of the inner limiting membrane (ILM) enable imaging the finer details of macular edema. They bring to frontal scan the possibility to obtain a retinal or choroidal section that follows the ILM curve and is parallel to it.

Frontal scans may be at will placed at any constant depth in the retina or choroid and are always parallel to ILM or RPE.

Clinicians obtain thus an optical *in vivo* dissection of the layer of the retina or choroid they want to study, the possibility to isolate a layer from the other layers. In this way clinicians study the features of retinal surface and of cystoid edema in the retinal layers.

Cystoid Diabetic Macular Edema may have Vascular or Tractional Causes

Vascular Cystoid Macular Edema

Long duration retinal edema results in damages of the Müller cells, leading to cystoid cavity formation in the retina. These spaces start in the outer plexiform layer, and subsequently penetrate the nuclear layers and the inner plexiform layer. There is a high correlation between fluorescein angiography and OCT in the pattern of hyperfluorescence.[1] Advanced cystoid edema brings residual tissue to atrophy (**Figures 1A to E**). It is important to quantify the edema by measuring its volume as well residual retinal tissue.[2,3]

Optical coherence tomography has shown that serous detachments are part of the final progression of diabetic edema. A small localized serous retinal detachment with optically blank cavity between the detached retina and the pigment epithelium can be seen.

En face OCT: The frontal scan placed at retina surface level shows a smooth surface in case of vascular edema. There are no retinal plaques or folds (**Figures 2A to E**).

The frontal scan placed inside the retina shows at the inner nuclear layer level numerous small petal-shaped cystoid cells. The frontal or coronal flower or honeycomb pattern is caused by the Henle fibers stellate structure. Cells are grossly ovoid with tips converging toward the fovea, flower or clover shaped.

In the outer nuclear layer we see regular, bigger cystoid cells, their shape is more polygonal than ovoid converging toward the fovea. Later in the evolution walls between cells disappear leading to large irregular chambers sustained by rare columns of residual retina (**Figures 3A to D**).

Traction Cystoid Macular Edema

It is seen when epiretinal membrane apply tension to retina leading to retraction of the inner limiting membrane. *En face* OCT enables us to detect easily epiretinal membranes (**Figures 4A and B**). These membranes, pulling on the retina, cause edema and sometimes serous detachments. It may lead to a syndrome of the vitreoretinal interface. The foveal depression disappears.

The frontal scan placed at retinal surface level shows retinal plaques and folds in case of tractional edema. These folds can take a parallel or stellate shape.

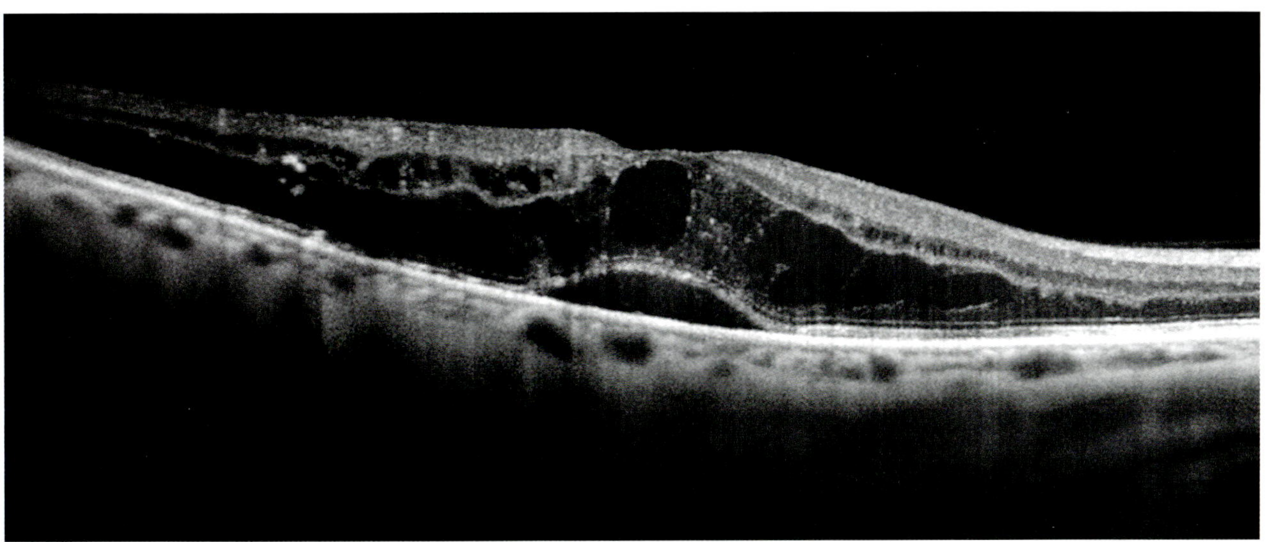

Figure 1A: Cystoid diabetic macular edema B scan. In this case of vascular edema two principal rows of cystoid cells are seen: Inner nuclear layer and outer nuclear layer; Small foveal detachment of retina; Some hard exudates (Optovue, RTVue)

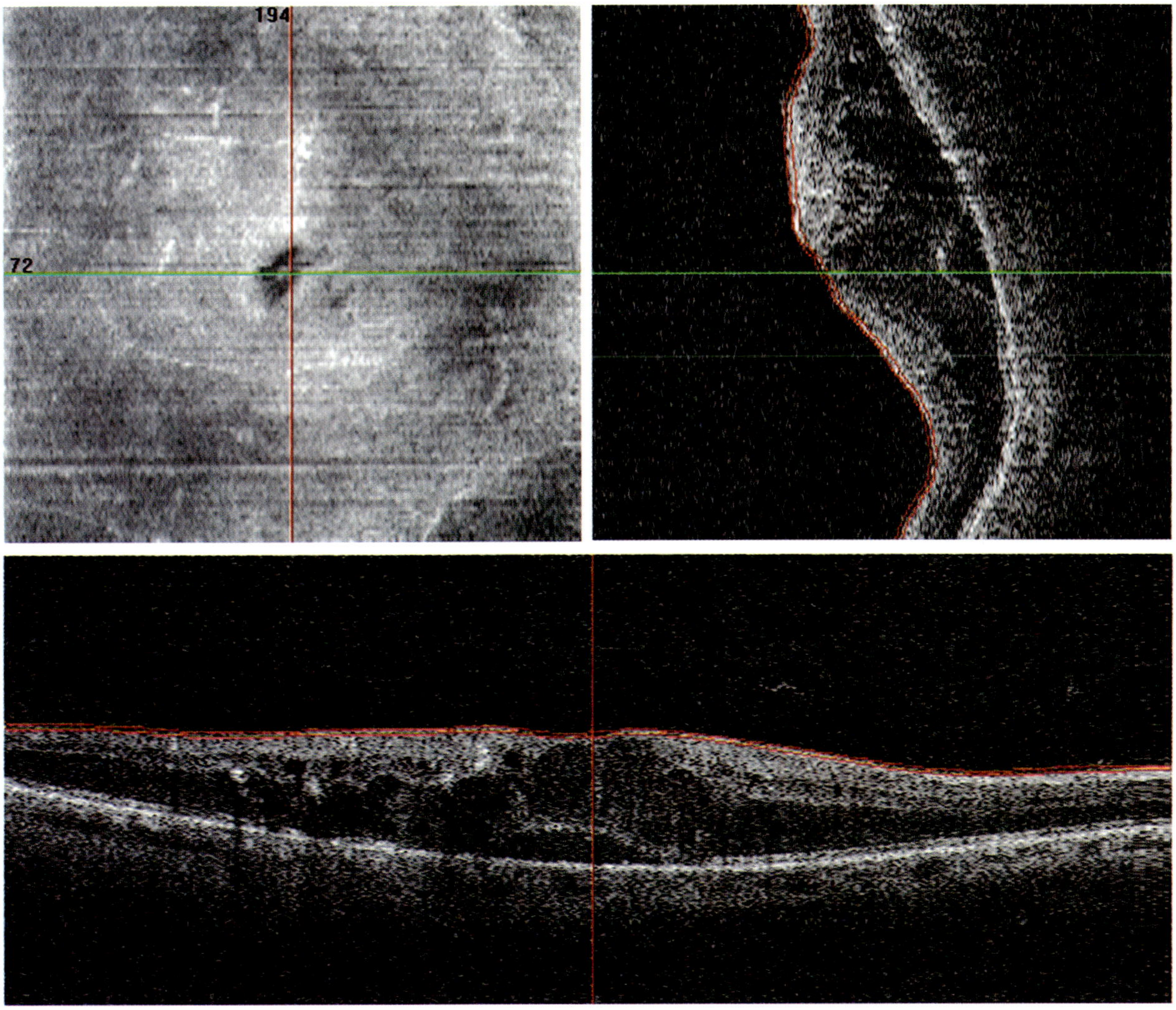

Figure 1B: Cystoid diabetic macular edema *en face* OCT: The frontal scan placed at: Internal limiting membrane (ILM) level shows a smooth surface in this case of vascular edema (Optovue, RTVue)

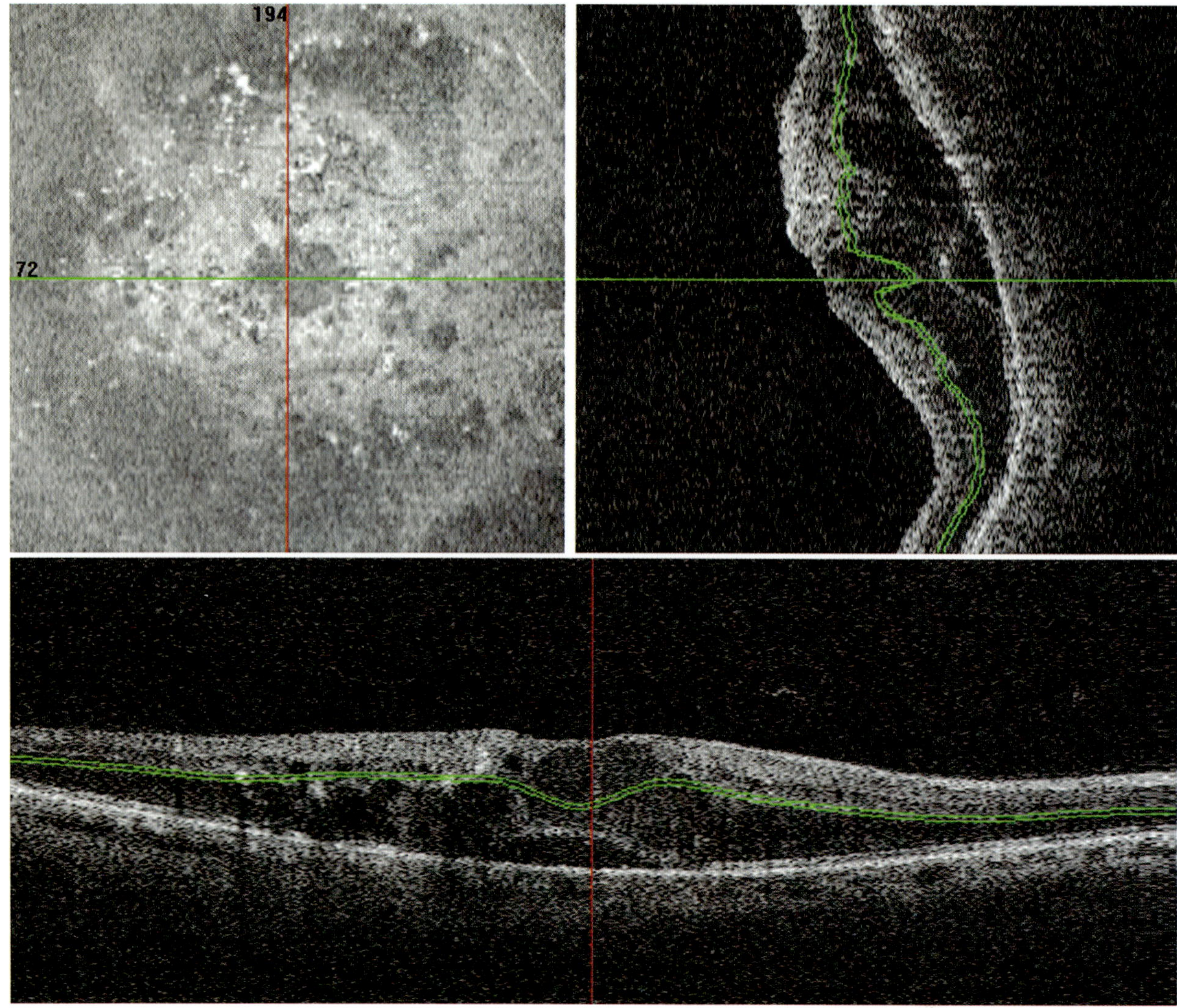

Figure 1C: Cystoid diabetic macular edema *en face* OCT: The frontal scan placed inside the retina, parallel to the ILM scan shows at the inner nuclear layer level numerous small petal-shaped cystoid cells. The honeycomb pattern is caused by the Henle fibers stellate structure. Cells are grossly ovoid with tips converging toward the fovea, flower or clover-shaped (Optovue, RTVue)

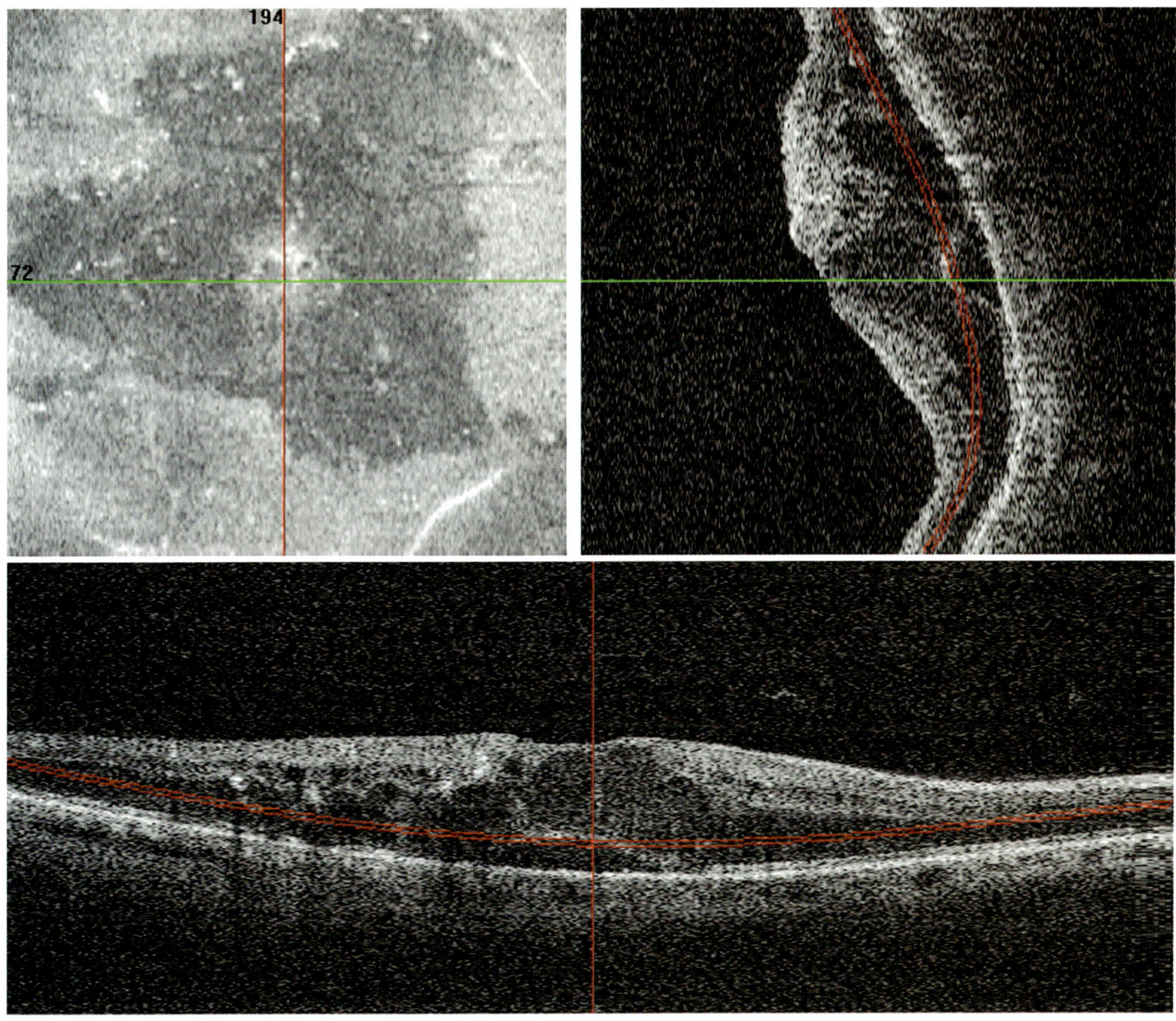

Figure 1D: Cystoid diabetic macular edema *en face* OCT: The frontal scan placed deeper inside the retina, parallel to the RPE scan shows at the outer nuclear layer level numerous big irregular trapezoid-shaped cystoid cells. The honeycomb pattern is difficult to recognize. Cells are grossly irregular converging toward the fovea, flower or clover-shaped (Optovue, RTVue)

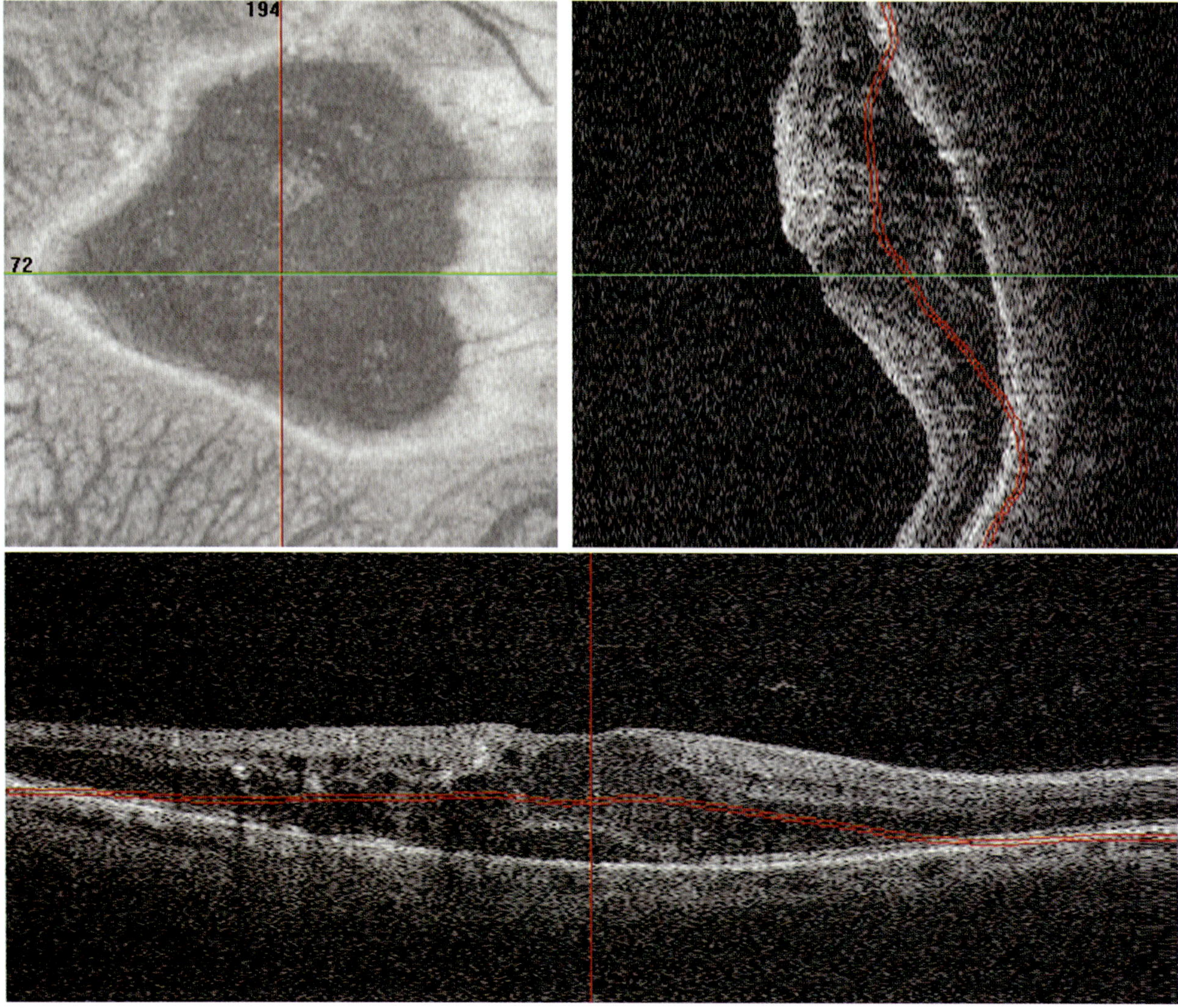

Figure 1E: Cystoid diabetic macular edema. The frontal scan placed deeper inside the retina parallel to the ILM and shows at the outer nuclear layer level numerous big irregular trapezoid-shaped cystoid cells. At the center a rounded cavity represents the foveal retinal detachment (Optovue, RTVue)

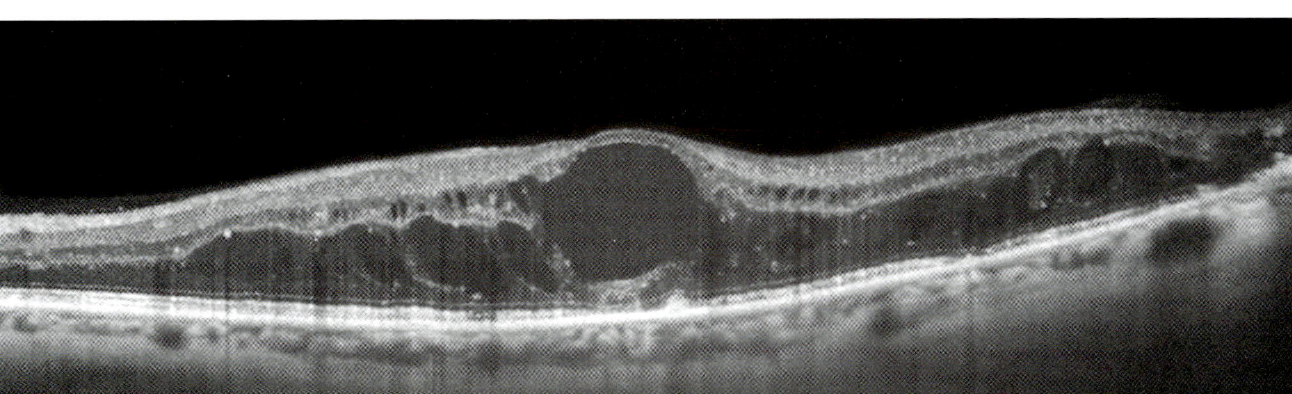

Figure 2A: Cystoid diabetic macular edema B scan. Vascular edema with two principal rows of cystoid cells are seen: inner nuclear layer and outer nuclear layer. A big rounded cell is seen centrally. No detachment of retina. Some hard exudates (Optovue, RTVue)

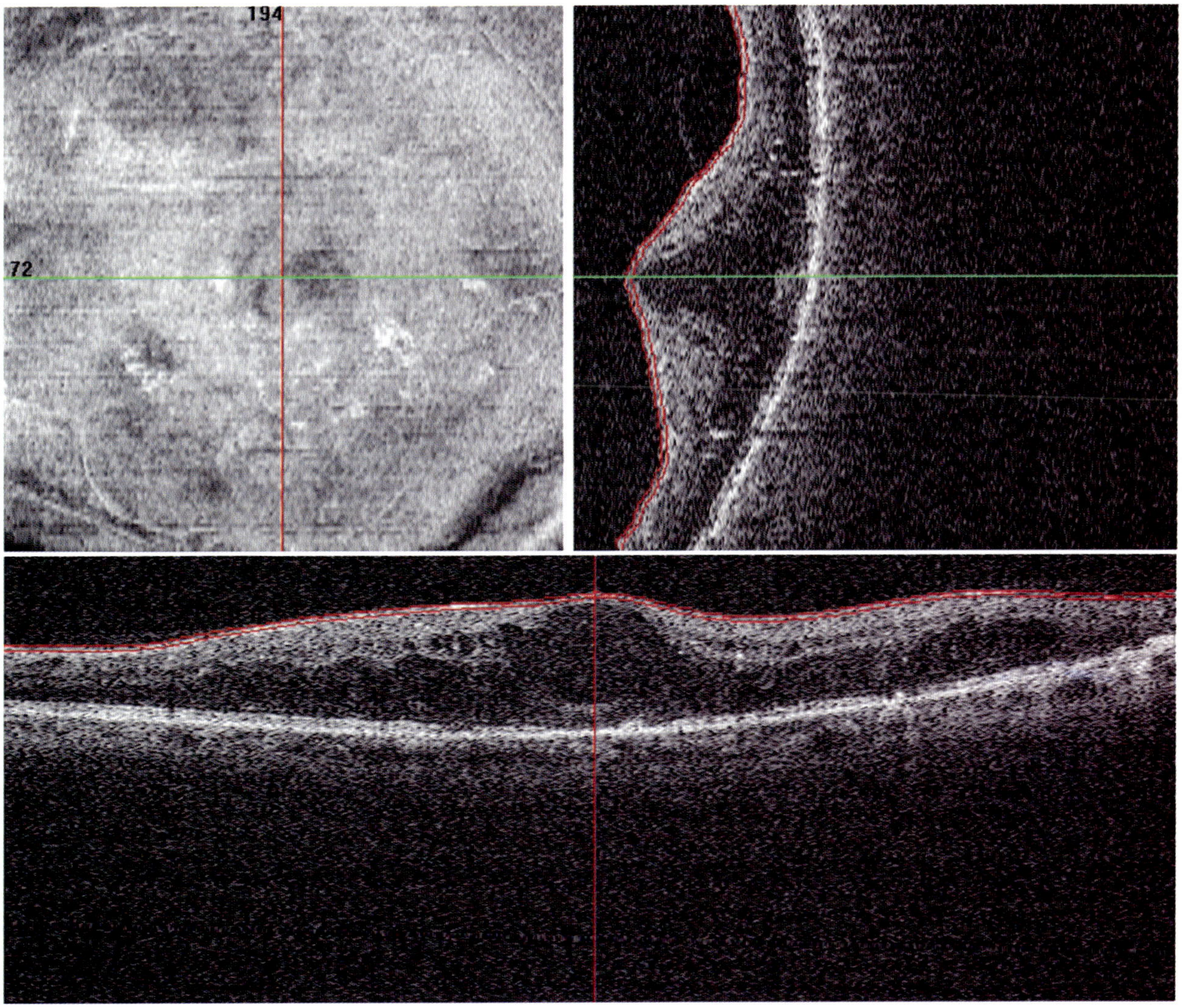

Figure 2B: Cystoid diabetic macular edema *en face* OCT: The frontal scan placed at ILM level shows a smooth surface in this case of vascular edema. Some surface irregularities are due to cystoid cells underneath the surface (Optovue, RTVue)

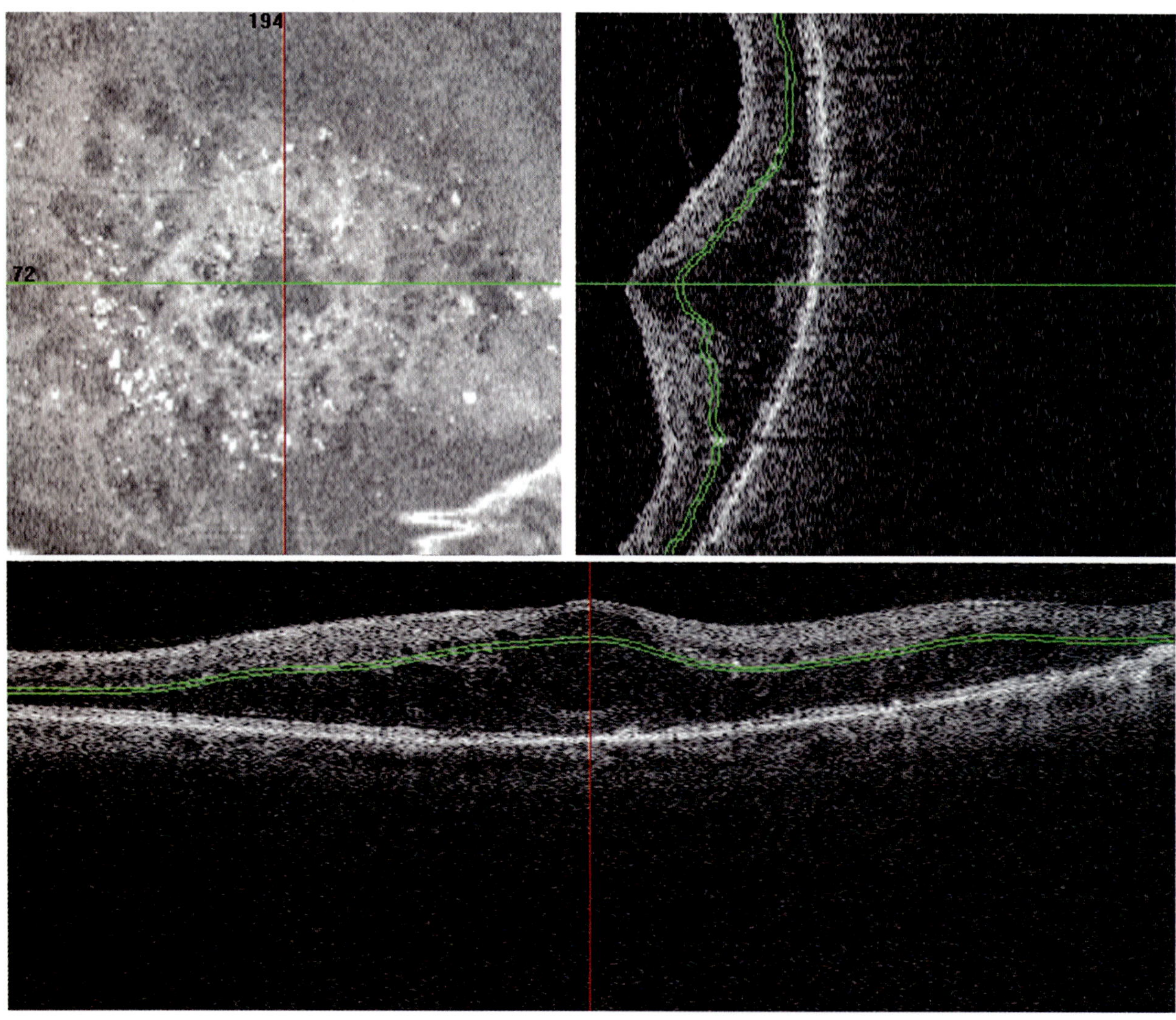

Figure 2C: Cystoid diabetic macular edema *en face* OCT: The frontal scan placed inside the retina, parallel to the ILM scan shows at the inner nuclear layer level numerous small irregular cystoid cells. The flower pattern is caused by the Henle fibers structure (Optovue, RTVue)

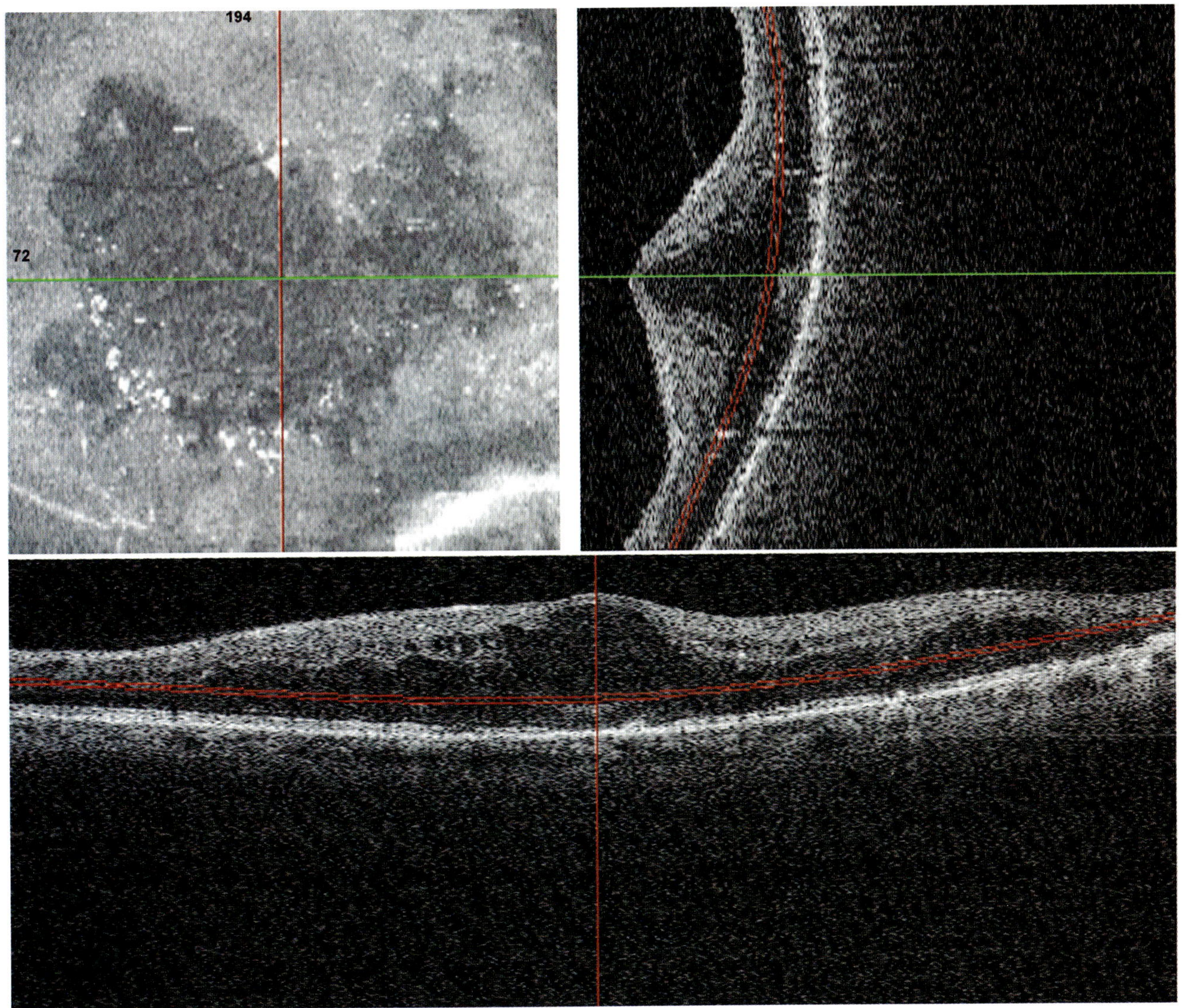

Figure 2D: Cystoid diabetic macular edema: The frontal scan placed deeper inside the retina parallel to the RPE shows at the outer nuclear layer level numerous big irregular trapezoid-shaped cystoid cells (Optovue, RTVue)

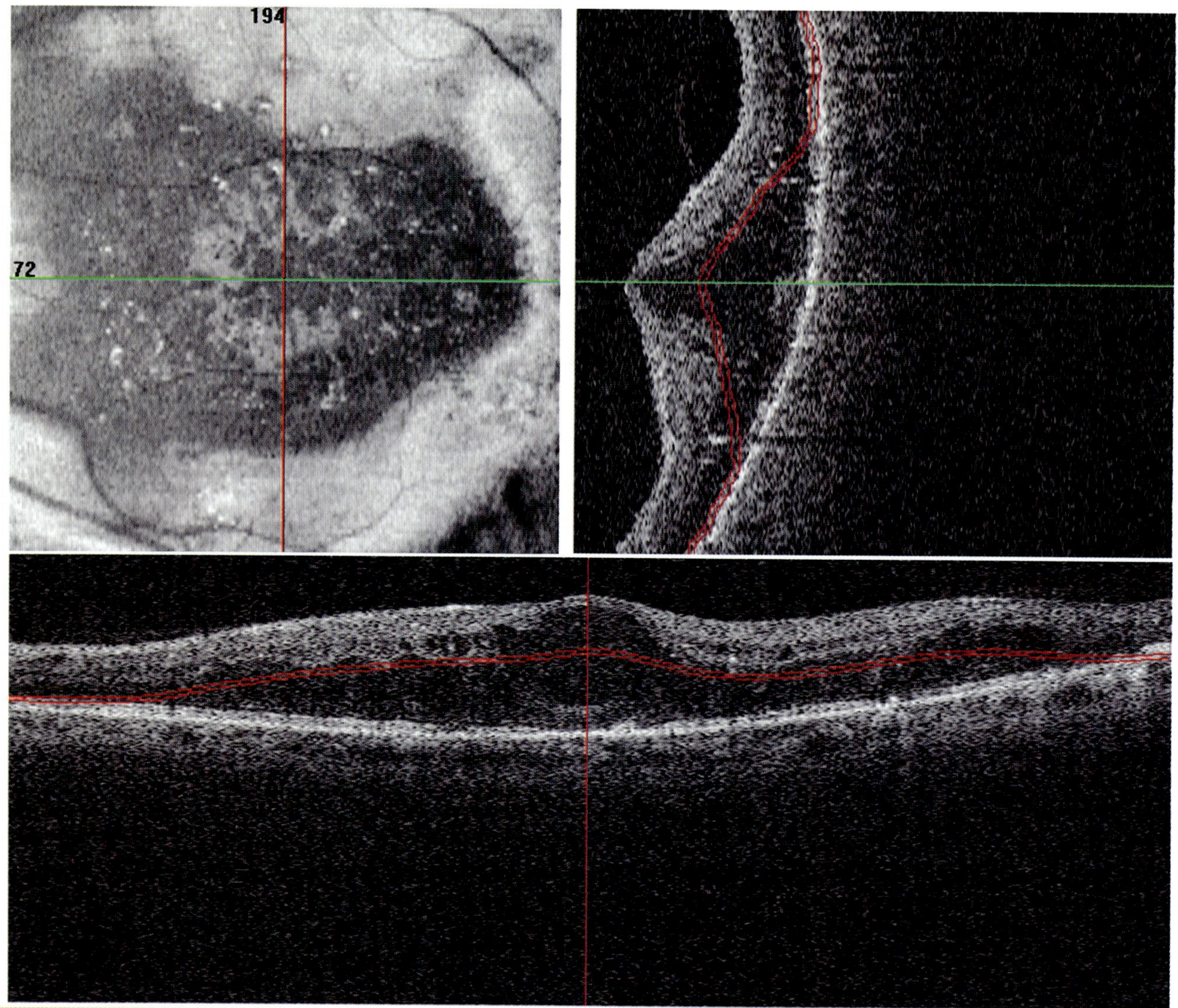

Figure 2E: Cystoid diabetic macular edema *en face* OCT: The frontal scan placed deeper inside the retina, parallel to the ILM scan shows at the outer nuclear layer level numerous big irregular cystoid cells. Cells are grossly irregular converging toward the fovea, flower or clover-shaped. Numerous hard exudates (Optovue, RTVue)

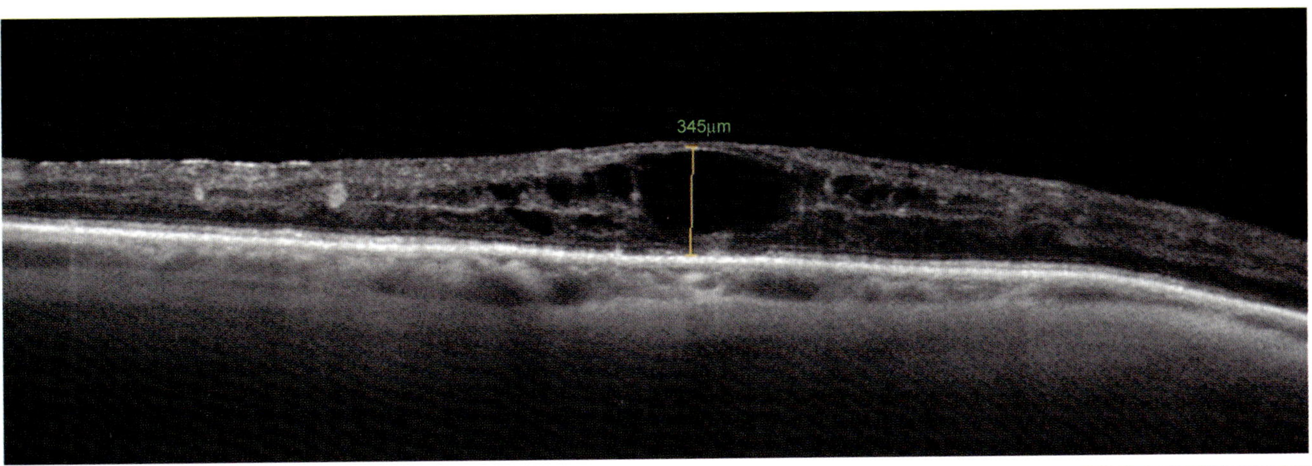

Figure 3A: Cystoid diabetic macular edema B scan. Vascular edema with two rows of cystoid cells are seen: inner nuclear layer and outer nuclear layer. A big horizontally elongated cell is seen at the fovea. No detachment of retina. Some hard exudates (Optovue, RTVue)

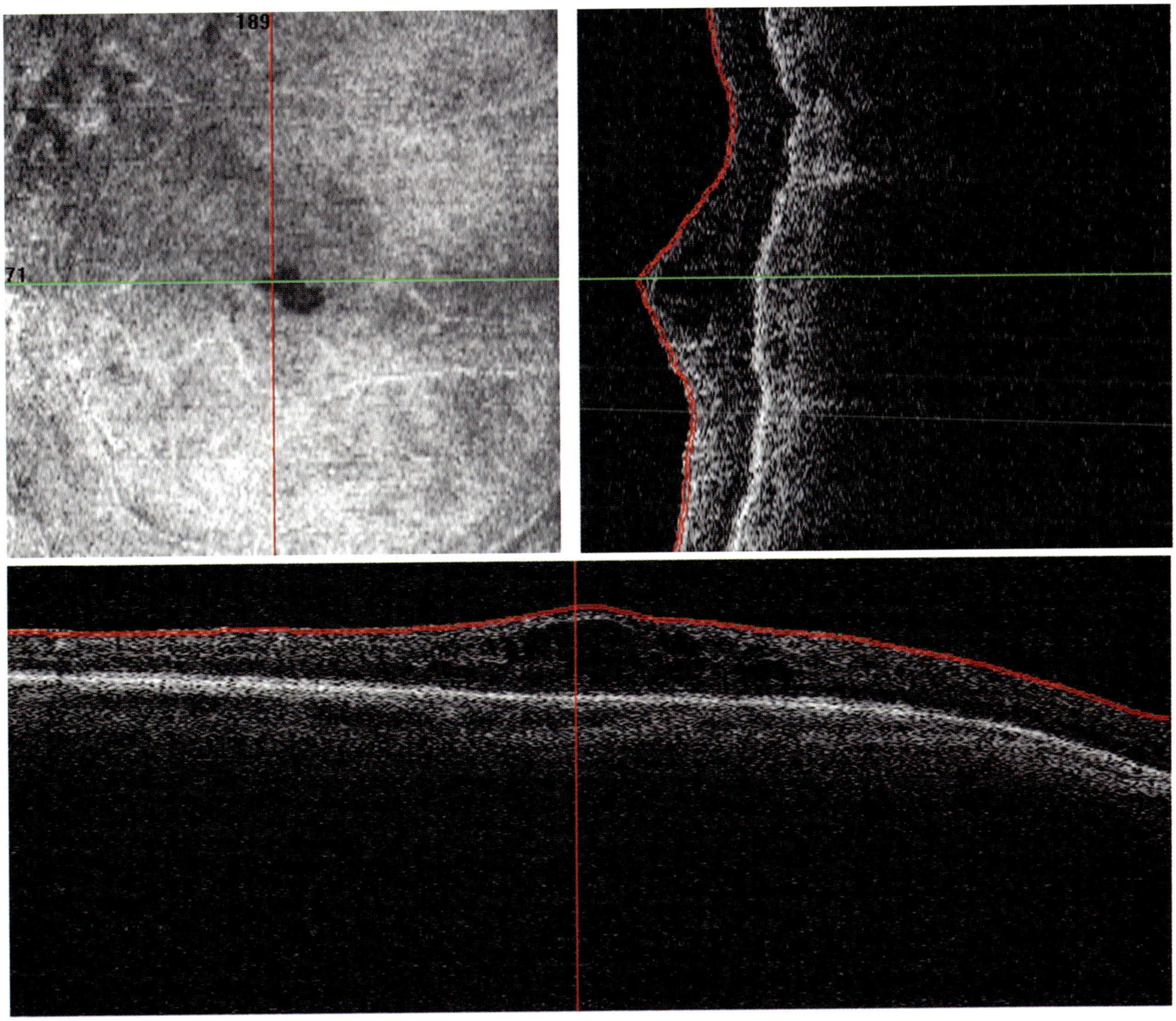

Figure 3B: Cystoid diabetic macular edema *en face* OCT: The frontal scan placed at ILM level shows a smooth surface in this case of vascular edema. Some surface irregularities are seen (Optovue, RTVue)

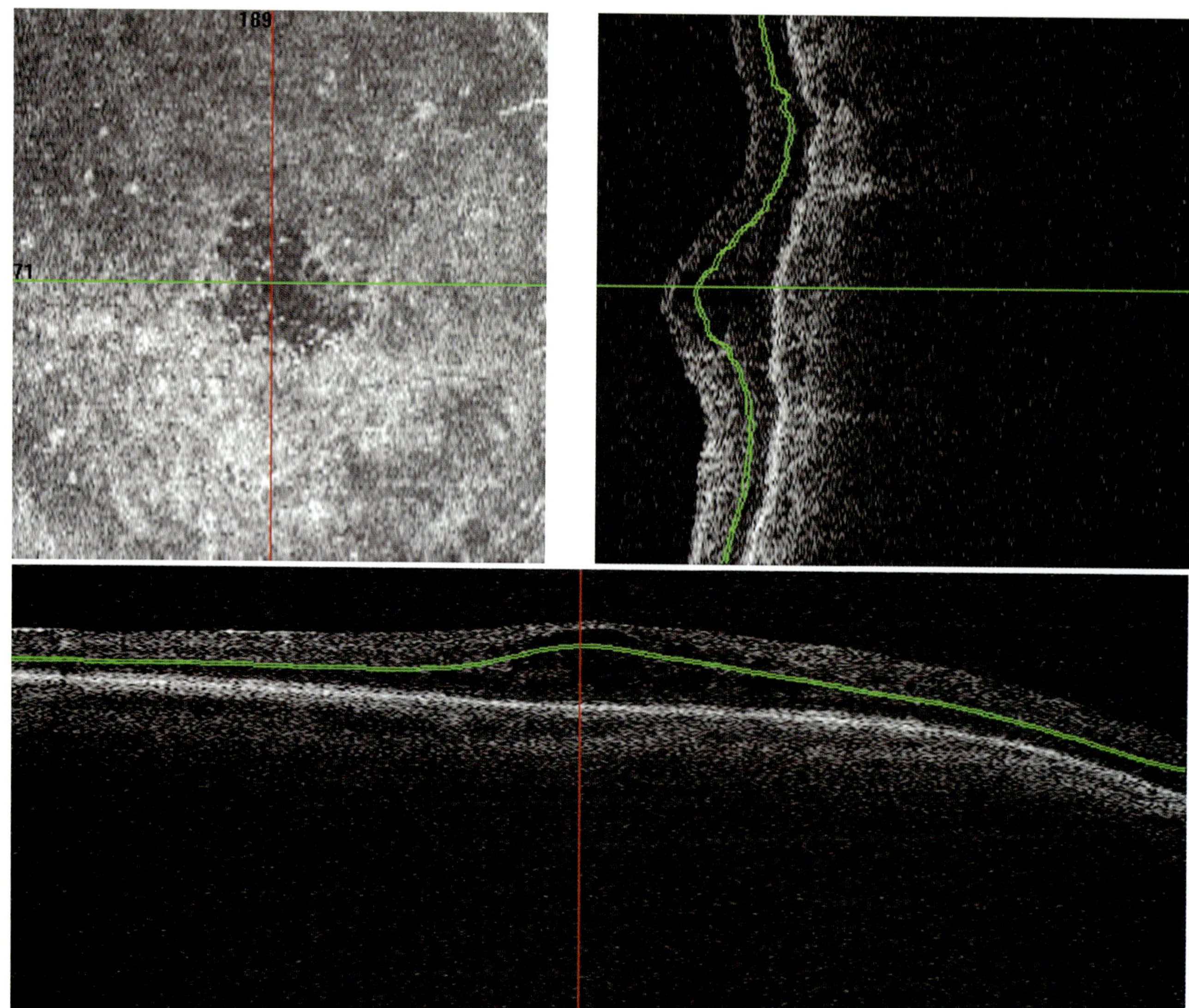

Figure 3C: Cystoid diabetic macular edema *en face* OCT: The frontal scan placed inside the retina, parallel to the ILM scan shows at the inner nuclear layer level numerous small petal shaped cystoid cells. A grossly polygonal and irregular cell is located at the fovea (Optovue, RTVue)

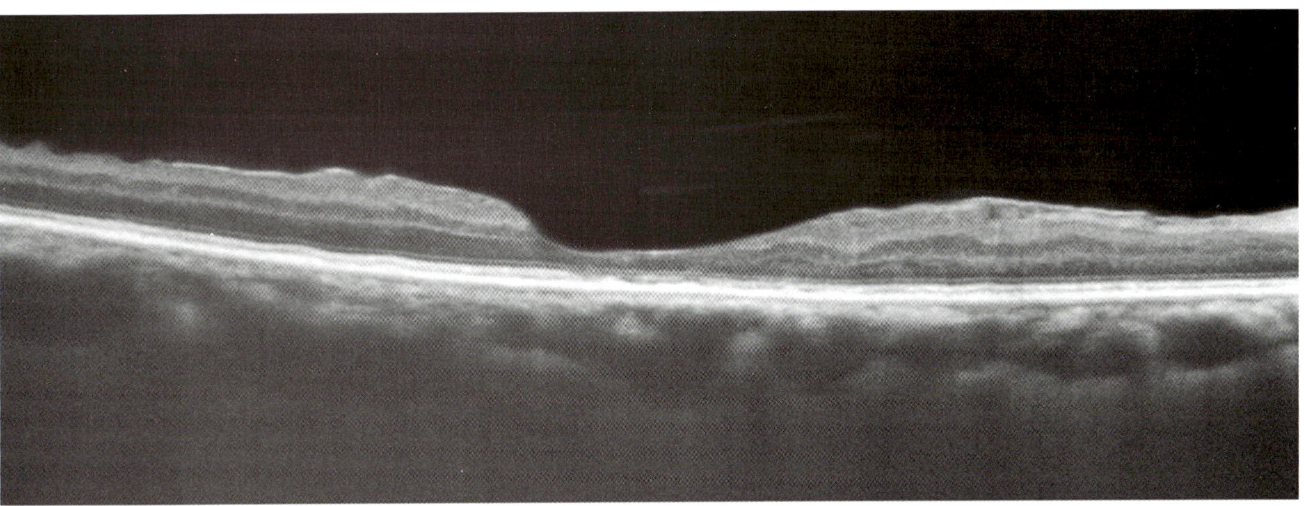

Figure 4A: Epiretinal membrane diabetic maculopathy B scan. Retina is thinned. An epiretinal membrane is very adherent to the retinal surface. Macular depression is irregular and asymmetric. Two small edema cells are seen close to the retinal surface (Optovue, RTVue)

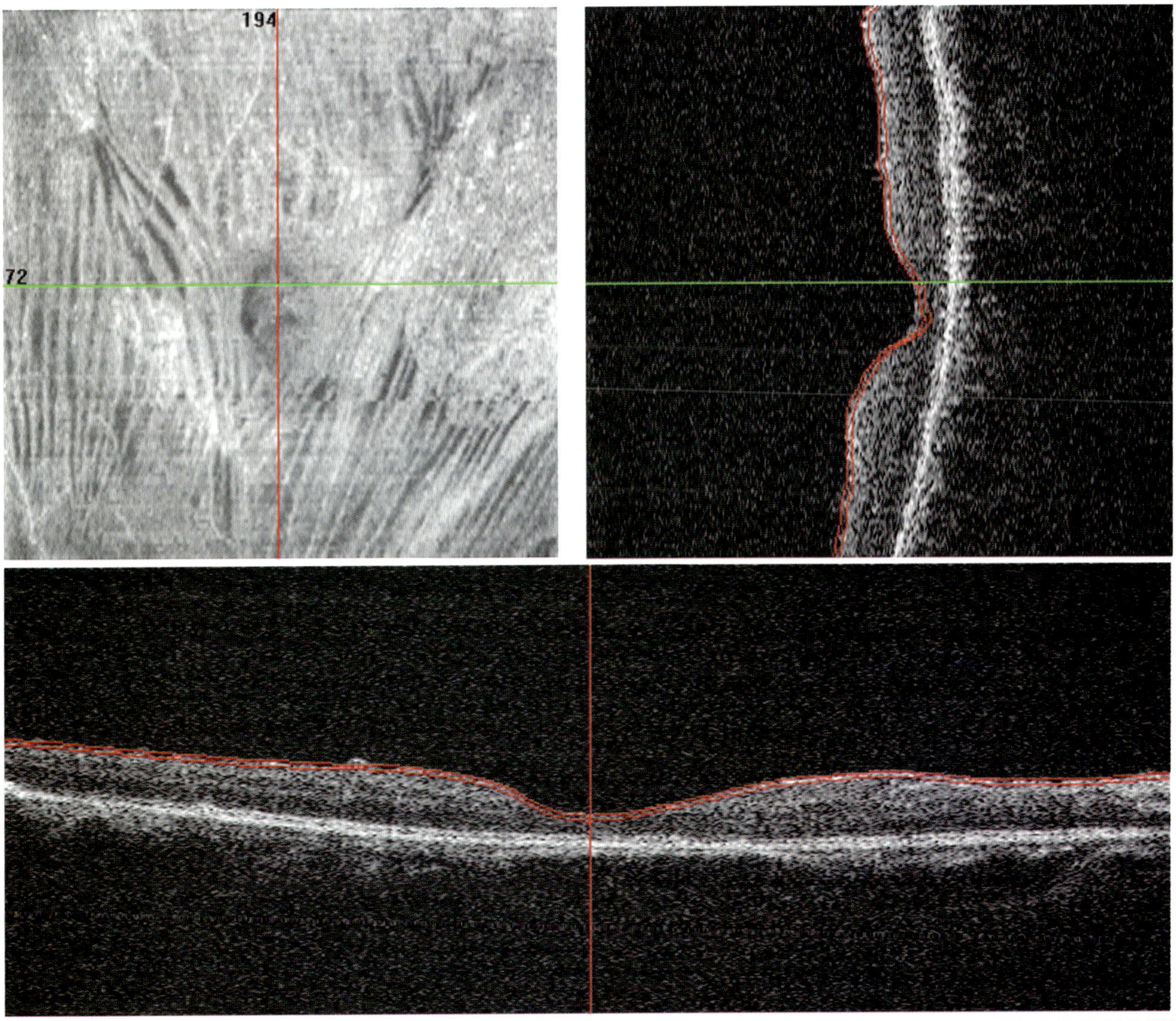

Figure 4B: Epiretinal membrane diabetic maculopathy: The frontal scan placed at retinal surface level shows retinal folds in case of tractional edema. These folds take in this case mainly a parallel vertical direction (Optovue, RTVue)

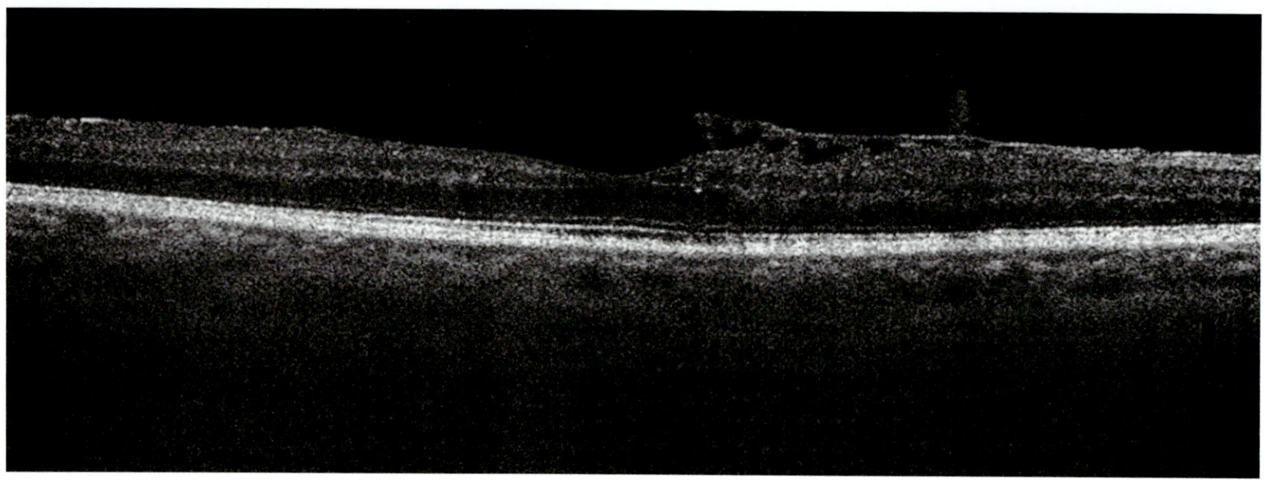

Figure 5A: Traction cystoid diabetic macular edema B scan: Retina thickness is irregular. An epiretinal membrane is loosely adherent to the retinal surface at the right hand side. Macular depression is irregular and asymmetric. Numerous folds are seen at the retinal surface (Optovue, RTVue)

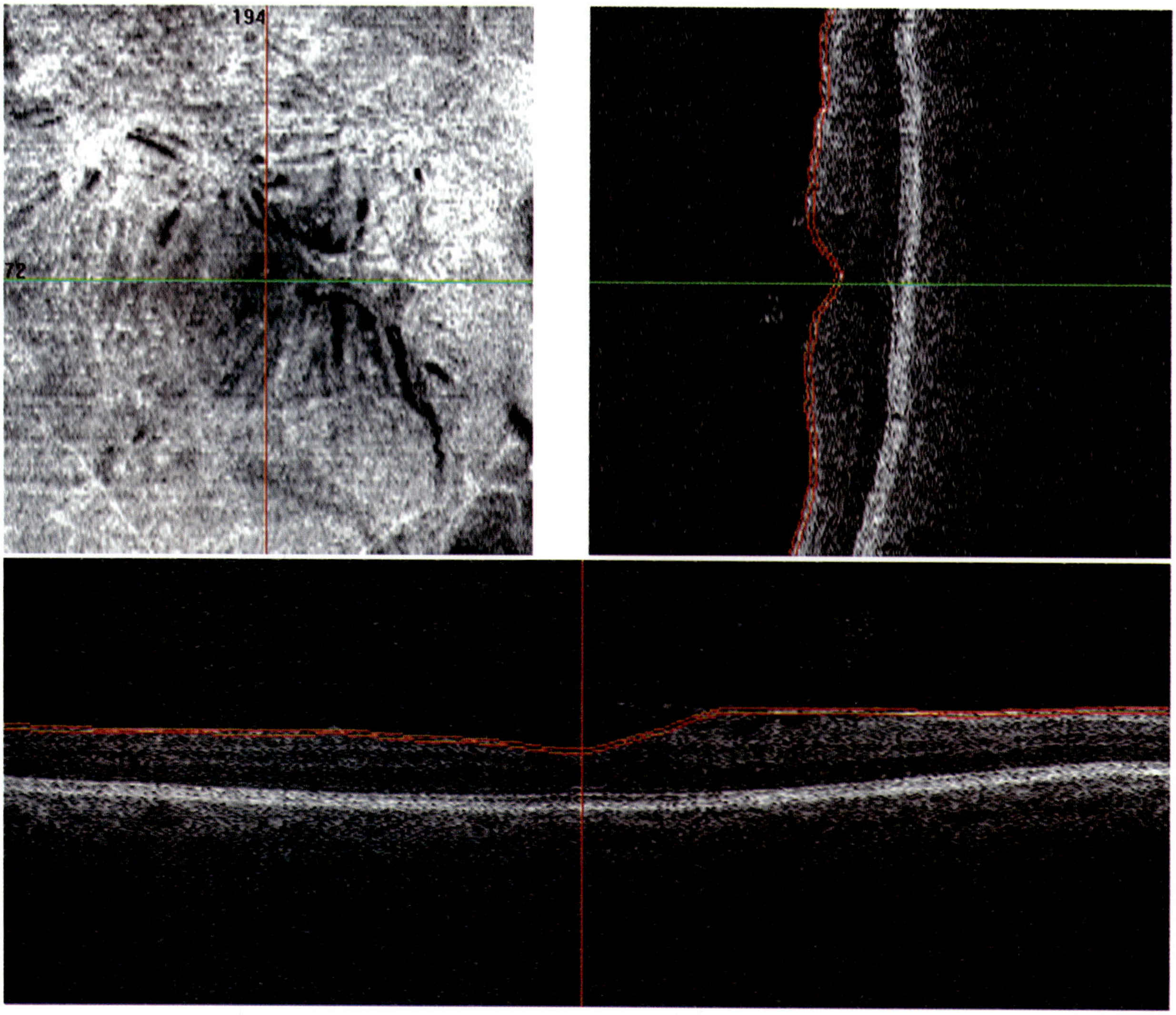

Figure 5B: Traction cystoid diabetic macular edema. The frontal scan placed at retinal surface level shows retinal folds in case of tractional edema. These folds show a stellate irregular shape (Optovue, RTVue)

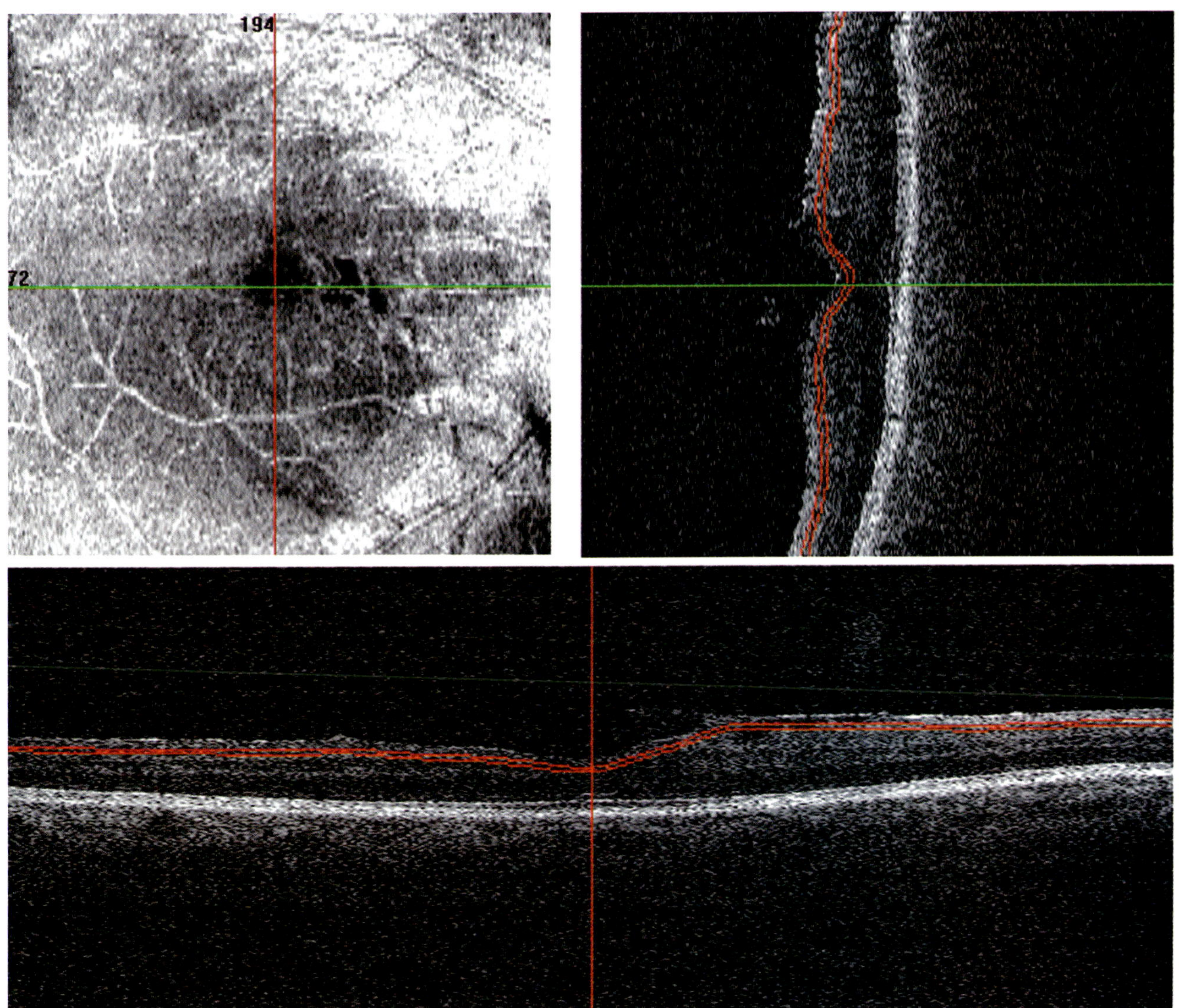

Figure 5C: Traction cystoid diabetic macular edema *en face* OCT: The frontal scan placed inside the retina, parallel to the ILM scan shows under the retinal surface few small irregular cystoid cells (Optovue, RTVue)

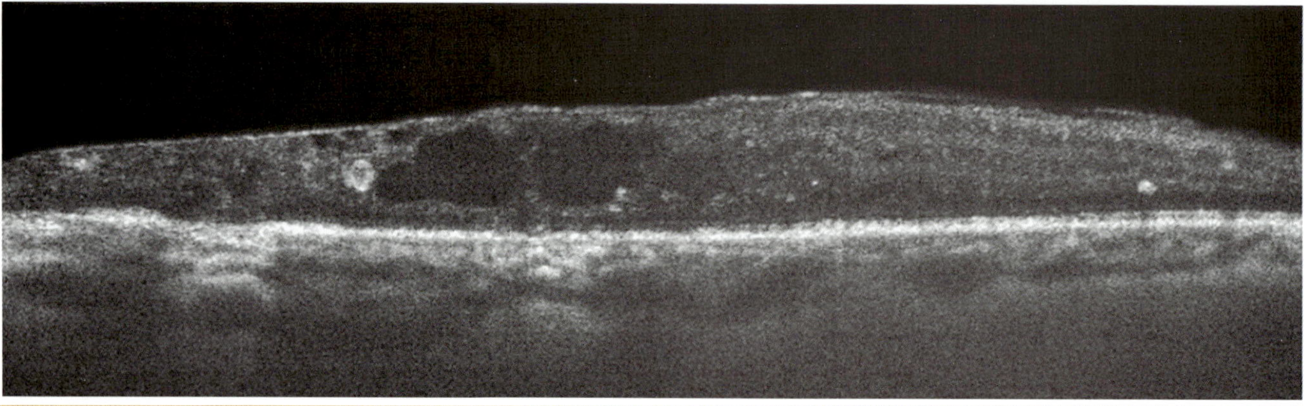

Figure 6A: Traction cystoid diabetic macular B scan: Retina has an irregularly increased thickness. An epiretinal membrane is tightly adherent to the retinal surface. Macular depression is not seen. Numerous folds at the retinal surface. Two big rectangular, irregular cystoid cells show that the edema evolution has lasted a long time (Optovue, RTVue)

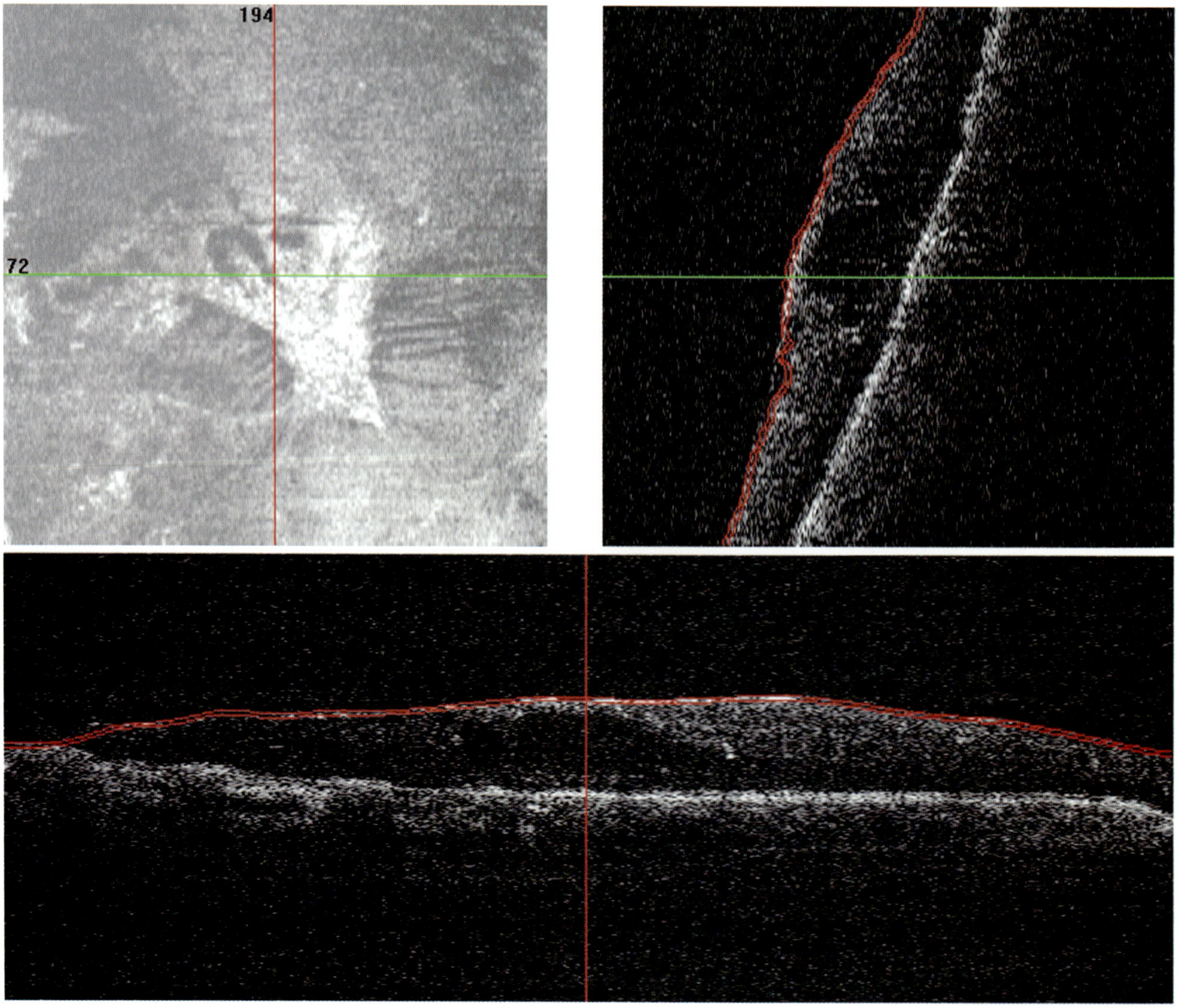

Figure 6B: Traction cystoid diabetic macular edema. The frontal scan placed at retinal surface level shows a central trapezoidal retinal plaque and numerous stellate folds (Optovue, RTVue)

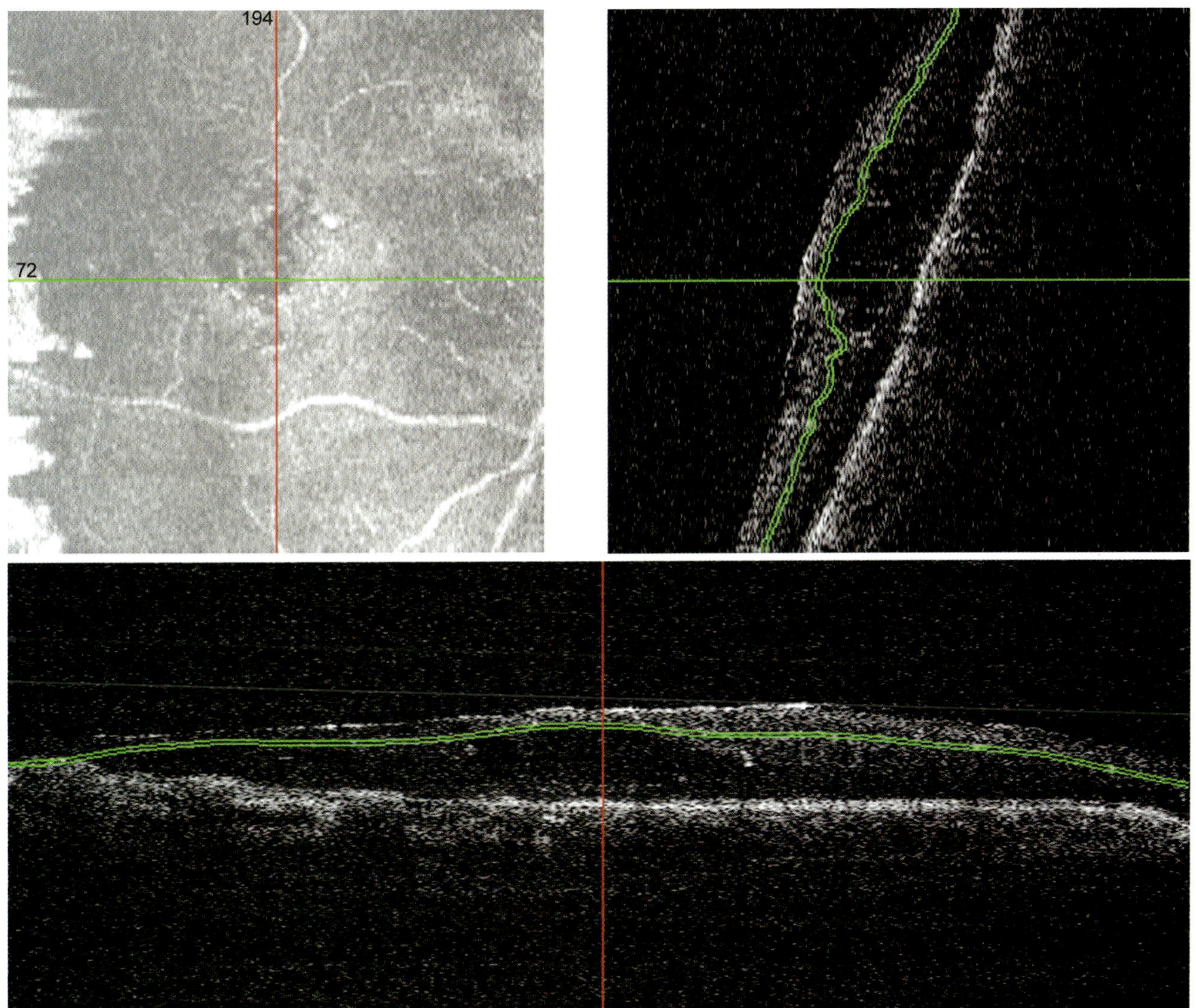

Figure 6C: Traction cystoid diabetic macular edema *en face* OCT: The frontal scan parallel to the ILM scan shows under the retinal surface few small irregular cystoid cells (Optovue, RTVue)

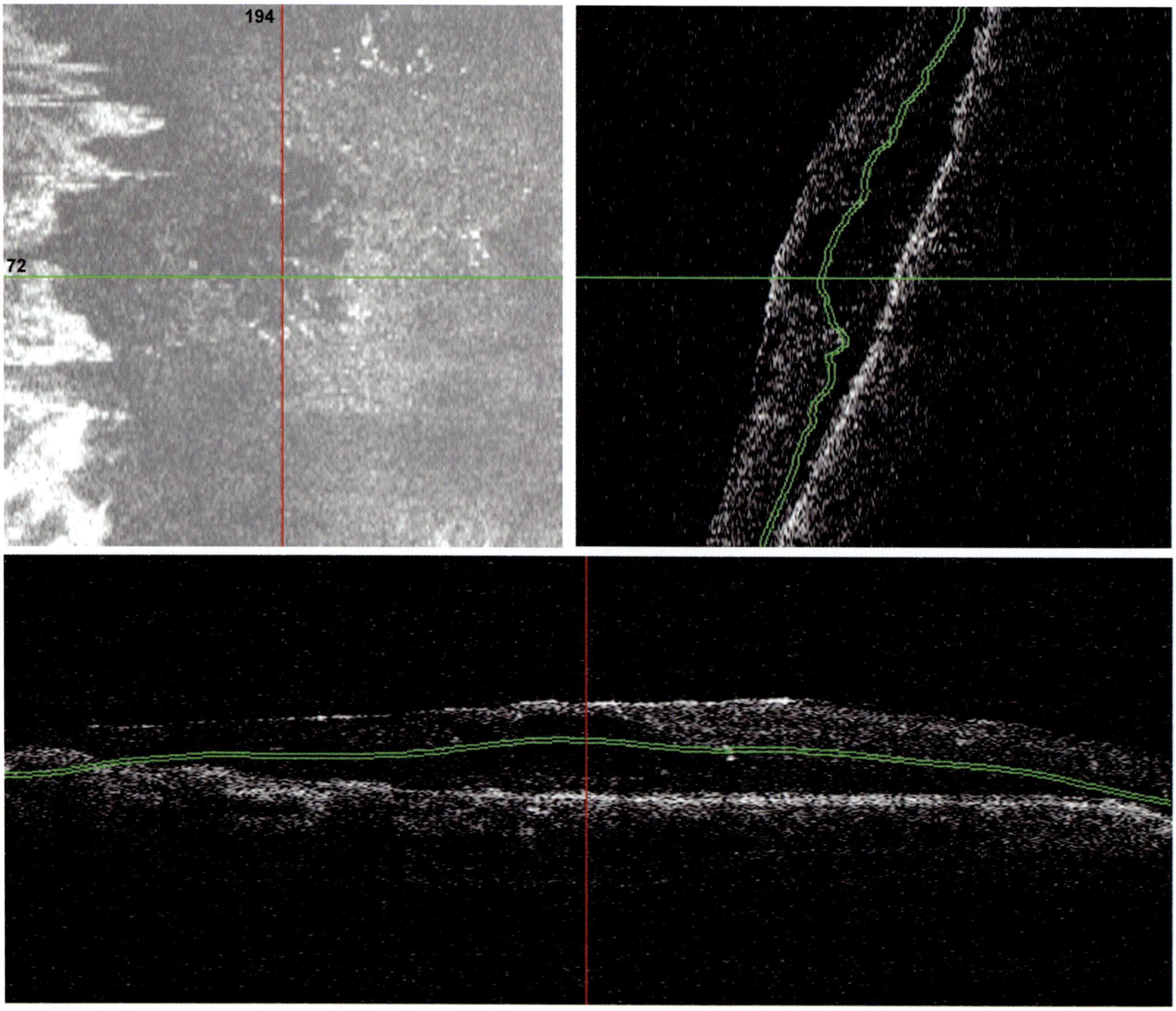

Figure 6D: Traction cystoid diabetic macular edema *en face* OCT: The frontal scan placed deeper inside the retina, parallel to the ILM scan shows at the inner nuclear layer level numerous big irregular shaped cystoid cells (Optovue, RTVue)

The frontal scan placed inside the retina under the epiretinal membranes shows at the inner nuclear layer level numerous small irregular cystoid cells. Cells are grossly ovoid, but irregular with tips converging toward the fovea.

In the outer nuclear layer bigger cystoid cells are seen, their shape is irregular and polygonal. Later in the evolution large irregular chambers with columns of residual retinal will appear **(Figures 5 and 6)**.

En face scan may follow the inner limiting membrane curvature or the pigment epithelium concavity. The profile should be selected according to the retinal or choroidal layers under study.

To study diabetic maculopathy inner limiting membrane scan will be used in case of vitreal or vitreoretinal anomalies; inner plexiform layer in case of edema or exudates. Pigment epithelium scan will be used to study outer retina, retinal exudative detachments or choroid problems.

En face technology can follow the irregularities of the inner limiting membrane. It will give tridimensional images useful to understand the lesion shape and dimensions.

References

1. Bolz M, Ritter M, Schneider M, et al. A systematic correlation of angiography and high-resolution optical coherence tomography in diabetic macular edema. Ophthalmology. 2009;116(1):66-72.
2. Pelosini L, Hull CC, Boyce JF, et al. Optical coherence tomography may be used to predict visual acuity in patients with macular edema. Invest Ophthalmol Vis Sci. 2011;52(5):2741-8.
3. Browning DJ, Apte RS, Bressler SB, et al. Association of the extent of diabetic macular edema as assessed by optical coherence tomography with visual acuity and retinal outcome variables. Retina. 2009;(3):300-5.

chapter 29

En Face Optical Coherence Tomography Scan in Inflammatory Disorders

Swapnil Parchand, Vishali Gupta, Amod Gupta

Introduction

In recent years, the important role of optical coherence tomography (OCT) in different uveitis conditions has been disclosed and the introduction of *en face* OCT scan has allowed a fine visualization of structural changes in retina or pigment epithelium.[1-7] Optical coherence tomography helps to define the extent, depth and thickness of the inflammatory lesions that helps the precise localization of the layer of retinochoroid harboring the lesion. It also helps in assessing the associated secondary changes including cystoid macular edema (CME), choroidal neovascular membrane, subretinal fluid, epiretinal membrane and subretinal fibrosis. The advantage of *en face* OCT scan over conventional OCT scan has already been discussed in previous chapters. In this chapter, the authors wish to elaborate the interpretation and utility of *en face* OCT scans in common inflammatory conditions.

Retinal Vasculitis

Retinal vasculitis is one of the important causes of vision loss in young adults. Two main causes of visual loss in vasculitis are CME and new blood vessel formation from retinal ischemia that leads to vitreous hemorrhage.[8] Optical coherence tomography is highly effective method in diagnosing CME and further assessing its response to treatment.[7]

Case Study

A 23-year-old woman presented with active vasculitis along inferotemporal arcade (green arrow) with CME (red arrow) **(Figure 1A)**. Fundus fluorescein angiography (FFA) showed profuse leakage of dye along the inferotemporal arcade suggestive of active vasculitis along with blocked fluorescence in the area of retinal hemorrhages **(Figure 1B)**. Horizontal scan passing through center of fovea shows large cystoid spaces (blue arrow) with retinal thickening at center and temporally to the fovea (yellow arrows) **(Figure 1C)**. The C scans of the right eye at presentation **(Figures 1D to F)** show an area of larger and smaller cysts (hyporeflective spaces) (blue arrow) with intervening septa (hyper-reflective bands) (red arrow) in the foveal region arranged in radial pattern. It thus allows fine visualization of the lateral extent of cystoid spaces in each scan which is not evident on conventional OCT scan. Because the foveal region is thickened by edema, the foveal pit is absent with massive serous exudation temporally (yellow arrow). Being Mantoux test positive, patient received full course of antitubercular treatment along with intravitreal injection Ozurdex. At 6 weeks of follow up **(Figure 1G)**, we can see resolution of cystoid spaces with normal foveal contour.

Inflammatory Choroidal Neovascular Membrane

Choroidal neovascular membrane (CNVM) is one of the causes for visual impairment in patients with uveitis. Many diseases like multifocal choroiditis, serpiginous choroiditis, toxoplasma retinochoroiditis, etc., can disrupt the homeostasis between the retinal pigment epithelium (RPE) and Bruch's membrane and lead to formation of CNVM.[9] Optical coherence tomography helps in documentation and precise location of CNVM with respect to various layers of retina.

Case Study

A 60-year-old woman who underwent pars plana vitrectomy for endogenous endophthalmitis presented with decreased

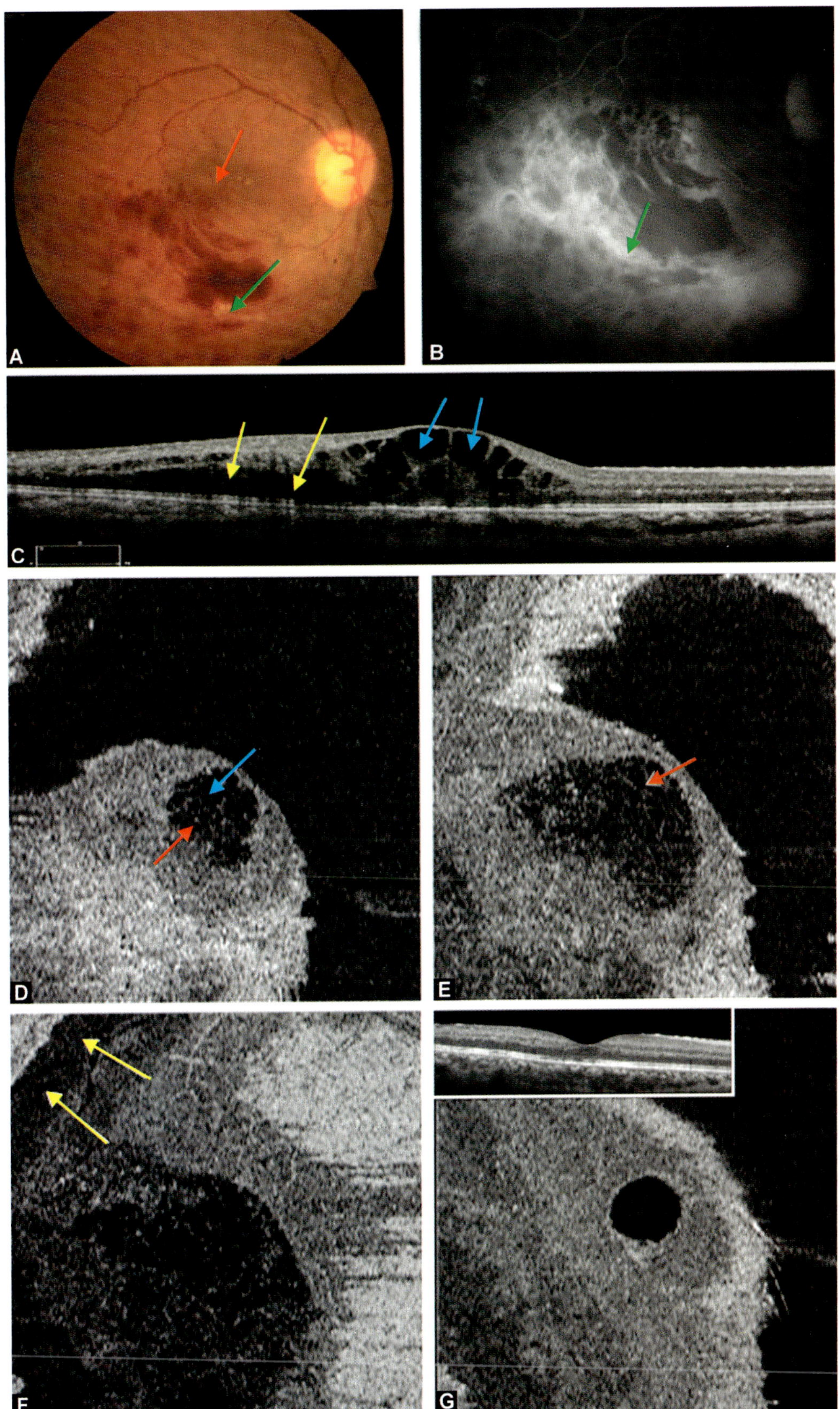

Figures 1A to G: Retinal vasculitis with cystoid macular edema: (A) Fundus picture of right eye; (B) FFA in late phase; (C) Horizontal scan passing through center of fovea; (D to F) Consecutive C scans at presentation; (G) *En face* OCT scan at 6 weeks

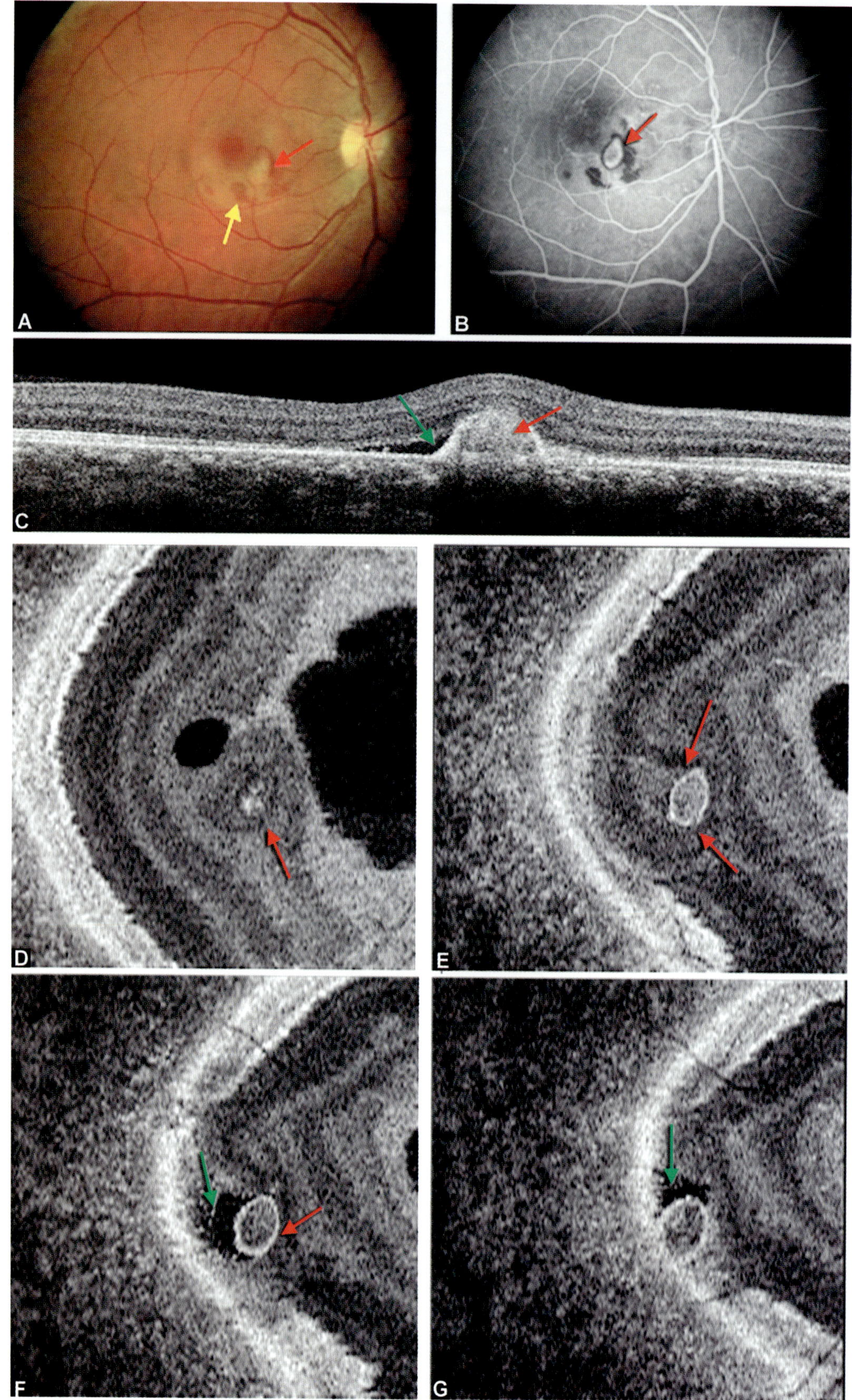

Figures 2A to G: Inflammatory choroidal neovascular membrane: (A) Fundus picture of right eye; (B) FFA in dye transit phase; (C) Raster line scan through the lesion; (D to G) Consecutive C scans

vision in the right eye. On ocular examination, right eye revealed inflammatory CNVM (red arrow) just inferonasal to fovea with subretinal bleed (yellow arrow) **(Figure 2A)**. Fundus FA showed initial mixed hyperfluorescence with late hyperfluorescence confirming CNVM **(Figure 2B)**. Raster line scan passing through center of lesion showing increased retinal thickening, nasal to fovea with increased reflectivity from the outer retinal layers suggestive of fibrovascular complex of CNVM with subretinal fluid (green arrow) **(Figure 2C)**. On consecutive C scan, hyper-reflective area (CNVM) (red arrow) is seen surrounded by relative hyporeflective area indicating the presence of fluid **(Figure 2D)**. On successive scans, circular fibrovascular CNVM is seen merging with retinal pigment epithelium and underlying choroid **(Figures 2E to G)**. Also, subretinal fluid can be seen adjacent to fibrovascular CNVM (green arrow) suggestive of active CNVM.

Vitreomacular Traction

In vitreomacular traction syndrome, an incomplete posterior vitreous detachment with persistent vitreous traction is present on the macula. This condition may determine formation of epiretinal membranes, macular pucker, macular edema and traction macular detachment. Optical coherence tomography coronal scans have allowed a fine visualization of the lateral extent and edges of the adherences of the posterior hyaloid, which appeared as a sigmoid hyper-reflective band in the black hyporeflective vitreous. Furthermore, coronal C scan images also clearly show the position of vitreoretinal adherences in relation to the structures of the posterior pole.[10]

Case Study

A 45-year-old man following pars plana vitrectomy for post cataract surgery endophthalmitis came with decreased vision in the left eye. On fundus examination, right eye showed cellophane reflex at fovea **(Figure 3A)**. On raster line scan, firm adherence of the posterior hyaloid (red arrow) to the retina is seen clearly causing traction at center with subfoveal serous detachment (blue arrow) **(Figure 3G)**. The *en face* scan (C scan) **(Figures 3B to F)** showing moderate hyper-reflective band (posterior hyaloid) (red arrow) in the hyporeflective vitreal chamber. On subsequent scans hyaloid is seen pulling the retina causing distortion of retinal tissue which is evident by serrated internal limiting membrane (yellow arrow). Since the scan is slightly tilted, the bottom of this circular structure shows its point of adhesion and traction to the retinal surface (green arrow) with different retinal layers seen within the same scan.

Epiretinal Membrane

Patients with posterior uveitis may develop thin translucent membrane on inner surface of retina in macular area (epiretinal membrane) which may contribute to the development of macular edema.[11,12] Optical coherence tomography helps in assessing the adhesiveness of the membranes to the retinal surface and changes seen in the underlying retina. Based on OCT, ERM have been classified as: (1) clearly separable where a clear space is visible between the ERM and inner retinal surface; and (2) globally adherent where no clear area of separation is seen between ERM and inner retinal surface. The C scan of ERM shows the complete structure of the membrane in the form of radial lines extending from the traction's epicenter with all its extensions in a radiating pattern along with retinal folds; this was not possible with the conventional B scan mode of OCT.[7] Thus, one can determine the areas of ERM where there is some space between it and the retinal surface. This may aid in the planning dissection sites for surgical removal of ERM.

Case Study

A 56-year-old man who was treated in past for intermediate uveitis with CME developed ERM on follow up after 4 years. Fundus picture and red free picture show cellophane reflex in macular area **(Figures 4A and B)**. On raster line scan fine hyper-reflective membrane (red arrow) is seen over fovea suggestive of ERM **(Figure 4C)**. Consecutive *en face* scans **(Figures 4D to G)** show ERM attached to inner surface of retina with fibrous tags (yellow arrow). Also, serrated internal limiting membrane indicating ERM pull at the retinal surface can be seen. This is type 1 ERM. The surface of the membrane was visible when the plane of the C scan was superficial at the level of vitreous-retina interface. As the plane of the C scan had travelled deeper (changing the Z coordinate), the ERM appeared less visible and the retinal layers started appearing as concentric rings in *en face* imaging. The *en face* imaging of ERM showed the complete structure of the membrane along with the traction's epicenter.

Vogt-Koyanagi-Harada Syndrome

Vogt-Koyanagi-Harada syndrome is characterized by anterior uveitis, exudative retinal detachment with yellowish white lesions. Optical coherence tomography is a useful tool to measure and monitor serous retinal detachment during acute and chronic stages of VKH disease.[13-16] It also detects RPE hypertrophy and fibrosis in the chronic phase of the disease.

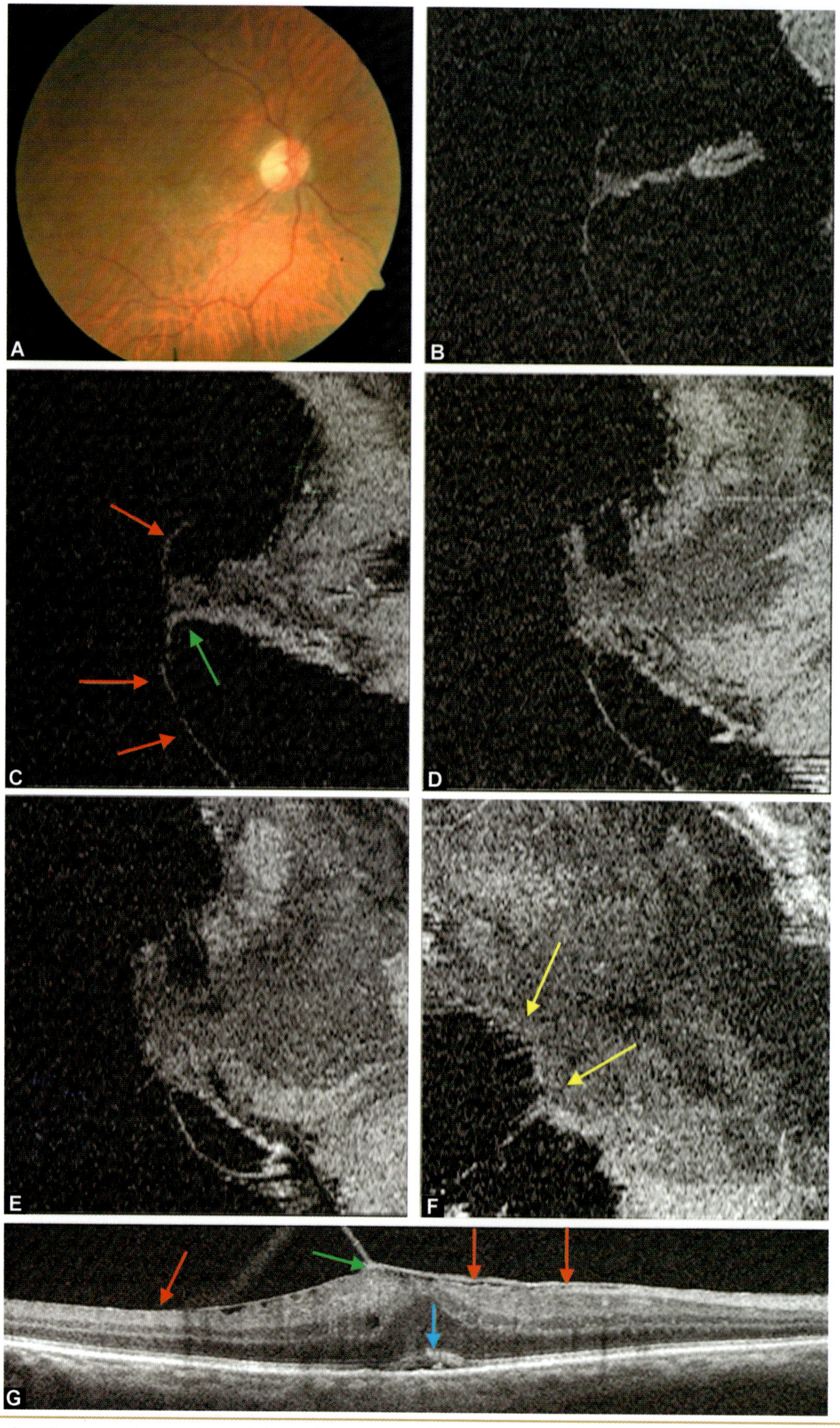

Figures 3A to G: Vitreomacular traction: (A) Fundus picture of right eye; (B to F) Consecutive C scans; (G) Raster line scan

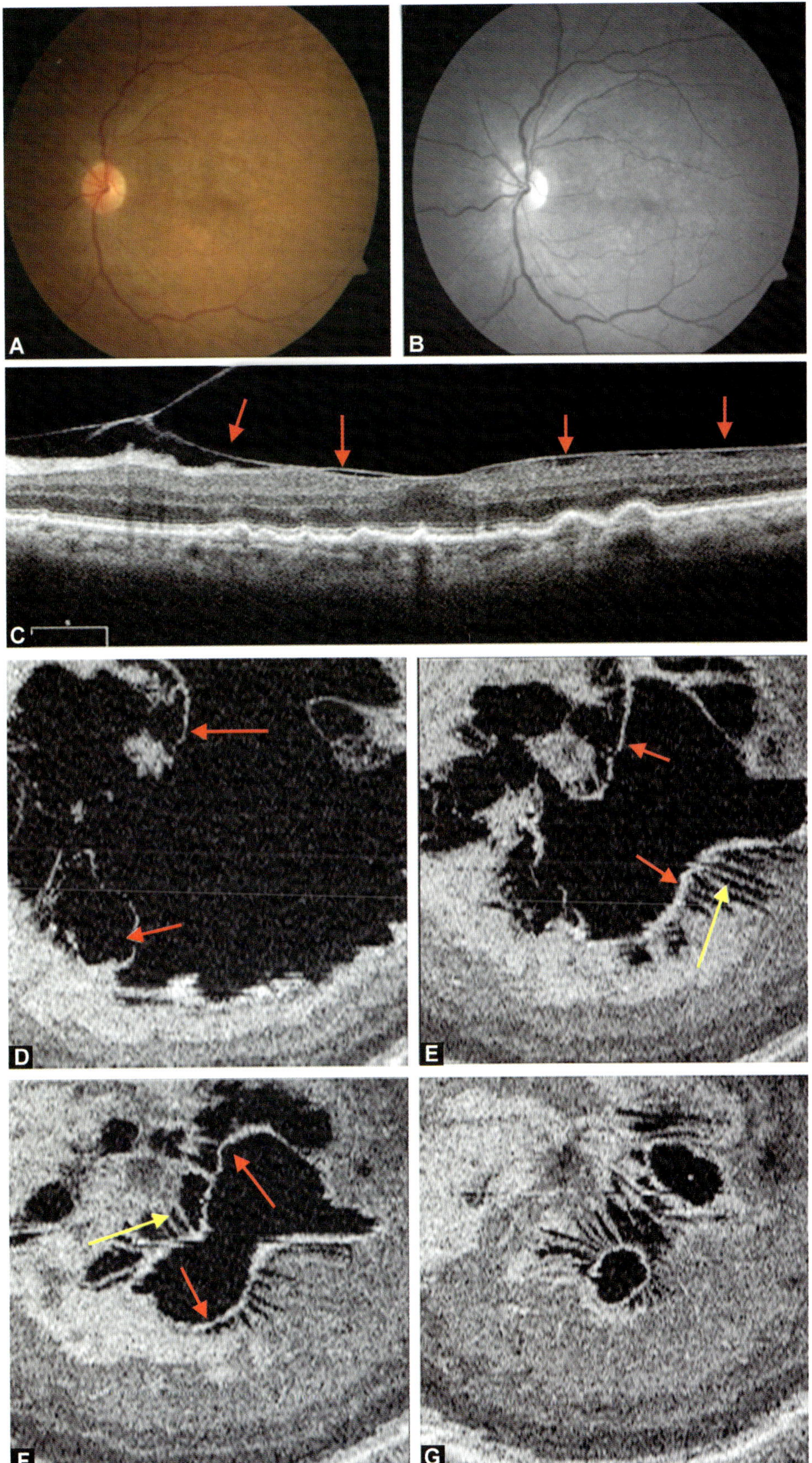

Figures 4A to G: Epiretinal membrane: (A) Fundus picture of left eye; (B) Red free picture highlighting the membrane; (C) Raster line scan; (D to G) Consecutive C scans

Case Study 1

Fundus picture of a 25-year-old woman showing multiple serous detachments of neurosensory and yellowish white lesions at posterior pole area (**Figure 5A**). Fundus FA showed multiple hyperfluorescent areas initially with pooling of dye in late phase confirming multiple detachments (**Figure 5B**). Raster line scan through center of fovea showed multiple areas of serous detachment (red arrow) with intraretinal pockets (green arrow) (**Figure 5C**). Consecutive C scans (**Figures 5D to F**) in depth indicate the extent of serous detachment and intraretinal pockets in the various areas. Note that the serous detachments are irregularly shaped. Patient received five doses of intravenous injection methylprednisolone followed by oral steroids with immunosuppression. At 2 weeks (**Figure 5G**), we can see resolution of serous detachment with normal architecture of retina.

Case Study 2

Fundus picture of 21-year-old woman shows hazy media due to vitritis with hyperemic disk and exudative retinal detachment (blue arrow) (**Figure 6A**). Fundus FA confirmed the diagnosis of VKH (**Figure 6B**). The raster line scan shows hyporeflective space between neurosensory retina (red arrow) and RPE (green arrow) indicating the presence of clear serous fluid (**Figure 6C**). On consecutive C scan, we can see wide separation of neurosensory retina from RPE which is not so evident on raster line scan (**Figures 6D to F**). This patient also received five doses of injection methylprednisolone followed by oral steroid with immuno-suppression. At 3 weeks follow up, we can still see some subretinal fluid (**Figure 6G,** blue arrow). At this point of time no hurry should be made to taper off steroids.

Case Study 3

A 32-year-old woman presented with vitritis, hyperemic disk and exudative retinal detachment in both the eyes (**Figure 7A**). Fundus FA confirmed the diagnosis of VKH (**Figure 7B**). Raster line scan passing through the center of fovea shows subretinal serous detachment with moderate back-scattering suggesting the presence of turbid fluid (**Figure 7C**). Also, visible are the moderate hyper-reflective area between neurosensory retina and RPE suggestive of deposition of subretinal fibrin. On *en face* OCT scan (**Figures 7D to F**), fibrin (yellow arrow) is more clearly seen between neurosensory retina and RPE surrounded by turbid fluid. Clear exudative fluid (green arrow) can also be seen at periphery of exudation. At 1 month follow up on oral steroid and immunosuppressives (**Figure 7G**), fibrin as well as exudative detachment has resolved.

Sympathetic Ophthalmia

Sympathetic ophthalmia is bilateral, diffuse granulomatous panuveitis that occurs after trauma or surgery in one or both of the eyes. Optical coherence tomography helps, in these patients, to detect associated CME and monitor the resolution of exudative retinal detachment in serial follow up.[5,17]

Case Study

An 18-year-old man with prior history of repaired corneal laceration in left eye 4 months back (**Figure 8C**) presented with sudden onset decreased vision in the right eye of 3 days duration. He had moderate anterior segment inflammation with vitritis. Fundoscopy of right eye showed hyperemic disk and exudative retinal detachment at posterior pole (**Figure 8A**). Fundus FA showed initial areas of delayed choroidal filling with late pooling of dye in peripapillary and posterior pole area (**Figure 8B**). Raster line scan passing through center of fovea showed multiple intraretinal (green arrow) and subretinal pockets of fluid (red arrow) with retinal thickening nasal to fovea (**Figure 8D**). Consecutive *en face* OCT scan showed lateral extent of serous detachment. Also multiple pockets of intraretinal fluid can be seen more clearly in deeper scans (**Figures 8E to G**). With intensive steroids and immunosuppression patient was managed successively (**Figure 8H**).

Behçet's Disease

Eye is the most commonly involved organ in Behçet's disease and typical form of involvement is relapsing and remitting panuveitis and retinal vasculitis. In Behçet's disease, OCT is used to detect and monitor macular edema. Other macular pathologies including serous retinal detachment, epiretinal membrane, macular hole and atrophy can also be diagnosed on OCT.[1,18]

Case Study

A 32-year-old man was seen with diffuse perivenous sheathing and hemorrhages all over the retina (**Figure 9A**). He had active oral and genital ulcer. Fundus FA showed diffuse capillary leakage (**Figure 9B**). Raster line scan passing through center of fovea showed retinal edema with serous retinal detachment (**Figure 9C**). *En face* scan at presentation (**Figures 9D and E**) shows diffuse retinal thickening (red arrow) with distorted retinal layers in the area of opacification with subretinal fluid (green arrow). Patient was treated with intensive systemic steroids with immunosuppressive treatment. On follow up at 4 weeks (**Figures 9F and G**), retinal thickness has decreased (red arrow) with resolution of exudative detachment (green arrow).

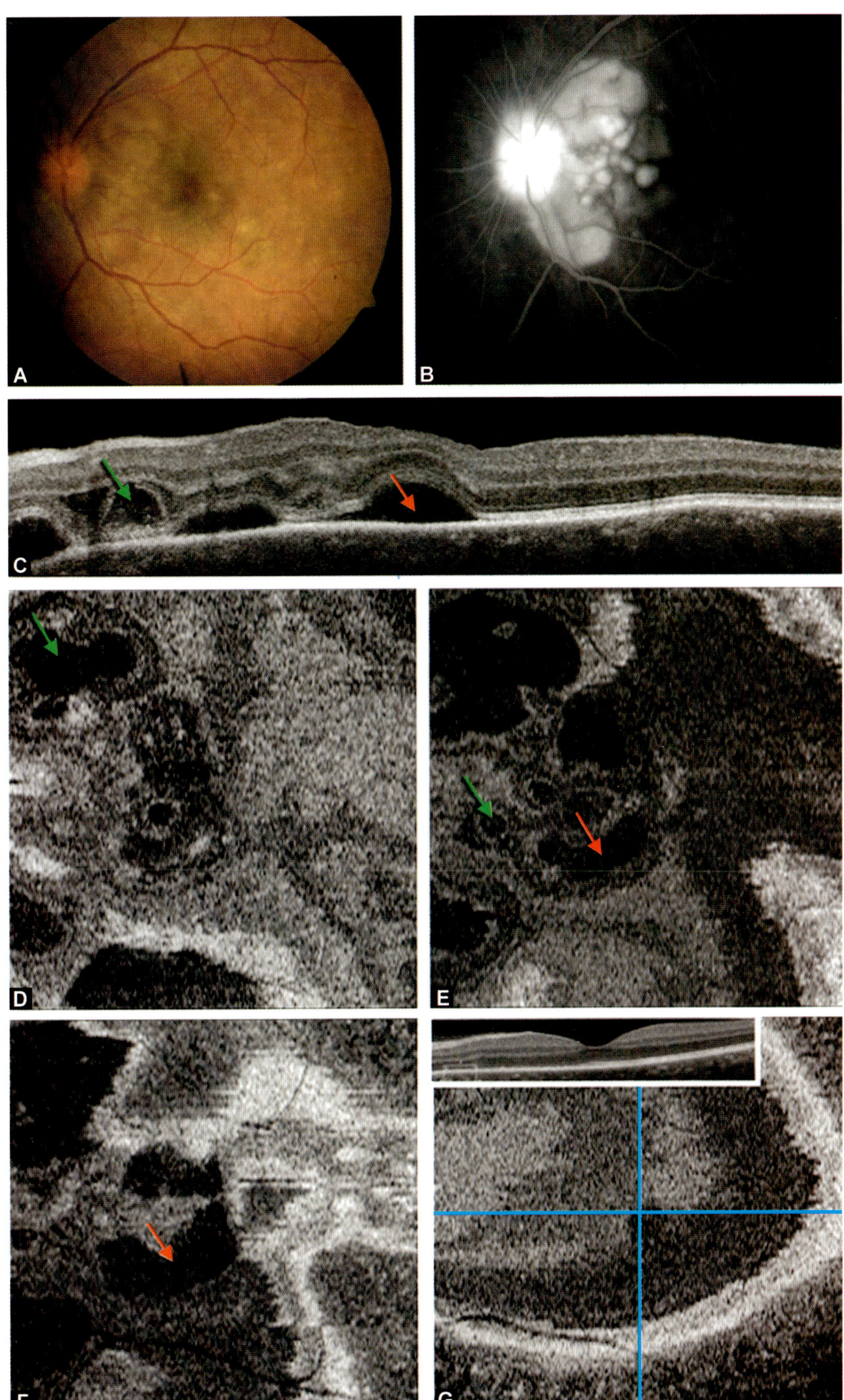

Figures 5A to G: Vogt-Koyanagi-Harada syndrome (Case 1): (A) Fundus picture of left eye; (B) FFA in late phase; (C) Raster line scan; (D to F) Consecutive C scans at presentation; (G) *En face* OCT scan at 2 weeks

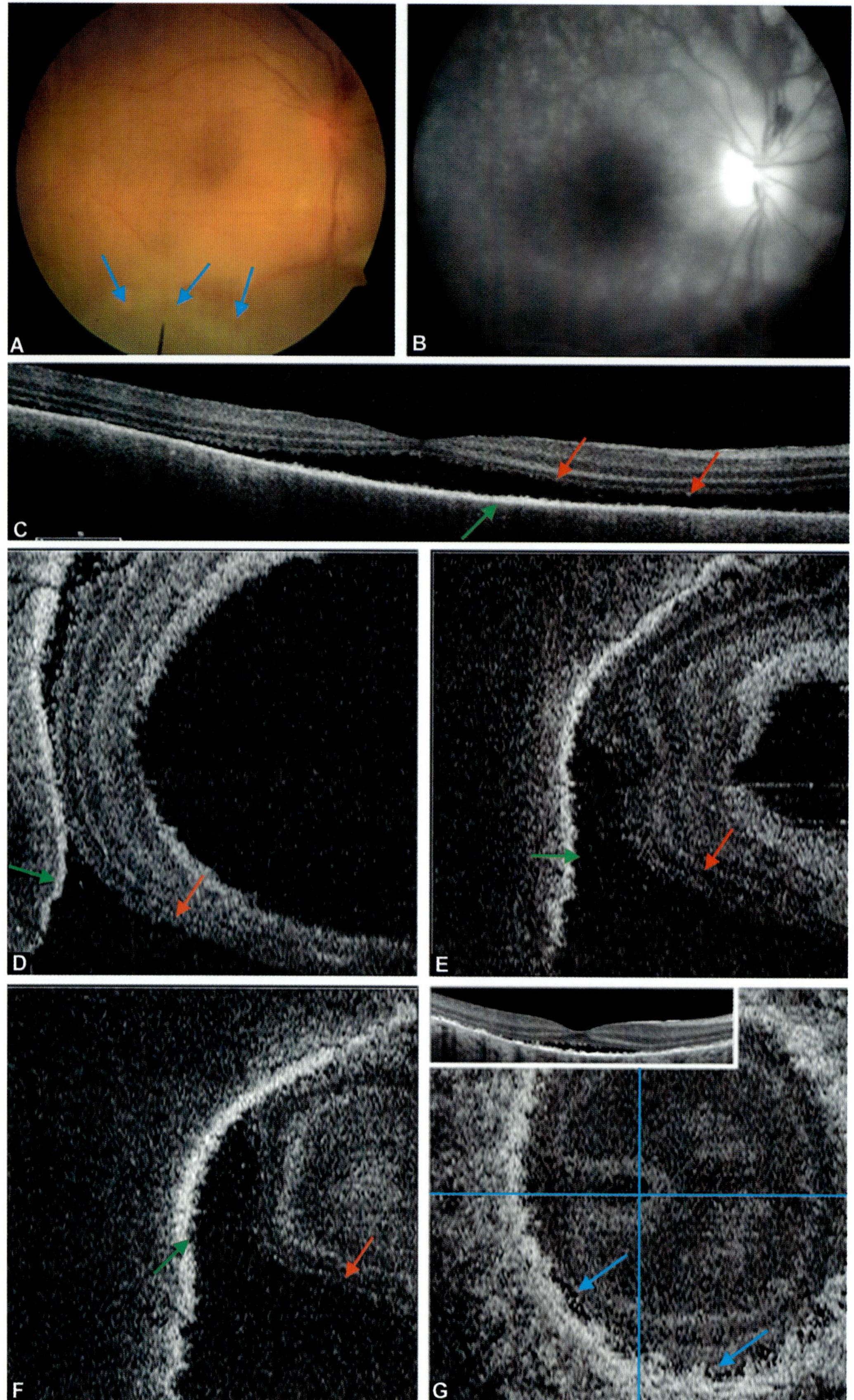

Figures 6A to G: Vogt-Koyanagi-Harada syndrome (Case 2): (A) Fundus picture of right eye; (B) FFA in late phase; (C) Raster line scan; (D to F) Consecutive C scans at presentation; (G) *En face* OCT scan at 3 weeks

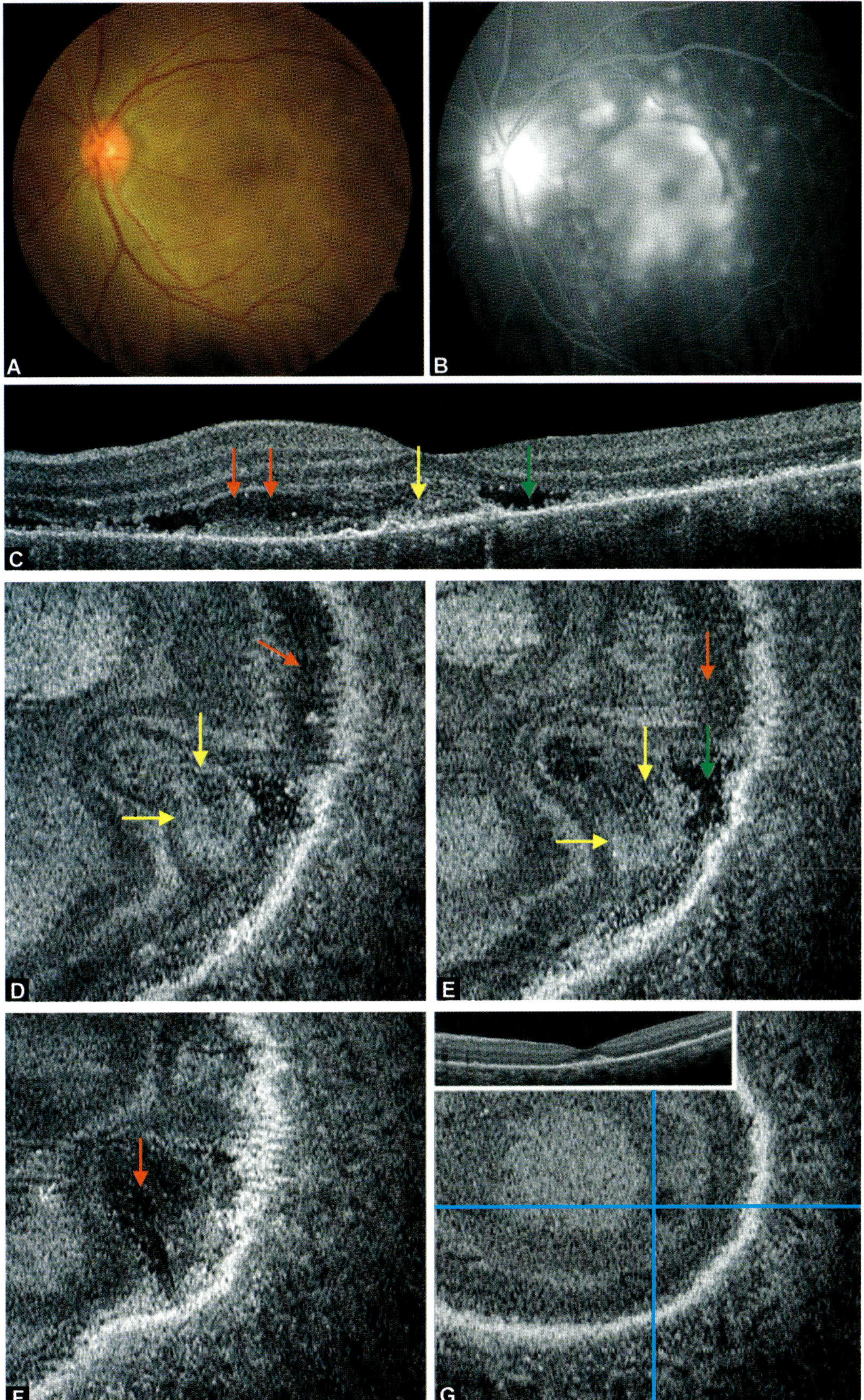

Figures 7A to G: Vogt-Koyanagi-Harada syndrome (Case 3): (A) Fundus picture of left eye; (B) FFA in late phase; (C) Raster line scan; (D to F) Consecutive C scans at presentation; (G) *En face* OCT scan at 1 month

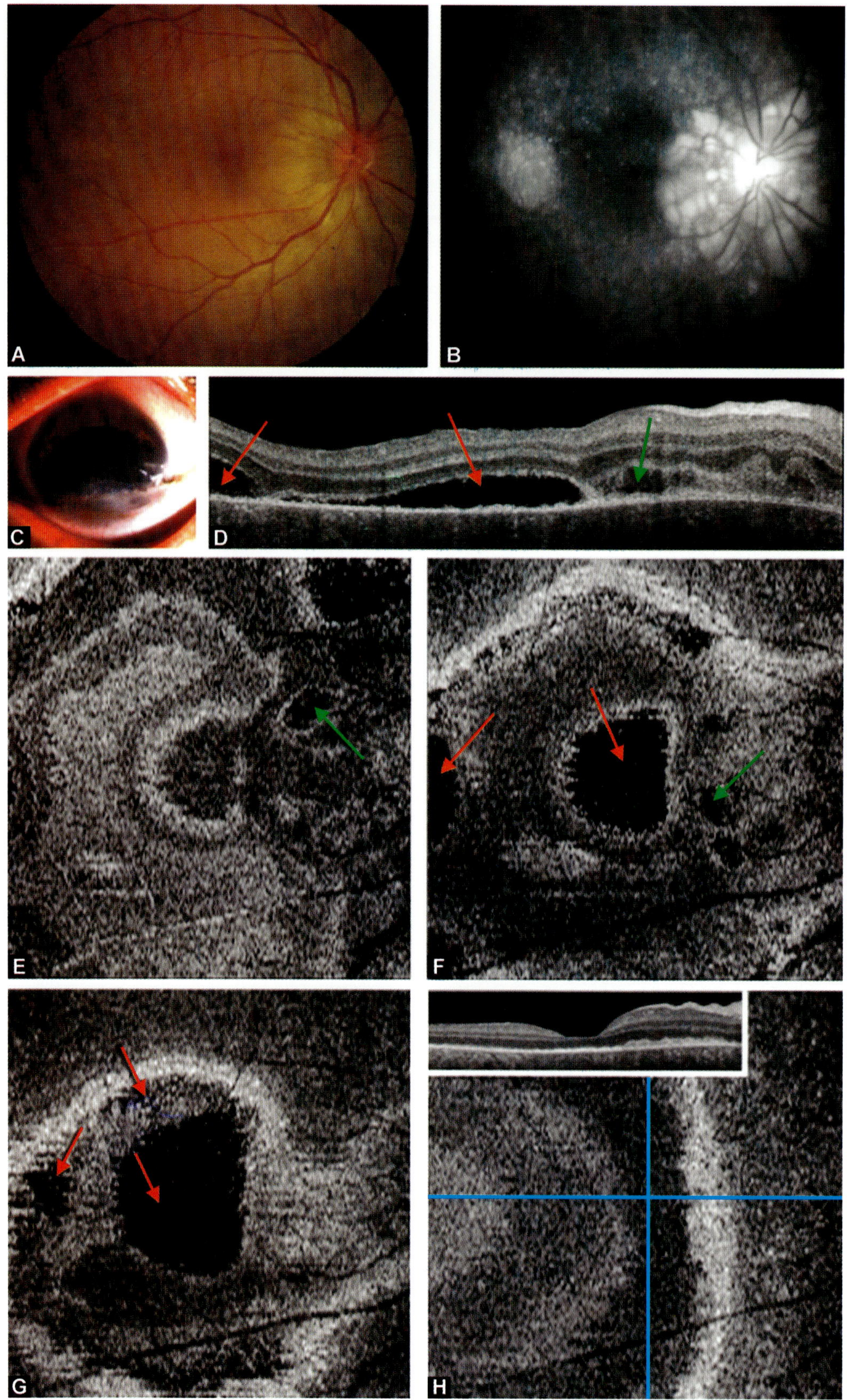

Figures 8A to G: Sympathetic ophthalmia: (A) Fundus picture of right eye; (B) FFA in late phase; (C) Anterior segment photograph of left eye showing repaired corneal laceration wound; (D) Raster line scan; (E to G) Consecutive C scans at presentation; (H) *En face* OCT scan at 4 weeks

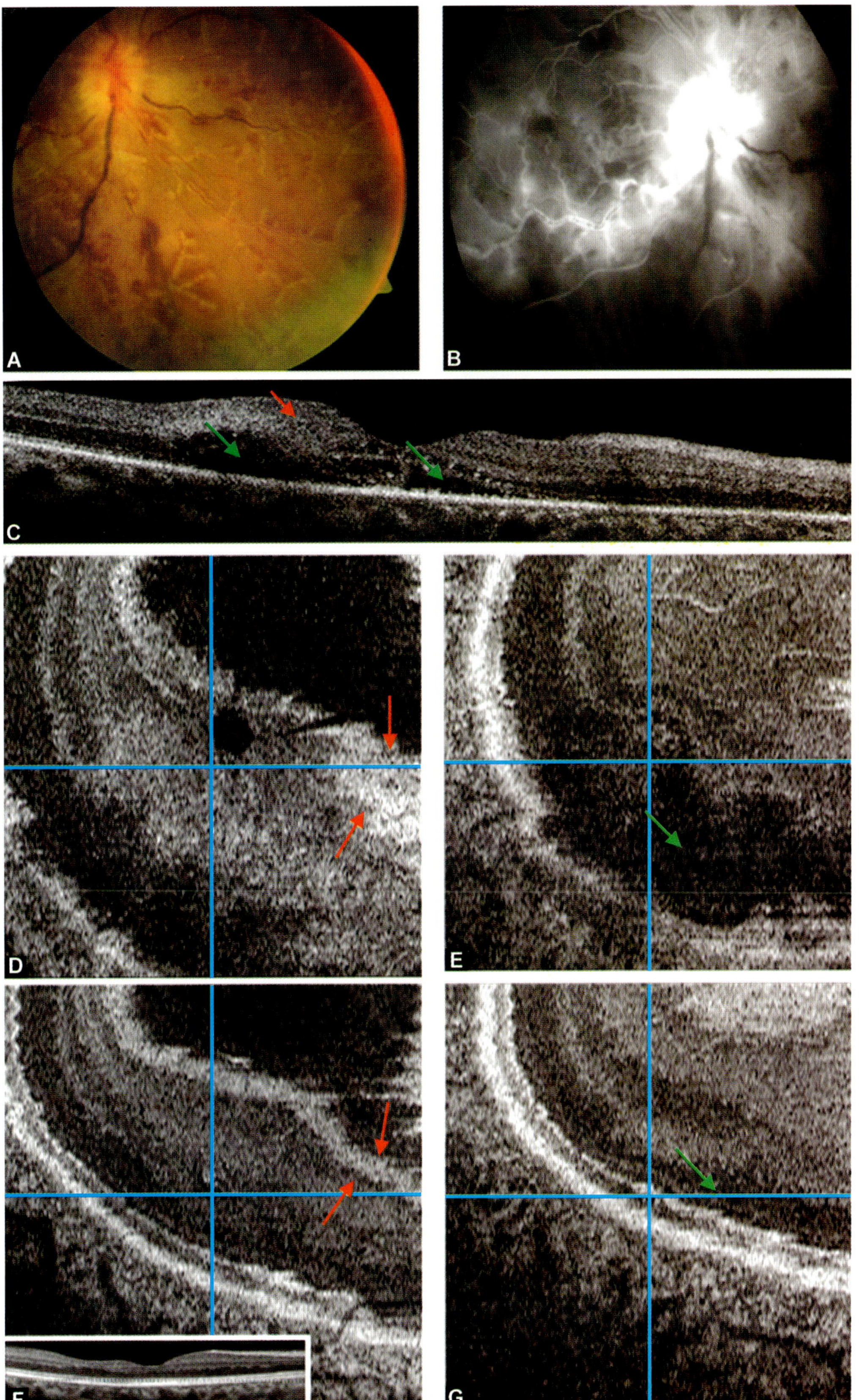

Figures 9A to G: Behcet's disease: (A) Fundus picture of right eye mainly showing inferonasal area; (B) FFA in late phase showing diffuse leakage; (C) Raster line scan; (D and E) Consecutive C scan at presentation; (F and G) *En face* OCT scan at 4 weeks

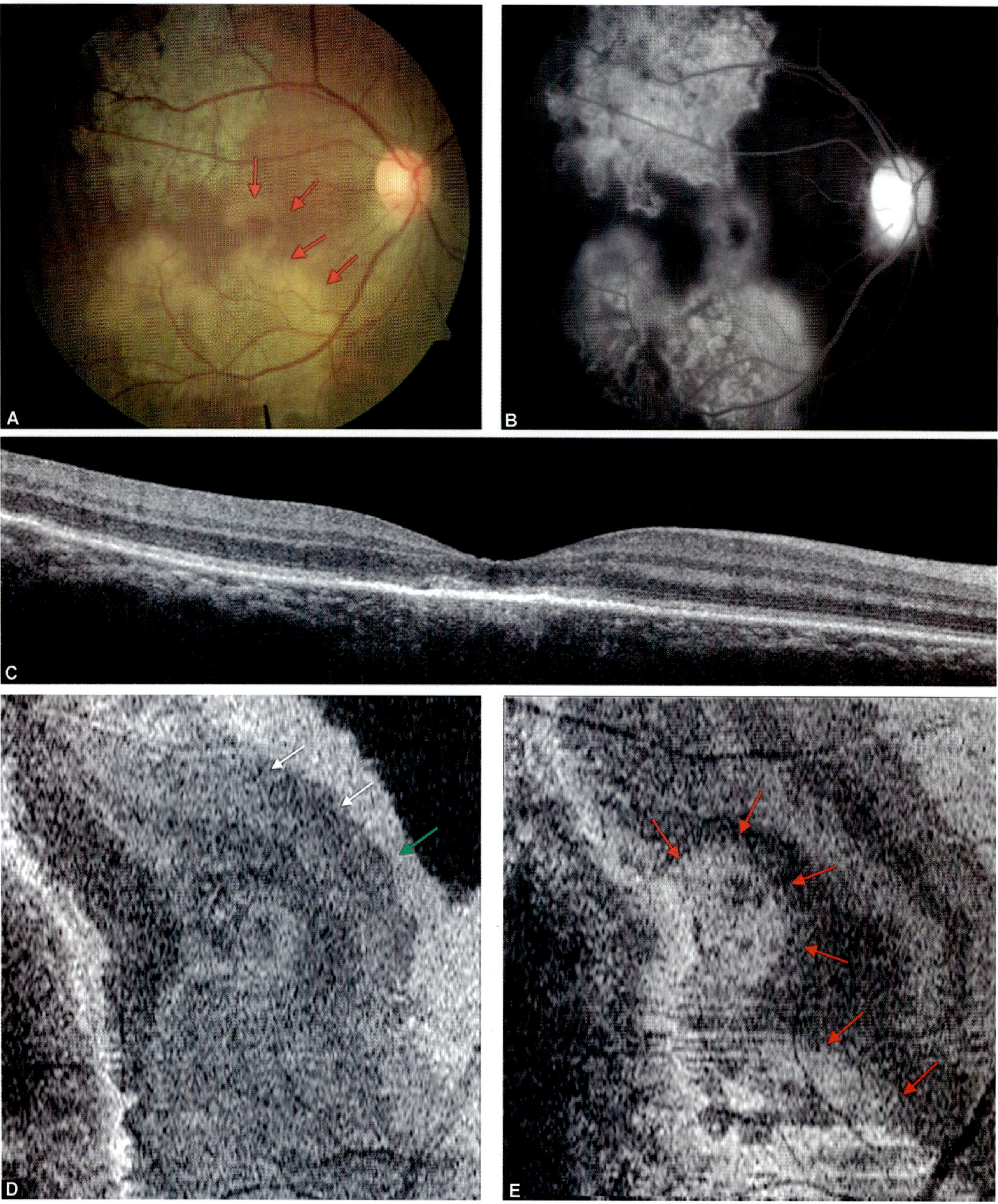

Figures 10A to E: Active phase of serpiginous choroiditis (Case 1): (A) Fundus picture of right eye showing active choroiditis lesions; (B) FFA in late phase; (C) Raster line scan; (D and E) Consecutive C scans

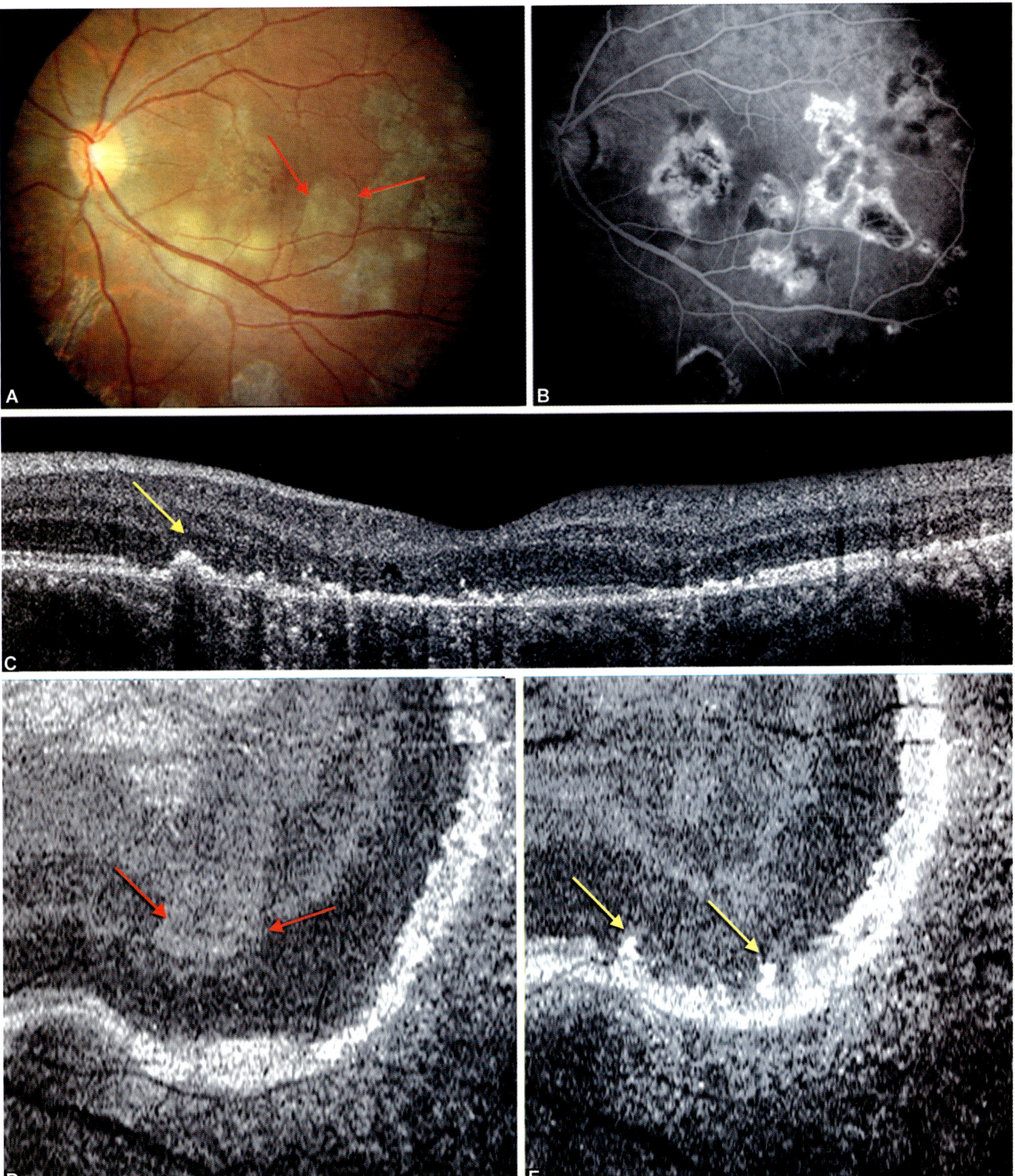

Figures 11A to E: Healing phase of serpiginous choroiditis (Case 2): (A) Fundus picture of left eye showing healing choroiditis leions; (B) FFA in late phase; (C) Raster line scan; (D and E) Consecutive C scans

Serpiginous Choroiditis

Serpiginous choroiditis (SC) is a progressive, chronic, recurrent inflammatory disease primarily affecting the inner choroid and RPE cell layer. They spread with an active edge and heal with destruction of choroid and overlying retina and pigment epithelium.[19,20] We can observe the structural changes on OCT scans occurring during the course of SC and follow a stepwise orderly sequence, similar to those as seen on the FAF images.[21]

Case Study 1

Fundoscopy of a patient with active serpiginous-like choroiditis (**Figure 10A**). Fundus FA showing active leakage of dye at the margin of lesion (**Figure 10B**). Raster line scan showing hyper-reflective area in the outer retina (**Figure 10C**). *En face* OCT scan (**Figures 10D and E**) showed a localized, fuzzy area of hyper-reflectivity (red arrow) in the outer retinal layers involving the RPE, photoreceptor outer segment tips (POST), photoreceptor inner segment/outer segment (IS/OS) junction, external limiting membrane (ELM) and the outer nuclear layer. The lesion was localized external to the outer plexiform layer with a mild distortion of the inner retinal layers (green arrow). Hyper-reflectivity in the outer retinal layers in an active SC lesion is believed to be suggestive of acute inflammation involving deeper retinal and choroidal structures.

Case Study 2

Fundoscopy and FFA of the patient showing healing serpiginous-like choroiditis lesion (**Figures 11A and B**). In this case, *en face* scan (**Figure 11D**) showed more compact hyper-reflective area corresponding to area of healing patch of choroiditis (red arrow). **Figures 11C and E** show irregular, hyper-reflective knobbly elevations of the outer retinal layers (yellow arrow). The RPE, the POST, IS/OS junction and the ELM could not be distinguished. At this stage, there was an increased reflectance from the choroidal layers due to attenuating RPE-photoreceptor complex. Following an acute inflammatory episode, the RPE cells undergo hyperplasia and hypertrophy which is evident as hyperautofluorescence on fundus autofluorescence due to increased collection of lipofuscin. This corresponds to the localized, knobbly elevations of the outer retinal layers which represents clumping of the inflamed RPE cells. Once these damaged RPE cells undergo atrophy, there is an irreversible loss of photoreceptors giving rise to the loss of the outer retinal layers on OCT.

References

1. Gupta V, Gupta A, Dogra MR. Inflammatory diseases of retino-choroid. In: Gupta V, Gupta A, Dogra MR (Eds). Atlas Optical Coherence Tomography Of Macular Diseases. New Delhi: Jaypee Brothers Medical Publishers (P) Ltd; 2010. pp. 458-540.
2. Gupta V, Gupta A. Time domain optical coherence tomography. In: Gupta A, Gupta V, Herbort C, Khairallah M (Eds). Uveitis Text and Imaging. New Delhi: Jaypee Brothers Medical Publishers (P) Ltd; 2009. pp. 180-222.
3. Velthoven M, Garcia P, Rosen R, et al. Optical coherence tomography and confocal ophthalmoscopy. In: Gupta A, Gupta V, Herbort C, Khairallah M (Eds). Uveitis Text and Imaging. New Delhi: Jaypee Brothers Medical Publishers (P) Ltd; 2009. pp. 201-11.
4. Gupta V, Gupta A. Spectral domain OCT. In: Gupta A, Gupta V, Herbort C, Khairallah M (Eds). Uveitis Text and Imaging. New Delhi: Jaypee Brothers Medical Publishers (P) Ltd; 2009. pp. 212-22.
5. Gallagher MJ, Yilmaz T, Cervantes-Castañeda RA, et al. The characteristic features of optical coherence tomography in posterior uveitis. Br J Ophthalmol. 2007;91(12): 1680-5.
6. Gupta V, Gupta P, Singh R, et al. Spectral-domain Cirrus high-definition optical coherence tomography is better than time-domain Stratus optical coherence tomography for evaluation of macular pathologic features in uveitis. Am J Ophthalmol. 2008;145(6):1018-22.
7. van Velthoven ME, Verbraak FD, Yannuzzi LA, et al. Imaging the retina by *en face* optical coherence tomography. Retina. 2006;26(2):129-36.
8. Palmer HE, Stanford MR, Sanders MD, et al. Visual outcome of patients with idiopathic ischaemic and non-ischaemic retinal vasculitis. Eye (Lond). 1996;10(Pt 3): 343-8.
9. Ciardella AP, Prall FR, Borodoker N, et al. Imaging techniques for posterior uveitis. Curr Opin Ophthalmol. 2004;15(6):519-30.
10. Forte R, Pascotto F, de Crecchio G. Visualization of vitreomacular tractions with *en face* optical coherence tomography. Eye (Lond). 2007;21(11):1391-4.
11. Kiryu J, Kita M, Tanabe T, et al. Pars plana vitrectomy for epiretinal membrane associated with sarcoidosis. Jpn J Ophthalmology. 2003;47(5):479-83.
12. Dev S, Mieler WF, Pulido JS, et al. Visual outcomes after pars plana vitrectomy for epiretinal membranes associated with pars planitis. Ophthalmology. 1999;106(6): 1086-90.
13. Maruyama Y, Kishi S. Tomographic features of serous retinal detachment in Vogt-Koyanagi-Harada syndrome. Ophthalmic Surg Lasers Imaging. 2004;35(3):239-42.
14. Parc C, Guenoun JM, Dhote R, et al. Optical coherence tomography in the acute and chronic phases of Vogt-Koyanagi-Harada disease. Ocul Immunol Inflamm. 2005;13(2-3):225-7.

15. Yamanaka E, Ohguro N, Yamamoto S, et al. Evaluation of pulse corticosteroid therapy for Vogt-Koyanagi-Harada disease assessed by optical coherence tomography. Am J Ophthalmol. 2002;134(3):454-6.

16. Gupta V, Gupta A, Gupta P, et al. Spectral-domain cirrus optical coherence tomography of choroidal striations seen in the acute stage of Vogt-Koyanagi-Harada disease. Am J Ophthalmol. 2009;147(1):148-53.

17. Gupta V, Gupta A, Dogra MR, et al. Reversible retinal changes in the acute stage of sympathetic ophthalmia seen on spectral domain optical coherence tomography. Int Ophthalmol. 2011;31(2):105-10.

18. Atmaca LS, Batioglu F, Müftüoglu O. Fluorescein angiography and optical coherence tomography in ocular Behçet's disease. A preliminary study. Adv Exp Med Biol. 2003;528:355-60.

19. Gupta V, Agarwal A, Gupta A, et al. Clinical characteristics of serpiginous choroidopathy in North India. Am J Ophthalmol. 2002;134(1):47-56.

20. Gupta V, Gupta, Arora S, et al. Presumed tubercular serpiginous like choroiditis: clinical presentations and management. Ophthalmology. 2003;110:1744-9.

21. Bansal R, Kulkarni P, Gupta A, et al. High-resolution spectral domain optical coherence tomography and fundus auto-fluorescence correlation in tubercular serpiginous like choroiditis. J Ophthalmic Inflamm Infect. 2011;1(4):157-63.

chapter 30

Outer Retina *En Face* OCT in Inflammatory Disorders

Massimo Accorinti, Bruno Lumbroso, Marco Rispoli, Marta Gilardi

Introduction

Ocular inflammations might affect all retinal layers, photoreceptors, pigment epithelium and choroid. In cross-sectional scans pigment epithelium may usually be thickened, while photoreceptor lesions may appear as localized areas of fuzziness or as horizontal pseudo-cavities, whose dimensions range from very small to medium. Their location is in the outer retina, close to pigment epithelium, and at the junction between inner and outer photoreceptor segment.

These lesions can also be easily seen in an *en face* scan passing exactly through the level of the junction between inner and outer segment of the photoreceptors. Due to the cup-shaped and not flat profile of the retina, a useful method for studying pathological changes at photoreceptors and RPE levels is an *en face* OCT adapted to the pigment epithelium contour. *En face* images adapted to retinal concavity are conceptually an improvement versus plane scans in the study of the retinal/pigment epithelium complex in ocular inflammatory diseases because they provide a frontal retinal section that, following RPE curve, is parallel to it at photoreceptors or IS/OS junction levels. Frontal scans adapted to pigment epithelium shape might be placed at any constant depth in the retina and choroid and are always parallel to RPE. With this approach, it is possible to obtain an optical *in vivo* dissection of the photoreceptor layer and to isolate this from the outer retinal layers.

Furthermore *en face* scans are able to ascertain whether there are single or multiple lesions: with this frontal sections it is possible to demonstrate that a clinical appearing single lesion is frequently an epiphenomenum of a wider disease. A single lesion is usually seen in acute retinitis, acute epithelitis and eclipse (solar) retinopathy, while multiple lesions can be detected in cases of multiple evanescent white dot syndrome (MEWDS), acute posterior multifocal placoid pigment epitheliopathy (APMPPE), tuberculosis, Vogt-Koyanagi-Harada disease, sympathetic ophthalmia and acute zonal occult outer retinopathy (AZOOR).

Multiple Evanescent White Dot Syndrome (MEWDS)

MEWDS is characterized by the onset at the posterior pole and in the mid-periphery of numerous small discrete white lesions deep in the retina or at the RPE level. The disease is usually unilateral and the etiology is unknown. Fluorescein angiography shows early hyperfluorescence with late staining while indocyanine green angiography shows hypofluorescent lesions throughout the posterior pole, which are more visible on ICG than is apparent on clinical examination.[1] Cross-section OCT scans show very limited lesions in the photoreceptor layer with segmentation or interruption of the junction between inner and outer photoreceptors segment **(Figures 1 and 3)**.

En face OCT scans passing exactly through the level of the junction between inner and outer segment of the photoreceptors show areas of more diffuse alterations thus giving a more detailed map of the lesions **(Figures 2, 4 and 5)**. Areas of decreased retinal sensitivity on microperimetry match exactly areas of junction disruption in the inner/outer segment junction seen on OCT images.

Acute Posterior Multifocal Placoid Pigment Epitheliopathy (APMPPE)

APMPPE is a syndrome characterized by a sudden onset of multiple large plaque-like lesions at the level of RPE, with possible choroidal vasculitis determining impaired filling of the choroidal vasculature, and a usually temporary visual loss **(Figure 6)**. Etiology is unknown, although a close association with viral prodrome has been reported.[2] In the

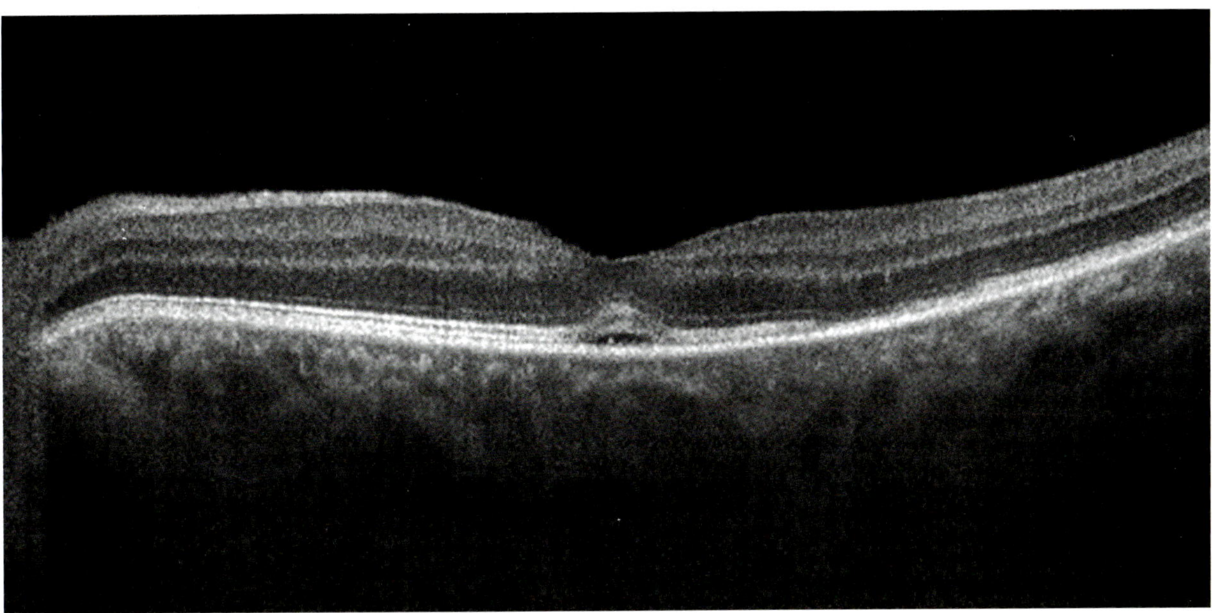

Figure 1: Multiple evanescent white dot syndrome (MEWDS). Foveal cross-section OCT scan showing changes of the junction between inner and outer segment of photoreceptors (Optovue, RTVue)

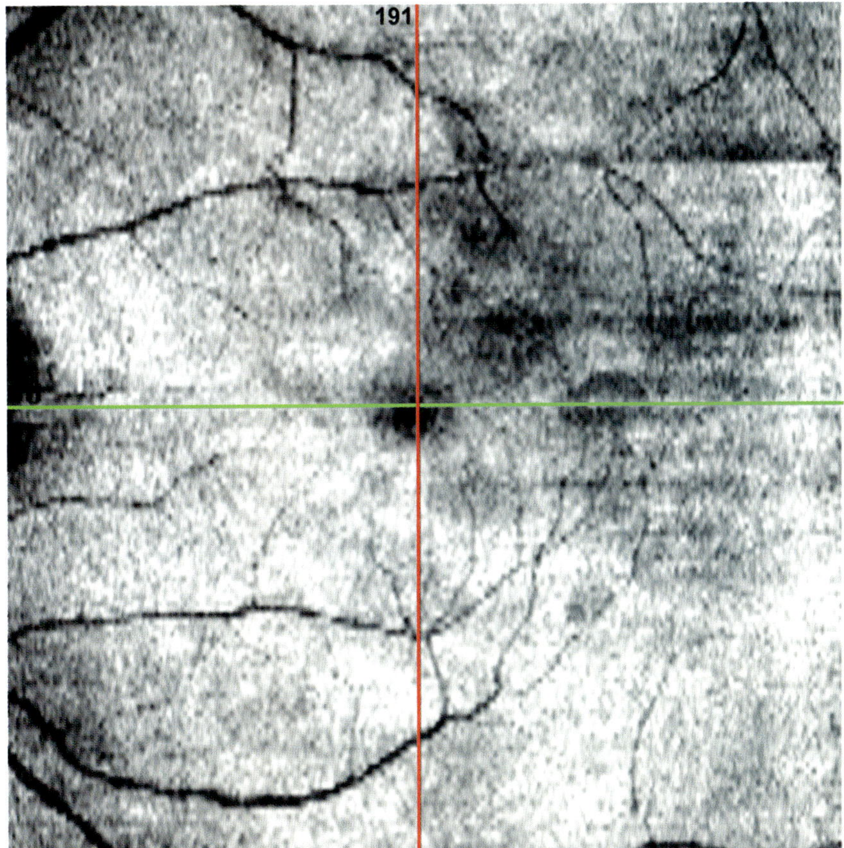

Figure 2: Multiple evanescent white dot syndrome (MEWDS). *En face* OCT scan passing through the level of the junction between inner and outer segment of the photoreceptors shows multiple areas of alterations and gives an accurate map of the lesions (Optovue, RTVue)

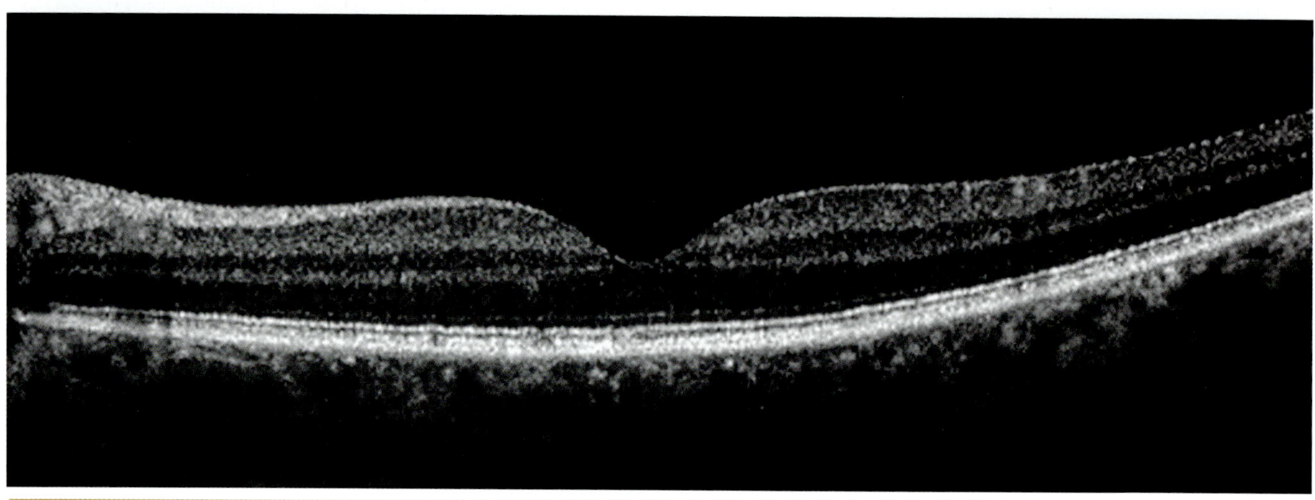

Figure 3: Multiple evanescent white dot syndrome (MEWDS). Cross-section OCT scan: localized changes of the junction between inner and outer segment of photoreceptors (Optovue, RTVue)

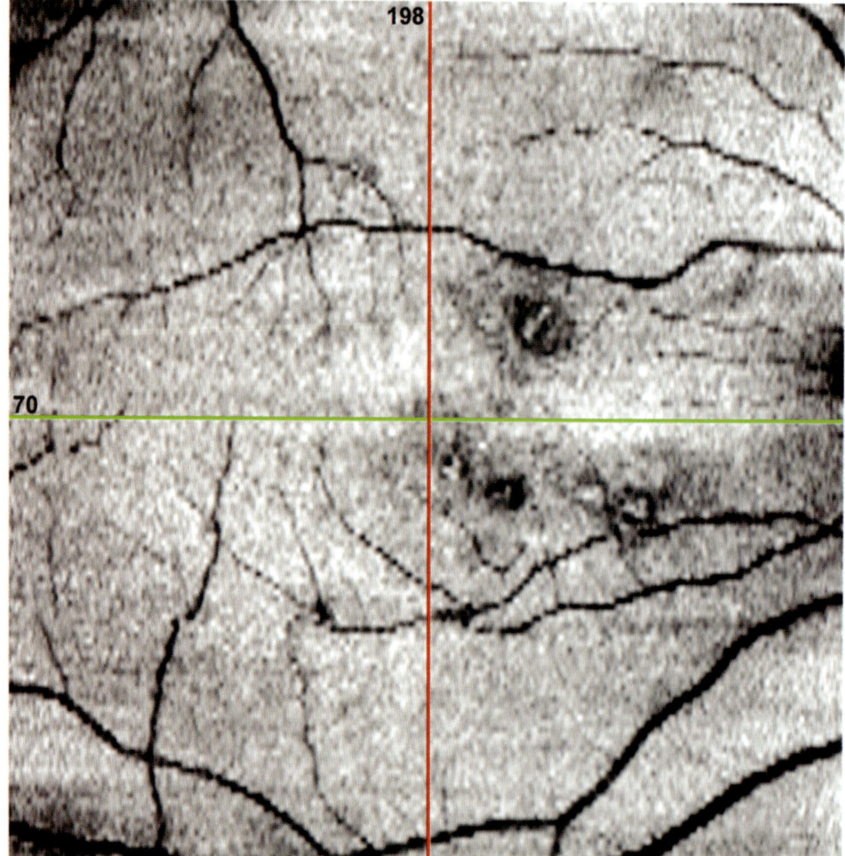

Figure 4: Multiple evanescent white dot syndrome (MEWDS). *En face* OCT scan: multiple irregular lesions at the level of the junction between inner and outer segment of photoreceptors of the same patient. Note the possibility to have an accurate map of the lesions (Optovue, RTVue)

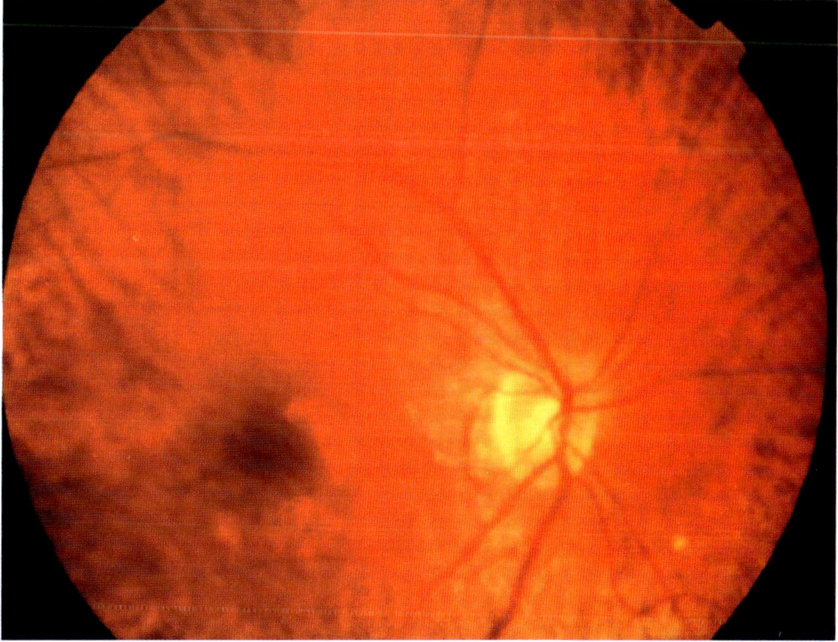

Figure 5: Multiple evanescent white dot syndrome (MEWDS). *En face* OCT scan: multiple irregular changes at the level of the junction between inner and outer segment of photoreceptors (Optovue, RTVue)

Figure 6: Acute posterior multifocal placoid pigment epitheliopathy (APMPPE). Fundus picture—late phase of the disease: multiple scattered lesions throughout the posterior pole

atrophic phase OCT scans show lesions in the photoreceptor layer with interruption of the IS/OS junction corresponding to the transmission defect in the RPE without leakage seen in fluorescein angiography (**Figures 7 and 8**). *En face* OCT scans passing exactly through the level of the junction between inner and outer photoreceptors segment give an exact map of the lesions (**Figure 9**).

Tuberculosis

Ocular involvement occurs in about 1-2% of patients with tuberculosis (TB), and the incidence of this infection is growing up in the western countries because of the immigration from endemic area and for the dissemination of HIV infection. TB lesions can be found at any ocular structure, including choroid and retina. In the acute phase a disseminated choroiditis is the most common presentation, and it is possible to observe numerous lesions at the posterior pole, even in different stages (**Figure 10**). Fluorescein angiography of chororetinal involvement presents an early fluorescence evolving in diffuse hyperfluorescence by the venous phase (**Figure 11**).[3] OCT cross-section can reveal hyper-reflective nodular fibrovascular lesions (**Figure 12**). *En face* OCT shows a hyper-reflective nodule inside an area of thickened retina. The granuloma in frontal section seems homogenous (**Figure 13**). In the chronic phase fundus picture shows extensive multiple scattered chorioretinal lesions and

scars at the posterior pole (**Figure 14**). Fluorescein angiography shows multiple scattered hypo-/hyper-pigmented lesions throughout the posterior pole appearing hypo- or hyperfluorescent according to the window defects or mask effects (**Figure 15**). OCT cross-section can easily demonstrate, within and area of atrophic retina, the presence of multiple chorioretinal lesions altering the retina profile along with edematous cystis in the macular area (**Figure 16**). *En face* OCT detects multiple scattered lesions with irregular shape containing heterogeneous elements (**Figure 17**).

Vogt-Koyanagi-Harada Disease

Vogt-Koyanagi-Harada disease is a systemic inflammatory condition that affects the eye, the meninges, the skin and the inner ear. It is common among pigmented race, especially Asian, and rarely found in Europe. The ocular involvement comprises, in the acute phase, the sudden onset of diffuse choroiditis, with or without papillitis, and numerous focal areas of subretinal fluid that might coalesce forming a bullous serous retinal detachment.[4] In the chronic and recurrent phase of the disease, a diffuse uveitis with a predominantly anterior segment involvement can be observed. In the quiescent phase a diffuse depigmentation of the fundus can be seen associated with RPE clumping and migration, numerous nummular chorioretinal scars and subretinal fibrosis (**Figures 18 and 19**).[5] In the chronic and in quiescent phases *en face* OCT

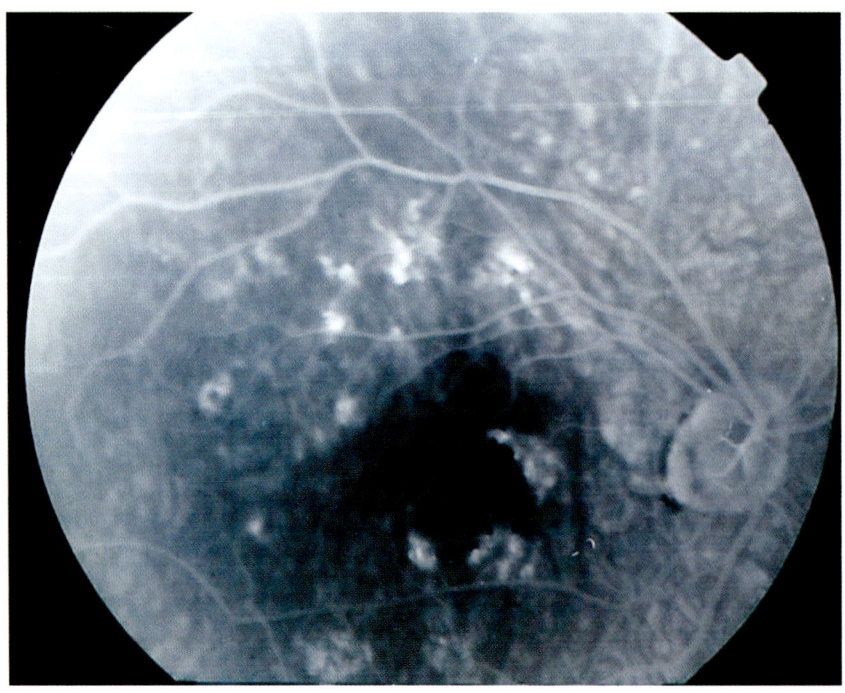

Figure 7: Acute posterior multifocal placoid pigment epitheliopathy (APMPPE). Fluorescein angiography—late phase of the disease: extensive hyperfluorescent lesions (window defects) disseminated at the posterior pole

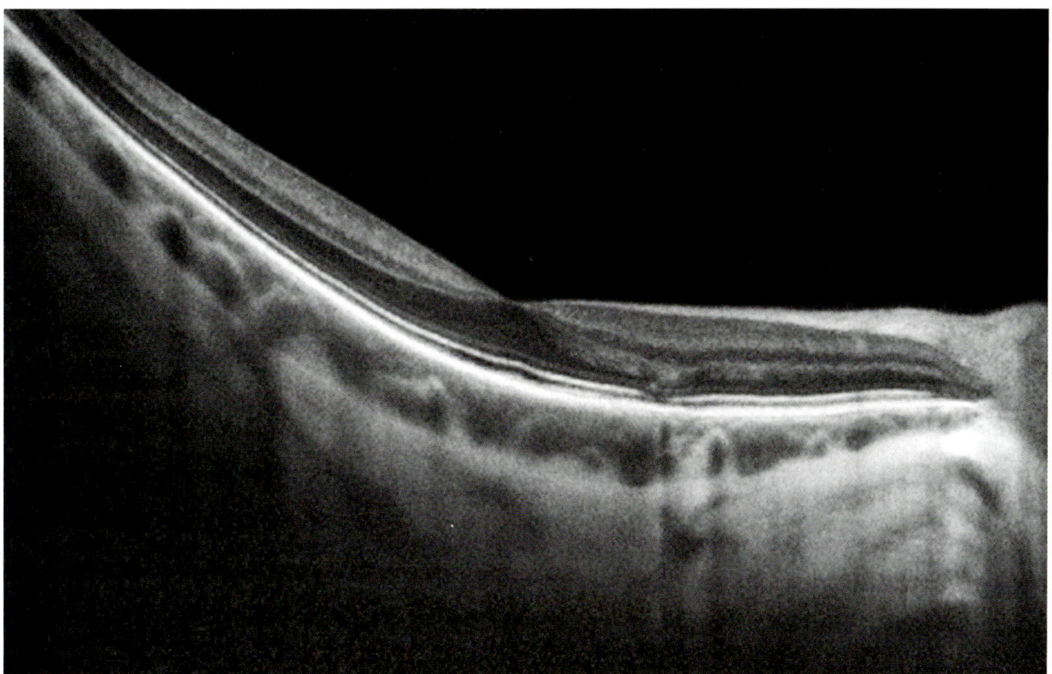

Figure 8: Acute posterior multifocal placoid pigment epitheliopathy (APMPPE). Cross-section OCT scan: lesions at the photoreceptor level with break of the junction between inner and outer segment of the photoreceptors that correspond with window defects present at fluorescein angiography (Optovue, RTVue)

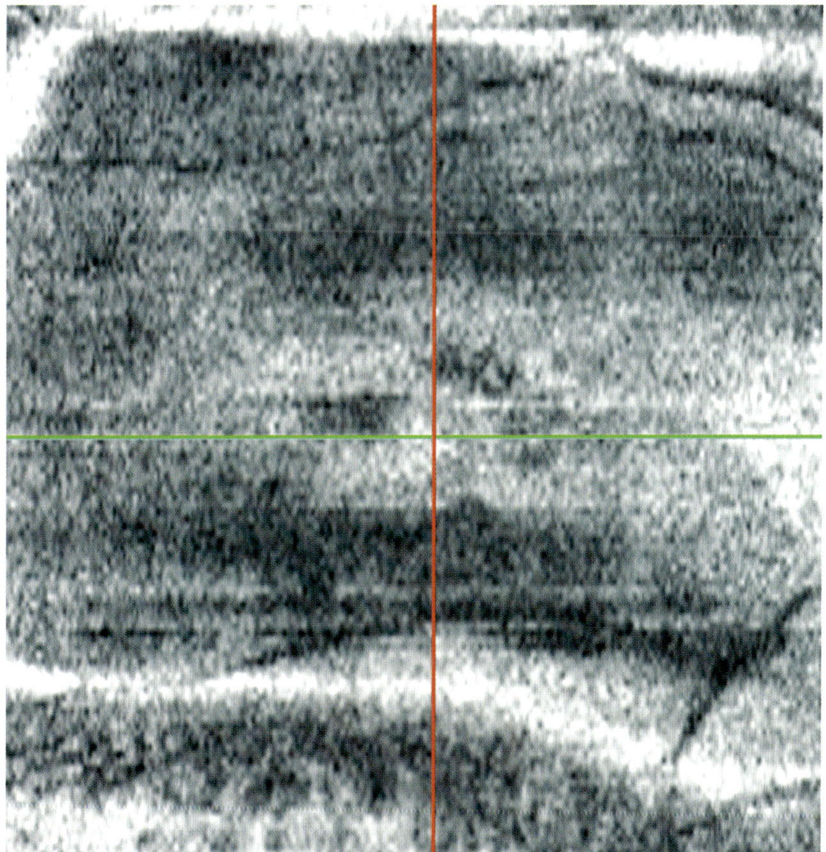

Figure 9: Acute posterior multifocal placoid pigment epitheliopathy (APMPPE). *En face* OCT scan passing exactly trough the level of the junction between inner and outer segment of the photoreceptors gives an accurate map of the alterations (Optovue, RTVue)

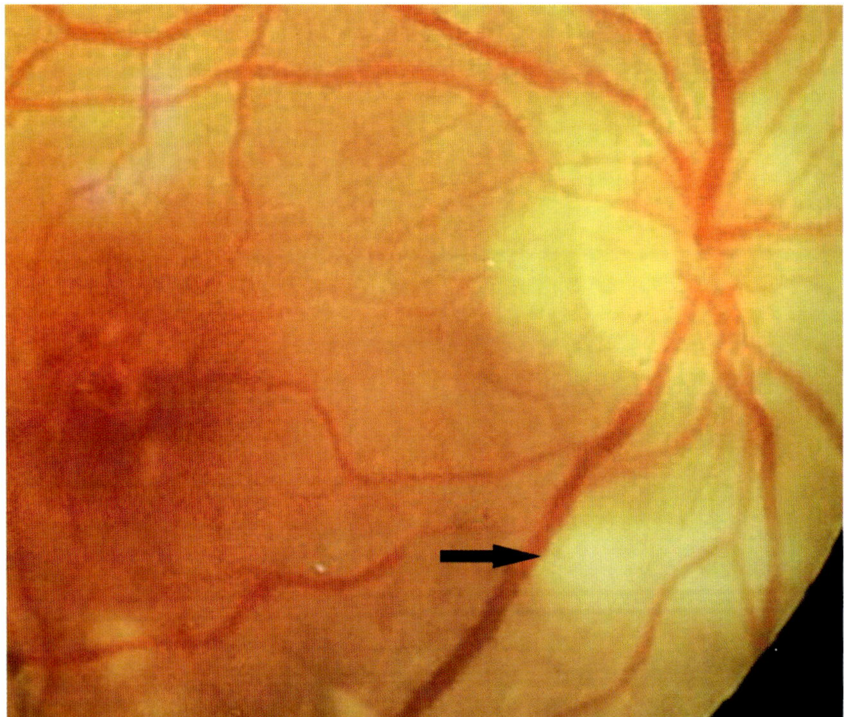

Figure 10: Tuberculosis. Fundus picture—active disease: choroidal granuloma

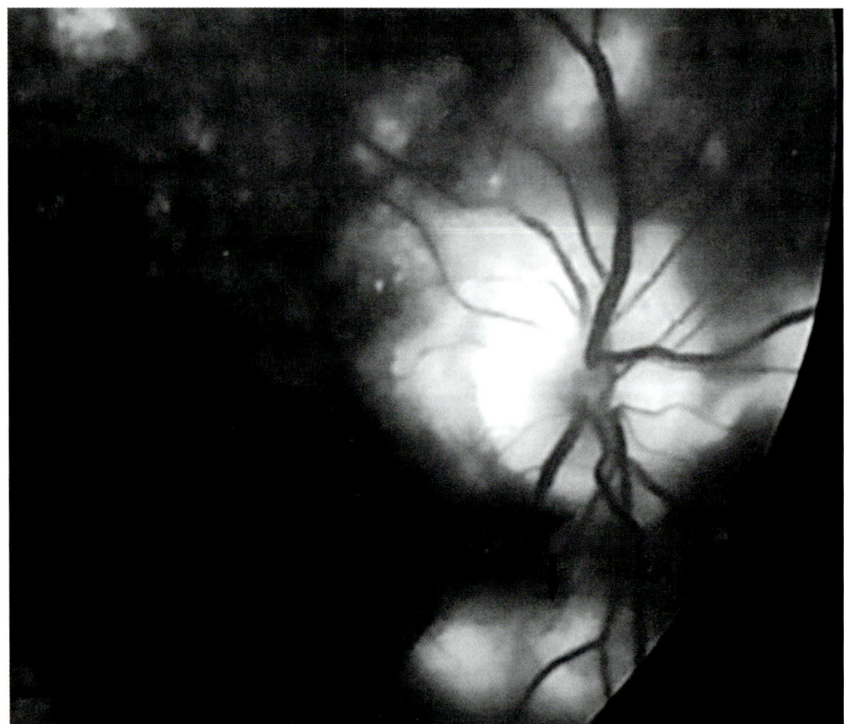

Figure 11: Tuberculosis. Fluorescein angiography: early hyperfluorescent subretinal lesion evolving in diffuse hyperfluorescence in the venous phase

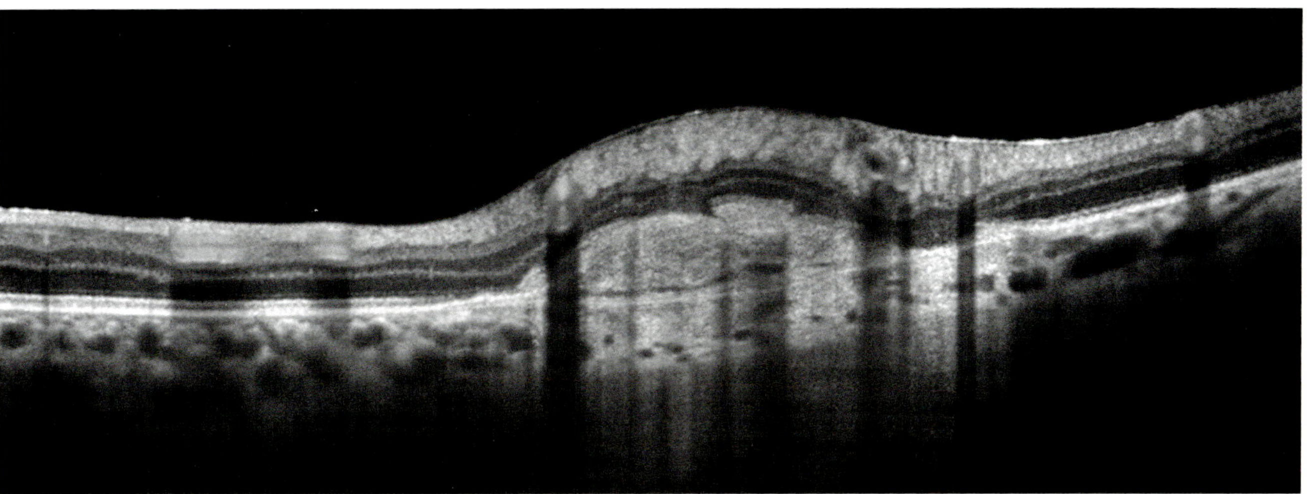

Figure 12: Tuberculosis. Cross-section OCT scan: chorioretinal hyper-reflective nodule deforming the retinal profile; thickness of the nerve fiber layer and retinal vessel walls. The nodule includes heterogeneous elements and is surrounded by a diffuse exudation in the sensory retina. Vessel diameters are reduced in the Sattler small vessel and Haller large vessel layers (Optovue, RTVue)

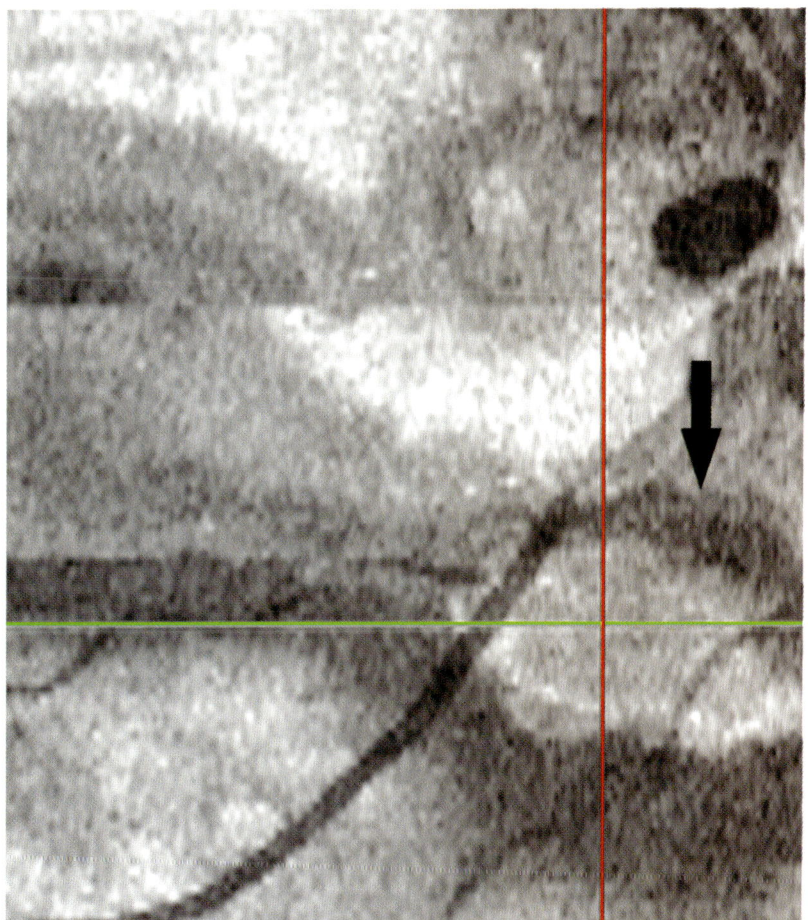

Figure 13: Tuberculosis. *En face* OCT scan: hyper-reflective nodule inside an area of thickened retina. The nodule in frontal section seems homogeneous (Optovue, RTVue)

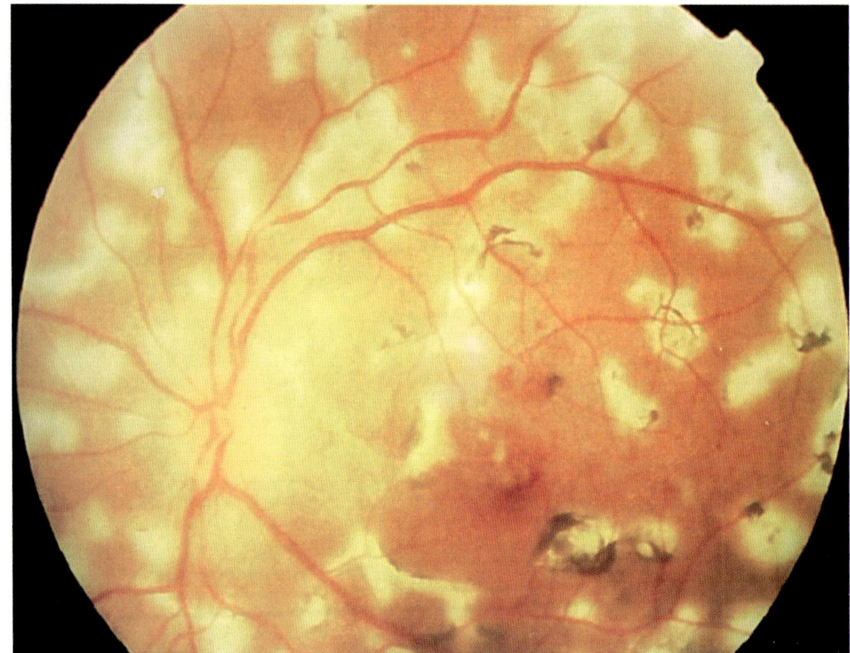

Figure 14: Tuberculosis. Fundus picture—late phase of the disease: multiple scattered chorioretinal lesions at the posterior pole

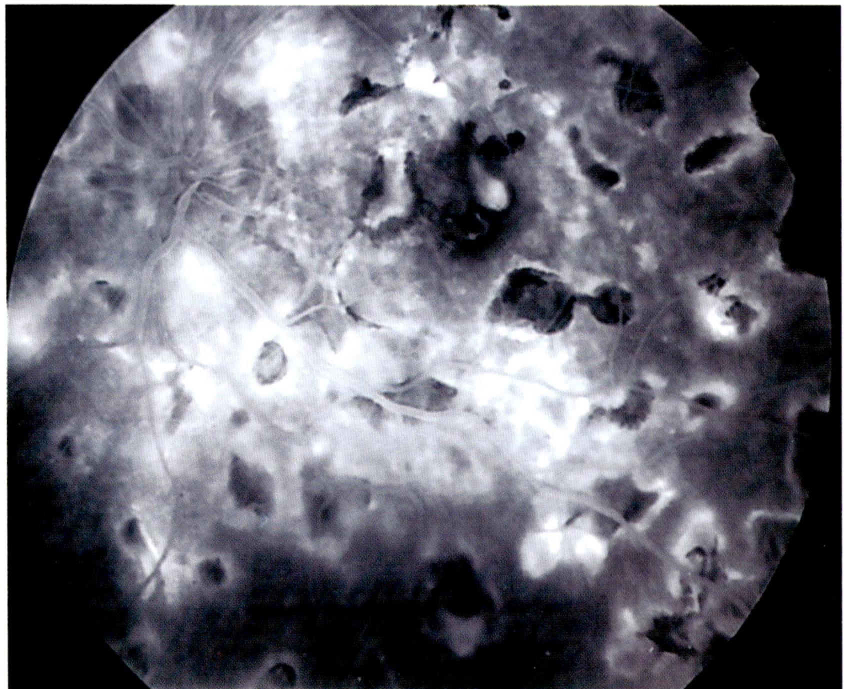

Figure 15: Tuberculosis. Fluorescein angiography—late phase of the disease: multiple scattered chorioretinal lesions with irregular shape at the posterior pole showing either hypofluorescence (pigment accumulation and scars) or hyperfluorescence (window defects)

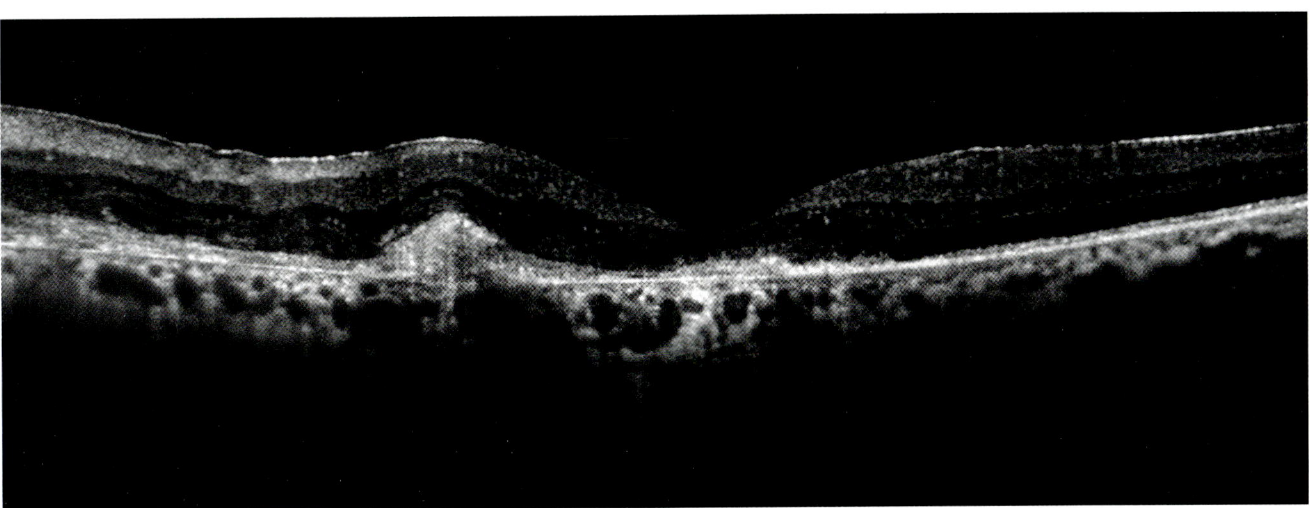

Figure 16: Cross-section OCT scan: chorioretinal lesions constituted by heterogeneous hyper-reflective areas surrounded by loss of retinal structures and decrease contrast between the layers. The lesions alter the normal retinal profile. Cystoid macular alterations and atrophy of the outer retinal layers are also detected (Optovue, RTVue)

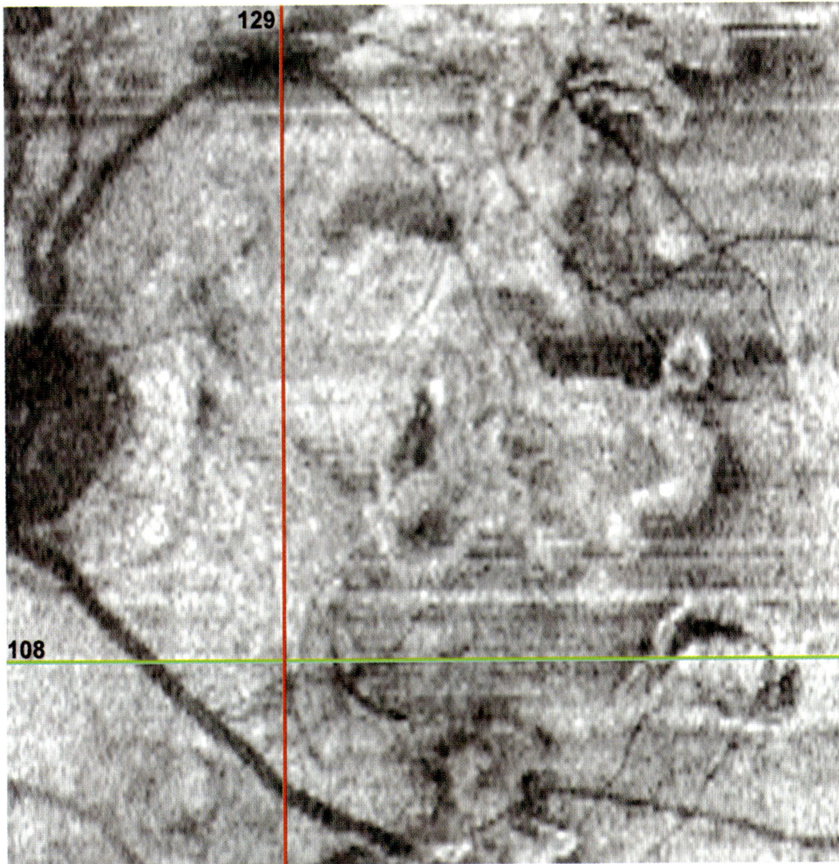

Figure 17: Tuberculosis. *En face* OCT scan at photoreceptor layer level reveals multiple fibrotic, irregularly shaped, hyper-reflective lesions containing heterogeneous elements (Optovue, RTVue)

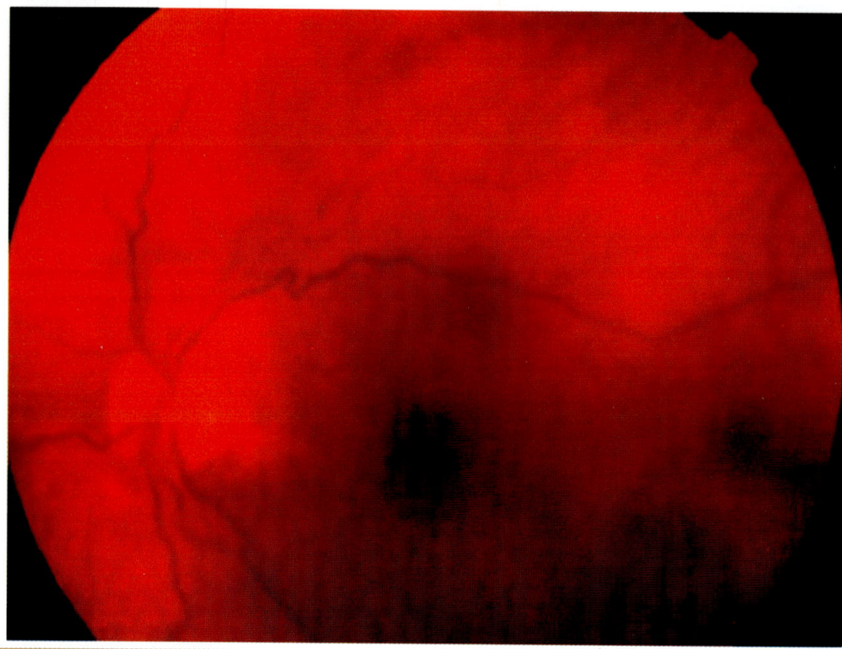

Figure 18: Vogt-Koyanagi-Harada disease. Fundus picture—quiescent phase of the disease: numerous scattered chorioretinal and pigment epithelium lesions at the posterior pole

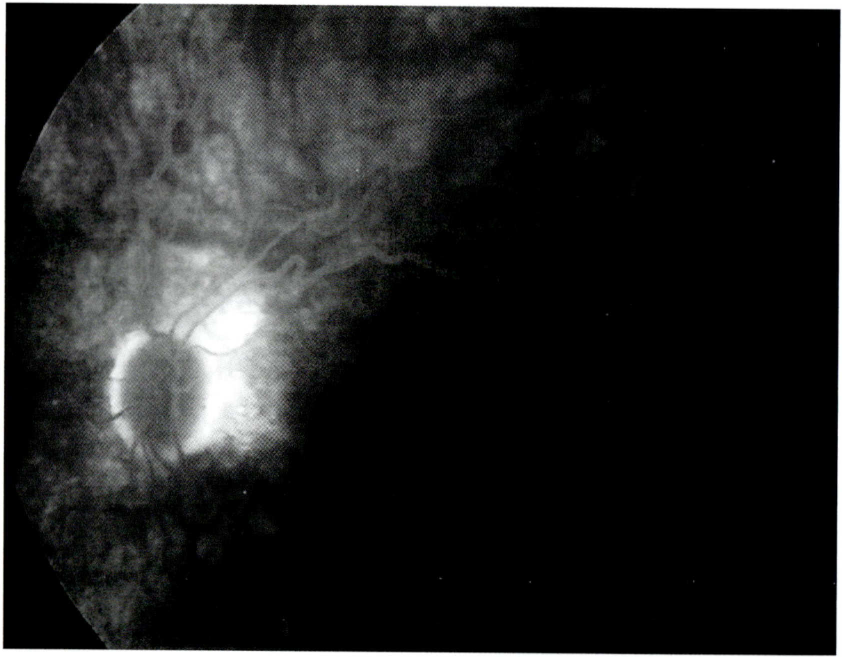

Figure 19: Vogt-Koyanagi-Harada disease. Fluorescein angiography—quiescent phase of the disease: hyperfluorescent lesions at the posterior pole expressing scattered pigment epithelium defects (window defects)

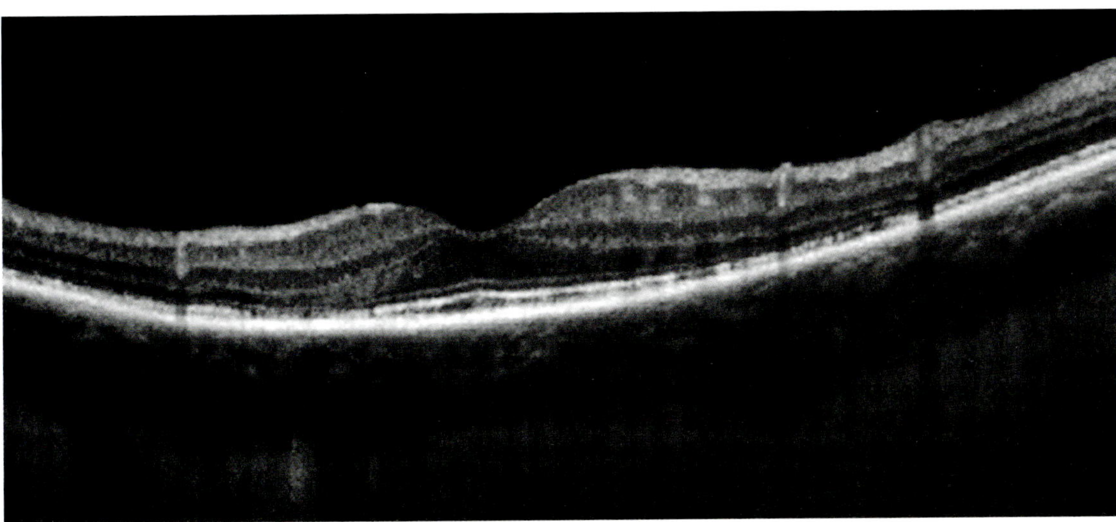

Figure 20: Vogt-Koyanagi-Harada disease. Cross-section OCT—quiescent phase of the disease: scattered retinal pigment epithelium lesions along with hypertrophy and fibrosis of the RPE. Choroid is thicker than normal and choroidal vessel diameters are increased both in Sattler and in Haller layer (Optovue, RTVue)

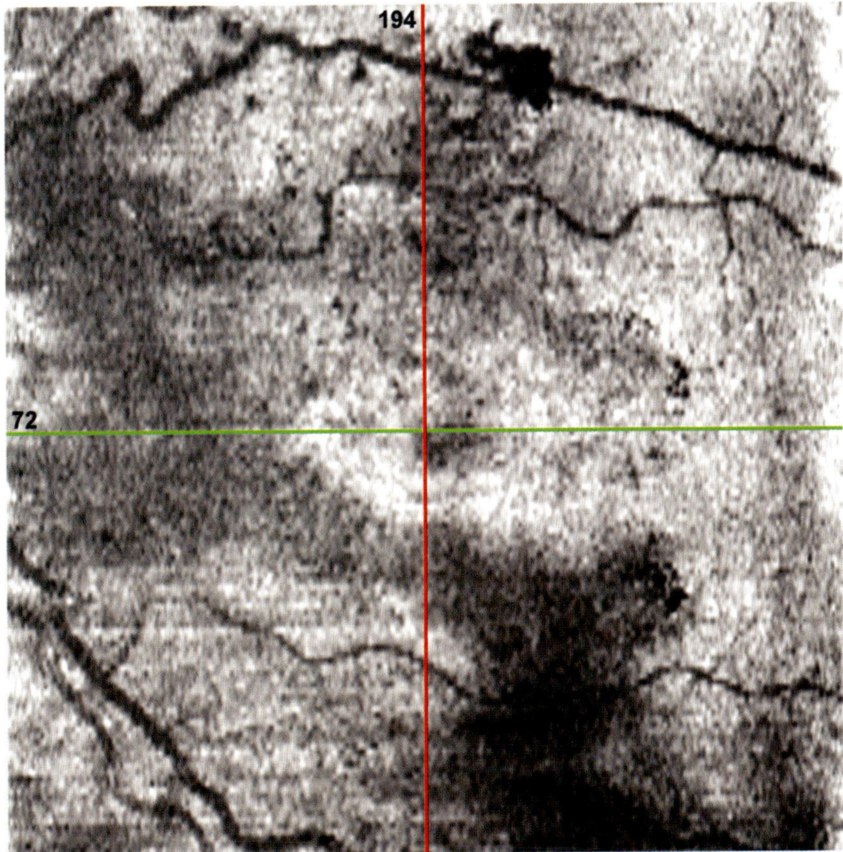

Figure 21: Vogt-Koyanagi-Harada disease. *En face* OCT—quiescent phase of the disease: scattered pigment epithelium hypertrophic and atrophic lesions with involvement of the outer retina (Optovue, RTVue)

may show retinal pigment epithelium hypertrophy and fibrosis, as well as involvement of the outer retina, corresponding clinically to areas of pigment epithelium scars **(Figures 20 and 21)**.

References

1. Abu-Yaghi NE, Hartono SP, Hodge DO, Pulido JS, Bakri SJ. White dot syndromes: a 20-year study of incidence, clinical features, and outcomes. Ocul Immunol Inflamm. 2011;19:426-30.
2. Goldenberg D, Habot-Wilner Z, Loewenstein A, Goldstein M. Spectral domain optical coherence tomography classification of acute posterior multifocal placoid pigment epitheliopathy. Retina. 2012;32:1403-10.
3. Tabbara KF. Tuberculosis. Curr Opin Ophthalmol. 2007; 18:493-501.
4. Ishihara K, Hangai M, Kita M, Yoshimura N. Acute Vogt-Koyanagi-Harada disease in enhanced spectral-domain optical coherence tomography. Ophthalmology. 2009;116: 1799-1807.
5. Fong AH, Li KK, Wong D. Choroidal evaluation using enhanced depth imaging spectral-domain optical coherence tomography in Vogt-Koyanagi-Harada disease. Retina. 2011;31:502-9.

chapter 31

En Face Optical Coherence Tomography Scan in Parasitosis

Swapnil Parchand, Vishali Gupta, Amod Gupta

Toxoplasmic Retinochoroiditis

Toxoplasmic retinochoroiditis is the most common identifiable cause of posterior uveitis in many parts of the world.[1] *Toxoplasma gondii*, an intracellular parasite can get transmitted to the fetus either *in utero*, i.e. congenital, or less commonly, retina can get involved in acquired variety due to ingestion of the organism.[2] In congenital toxoplasmosis, bilateral macular involvement is present at birth and is characterized by the presence of a large, atrophic, excavated scar. Acquired form is characterized by presence of focal necrotizing retinitis with involvement of inner retinal layers and overlying vitritis. Retinal thickening in the main focus and retinal edema can be easily demonstrated during acute phase on optical coherence tomography (OCT). OCT also helps in the diagnosis and follow-up of the complications such as epiretinal membranes, vitreoretinal traction, cystoid macular edema and choroidal neovascular membrane (CNVM).[3-8]

Case Study 1

A 20-year-old male presented with low vision in both eyes since childhood. On examination, fundus picture of both eyes showed congenital toxoplasmic scar. The scar typically showed three zones: (1) outer white zone (white arrow), (2) intermediate zone with pigmentary hyperplasia (red arrow) and (3) inner dark zone of atrophy (blue arrow) (**Figure 1A**). Red free picture typically highlighted this scar (**Figure 1B**). Five-line raster scan through central zone shows total absence of neurosensory retina over central zone (**Figure 1C**). *En face* OCT scan passing through intermediate zone shows atrophy of neurosensory retina though some redundant tissue still persistent along with retinal pigment epithelium (RPE) hyperplasia (**Figure 1D**). Deeper scan through inner dark zone shows total absence of neurosensory retina with disorganized RPE (**Figure 1E**).

Case Study 2

A 26-year-old woman presented with blurring of vision in right eye since 2 weeks. Fundoscopy of right eye revealed patch of focal retinochoroiditis in perifoveal region with overlying vitritis (**Figure 2A**). Red free picture highlighting the same area of active retinochoroiditis lesion (**Figure 2B**). Raster line scan passing through the lesion shows hyper-reflectivity confined to inner layers with back shadowing along with overlying vitritis (white arrow) (**Figure 2C**). Also, serous retinal detachment with pocket of fluid can be seen in the outer retina; outer to external limiting membrane. Internal limiting membrane slab (white arrows) passing through inner layer of retina (**Figure 2D**) shows hyper-reflective area corresponding to active lesion on overlay map (**Figure 2E**). *En face* OCT scan (**Figures 2F and G**) through active area showed hyper-reflectivity within inner retinal layer of retina along with distortion and lack of demarcation of the inner layers (white arrows) as compared to surrounding area. Also, cystoid spaces with subretinal exudation (red arrow) can be seen on deeper scans. Serology for Toxoplasma was positive and patient was successfully managed on oral clindamycin and septran with systemic steroid.

Case Study 3

A 34-year-old female treated in past for toxoplasma retinochoroiditis complained of further decreased vision in left eye. Fundoscopy revealed healed toxoplasmosis scar and area of grayish discoloration of the retina adjacent to it (white arrows) (**Figure 3A**). During the late phase of fundus fluorescein angiography, lacy network pattern of hyper-fluorescence in the area corresponding to the grayish discoloration of the retina was seen indicating the presence of CNVM (**Figure 3B**). Horizontal OCT scan through the same area showed vitreomacular traction (red arrows) with underlying CNVM lesion (**Figure 3C**). Consecutive *en face*

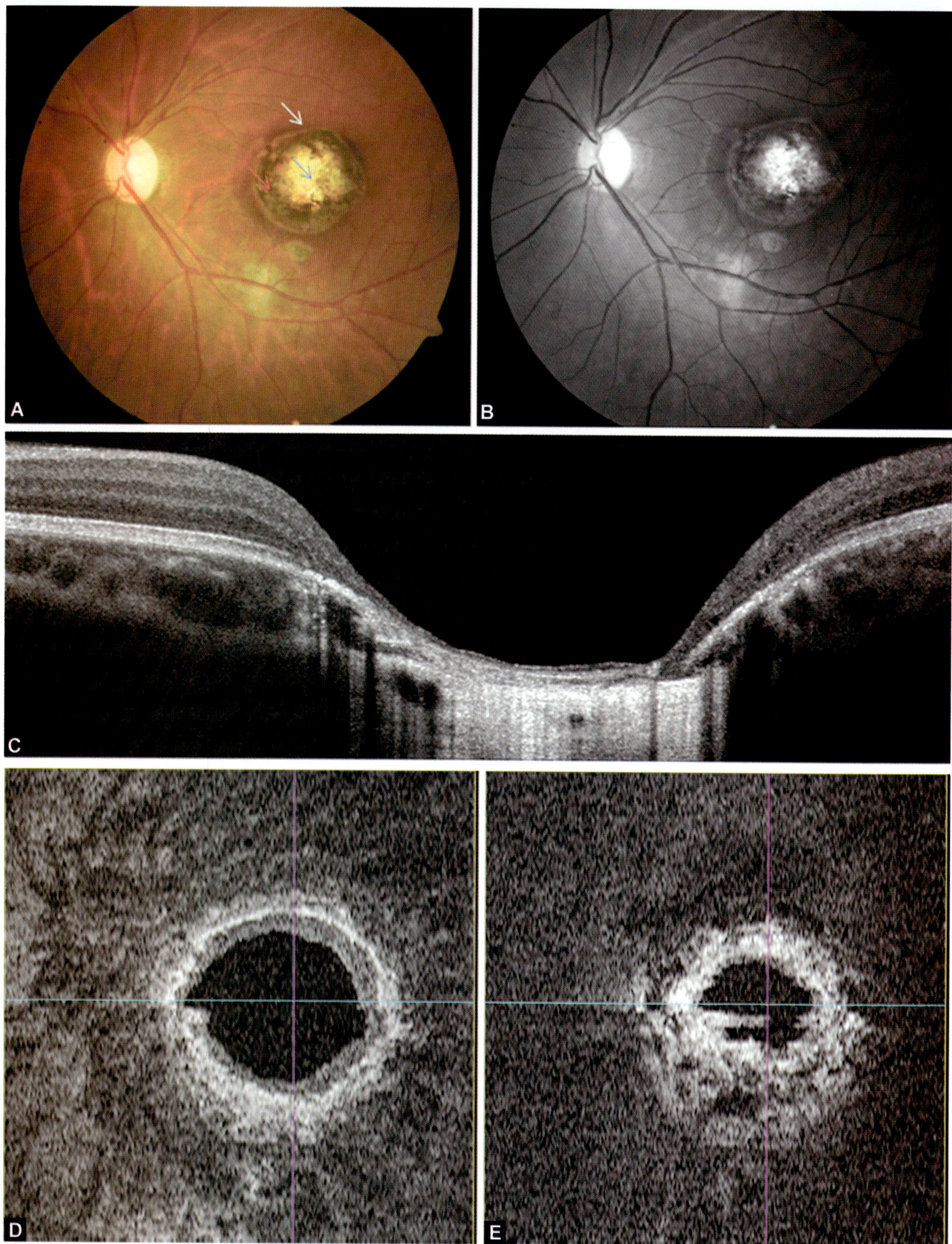

Figures 1A to E: Congenital toxoplasmosis: (A) Fundus photograph of left eye mainly showing congenital toxoplasmic scar; (B) Red free picture; (C) Raster line scan through scar; (D and E) Consecutive C scans

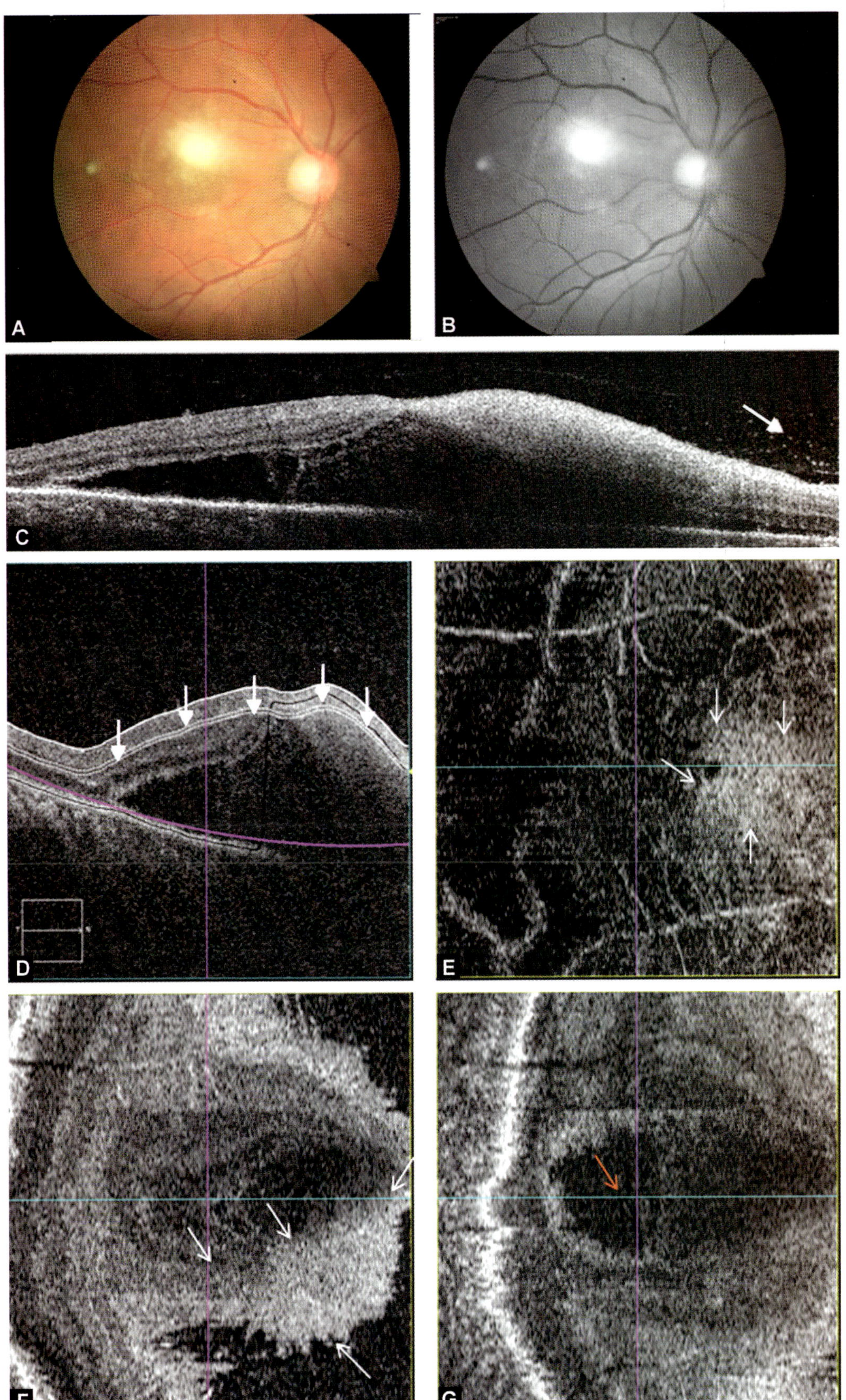

Figures 2A to G: Acquired toxoplasmosis: (A) Fundus photograph of right eye mainly showing active retino-choroiditis toxoplasmic lesion; (B) Red free picture; (C) Raster line scan through the lesion; (D and E) Overlay scan; (F and G) *En face* OCT scans

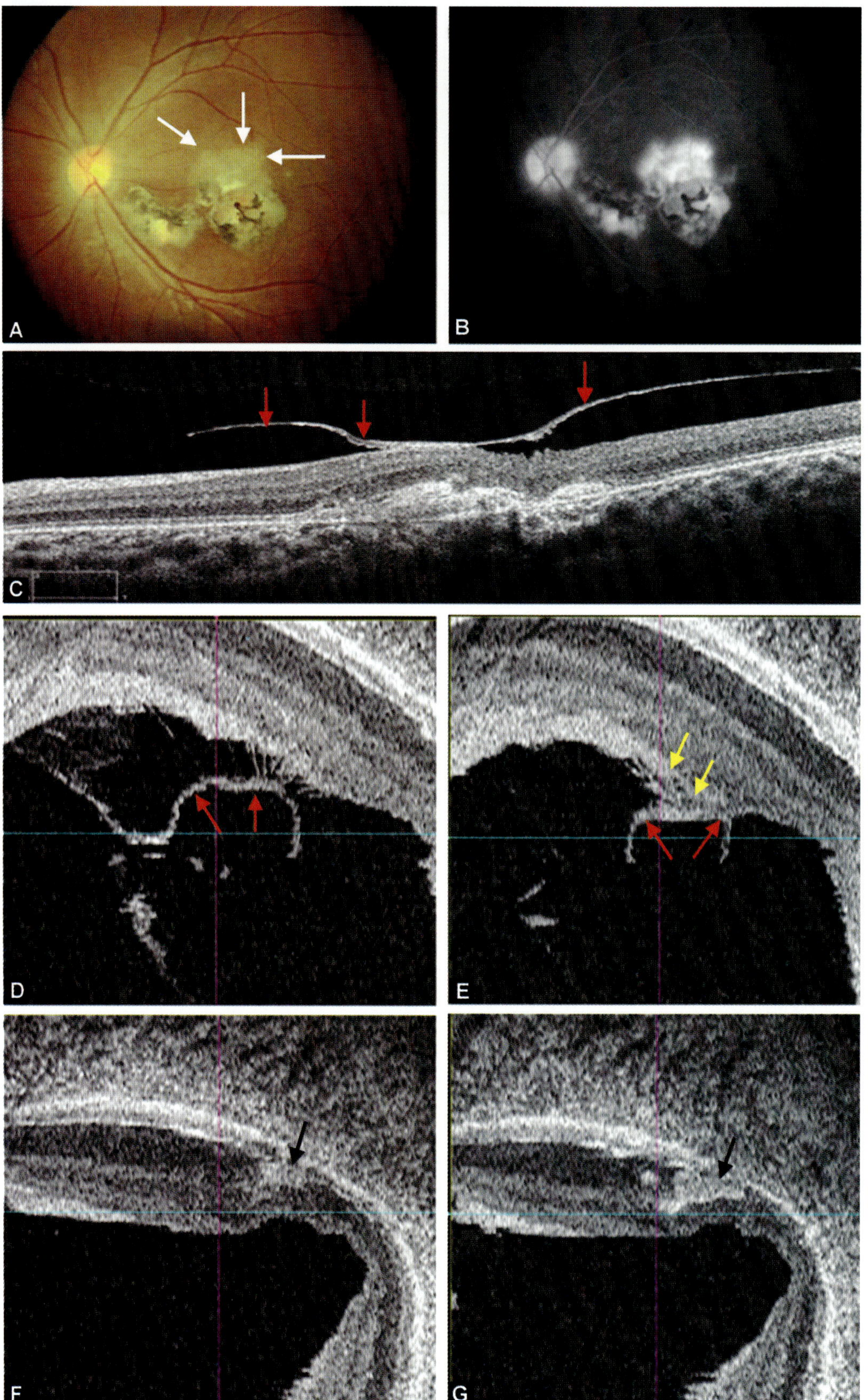

Figures 3A to G: Healed toxoplasmic retino-choroiditis lesion associated with choroidal neo-vascular membrane and vitreomacular traction: (A) Fundus photograph of left eye; (B) FFA in late phase; (C) Raster line scan; (D to G) Consecutive C scan at presentation

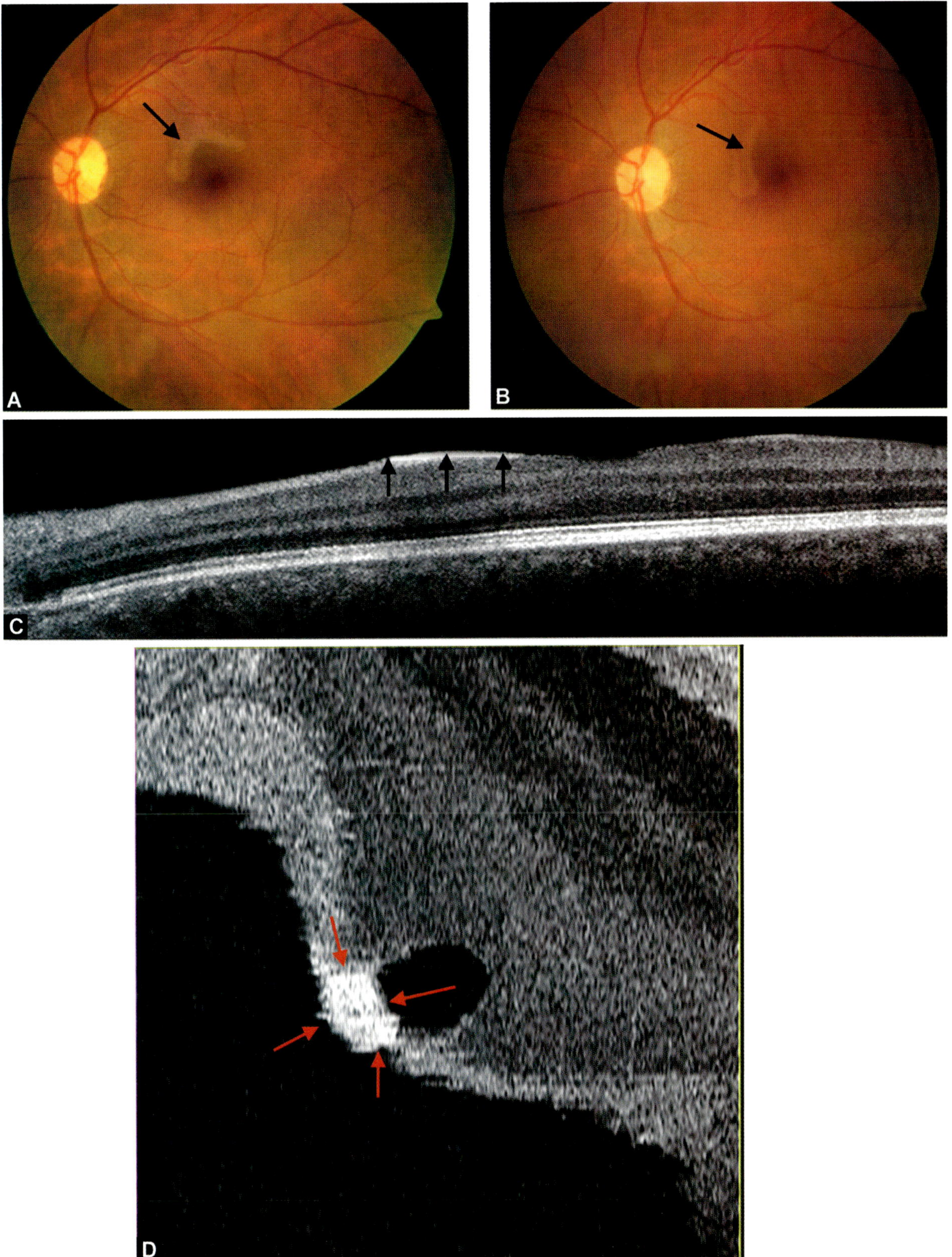

Figures 4A to D: Diffuse unilateral subacute neuroretinitis: (A and B) Fundus photographs of left eye showing mobile worm; (C) Raster line scan passing through the worm; (D) *En face* OCT scan showing exact position of worm

OCT scans (C scan) (**Figures 3D to G**) showing moderate hyper-reflective band (posterior hyaloid) (red arrows) in the hyporeflective vitreal chamber. On subsequent scans hyaloid is seen pulling the retina causing distortion of retinal tissue which is evident by serrated internal limiting membrane (yellow arrows). We can distinctly see fibrous strands between hyaloid and underlying retina. Further deeper scan (**Figures 3F to G**) shows hyper-reflective CNVM lesion (black arrows) in continuation with underlying RPE and choroid.

Diffuse Unilateral Subacute Neuroretinitis

Diffuse unilateral subacute neuroretinitis is a clinical syndrome characterized initially by visual loss, vitritis, papillitis, retinal vasculitis and recurrent crops of evanescent gray-white outer retinal lesions and later, by progressive visual loss, optic atrophy, retinal vessel narrowing and diffuse RPE degeneration occurring in one eye of otherwise healthy patients. Optical coherence tomography helps in serial evaluation of retinal nerve fiber layer thickness and central macular thickness in these cases. It also helps in precise localization of the worm with respect to different layers of retina.[9-11]

Case Study 4

A 50-year-old female who was being treated for intermediate uveitis complained of persistent floaters in left eye. Fundoscopy of left eye revealed perifoveal mobile comma shaped lesion (large worm) (black arrows) (**Figures 4A and B**). Horizontal scan passing through the lesion showed hyper-reflective area in preretinal region (black arrows) (**Figure 4C**). But, *en face* OCT scan precisely located same hyper-reflective lesion in inner most layers of retina identifying correctly the exact position of worm (red arrows) (**Figure 4D**).

References

1. Petersen E, Kijlstra A, Stanford M. Epidemiology of ocular toxoplasmosis. Ocul Immunol Inflamm. 2012;20(2):68-75.
2. Pavesio C. Parasitic infection: Toxoplasmosis. In: Gupta A, Gupta V, Herbort C, et al (Eds). Uveitis Text and Imaging. New Delhi: Jaypee Brothers Medical Publishers (P) Ltd; 2009. pp. 201-11.
3. Gupta V, Gupta A, Dogra MR. Inflammatory diseases of retino-choroid. In: Gupta V, Gupta A, Dogra MR (Eds). Atlas Optical Coherence Tomography of Macular Diseases. New Delhi: Jaypee Brothers Medical Publishers (P) Ltd; 2010. pp. 458-540.
4. Oréfice JL, Costa RA, Campos W, et al. Third-generation optical coherence tomography findings in punctate retinal toxoplasmosis. Am J Ophthalmol. 2006;142(3):503-5.
5. Garg S, Mets MB, Bearelly S, et al. Imaging of congenital toxoplasmosis macular scars with optical coherence tomography. Retina. 2009;29(5):631-7.
6. Diniz B, Regatieri C, Andrade R, et al. Evaluation of spectral domain and time domain optical coherence tomography findings in toxoplasmic retinochoroiditis. Clin Ophthalmol. 2011;5:645-50.
7. Monnet D, Averous K, Delair E, et al. Optical coherence tomography in ocular toxoplasmosis. Int J Med Sci. 2009;6(3):137-8.
8. Oréfice JL, Costa RA, Oréfice F, et al. Vitreoretinal morphology in active ocular toxoplasmosis: a prospective study by optical coherence tomography. Br J Ophthalmol. 2007;91(6):773-80.
9. Garcia Filho CA, Soares AC, Penha FM, et al. Spectral domain optical coherence tomography in diffuse unilateral subacute neuroretinitis. J Ophthalmol. 2011;285-96.
10. Cunha LP, Costa-Cunha LV, Souza EC, et al. Intraretinal worm documented by optical coherence tomography in a patient with diffuse unilateral subacute neuroretinitis: case report. J Ophthalmol. 2010;73(5):462-3.
11. Casella AM, Farah ME, Souza EC, et al. Retinal nerve fiber layer atrophy as relevant feature for diffuse unilateral subacute neuroretinitis (DUSN): case series. Arq Bras Oftalmol. 2010;73(5):182-5.

chapter 32

En Face OCT Imaging in Ocular Toxoplasmosis

Andre Romano, Roberta Velletri
Rubens N Belfort, Rubens Belfort Jr.

Introduction

Toxoplasmic retinochoroiditis is the most common form of posterior uveitis in otherwise healthy individuals, and *Toxoplasma gondii* infection is distributed worldwide.[1]

It is transmitted usually by the ingestion of undercooked lamb, pork and chicken as well as food and water contaminated by the feces of infected cats.[2]

The focus of infection is established, if a parasite reaches the eye. It progresses from retinitis to secondarily involve the choroid. The host's immune response appears to induce the conversion of the tachyzoite to bradyzoite and encystment in the Toxoplasma life cycle, and a large number of T cells are found in retinal lesions and in the choroid. Infiltrating T lymphocytes may play a role in the early recognition of Toxoplasma in the eye as well as in the chronicity and recurrences. Healing of the lesion occurs with control of the acute infection and scar formation.

The cyst may remain inactive in the scar or adjacent to it for a period of years. Ultimately, the cyst wall may rupture, releasing organisms into the surrounding retina and resulting in recurring retinitis.[6] As a result, the initial lesion can cause damage to the inner retinal layers adjacent to an old chorioretinal scar and can be accompanied by vitreitis.[3]

The rupture of tissue cysts elsewhere has also been implicated in the pathogenesis of the recurrences.

Ocular toxoplasmosis in immunocompetent patients is characterized by an acute inflammatory granulomatous chorioretinal necrotizing inflammation of the retina and choroid. It can be widespread in the eye and involve also the vitreous, ciliary body, iris, anterior chamber, cornea and trabecular meshwork.[4]

Imaging in ocular toxoplasmosis contributes to the right characterization of the different aspects of the lesions secondary to the infection and inflammation complications, and it is important for follow-up also.

Optical coherent tomography (OCT), Ultra-sound (US), Confocal scanning laser Ophthalmoscopy (CSLO), Fluorescent angiography (FA), Fundus autofluorescence (FAF) and Indocyanine green angiography (ICGA) may be necessary also to evaluate complications that include macular edema, retinal neovascularization, vascular occlusion and vitreoretinal lesions such as vitreous hemorrhage and subretinal neovascular and epiretinal membranes.[5] Retinal detachments may occur as well as optic nerve atrophy, glaucoma and cataracts and the pertinent imaging techniques applied to its diagnosis and management.

The following description of *en face* OCT in toxoplasmosis was obtained with RTVue OCT (Optovue, Fremont, California).

Description of Vitreous, Retinal and Choroidal Changes

Acute and new lesions are usually intensely white, focal lesions with overlying vitreous inflammatory haze and will occasionally develop retinal vasculitis with vascular sheathing and hemorrhages (**Figures 1 and 2**).

In **Figures 1A to C**, color photograph depicts both acute (green arrow) and cicatricial (white arrow) lesions (**Figure 1A**). Tridimentional scan (**Figure 1B**) shows vitreous retinal traction that can also be seen in both color photograph and B scan (yellow arrows). Intensive inflammatory reaction can also be observed (red stars) (**Figures 1B and C**).

En face image at the level of the inner nuclear layer depicts presumed vascular sheathing (blue arrows) (**Figure 2**).

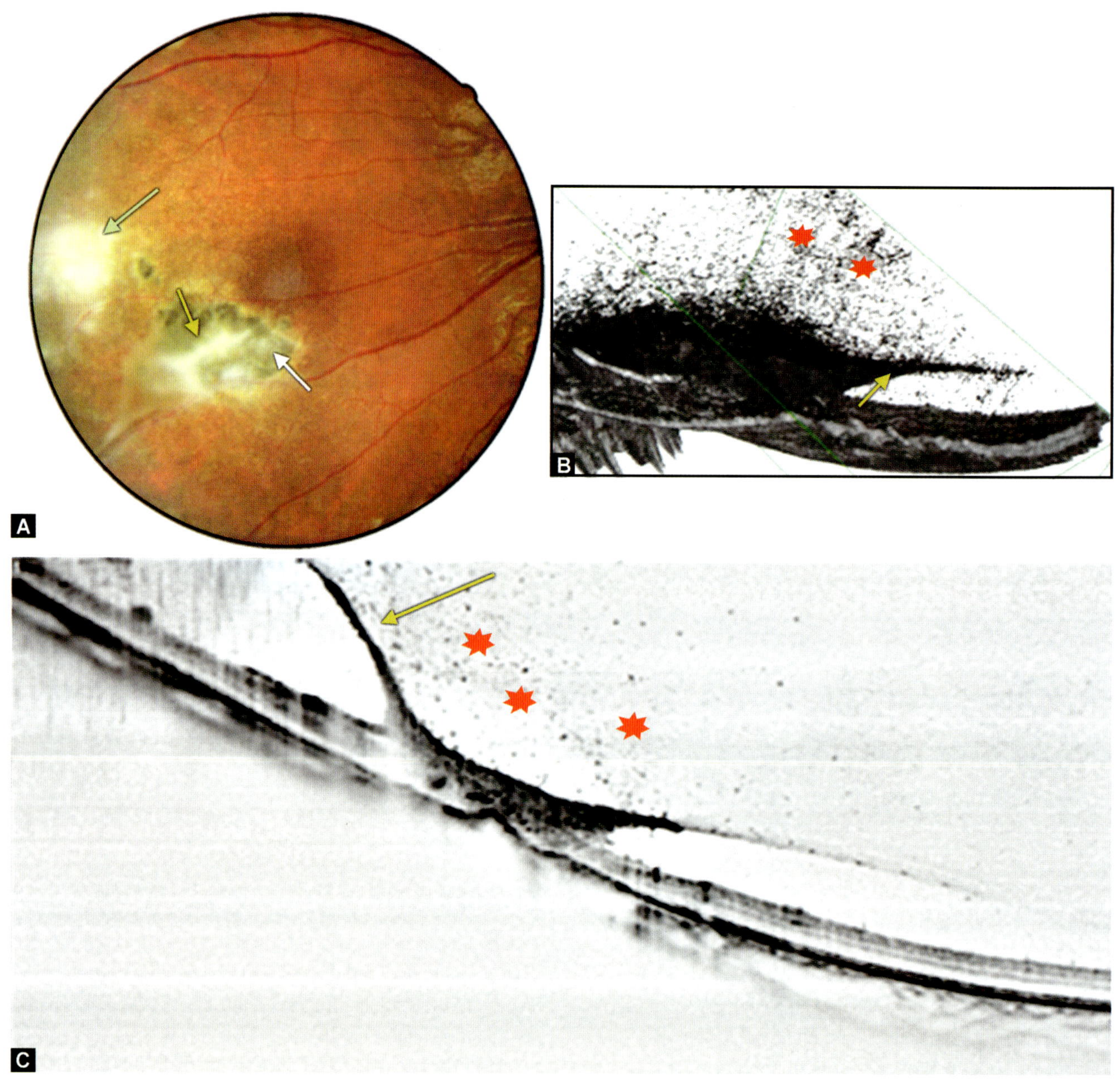

Figures 1A to C: Color photograph depicts both acute (green arrow) and cicatricial (white arrow) lesions (A); Tridimensional scan; (B) shows vitreous retinal traction that can also be seen in both color photograph and B scan (yellow arrows) (C) intensive inflammatory reaction can also be observed (red stars)

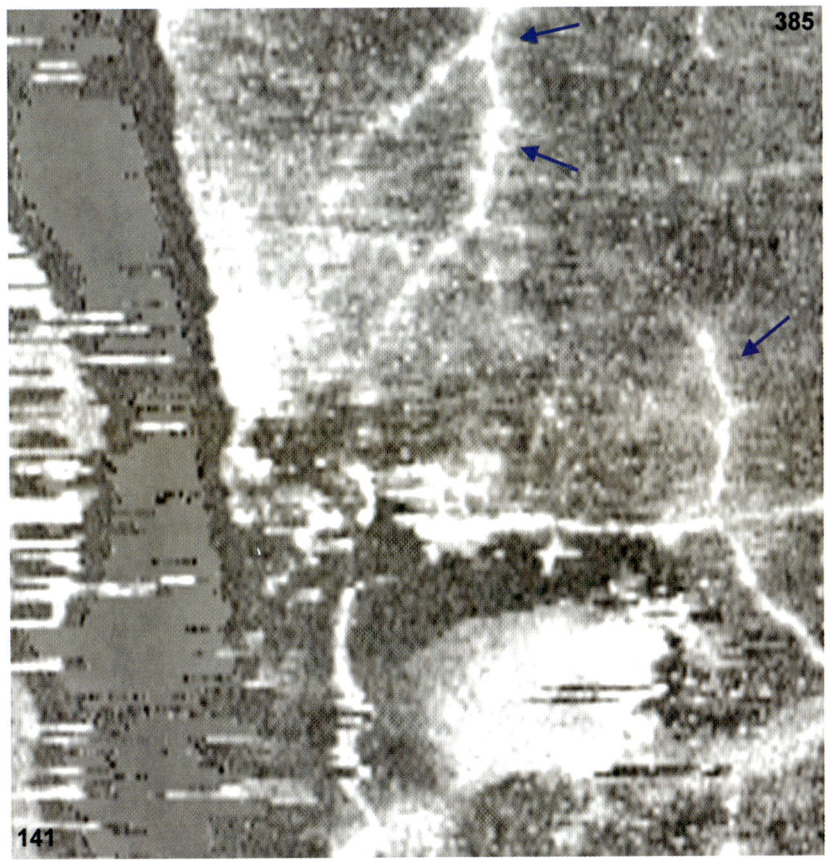

Figure 2: *En face* image at the level of the inner nuclear layer depicts presumed vascular sheathing (blue arrows)

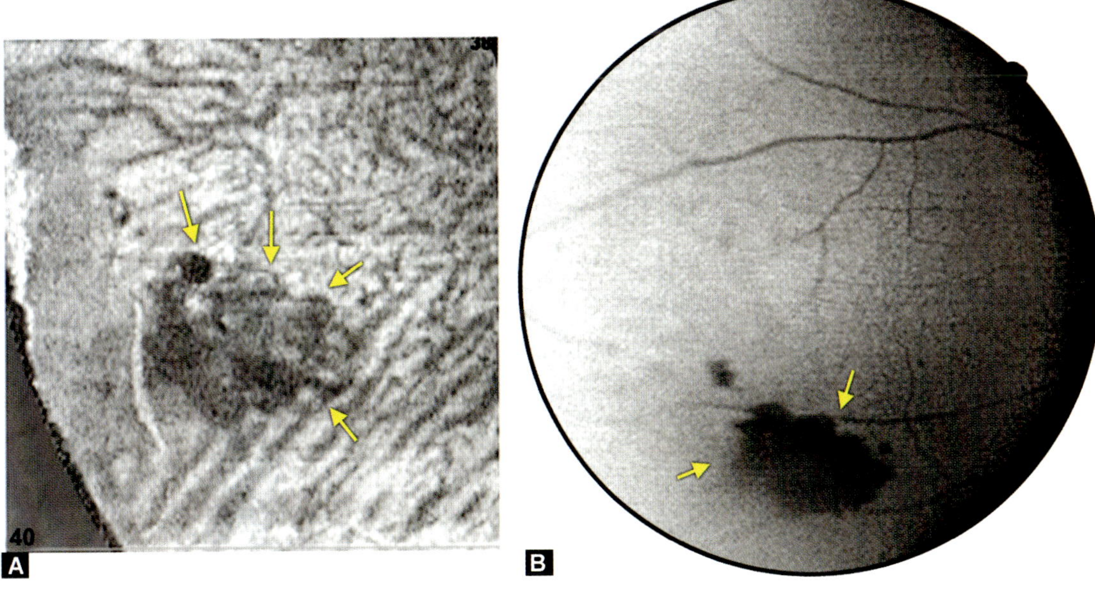

Figures 3A and B: Autofluorescence image shows hipoautofluorescence scar (yellow arrows) (A), which also can be observed in *en face* OCT imaging using the RPE as a reference plane (yellow arrows) (B)

In ocular toxoplasmosis, autofluorescence may be observed an extensive granulomatous inflammatory infiltration of the retinal pigment epithelium (RPE) and choroid leading to a considerable subretinal fibrosis. The FAF signal may vary depending on the stage and level of activity of the disease.

In **Figure 3**, autofluorescence image shows hipoautofluorescence scar (yellow arrows) **(Figure 3A)**, which also can be observed in *en face* OCT imaging using the RPE as a reference plane **(Figure 3B)**.

References

1. McCannel CA, Holland GN, Helm CJ, et al. UCLA Community-Based Uveitis Study Group. Causes of uveitis in the general practice of ophthalmology. Am J Ophthalmol. 1996;121:35-46.
2. Commodaro AG, Belfort RN, Rizzo LV, et al. Ocular toxoplasmosis: an update and review of the literature. Mem Inst Oswaldo Cruz. 2009;104:345-50.
3. Pierce EA, D'amico DJ. Ocular toxoplasmosis: pathogenesis, diagnosis, and management. Semin Ophthalmol. 1993;8:40-52.
4. Rothova A. Ocular manifestations of toxoplasmosis. Curr Opin Ophthalmol. 2003;14:384-8.
5. Lavinsky D, Romano A, Muccioli C, Belfort R Jr. Imaging in ocular toxoplasmosis. Int Ophthalmol Clin. 2012;52(4): 131-43.
6. Silveira C, Vallochi AL, Rodrigues da Silva U, Muccioli C, Holland GN, Nussenblatt RB, et al. Toxoplasma gondii in the peripheral blood of patients with acute and chronic toxoplasmosis. Br J Ophthalmol. 2011;95(3): 396-400.

Section 8

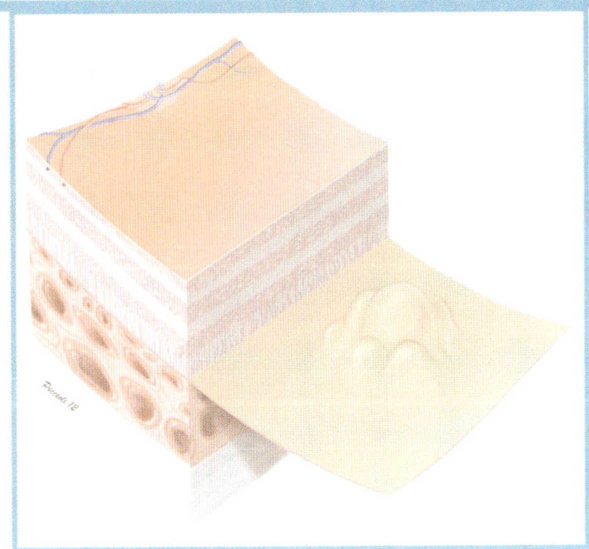

Myopia and Pathologic Myopia

chapter 33

En Face Optical Coherence Tomography in High Myopia

Gilda Cennamo, Raimondo Forte, Giuseppe de Crecchio

Introduction

Degenerative myopia, also called pathologic or high myopia, is defined as a myopic refractive error of more than 6 diopters associated with degenerative fundus changes.

The combination of retinal tractions, posterior staphyloma, and progressive global scleral stretching frequently leads to posterior pole abnormalities, such as myopic foveoschisis (**Figures 1 and 2**), macular holes[1] (**Figures 3 to 5**), posterior retinal detachment[2,3] (**Figures 6A to C**), detachment of the internal limiting membrane,[4] peripapillary detachment of the pigment epithelium,[5-7] choroidal neovascularization (**Figures 7A and B**), epiretinal membranes (**Figures 8 and 9**), vascular tractions with retinal microfolds (**Figures 10A and B**), paravascular intraretinal cysts[8,9] and dome shaped macula (**Figures 11A and B**).

En face optical coherence tomography (OCT) provides an accurate imaging of retinal changes of the posterior pole in high myopia and allows a prompt recognition of their localization. In fact the OCT C scans are represented as two-dimensional transversal slices at any given depth through the retina, enabling to visualize the lateral extent of structures.[10-14]

Furthermore, OCT B scans provide high quality images of the retinal layers.

In cases with posterior retinal detachment the OCT C scan image has been used to determine the relationships between the detachment and the staphyloma.[11]

References

1. Siam A. Macular hole with central retinal detachment in high myopia with posterior staphyloma. Br J Ophthalmol. 1969;53(1):62-3.
2. Takano M, Kishi S. Foveal retinoschisis and retinal detachment in severely myopic eyes with posterior staphyloma. Am J Ophthalmol. 1999;128(4):472-6.
3. Baba T, Ohno-Matsui K, Futagami S, et al. Prevalence and characteristics of foveal retinal detachment without macular hole in high myopia. Am J Ophthalmol. 2003;135(3):338-42.
4. Sayanagi K, Ikuno Y, Tano Y. Tractional internal limiting membrane detachment in highly myopic eyes. Am J Ophthalmol. 2006;142(5):850-2.
5. Freund KB, Ciardella AP, Yannuzzi LA, et al. Peripapillary detachment in pathologic myopia. Arch Ophthalmol. 2003;121(2):197-204.
6. Toranzo J, Cohen SY, Erginay A, et al. Peripapillary intrachoroidal cavitation in myopia. Am J Ophthalmol. 2005;140(4):731-2.
7. Shimada N, Ohno-Matsui K, Yoshida T, et al. Characteristics of peripapillary detachment in pathologic myopia. Arch Ophthalmol. 2006;124(1):46-52.
8. Sayanagi K, Ikuno Y, Gomi F, et al. Retinal vascular microfolds in highly myopic eyes. Am J Ophthalmol. 2005;139(4):658-63.
9. Ikuno Y, Gomi F, Tano Y. Potent retinal arteriolar traction as a possible cause of myopic foveoschisis. Am J Ophthalmol. 2005;139(3):462-7.
10. van Velthoven ME, Verbraak FD, Yannuzzi LA, et al. Imaging the retina by *en face* optical coherence tomography. Retina. 2006;26(2):129-36.
11. Forte R, Pascotto F, Soreca E, et al. Posterior retinal detachment without macular hole in high myopia: visualization with *en face* optical coherence tomography. Eye (Lond). 2007;21(1):111-3.
12. Forte R, Pascotto F, Napolitano F, et al. *En face* optical coherence tomography of macular holes in high myopia. Eye (Lond). 2007;21(3):436-7.
13. Forte R, Pascotto F, Cennamo G, et al. Evaluation of peripapillary detachment in pathologic myopia with *en face* optical coherence tomography. Eye (Lond). 2008;22(1):158-61.
14. Forte R, Cennamo G, Pascotto F, et al. *En face* optical coherence tomography of the posterior pole in high myopia. Am J Ophthalmol. 2008;145(2):281-8.

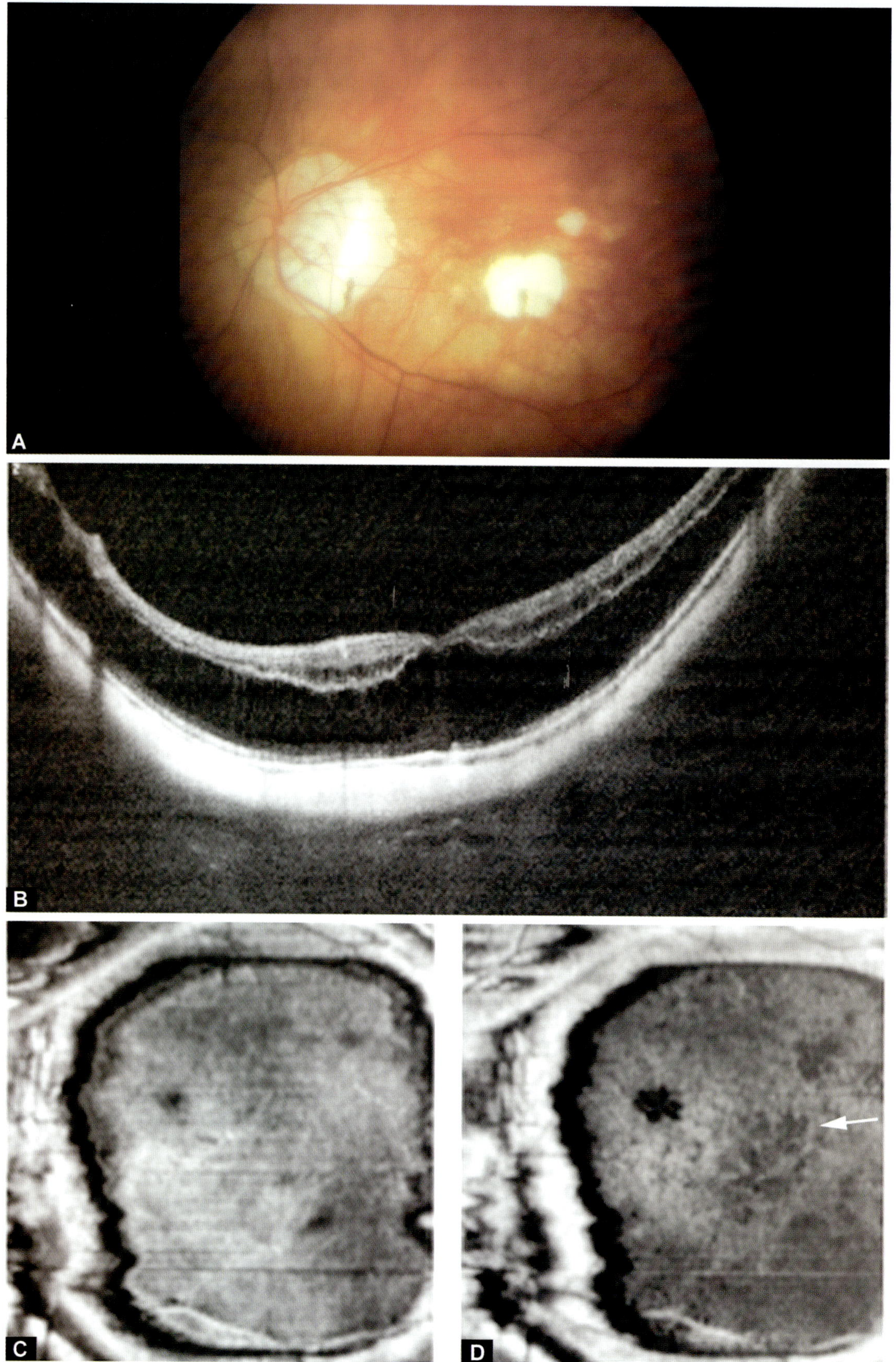

Figures 1A to D: Myopic foveoschisis indicated in (A) color fundus image and (B) longitudinal B scan; (C and D) On *en face* C scans, the intraretinal schisis shows a honeycomb pattern (arrow) (Optovue Inc, Fremont, CA, USA)

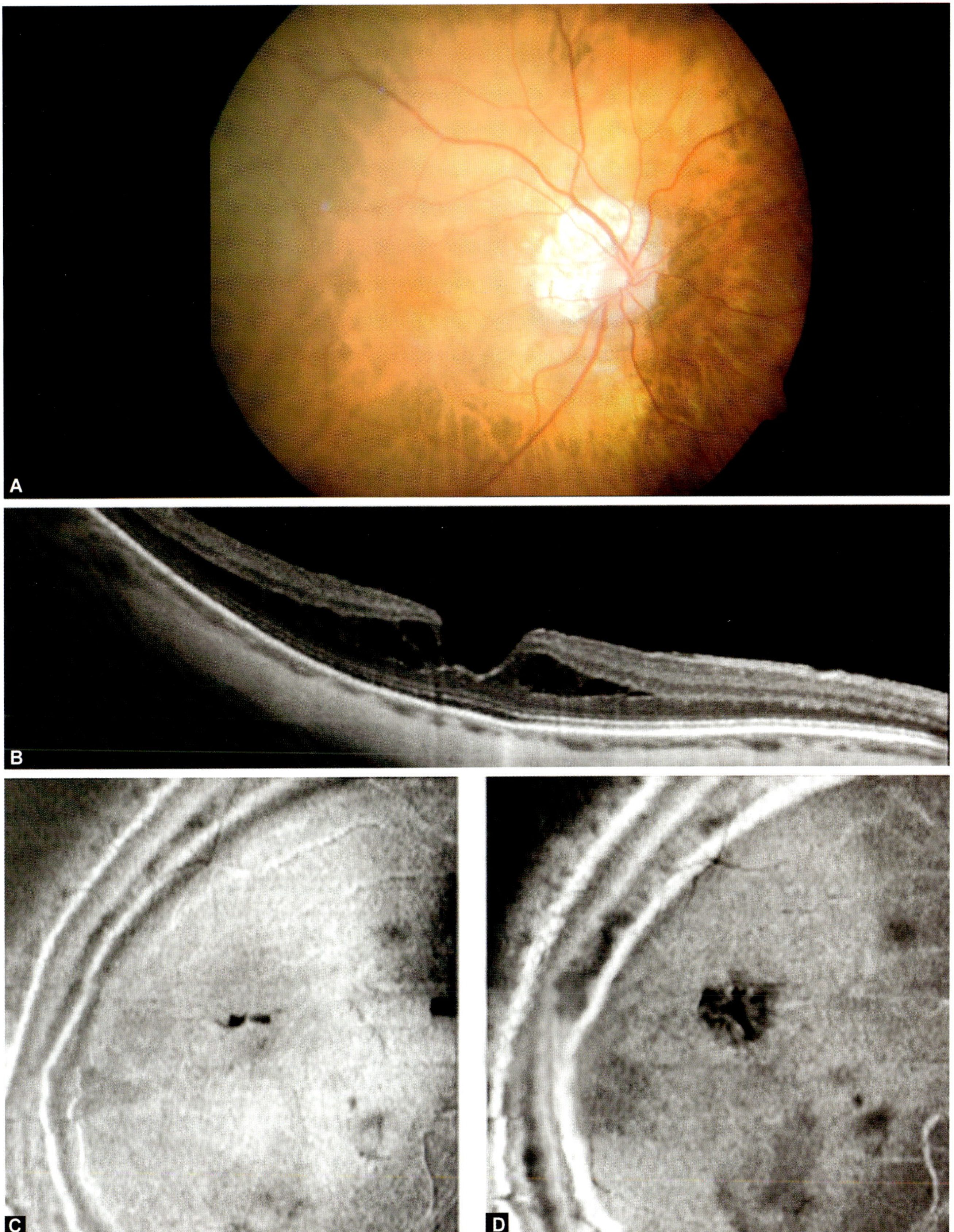

Figures 2A to D: Lamellar macular hole and myopic foveoschisis at (A) color fundus image, (B) longitudinal B scan and (C and D) consecutive anteroposterior *en face* C scans (Optovue Inc, Fremont, CA, USA)

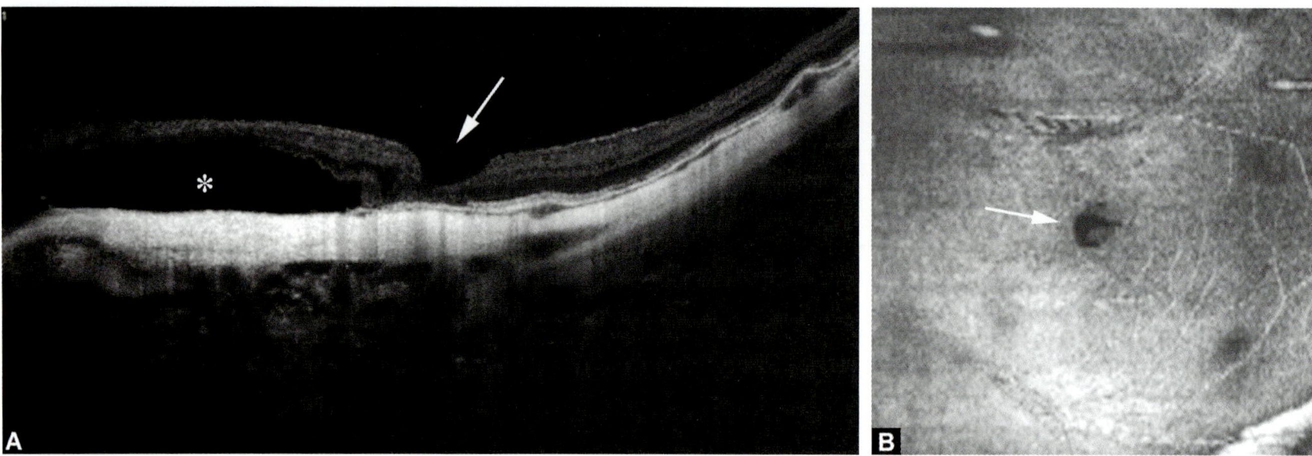

Figures 3A and B: Lamellar macular hole (arrow) and schisis of the outer retinal layers (asterisk) in high myopia as shown by (A) longitudinal B scan and (B) *en face* C scan. Epiretinal membrane is present (Optovue Inc, Fremont, CA, USA)

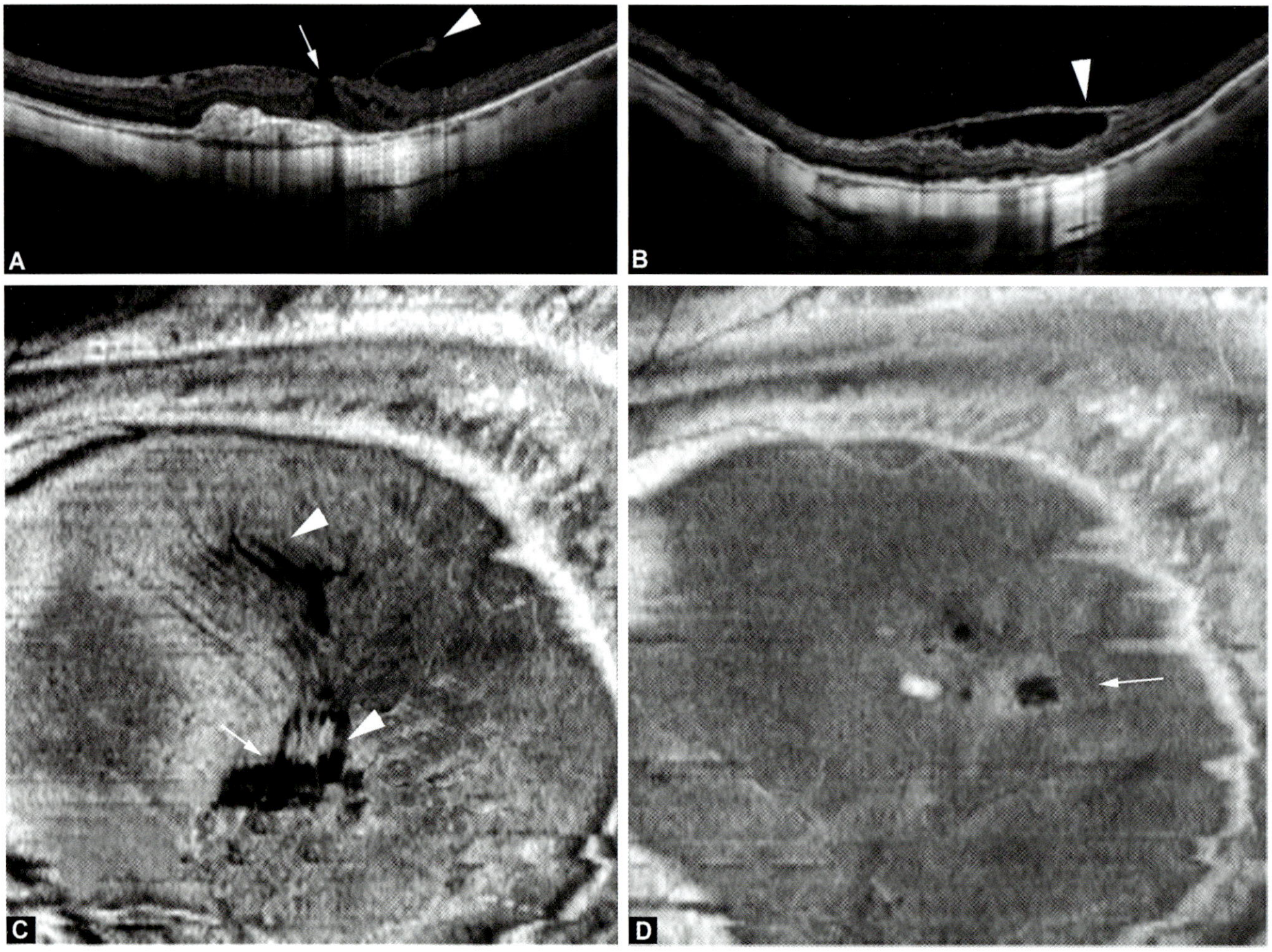

Figures 4A to D: (A) Lamellar hole with thin residual retina (arrow) and epiretinal membrane (B, arrowhead) in high myopia at longitudinal B scans and at (C and D) consecutive anteroposterior *en face* scans (Optovue Inc, Fremont, CA, USA)

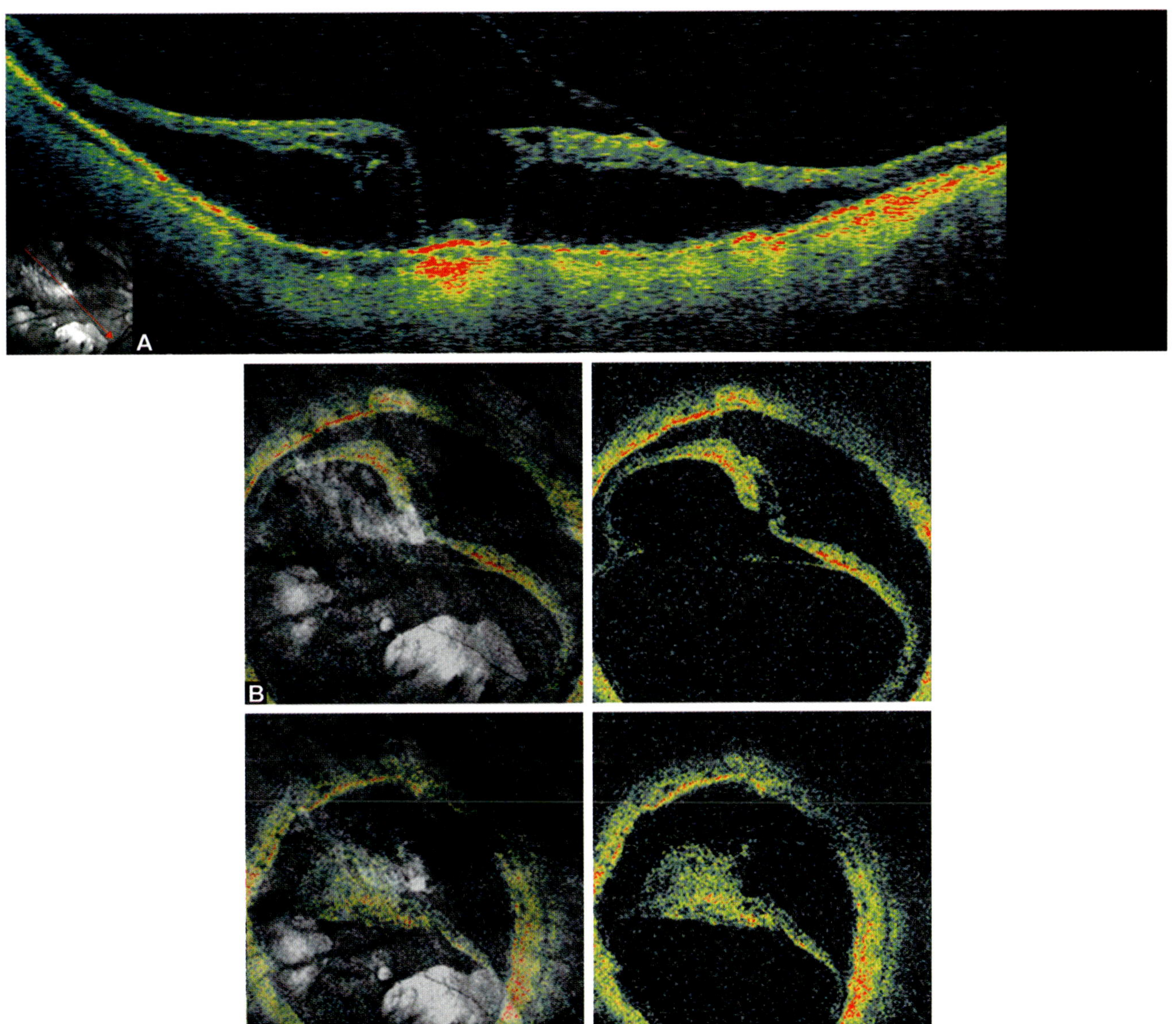

Figures 5A to C: Myopic macular hole with thin residual retina as shown by (A) longitudinal B scan showing outer retinoschisis and hyaloidal traction; (B and C) Anteroposterior (left) overlaid scanning laser ophthalmoscopy (SLO) image/C scan and (right) C scan images of the posterior pole showing the edges of the macular hole (OCT/SLO; OPKO/OTI, Miami, FL)

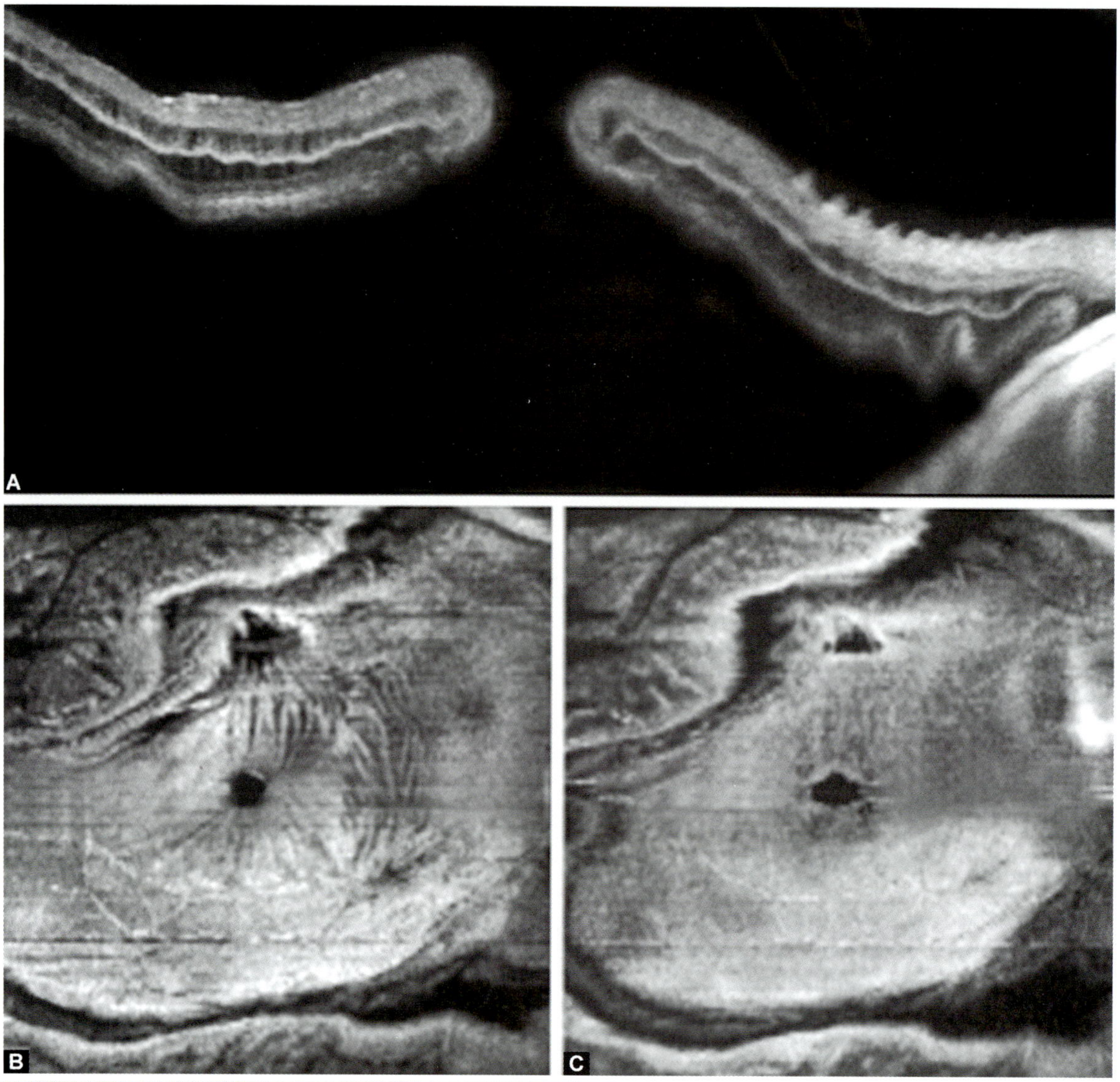

Figures 6A to C: Posterior retinal detachment and full-thickness macular hole in a highly myopic eye as shown by (A) longitudinal B scan and (B and C) consecutive anteroposterior *en face* scans. Epiretinal membrane is present (Optovue Inc, Fremont, CA, USA)

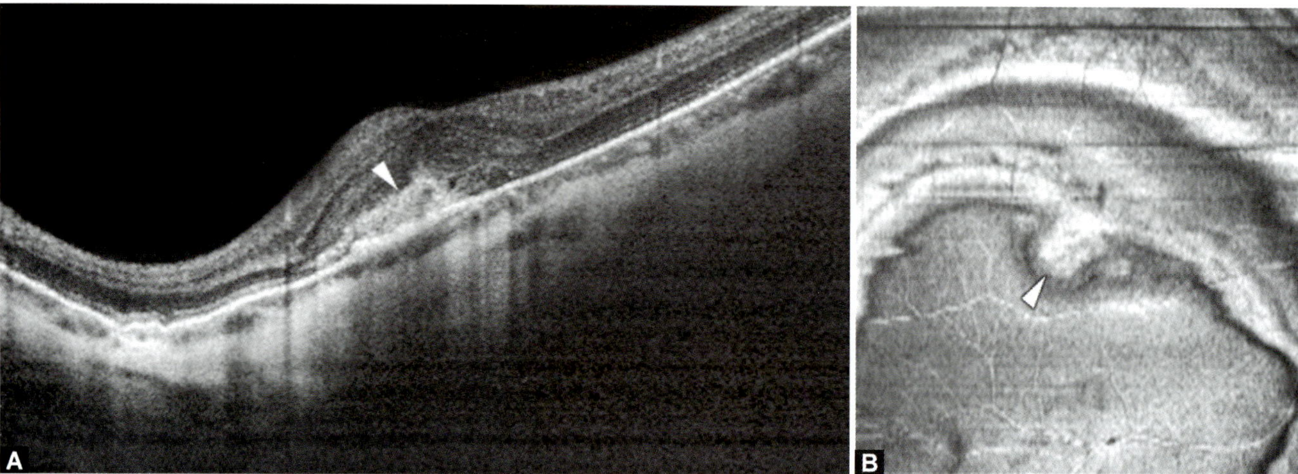

Figures 7A and B: Subfoveal choroidal neovascularization (arrowhead) in high myopia as shown by (A) longitudinal B scan and (B) en face scan (Optovue Inc, Fremont, CA, USA)

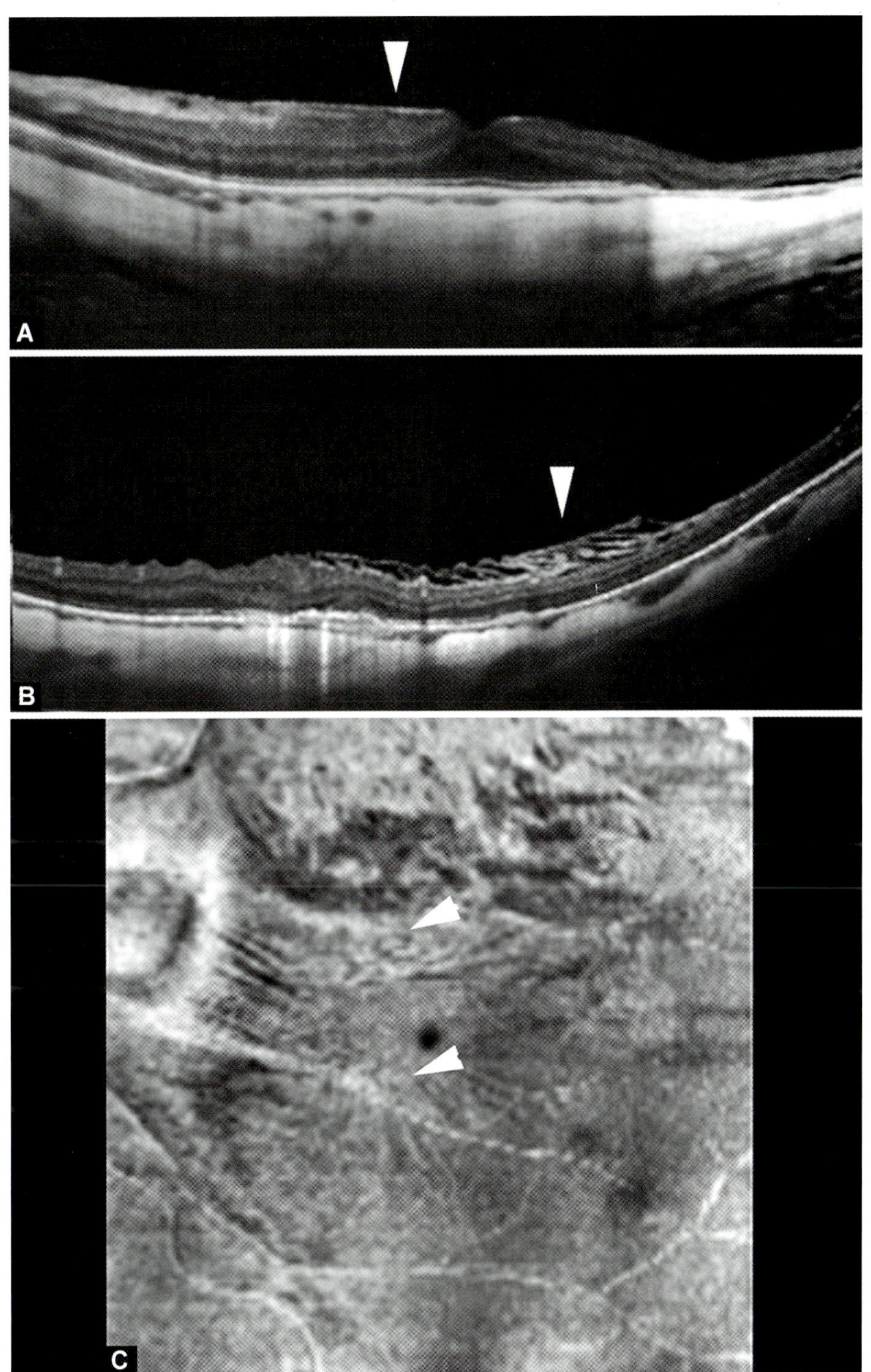

Figures 8A to C: Epiretinal membrane (arrowhead) in high myopia as shown by (A) longitudinal B scans and by (B and C) consecutive anteroposterior *en face* scans (Optovue Inc, Fremont, CA, USA)

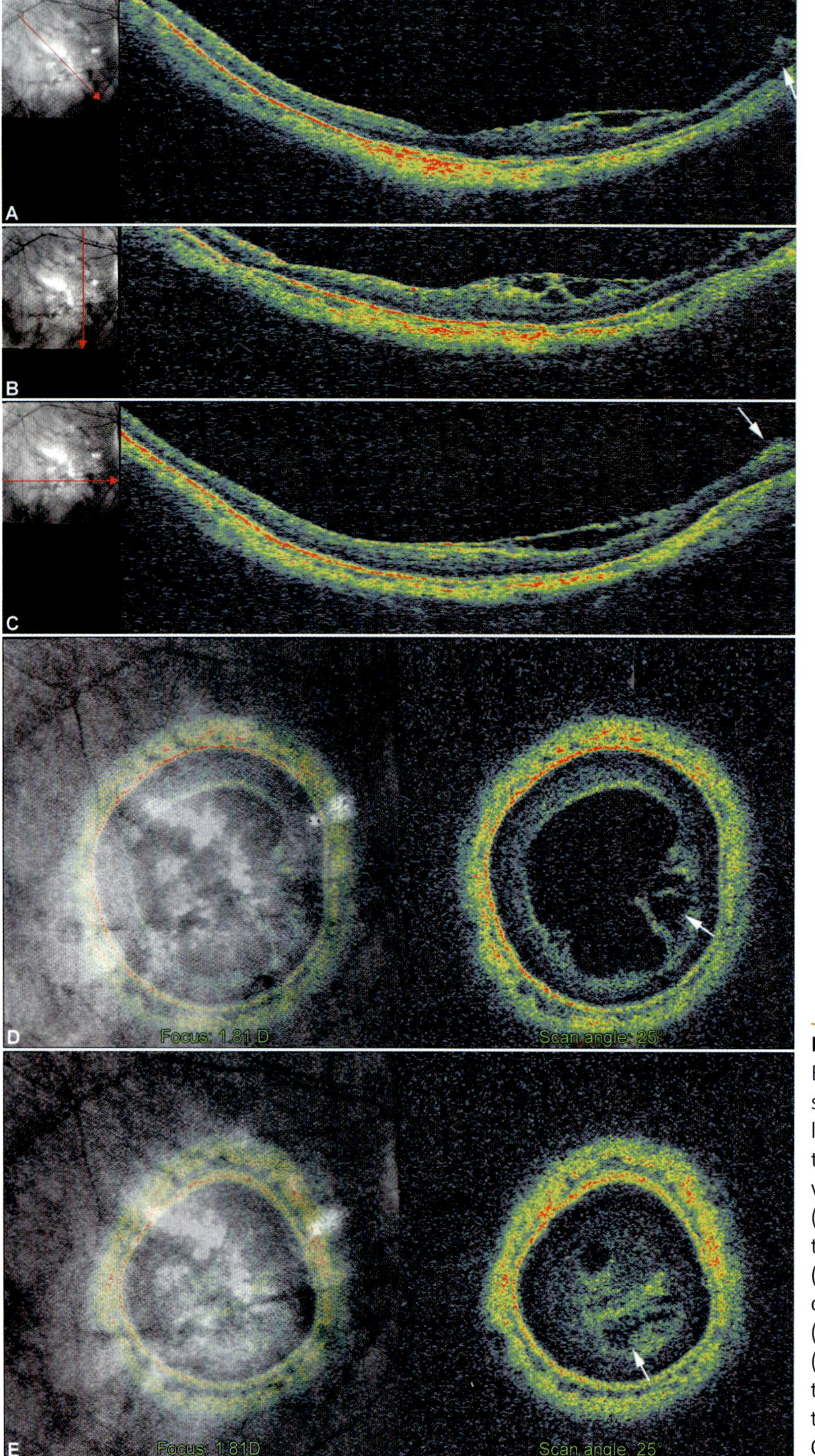

Figures 9A to E: (A to C) Longitudinal B scan images showing inner retinoschisis and epiretinal membrane located among nasal retinal vessels at the edge of peripapillary atrophy. A vascular retinal microfold is detectable (arrow). Irregular hyper-reflectivity of the choroid is present in macular area; (D and E) (left) overlay of scanning laser ophthalmoscopy image and C scan and (right) C scan image showing the schisis (arrow) which extends among the temporal retinal vessels at the edge of the peripapillary staphyloma (OCT/SLO; OPKO/OTI, Miami, FL)

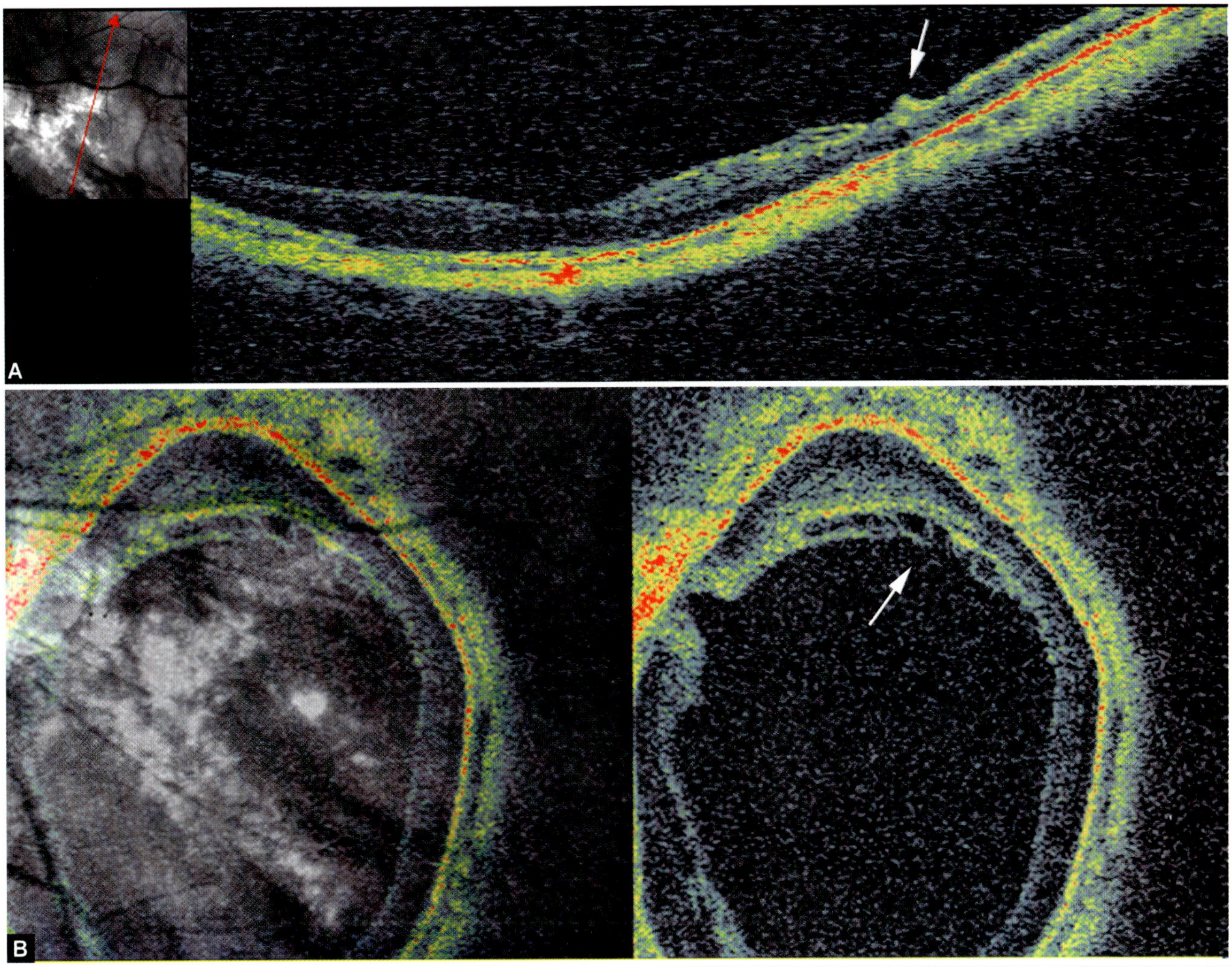

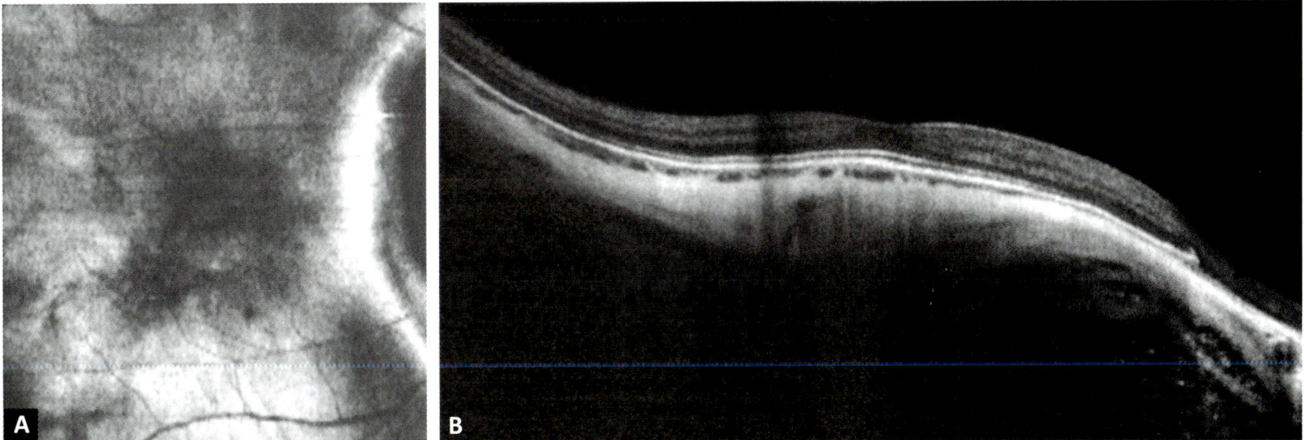

Figures 10A and B: (A) Longitudinal cross-sectional B scan showing a retinal microfold (arrow). Low-grade choroidal hyper-reflectivity is present in the macula; (B) (left) overlaid scanning laser ophthalmoscopy (SLO) image/C scan and (right) C scan image. The retinal microfold (arrow) is clearly detectable (OCT/SLO; OPKO/OTI, Miami, FL)

Figures 11A and B: Dome shaped macula within a posterior myopic staphyloma. Visual acuity is 20/20. (A) *En face* and (B) Longitudinal B scan image. Scleral thickening is present in the macular region (Optovue Inc, Fremont, CA, USA)

Section 9

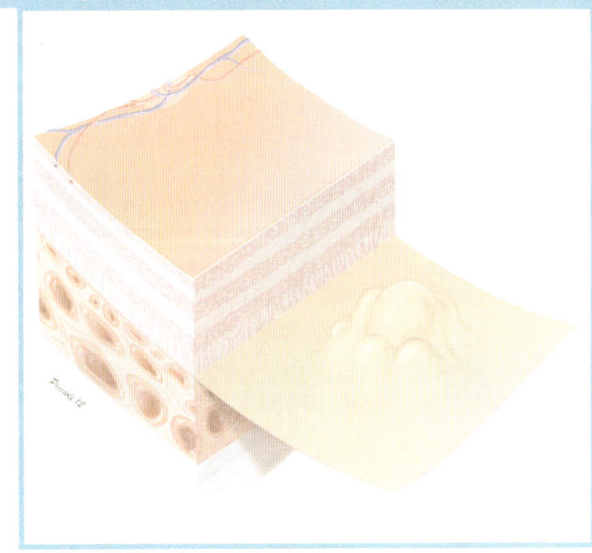

Vitreoretinal Interface: Macular Holes, Pseudoholes and Lamellar Holes

Vitreomacular Interface Alteration: A New Semiology with *En Face* Optical Coherence Tomography

Jean-Francois Le Rouic, Marco Rispoli

Introduction

Vitreomacular interface disorders include a variety of macular diseases such as vitreomacular traction with or without epiretinal membrane (ERM) formation, macular hole and isolated ERM. These conditions become more common with age.[1] So far, imaging of these pathologies lay mainly on: (1) color or blue filter frames which provided a global overview of the posterior fundus and confirmed the diagnosis of ERM, and (2) standard longitudinal optical coherence tomography (OCT) sections which assessed possible traction or adherence of the vitreous on the posterior retina and detected associated intraretinal alterations such as cystoid macular edema, foveal schisis, or macular hole.

En face OCT of the retinal surface, now available, thanks to the development of spectral domain optical coherence tomography (SD-OCT), allows three-dimensional reconstruction and visualization of the retinal surface following the concavity of the posterior pole of the eye with high quality imaging that would not be obtained from longitudinal scans alone. *En face* OCT of the retinal surface is a new way of analyzing the inner retina and opens the door to a new semiology.[2-4] In this chapter, the authors will present the main characteristics disclosed by an *en face* OCT of the inner face of the retina in patients presenting with alterations of retinovitreal relationships.

En Face Spectral Domain Optical Coherence Tomography Picture of the Retinal Surface

All the figures, shown below by the authors have been obtained with the same technique using the Optovue RTVue 100. This SD-OCT machine equipped with the software version 5.1.090 analyzes 141 horizontal, parallel B scans centered on the macula and spaced 0.49 mm. Each scan is 7 mm long on the horizontal axis. Each B scan is made of 385 A scans (one A scan every 0.018 mm).

We thus obtain an analysis grid made of 54285 A scans. The "macular cube" is 7 mm by 7 mm wide by 2 mm high. During the 4 seconds of acquisition time, the patient is asked to maintain fixation without blinking.

Then, the segmentation algorithm determines automatically in each of the 141 B scans the inner retinal surface. The *en face* section (slice) can be 9–30 μm thick as needed. The *en face* slice is performed at internal limiting membrane (ILM) line level. The ILM line is given by the software. Herein, the operator used a slice 30 μm thick. The authors always used the automatic software detection and never manually corrected irregularities.[4]

Vitreomacular Traction

The segmentation algorithm of *en face* OCT focuses on a single layer, after determining the ideal line for the retinal surface. In eyes with vitreomacular traction or adherence, the retinal surface has three different textures: (1) in the most central area the posterior hyaloid is tightly adherent to the retina, (2) in periphery where the vitreous is detached, the retina may appear normal or be folded radially and (3) at the edge of these two areas a hyper-reflective curved line can be visualized. When comparing the *en face* OCT with longitudinal scan this curved hyper-reflective line is due to the posterior hyaloid leaving steeply the plane of the retinal surface (**Figure 1**).

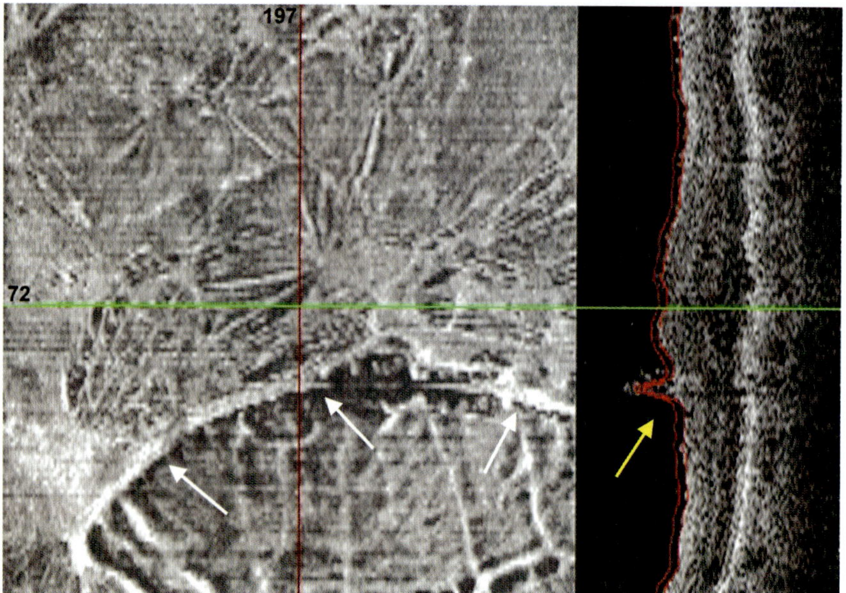

Figure 1: *En face* optical coherence tomography (OCT) scan of an eye with an epiretinal membrane and vitreomacular traction. The curved hyper-reflective line (white arrows) correlates with the posterior hyaloid leaving the retinal surface on longitudinal OCT sections (yellow arrow)

Classification of Epiretinal Membrane with *En Face* Optical Coherence Tomography of the Retinal Surface

Gass Classification

A classification of ERM severity taking into account the reflection of the retinal surface and the distortion of the retina have been proposed by Gass who described the three stages as follows:[5]

- Stage 0: consists in a cellophane maculopathy with a brilliant aspect and few retinal distortions
- Stage 1: consists in a wrinkled cellophane maculopathy with irregular wrinkling of the retinal surface
- Stage 2: consists in a macular pucker with a thick and opaque membrane covering the retina

Following this classification, an OCT *en face* of the retinal surface classification of ERMs according to the severity of the folds also seems possible (**Figures 2A to C**).

Differentiating the Main *En Face* Optical Coherence Tomography Patterns

The authors retrospectively studied the aspects of the retinal surface with *en face* OCT in a consecutive series of 90 eyes of 85 patients who consulted at their institution and were diagnosed with idiopathic ERM. In this series, the aspect of the retinal surface could be divided into some main patterns, whose frequency appears as follows:

- Plaque (33%): Plaques are the most common feature in patients with ERM. In almost every case they are surrounded by radiating folds. These single or multiple plaques can be of variable size.

  Comparison of *en face* SD-OCT retinal surface images with standard OCT sections reveals that plaques are the results from the focus of the segmentation algorithm on the membrane rather than on the retina. Hence, plaques correspond generally to localized areas of tight adherence between the retina and the ERM or the posterior hyaloid. Retinal folds follow the serrated pattern of the vitreal face of the retina; they are generally associated with subtle detachment of the membrane (**Figures 3 and 4**).

- Retinal starfolds (12%): Starfolds are less common than plaques in patients with ERM. Single or multiple starfolds can be observed. They can be classified according to their location: juxta or extrafoveolar (**Figure 5**). Folds can sometimes involve the fovea (**Figure 6**). It is possible that starfolds are the first step and will progress into plaques.

- Diffuse folding of the retina (10%): Folds of the retina can also take a grossly parallel pattern and involve a wide area. In such cases, diffuse retinal folds are not radiating from an epicenter (starfold) or a plaque.

  On longitudinal OCT section, the authors never observed vitreous attachment in the area affected with this type of fold (**Figure 7**).

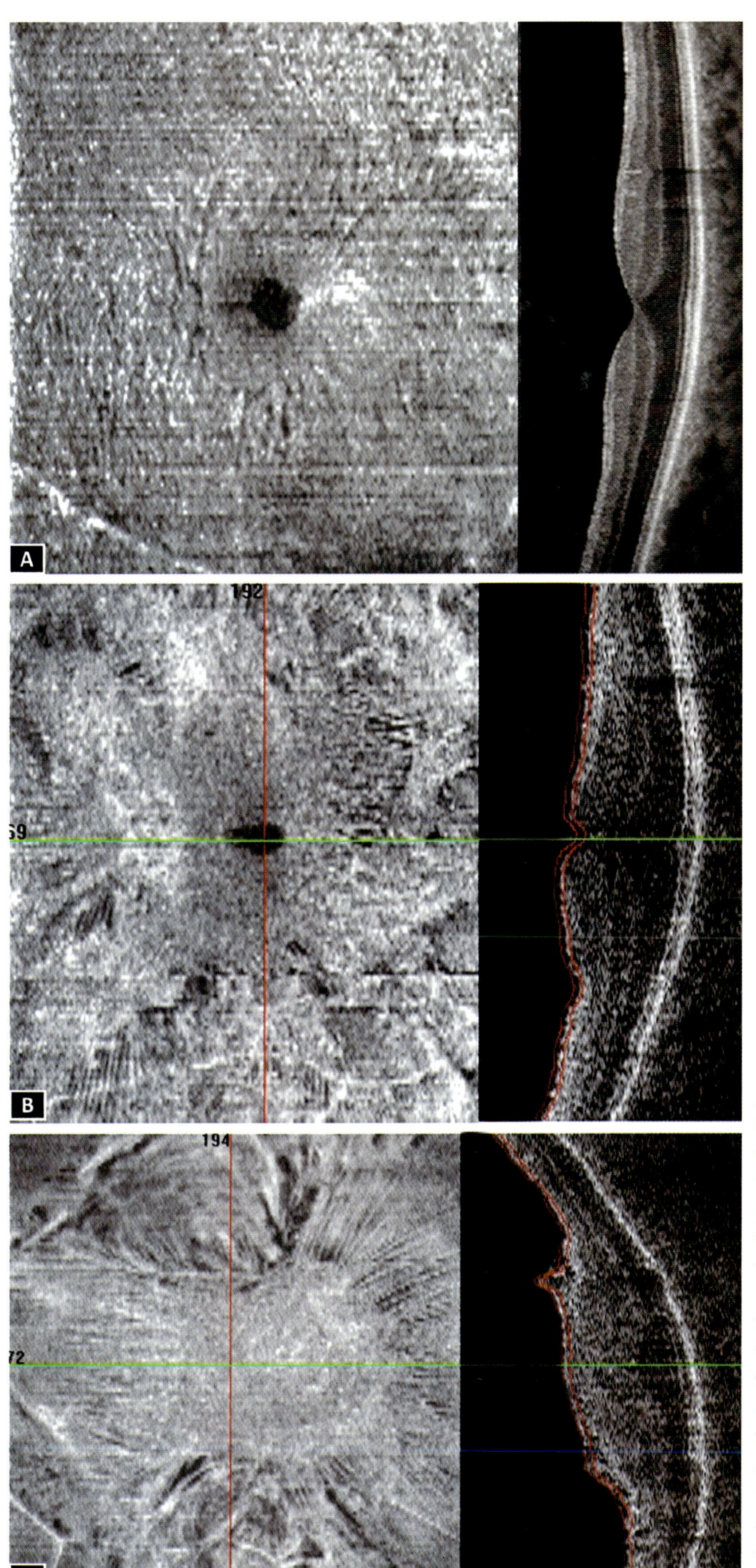

Figures 2A to C: *En face* optical coherence tomography (OCT) of the retinal surface in three patients presenting with epiretinal membrane (ERM) and various amount of folding of the inner face of the retina. Similar to Gass classification of ERMs, (A) would be stage 0 with normal longitudinal section and faint and diffuse folds on *en face* OCT; (B) would be stage 1 with increased central thickness, slightly altered foveal depression on OCT section and central plaque pattern with small radiating folds on *en face* OCT and (C) would be stage 2 with increased retinal thickness on OCT longitudinal section, and a thick central plaque surrounded by clearly visible folds on *en face* OCT. The foveal depression is not visible

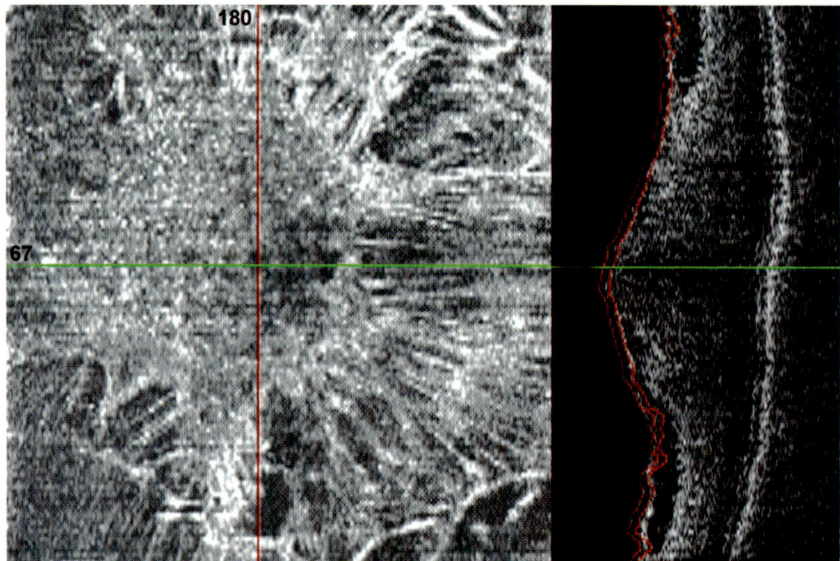

Figure 3: The most common aspect of epiretinal membrane is a plaque surrounded by folds (mainly seen in the left and in the superior part of the picture). When compared with the optical coherence tomography section, the plaque is an area of tight adherence between the retina and the membrane

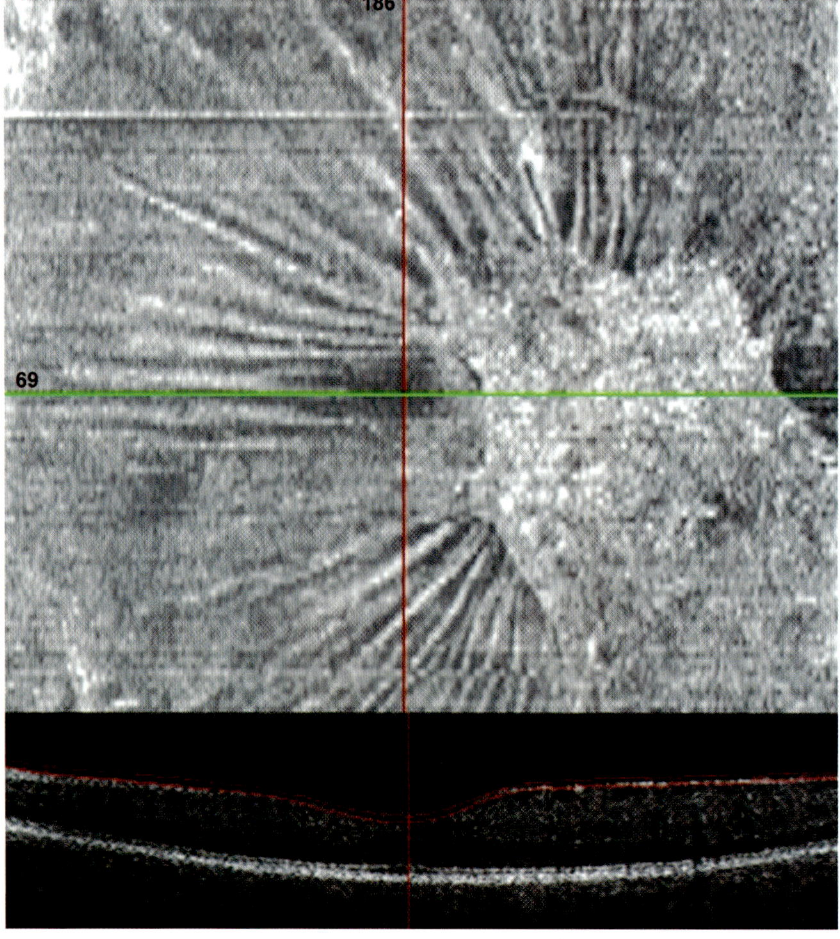

Figure 4: Plaques can involve the entire macula or be smaller and be located outside the fovea such as in this case

Figure 5: Epiretinal membranes may take the appearance of starfolds on *en face* optical coherence tomography. In this case two juxtafoveal folds can be seen

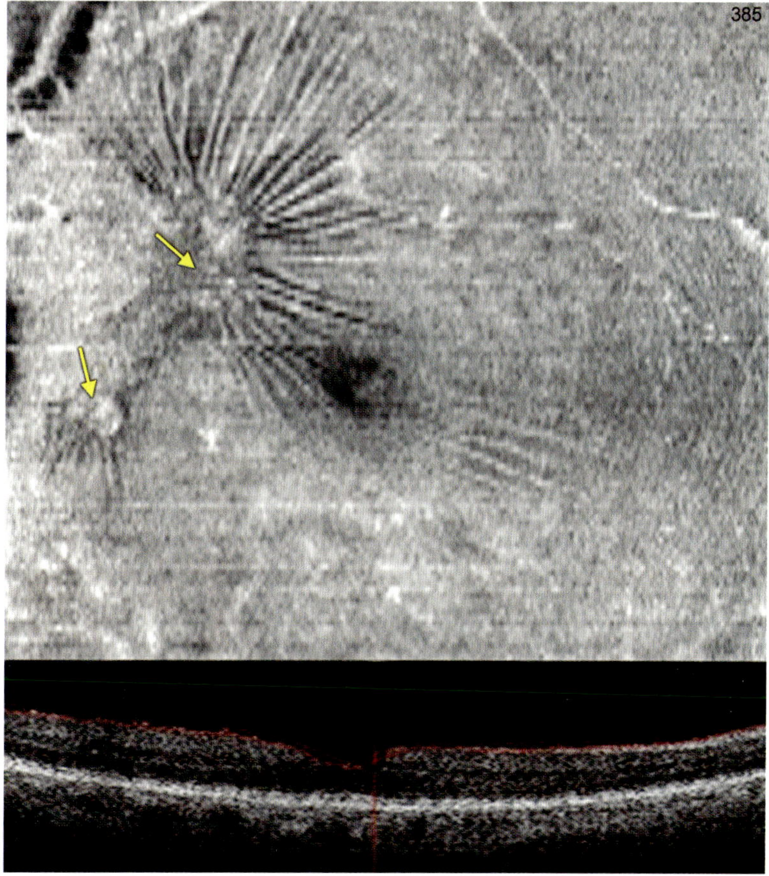

Figure 6: Two extrafoveal folds are present (arrows). Folds extending from the superior starfold involve the fovea

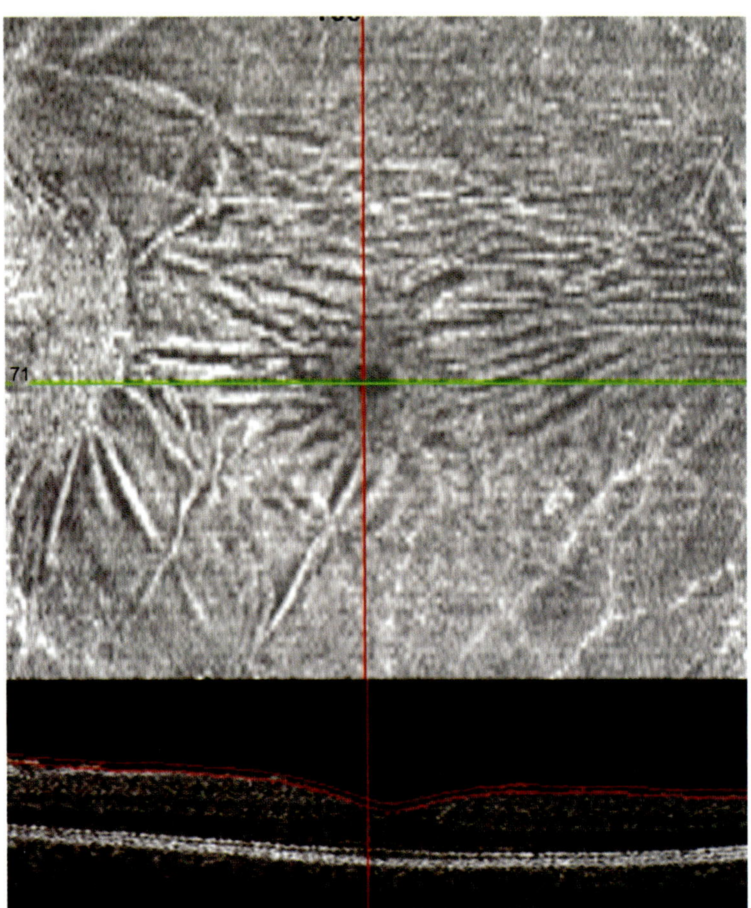

Figure 7: Epiretinal membrane on *en face* optical coherence tomography of the retinal surface with diffuse and grossly parallel folds of the retina

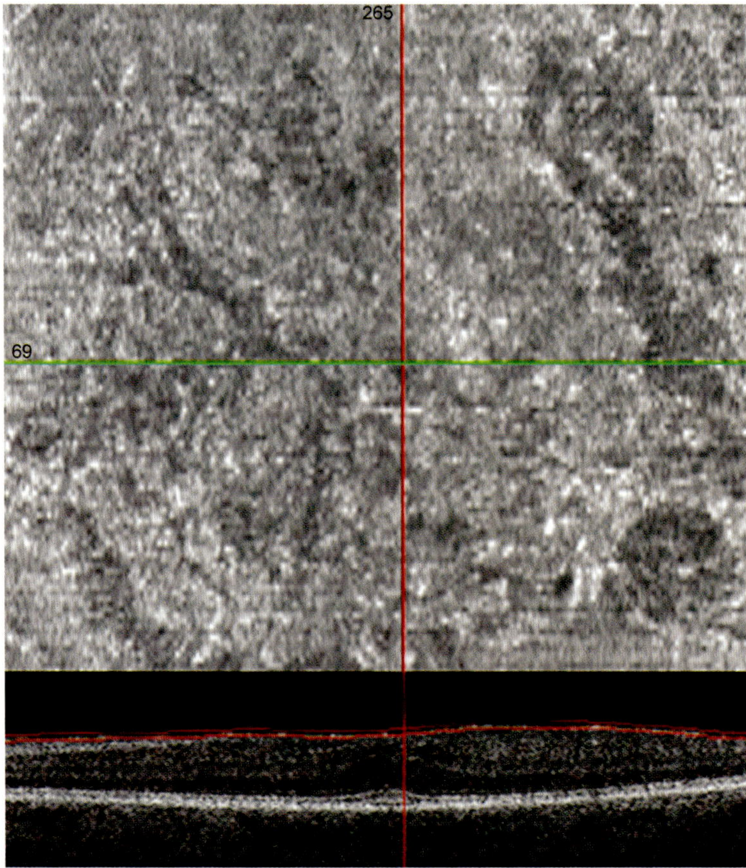

Figure 8: *En face* optical coherence tomography (OCT) of a patient with epiretinal membrane on fundus examination. The image seems foggy and lacking of details of the retinal surface. On longitudinal OCT section, a membrane covering the entire retinal surface can be observed. The *en face* OCT is actually focused on the posterior hyaloid still attached

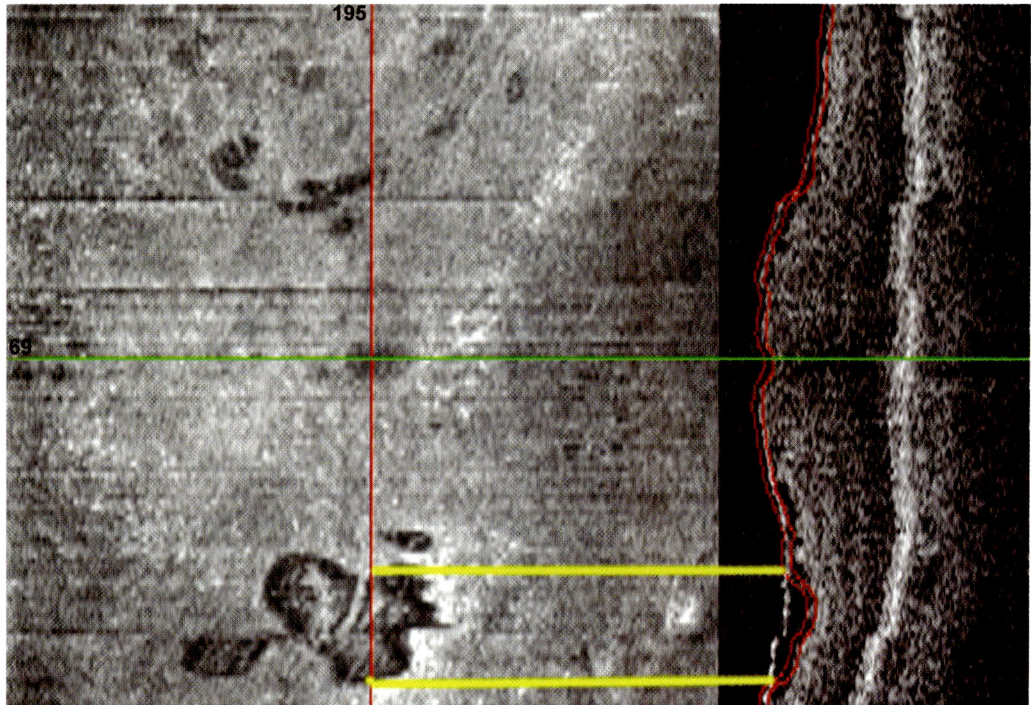

Figure 9: *En face* optical coherence tomography disclosing "retinal windows". The segmentation algorithm is focused on the attached posterior hyaloid except in areas where it is detached from the retinal surface (yellow lines). Retinal windows appear as well limited areas generally covered with streaks

- Focus on the posterior hyaloid (14%): This pattern gives a cloudy or foggy appearance of the retinal surface with *en face* OCT. At first, this image seems poor in information and needs to be compared with longitudinal OCT sections. Here, a thick linear membrane diffusely adherent to the inner face of the retina can be observed **(Figure 8)**. The automated detection of the ideal line of the retinal surface follows this thick membrane and produces a pattern similar to a plaque covering the entire analyzed area. Intra-operatively, it appears that this pattern is due to the persistent adherence of the posterior hyaloid on the posterior retina.[6]
- Focus on the posterior hyaloid with "retinal windows" (13%): An additional feature can be added to the previous pattern: well-defined areas covered with streaks. When compared with OCT sections, these areas are due to localized detachment of the membrane/hyaloid. The segmentation algorithm will then run from the membrane to the retinal surface and back to the membrane. Localized areas of detachment of the membrane from the retinal surface, which appears as "retinal windows" on *en face* OCT, are probably the safer zone to initiate the grasping during ERM surgery **(Figure 9)**.

- Mixed features (18%): Different patterns can be associated on the retinal surface in patients presenting with ERM. An example is presented in **Figure 10**.

Secondary Patterns

Beside the main patterns due to vitreoretinal relationship alterations, *en face* OCT of the retinal surface can disclose other noteworthy information such as:
- Foveal depression: In patients with ERM, the foveal depression can be present, distorted, or absent **(Figures 11A to C)**.
- Retraction of the ERM: In two cases, the authors observed at the edge of a plaque an area dotted with small craters and pits. This pattern, looking like the moon surface, gave them the impression that an area of retinal nerve fiber layer was exposed after tearing of the ILM during spontaneous detachment of the ERM **(Figure 12)**. In a series by Bovey and Uffer,[7] including more than 200 ERM peeling, they observed such tearing and folding of the ILM in 8.6% of patients. Grasping the retina with a forceps in this region should be avoided as it would result in the nerve fiber layer damage.

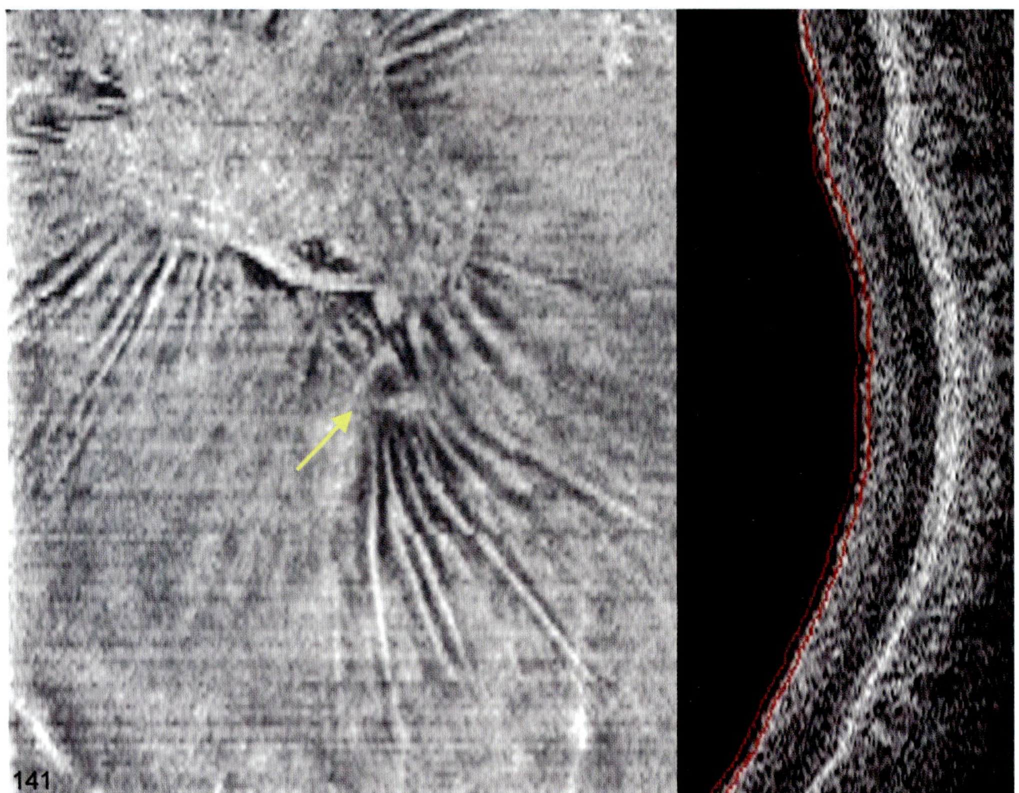

Figure 10: *En face* optical coherence tomography of an epiretinal membrane with an aspect of plaque associated with a starfold (arrow)

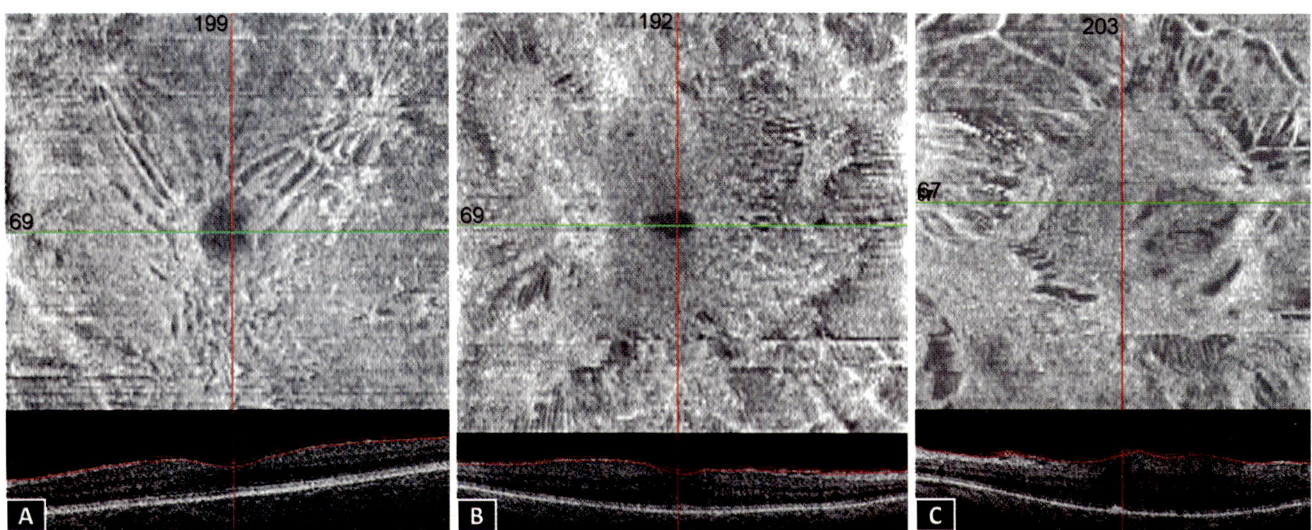

Figures 11A to C: In eyes with epiretinal membrane, *en face* optical coherence tomography of the retinal surface can give information on the foveal depression which can be normal (A), distorted (B) or absent (C)

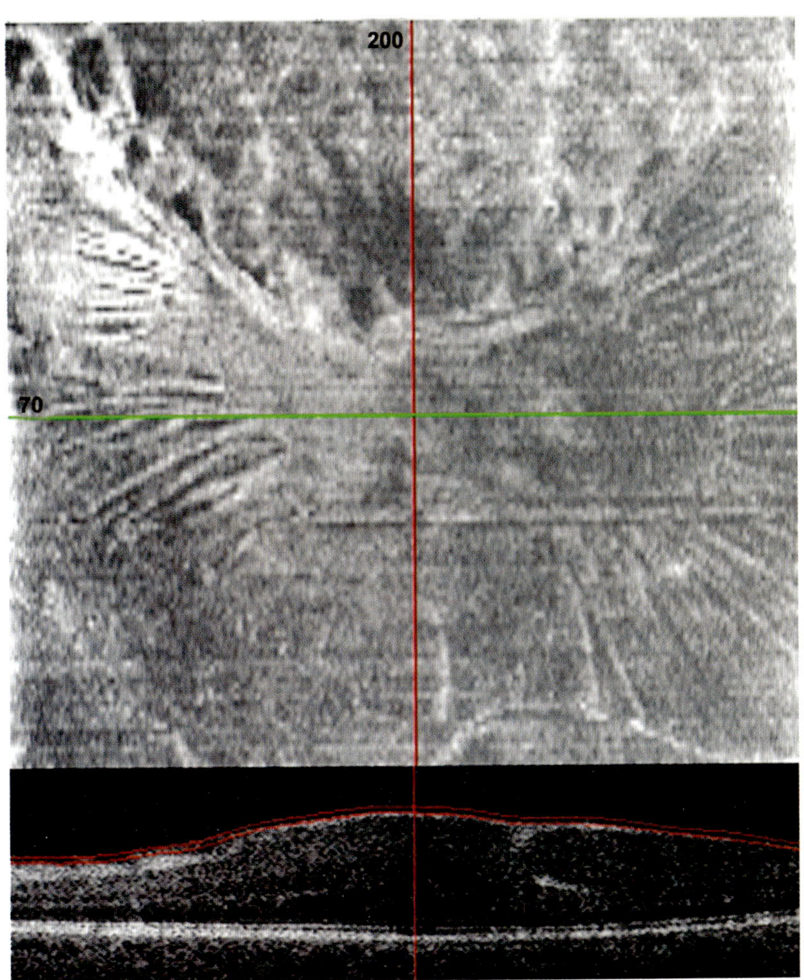

Figure 12: *En face* optical coherence tomography of the retinal surface disclosing on top of the picture a circumscribed area covered with pits and craters looking like the moon surface. This feature could be due to retinal nerve fiber layer exposure after internal limiting membrane rupture due to epiretinal membrane contraction. A plaque pattern is observed in the center of the picture

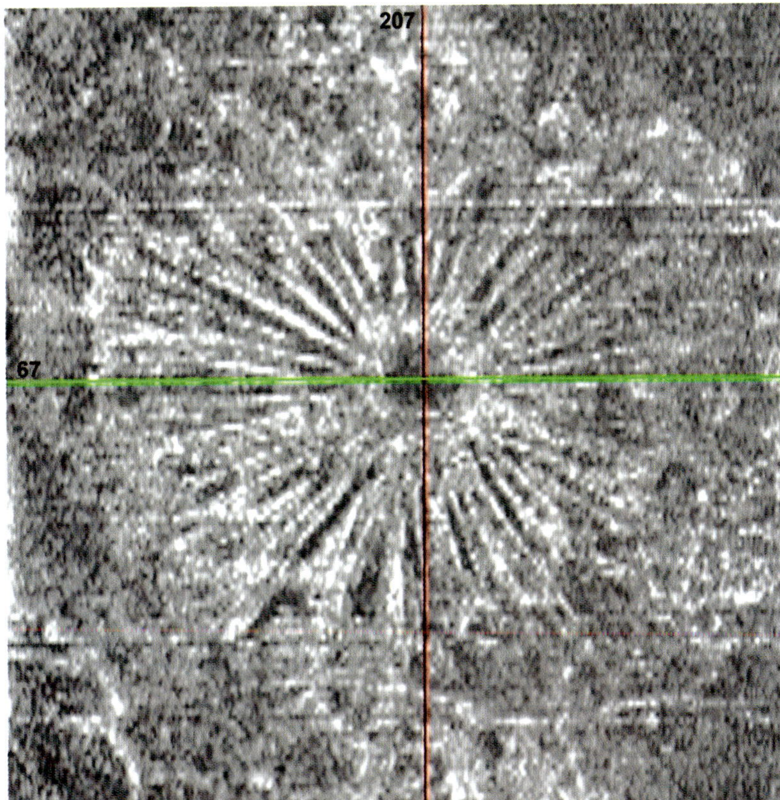

Figure 13: *En face* optical coherence tomography of the retinal surface in a patient with a perifoveal form of epiretinal membrane. Folds radiating from the fovea imitating the sunlight can be seen

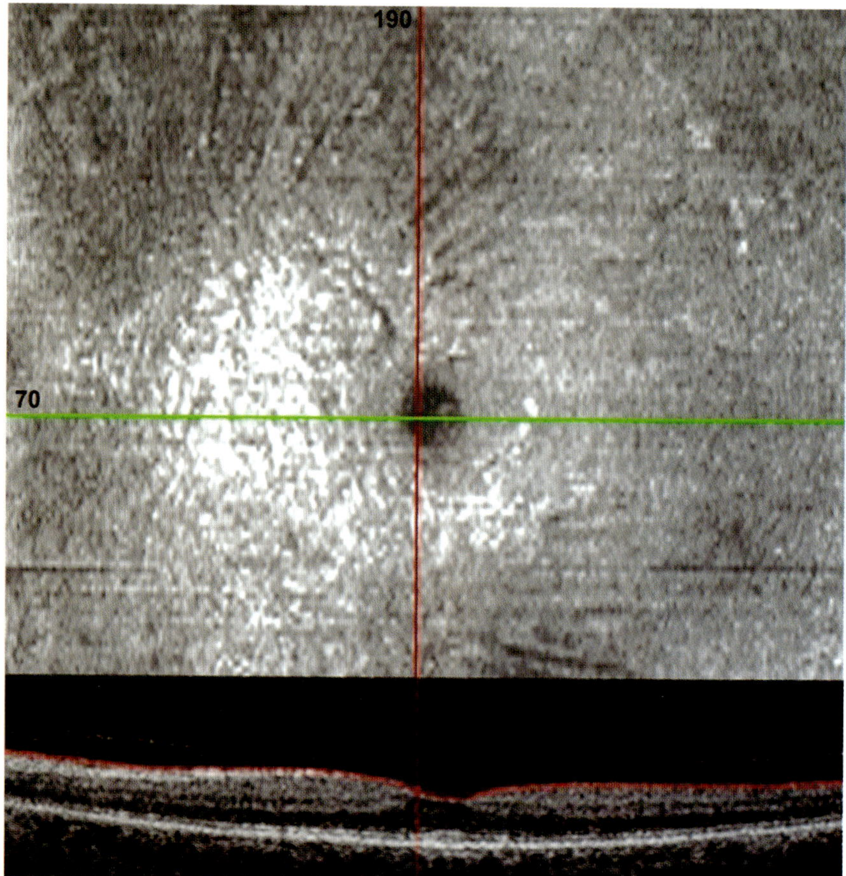

Figure 14: *En face* optical coherence tomography (OCT) of the retinal surface disclosing mild folds. The longitudinal OCT scan demonstrates partial vitreous detachment with foveal adherence. The folds might thus interest the internal limiting membrane

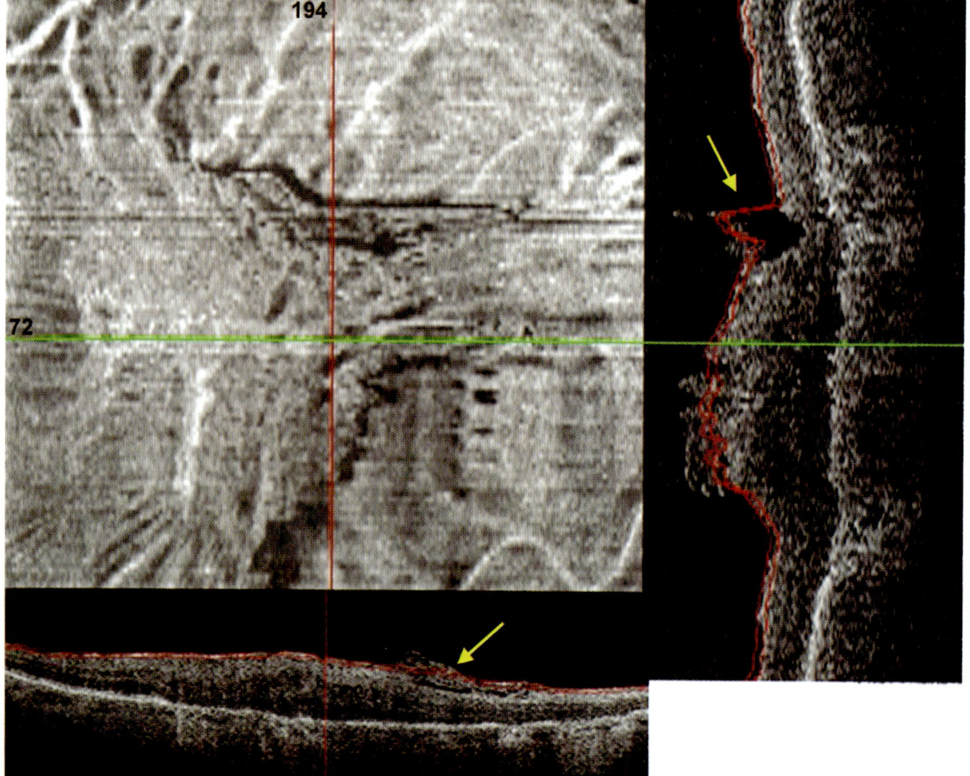

Figure 15: *En face* optical coherence tomography and longitudinal section in a case of vitreomacular traction. At some point, the automatic detection of the ideal line of the retinal surface erroneously follows the thick posterior hyaloids (arrows)

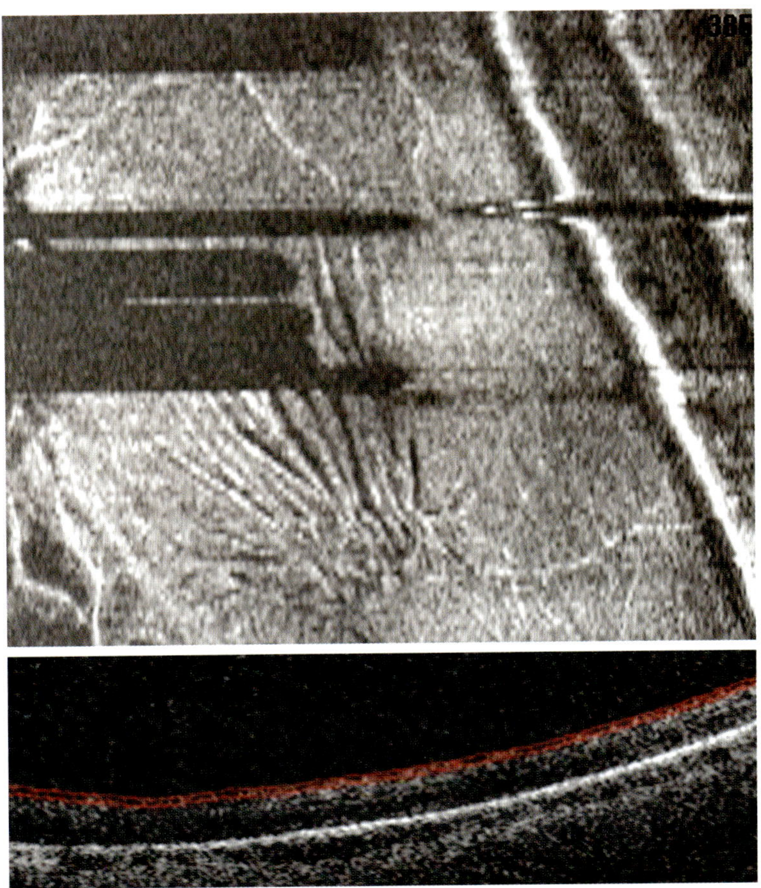

Figure 16: For an entire capture of a 7 by 7 mm wide area, the patient should fixate without blinking for 4 seconds. On this *en face* optical coherence tomography scan, the patient could not maintain fixation

- Perifoveal form: A peculiar form centered on the fovea with radiating retinal folds was noted in two eyes. This pattern mimicking the sunlight was called perifoveal form **(Figure 13)**.
- Folds of the ILM and posterior hyaloid detachment: In one case, OCT section disclosed partial detachment of the posterior hyaloid with foveal attachment. On *en face* OCT, the retinal surface is covered with small folds. In the presence of a vitreous detachment, these folds are likely interesting the ILM **(Figure 14)**.

Limits and Shortcomings of *En Face* Optical Coherence Tomography of the Retinal Surface

In eyes with thickened and partially adherent posterior hyaloid, the automatic detection may erroneously follow the vitreous instead of the retinal surface **(Figure 15)**.

The capture time is approximately 4 sec, and patients need to fixate without blinking. In the authors' series of four patients (5%) had an incomplete capture preventing the precise analysis of the retinal surface **(Figure 16)**.

References

1. Abdelkader E, Lois N. Internal limiting membrane peeling in vitreoretinal surgery. Surv Ophthalmol. 2008;53(4): 368-96.
2. Lumbroso B, Savastano MC, Rispoli M, et al. Morphologic differences, according to etiology, in pigment epithelial detachments by means of *en face* optical coherence tomography. Retina. 2011;31(3):553-8.
3. Alkabes M, Salinas C, Vitale L, et al. *En face* optical coherence tomography of inner retinal defects after internal limiting membrane peeling for idiopathic macular hole. Invest Ophthalmol Vis Sci. 2011;52(11): 8349-55.
4. Rispoli M, Le Rouic JF, Lesnoni G, et al. Retinal surface *en face* optical coherence tomography: A new imaging approach in epiretinal membrane surgery. Retina. 2012 (under publication).
5. Gass JD. Stereoscopic atlas of macular diseases: diagnostic and treatment. In: Ryan SJ (Ed). Retina: Basic Science and Inherited Retinal Disease. St Louis: CV Mosby Company; 1989.
6. Yamashita T, Uemura A, Sakamoto T. Intraoperative characteristics of the posterior vitreous cortex in patients with epiretinal membrane. Graefes Arch Clin Exp Ophthalmol. 2008;246(3):333-7.
7. Bovey EH, Uffer S. Tearing and folding of the retinal internal limiting membrane associated with macular epiretinal membrane. Retina. 2008;28(3):433-40.

chapter 35

Vitreoretinal Interface Before and After Macular Surgery

Marco Rispoli, Jean-Francois Le Rouic

En face analysis of the vitreoretinal interface is a relatively recent acquisition that adds precious qualitative data to the physician and to the surgeon.[1,2]

Bidimensional approach (traditional B scan) to the vitreoretinal interface gives a limited point of view due to extremely localized examination. In this way it is very difficult to rebuild a three dimensional (3D) structure by viewing bidimensional images (**Figures 1A and B**). Contrarily, the raster acquisition (several parallel B scans on the macula, **Figure 2**) allows 3D reconstruction of the macular cube from which all main layers can be extracted based on tissue reflectivity. The instrument software is able to recognize at least inner limiting membrane (ILM), inner plexiform layer (IPL) and retinal pigment epithelium (RPE) for each B scan that compose the macular cube (retinal segmentation). All segmentation lines are put together by software on a three dimensional virtual multilayer image. Operator may adjust the profile cut, the thickness cut and the cut deepness.[3]

The *en face* study of the vitreoretinal interface is very useful before and after macular surgery.[4] Some typical features resulting from macular peeling procedure are now well highlighted with *en face* view,[5,15] completing and integrating traditional B scan. Analyzing the macular pucker before the surgery,[6] *en face* cut gives a high relief of pathological structures and indicates with great accuracy the dimensions, thicknesses, folds and going deeper, the tractional edema features (**Figure 3**).[7,8]

After macular pucker surgery with ILM peeling, a characteristic feature of the peeled ILM area named "dissociated optic nerve fiber layer" (DONFL) has frequently been observed (**Figures 4A and B**).[9,10] The area covered by dimples had different patterns: oval, centered by the fovea, crescent-shaped skirting the fovea or distant from the fovea.[11-13]

In 15% of cases, *en face* spectral domain optical coherence tomography (SD-OCT) clearly shows an increase of dimples in number and size during postoperative follow-up. Those arcuate lines develop progressively after surgery in the peeled area.

En face reconstruction of the retinal surface follows the concavity of the inner retinal surface (**Figure 5**), which was not possible on all commercialized SD-OCT machines so far.

En face SD-OCT of the retinal surface performed within couple of weeks after surgery, reveals a rough aspect of the peeled ILM area. Dimples appear rarely at this time. During the follow-up after 2 weeks these curved dips can be observed by *en face* view adapted to ILM (**Figures 6A to D**).

This pattern could be due to the exposure of a rough surface composed of optic nerve fibers surrounded by Müller cell processes or more probably to the early and transient swelling of the retinal nerve fiber layer. Three months or more after surgery, dimples of the retinal surface were noted in 87% of cases (**Figure 7**).[14]

After ILM removal, several OCT studies observed dimples limited to the retinal nerve fiber layer corresponding to retinal striae on blue light retinographies. The correlation between *en face* and blue light retinography aspects is very high (**Figures 8A to C**).

The Optovue RTVue 100 is one of the few OCT devices that is able to analyze the retina by *en face* scans (141 horizontal parallel B scans centered on the macula and spaced 0.49 mm). Each scan is 7 mm long on the horizontal axis. Each B scan is made of 385 A scans (one A scan every 0.018 mm). System gives an analysis grid made of 54285 A scan. The "macular cube" is 7 mm by 7 mm wide by 2 mm high. Software determines automatically, in each of the 141 B scans, the inner retinal surface. The *en face* section can be 10 μm (or less) to 30 μm (or more) thick as needed. The *en face* slice is performed at ILM line level.

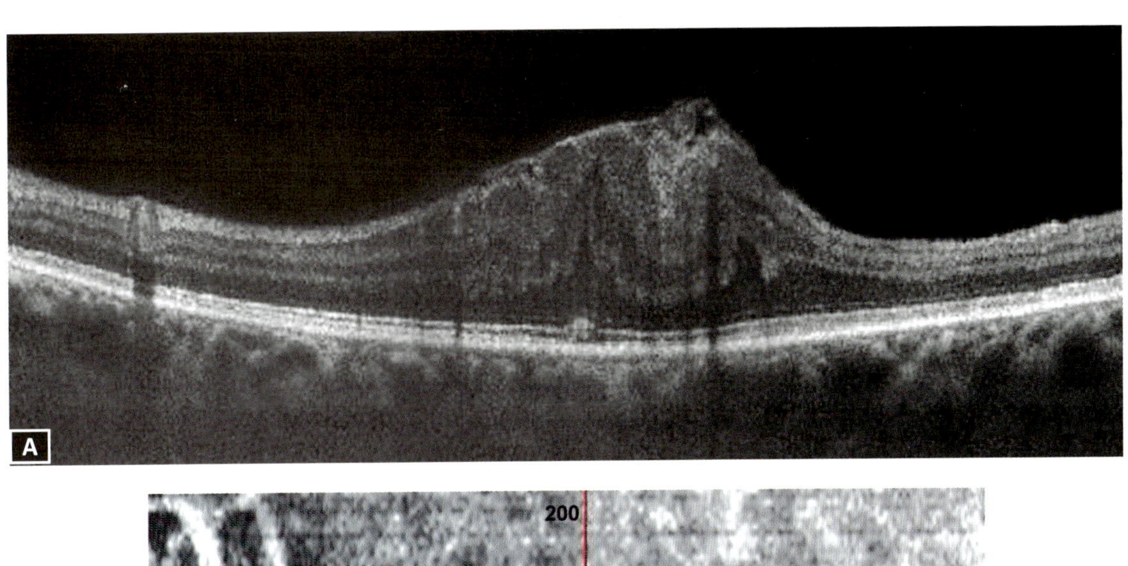

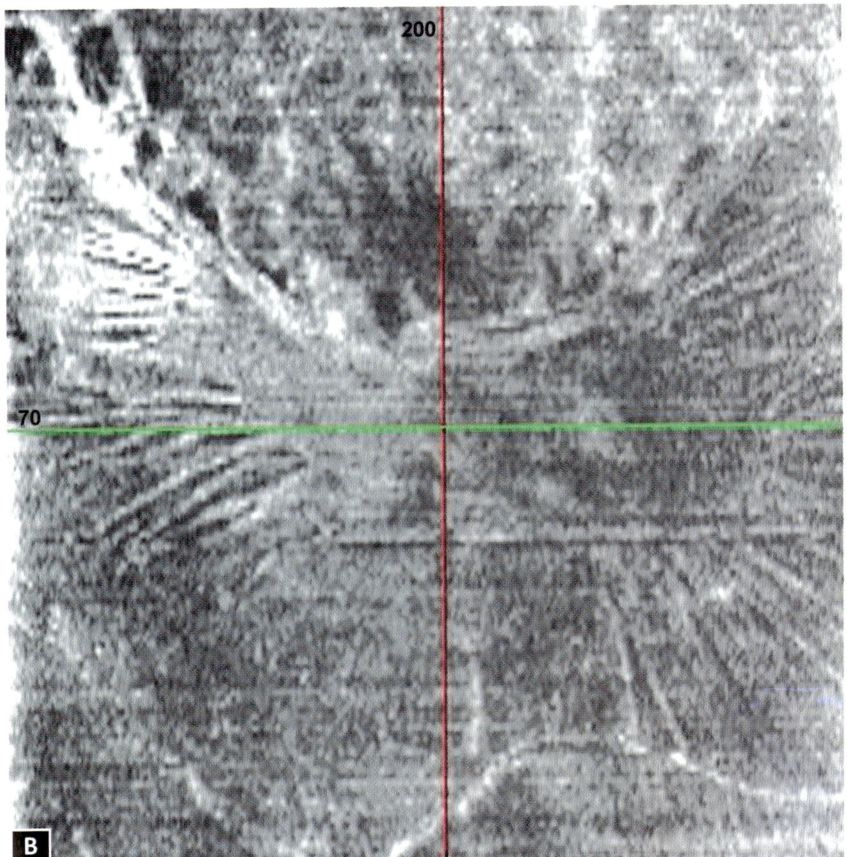

Figures 1A and B: Difference between a (A) traditional B scan and (B) an *en face* view of vitreoretinal interface. *En face* view allows us to see the entire pucker size while B scan shows intraretinal alterations (edema)

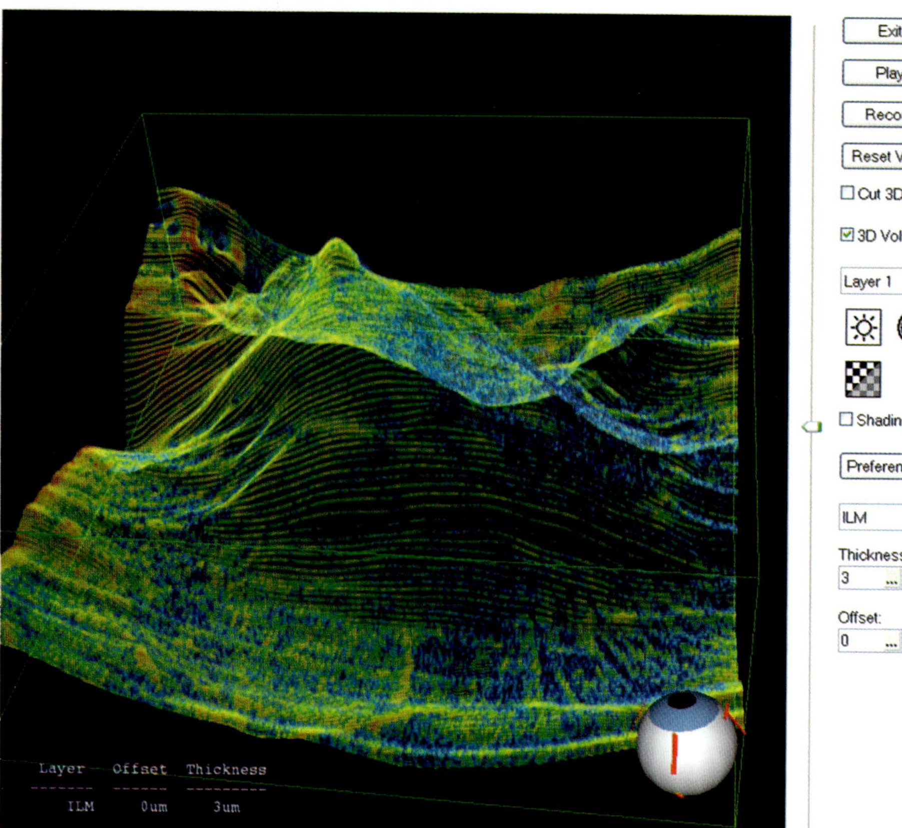

Figure 2: Evidence of tridimensional image matrix. Several horizontal B scans, parallel, concur to build a new three-dimensional surface. This new image lies on a coronal plane as compared to B scan

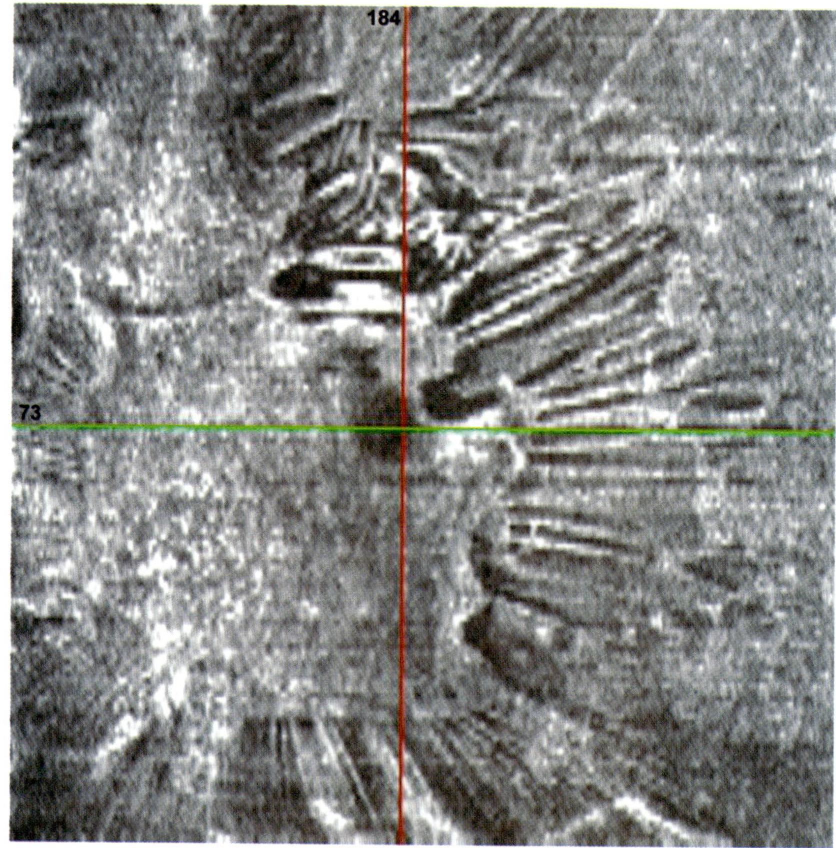

Figure 3: *En face* scan of a macular pucker. This scan allows us to study plaque size, borders and retinal folds. Surgical interest comes from evidence of plaque detached limit, useful to start grabbing by Eckardt forceps

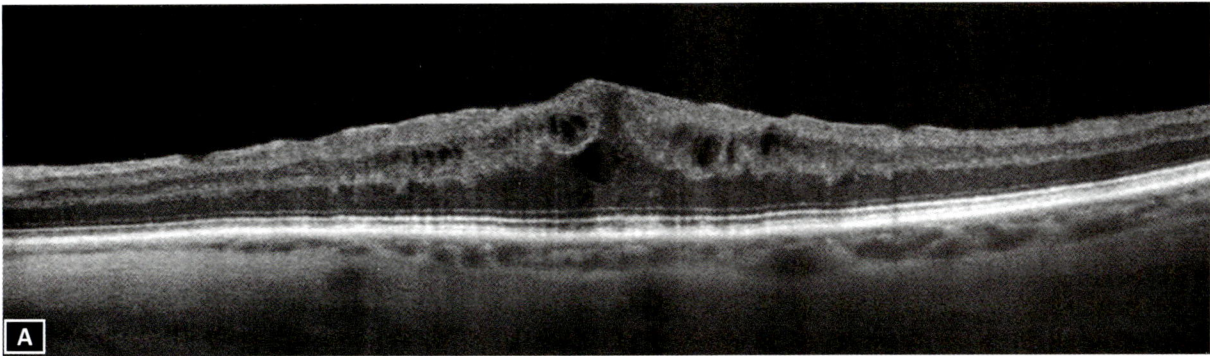

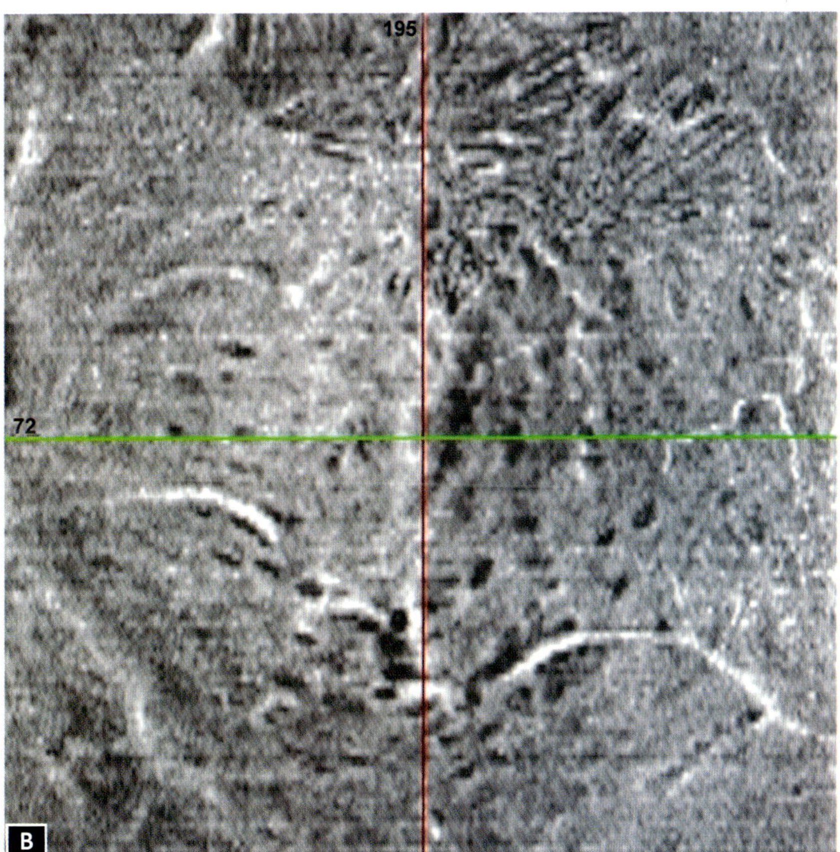

Figures 4A and B: (A) B scan and internal limiting membrane (ILM) adapted (B) *en face* scan of postoperative dissociated optical nerve fiber layer 30 days after macular surgery with ILM removal. Several dimples (dips) appear in the area that underwent surgery

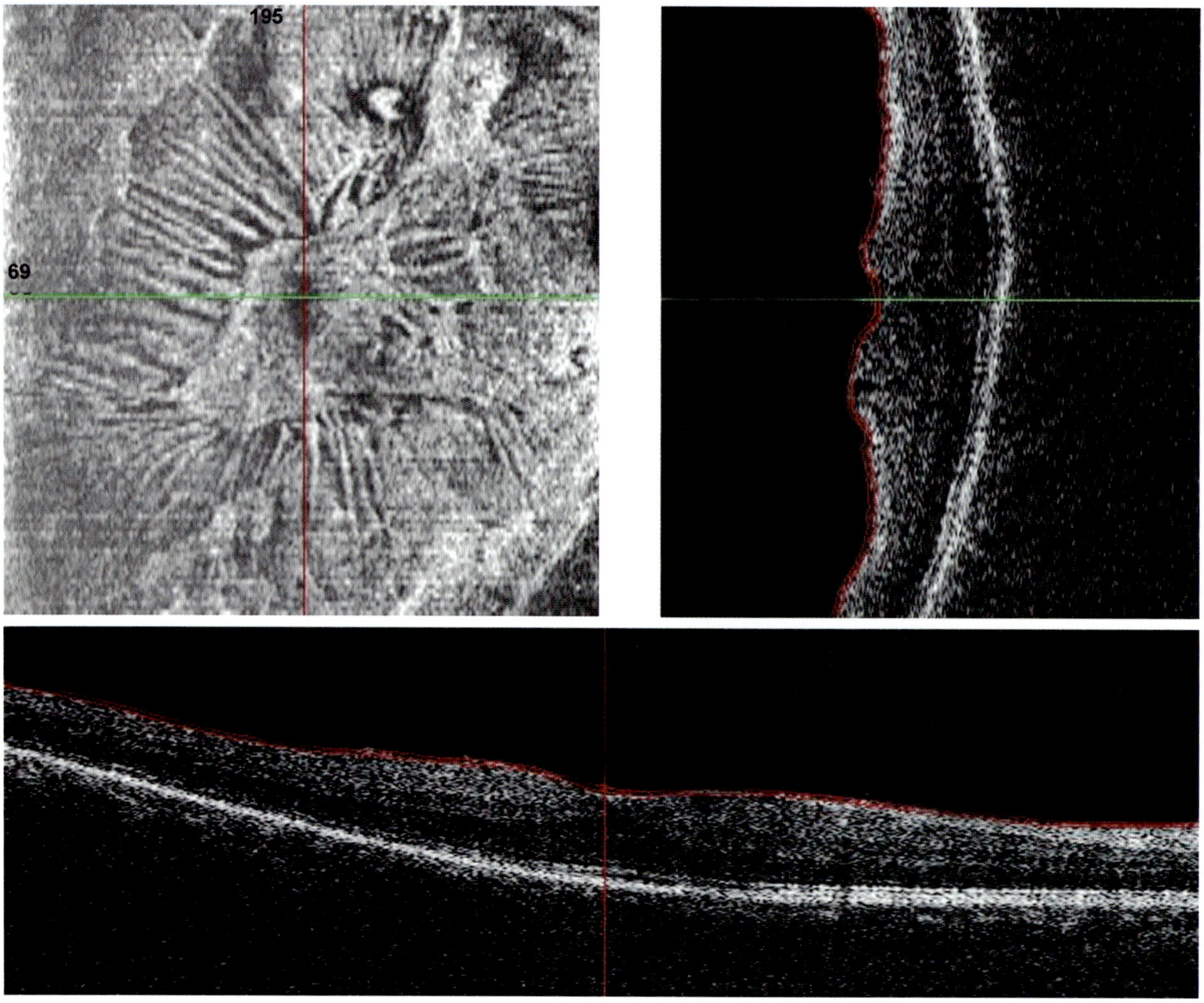

Figure 5: Example of correct internal limiting membrane (ILM) *en face* section. The red marker on the B scan must follow the ILM and its thickness is in this case about 20 microns, in any case not thicker than ILM. *En face* view will show the epiretinal membrane features

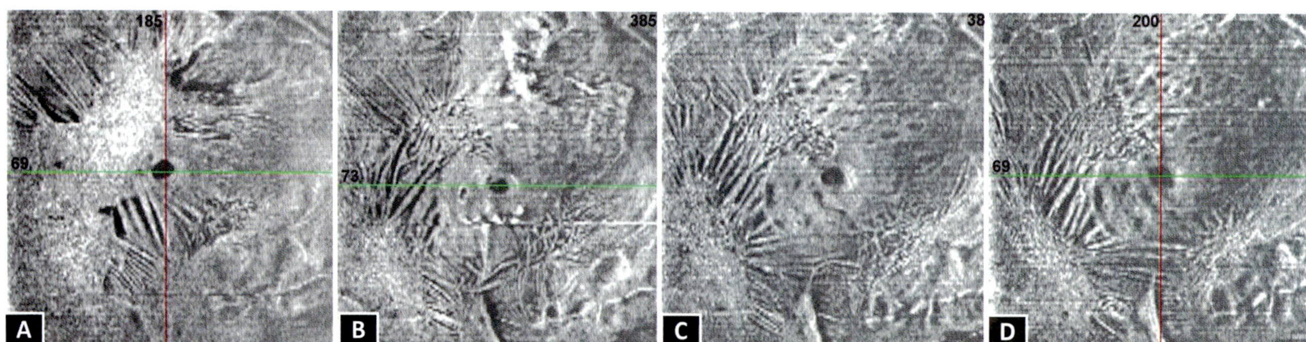

Figures 6A to D: *En face* internal limiting membrane (ILM) study (A) preoperatively, (B) after 7, (C) 30 and (D) 90 days macular surgery with ILM removal. Evidence of dimples increase during optical coherence tomography follow-up

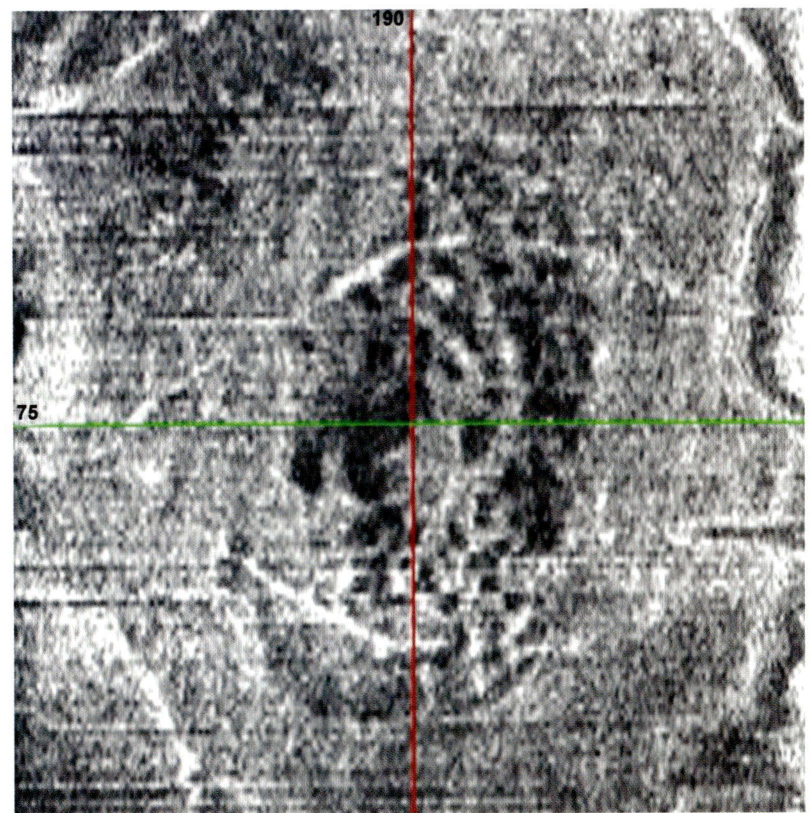

Figure 7: *En face* internal limiting membrane adapted scan of a case that underwent surgery 14 years earlier. Dissociated optic nerve fiber layer is well defined in the peeled area (*Courtesy* of Cristina Savastano)

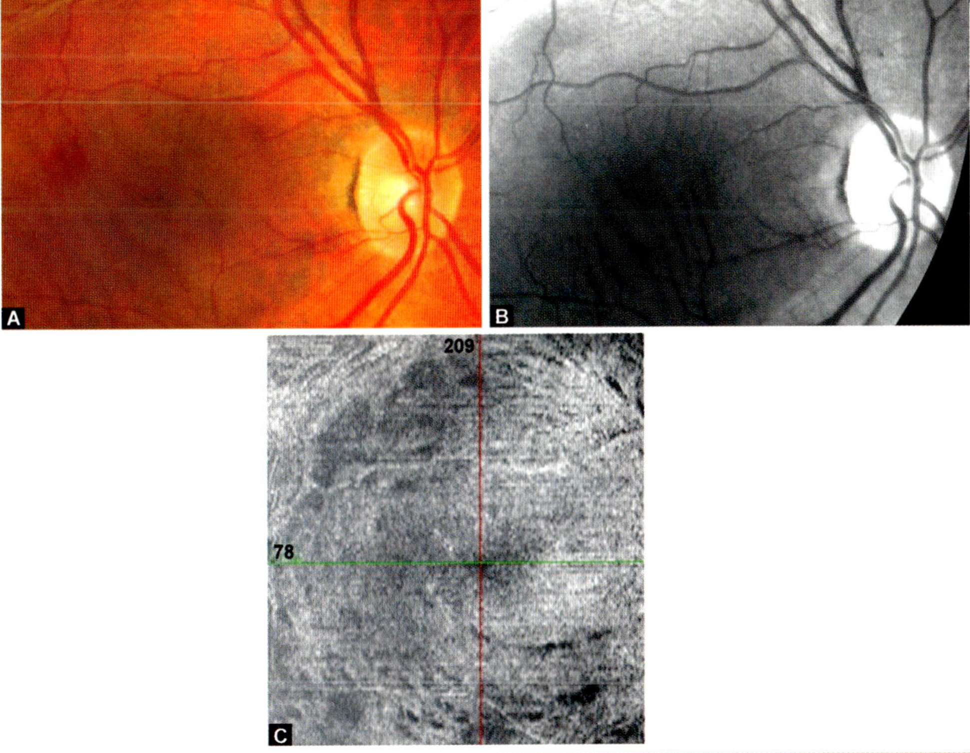

Figures 8A to C: (A) Color retinography, (B) blue light retinography, (C) *en face* internal limiting membrane (ILM) adapted, 180 days after macular surgery with ILM removal. *En face* view seems to be more sensitive than blue light retinography in enhancing dissociated optic nerve fiber layer

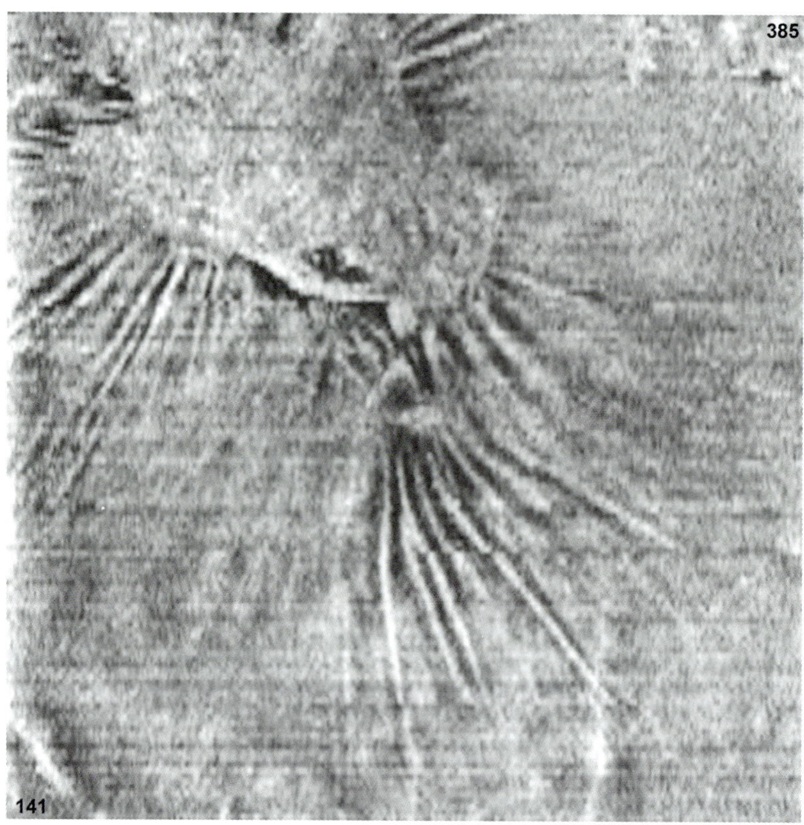

Figure 9: *En face* scan enhancing internal limiting membrane contraction

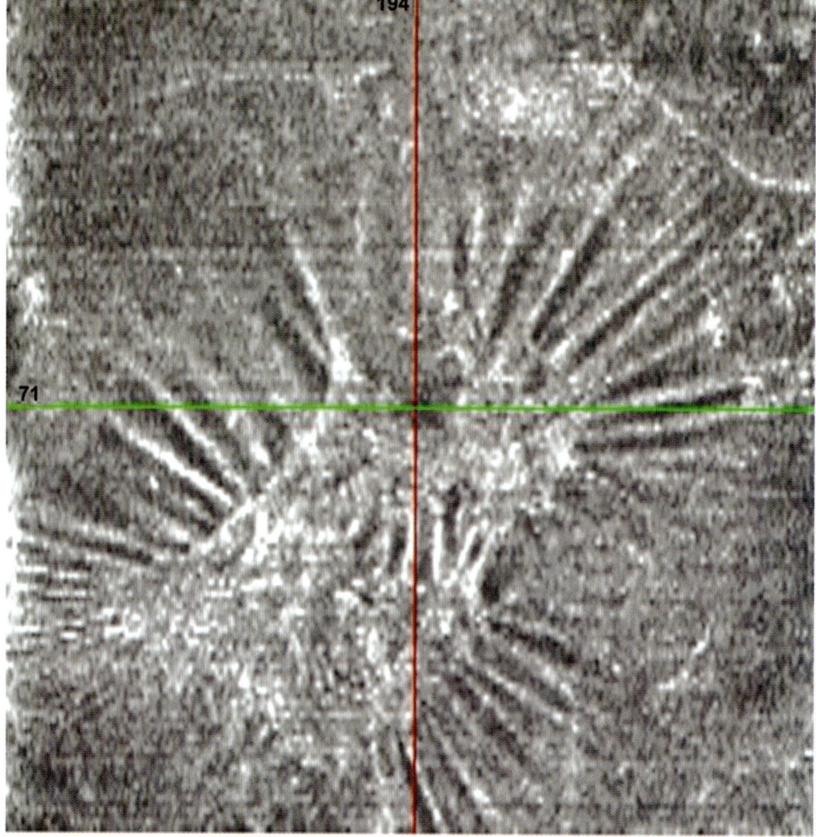

Figure 10A

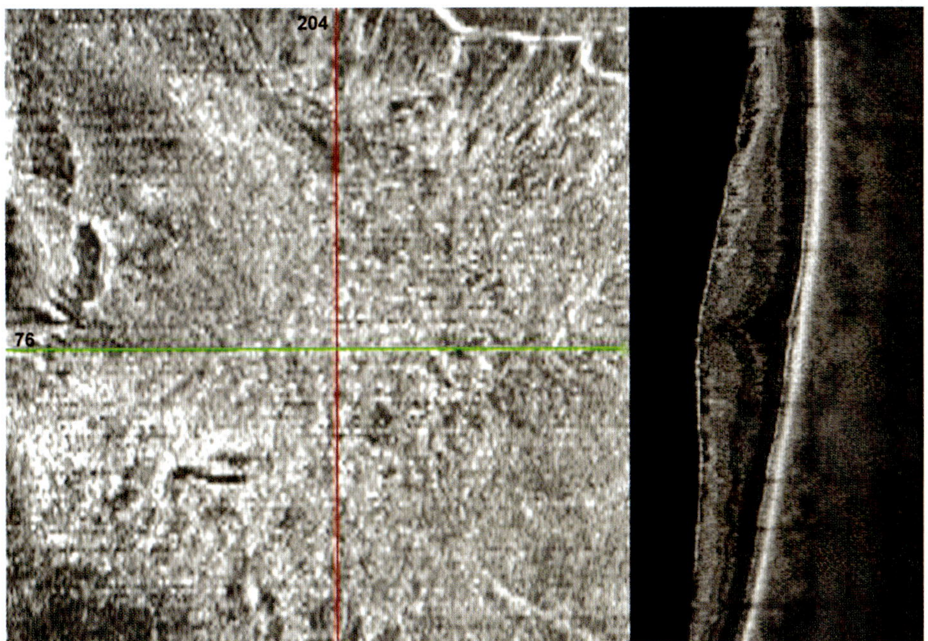

Figure 10B

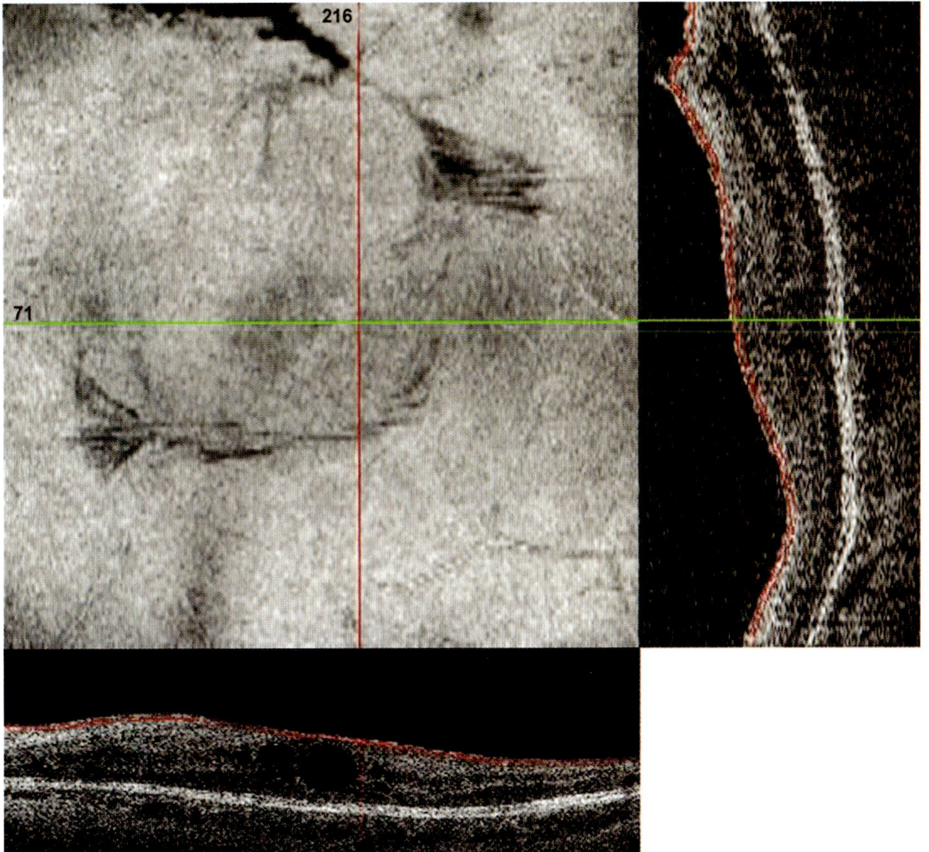

Figure 10C

Figures 10A to C: (A) Light adherent epiretinal membrane. It is easy to evidence all the alterations as plaque and folds. (B) Tight adherent epiretinal membrane, surface adapted scan. It is very difficult to enhance the density and the extension of plaque. It might be necessary to scan deeper in order to find retinal folds. (C) This view gives an indirect image of the plaque based on folds valleys

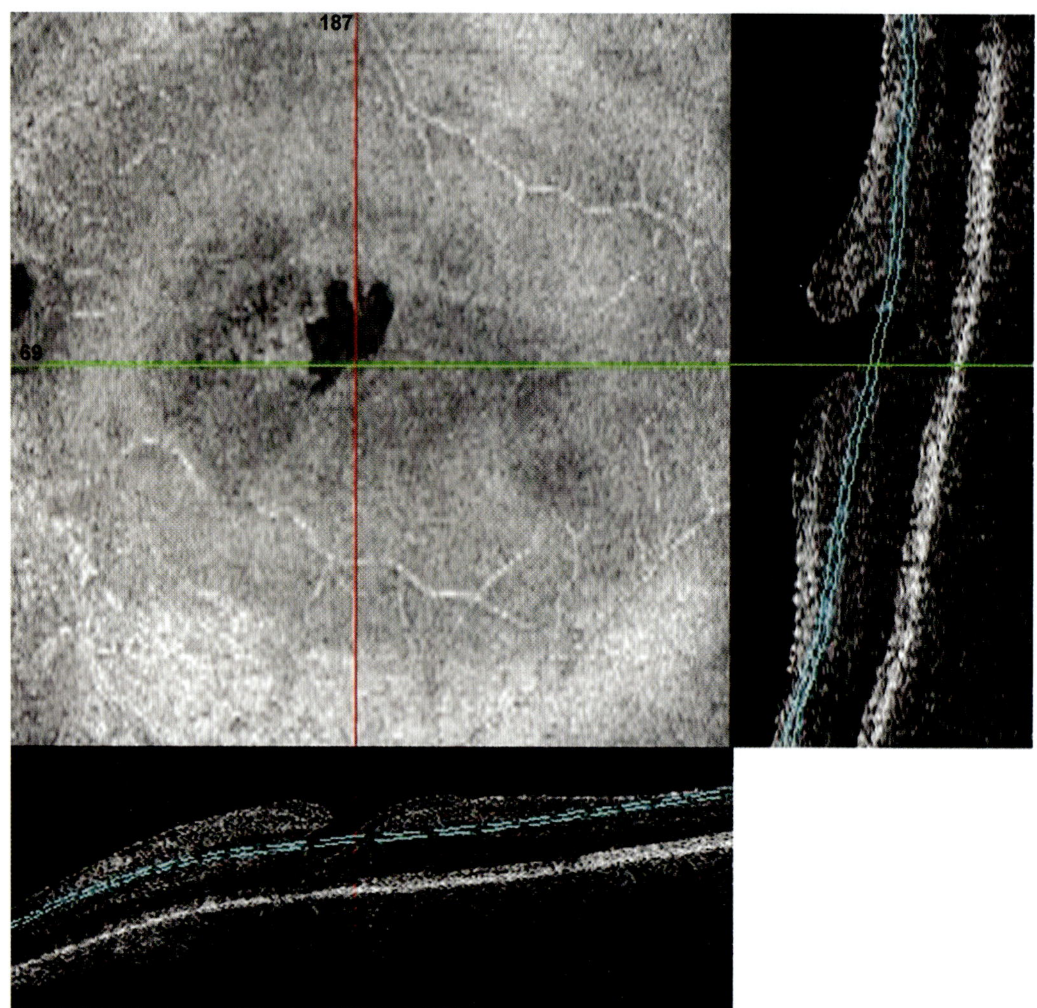

Figure 11: Lamellar hole shape in *en face* view

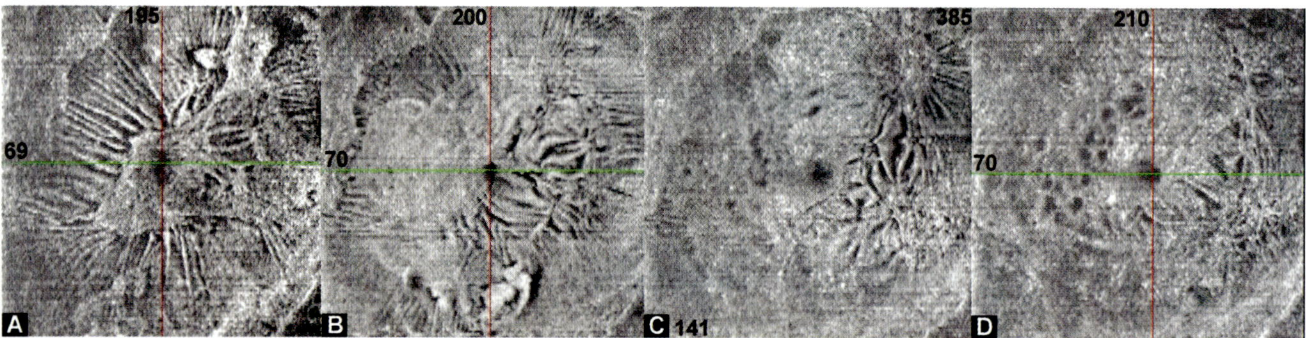

Figures 12A to D: Dissociated optic nerve fiber layer progression from (A) preoperative (B to D) up to 180 days after surgery

Taking a correct *en face* scan on vitreoretinal interface needs some particular attentions. Scanning profile must be real, adapted to ILM profile. Best scanning thickness is about 15–20 microns, or in any case not thicker than the vertical membrane extension. A correct analysis should start from vitreal side going toward the retina. In this way it will be possible to observe and study some posterior vitreous relationships with ILM. Proceeding on surface, the entire ILM contraction will be clearly visualized (**Figure 9**).

Enhancing vitreoretinal membranes will be easy for membranes that are not tightly adhering to the retinal surface (**Figures 10A to C**). So it will be possible to study all membrane features and going deeper, all retinal folds or tractional delamination (lamellar holes, macular holes, schisis) (**Figure 11**).

Dissociated optic nerve fiber layer morphology changes during the long time follow-up. During the first 3 months we can observe light dips with acute watersheds. After 6 or more months dimples appear more deep and the watersheds between one dimple and another will become flatter (**Figure 12**).

References

1. Mirza RG, Johnson MW, Jampol LM. Optical coherence tomography use in evaluation of the vitreoretinal interface: a review. Surv Ophthalmol. 2007;52(4):397-421.
2. Treumer F, Wacker N, Junge O, et al. Foveal structure and thickness of retinal layers long-term after surgical peeling of idiopathic epiretinal membrane. Invest Ophthalmol Vis Sci. 2011;52(2):744-50.
3. Lumbroso B, Savastano MC, Rispoli M, et al. Morphologic differences, according to etiology, in pigment epithelial detachments by means of *en face* optical coherence tomography. Retina. 2011;31(3):553-8.
4. Bovey EH, Uffer S, Achache F. Surgery for epimacular membrane: impact of retinal internal limiting membrane removal on functional outcome. Retina. 2004;24(5):728-35.
5. Rispoli M, Le Rouic JF, Lesnoni G, et al. Retinal surface *en face* optical coherence tomography: A new imaging approach in epiretinal membrane surgery. Retina. 2012, manuscript number 211-779R1 on print.
6. Tadayoni R, Paques M, Massin P, et al. Dissociated optic nerve fiber layer appearance of the fundus after idiopathic epiretinal membrane removal. Ophthalmology. 2001;108(12):2279-83.
7. Mitamura Y, Ohtsuka K. Relationship of dissociated optic nerve fiber layer appearance to internal limiting membrane peeling. Ophthalmology. 2005;112(10):1766-70.
8. Mitamura Y, Suzuki T, Kinoshita T, et al. Optical coherence tomographic findings of dissociated optic nerve fiber layer appearance. Am J Ophthalmol. 2004;137(6):1155-6.
9. Ito Y, Terasaki H, Takahashi A, et al. Dissociated optic nerve fiber layer appearance after internal limiting membrane peeling for idiopathic macular holes. Ophthalmology. 2005;112(8):1415-20.
10. Miura M, Elsner AE, Osako M, et al. Dissociated optic nerve fiber layer appearance after internal limiting membrane peeling for idiopathic macular hole. Retina. 2003;23(4):561-3.
11. Srinivasan VJ, Wojtkowski M, Witkin AJ, et al. High-definition and 3-dimensional imaging of macular pathologies with high-speed ultrahigh-resolution optical coherence tomography. Ophthalmology. 2006;113(11):2054.e1-14.
12. Hangai M, Ojima Y, Gotoh N, et al. Three-dimensional imaging of macular holes with high-speed optical coherence tomography. Ophthalmology. 2007;114(4):763-73.
13. Lois N, Burr J, Norrie J, et al. Internal limiting membrane peeling versus no peeling for idiopathic full-thickness macular hole: a pragmatic randomized controlled trial. Invest Ophthalmol Vis Sci. 2011;52(3):1586-92.
14. Nakamura T, Murata T, Hisatomi T, et al. Ultrastructure of the vitreoretinal interface following the removal of the internal limiting membrane using indocyanine green. Curr Eye Res. 2003;27(6):395-9.
15. Alkabes M, Salinas C, Vitale L, et al. *En face* optical coherence tomography of inner retinal defects after internal limiting membrane peeling for idiopathic macular hole. Invest Ophthalmol Vis Sci. 2011;52(11):8349-55.

chapter 36

Vitreoretinal Interface Aspects After Macular Hole Surgery

Micol Alkabes, Paolo Nucci, Carlos Mateo

Internal Limiting Membrane Peeling: The Rationale

The internal limiting membrane (ILM) is a 10 µ-thick transparent structure formed by the basement membrane of the retinal Müller cells and composed mainly of collagen fibers, glycosaminoglycans (GAGs), laminin and fibronectin,[1] which are responsible for the biochemical properties of the retina, as demonstrated by Wallensack et al.[2] Analyzing several retinal specimens they observed a remarkably plastic biomechanical behavior of the retina providing a certain protective mechanism against tear formation. Moreover, their results showed that after ILM removal the mean force of the central retina was reduced significantly by 53.6% with respect to the unpeeled retinal specimens, demonstrating that the ILM is the structure which mostly contributes to the biochemical strength of the retina.[3]

It is well known that forces between retina and vitreous body are transmitted via the ILM and for this reason it seems to play a great role in the pathogenesis of various retinal disorders such as full-thickness macular holes (FTMH).

Nevertheless, the ILM received virtually no clinical attention until 1980s when Dr Didier Ducournau, during a vitrectomy removal of epimacular proliferations (EMP), pioneered an "unintentionally" new technique: the ILM peeling.[4]

However, the controversial issue of intentional ILM peeling first emerged in the early 1990s, following Gass' theory of macular hole formation pathogenesis[5] and coinciding with the advent of macular hole (MH) surgery.[6]

Thinking of the ILM as a scaffold for cellular proliferation on which glial cells may migrate creating a further tangential contractile force; ILM peeling was therefore widely accepted to be an effective treatment option to achieve anatomic MH closure and functional recovery.[7]

Several studies have been published in literature to assess the value of ILM peeling in MH surgery for its potential anatomical and visual success. Since addressing this issue is not the aim of this chapter, the authors would try to describe what occurs on the inner retinal surface after ILM peeling in MH surgery.

En Face Optical Coherence Tomography After Macular Hole Surgery with Internal Limiting Membrane Peeling

Due to its properties, the *en face* OCT technique is, in our opinion, one of the most useful imaging procedures to analyze vitreoretinal disorders that affect the inner retinal layers.

At present, several available spectral domain OCT (SD-OCT) instruments include in their software a particular acquisition protocol that allows to create a transversal *en face* OCT C scan.

Cirrus HD-OCT 4000 version 5.0 (*Carl Zeiss Meditec, Dublin, CA*) is one of these commercial SD-OCTs that acquires images at 27,000 axially oriented A scans per second. Moreover, it has a three-dimensional (3D) macular cube scan (128 raster cross-sectional B scans with 512 A scans each, within a 6 × 6 mm area for an axial imaging depth range of 2 mm) in which every OCT C scan is represented as two-dimensional (2D) transversal slice at any given depth through the retina.

Using this OCT instrument and selecting the type of analysis as shown in **Figures 1A to D**, the authors retrospectively evaluated 36 eyes of 36 patients who underwent pars plana vitrectomy with ILM peeling for idiopathic MH (stage 3 or 4), to describe the appearance of some postoperative inner retinal defects on the *en face* OCT images. The design

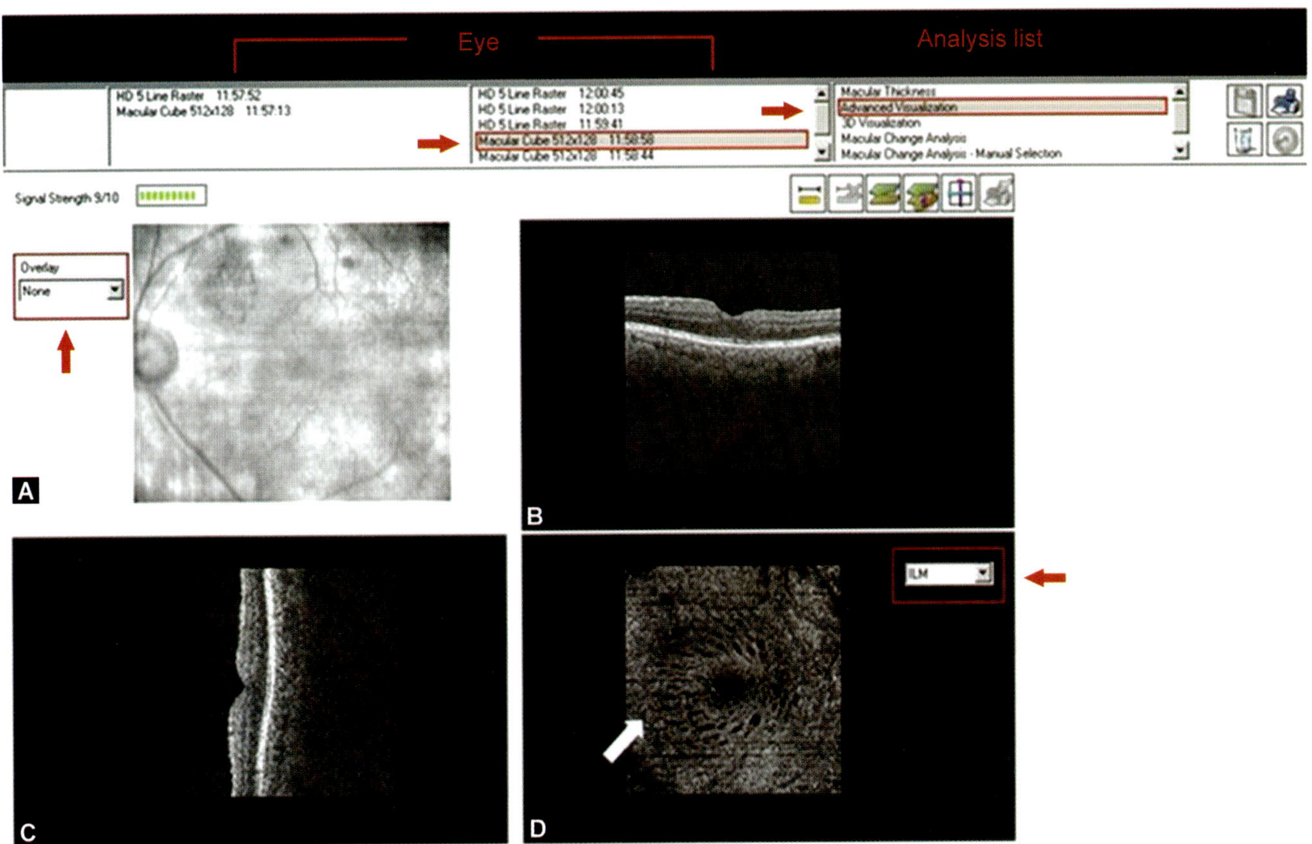

Figures 1A to D: Image captured on computer screen of Cirrus HD-OCT 4000 (Carl Zeiss Meditec, Dublin, CA). C scan was acquired using the *Macular Cube 512 x 128* to create the *en face* image. Advanced visualization was then selected in the analysis list as reported. (A) In the screenshot obtained, the upper left viewport showed the fundus image whereas the other three viewports showed cross-sectional scan images in three planes. Images are shown in the viewports as planes parallel (B) to the front (X plane, upper right viewport); (C) to the side of a hypothetical cube (Y plane, lower left viewport) and (D) to the top (Z plane, lower right viewport). Then, on the overlay drop-down options, none was selected to show the corresponding saved fundus image without slices (upper left image). Knowing that cube scan analyses incorporate an algorithm to automatically find and display the inner limiting membrane (ILM), in the lower right viewport and on the drop-down options, ILM must be selected by changing the default setting (*Slice → ILM*). This image corresponds to the *en face* C scan on the Z plane of the macular cube. Finally, to improve image quality, grayscale of slices was preferred
[*Courtesy:* Cirrus HD-OCT 4000 (Carl Zeiss Meditec, Dublic, CA); IMO (Instituto de Microcirugia Ocular), Barcelona, Spain]

of this study and its results have been published in IOVS in 2011.[8] In this series, a typical OCT pattern that was called concentric macular dark spots (CMDS), has been observed from the third month on the *en face* C scans after ILM removal **(Figure 2)**. This acronym refers in a practical manner to the features shown on tomographic images, in regard to its distribution, localization and reflectivity, but does not address the underlying nature of these changes on the retinal surface. Thus, where do these CMDS originate from?

Performing the ILM peeling the authors do not remove only the basement membrane of the Müller cells (the true so-called "ILM"), but also their cell endfeet, which are in close contact with the nerve fibers, as confirmed by Wolf et al in 2004.[9] This results in a substantial ultrastructural damage to the inner retinal surface that can be observed on the *en face* OCT images as arcuate dark defects in the same course of the optic nerve fibers **(Figures 3A and B)** and which are due to shallow dimples within the thickness of the retinal nerve fibers layer (RNFL), as shown on cross-sectional OCT B scans[10] **(Figures 4 to 9)**.

These CMDS are actually the tomographic feature of the dissociated optic nerve fiber layer (DONFL) described firstly by Tadayoni, et al in 2001,[11] who reported the characteristic appearance of some arcuate, slightly dark striae

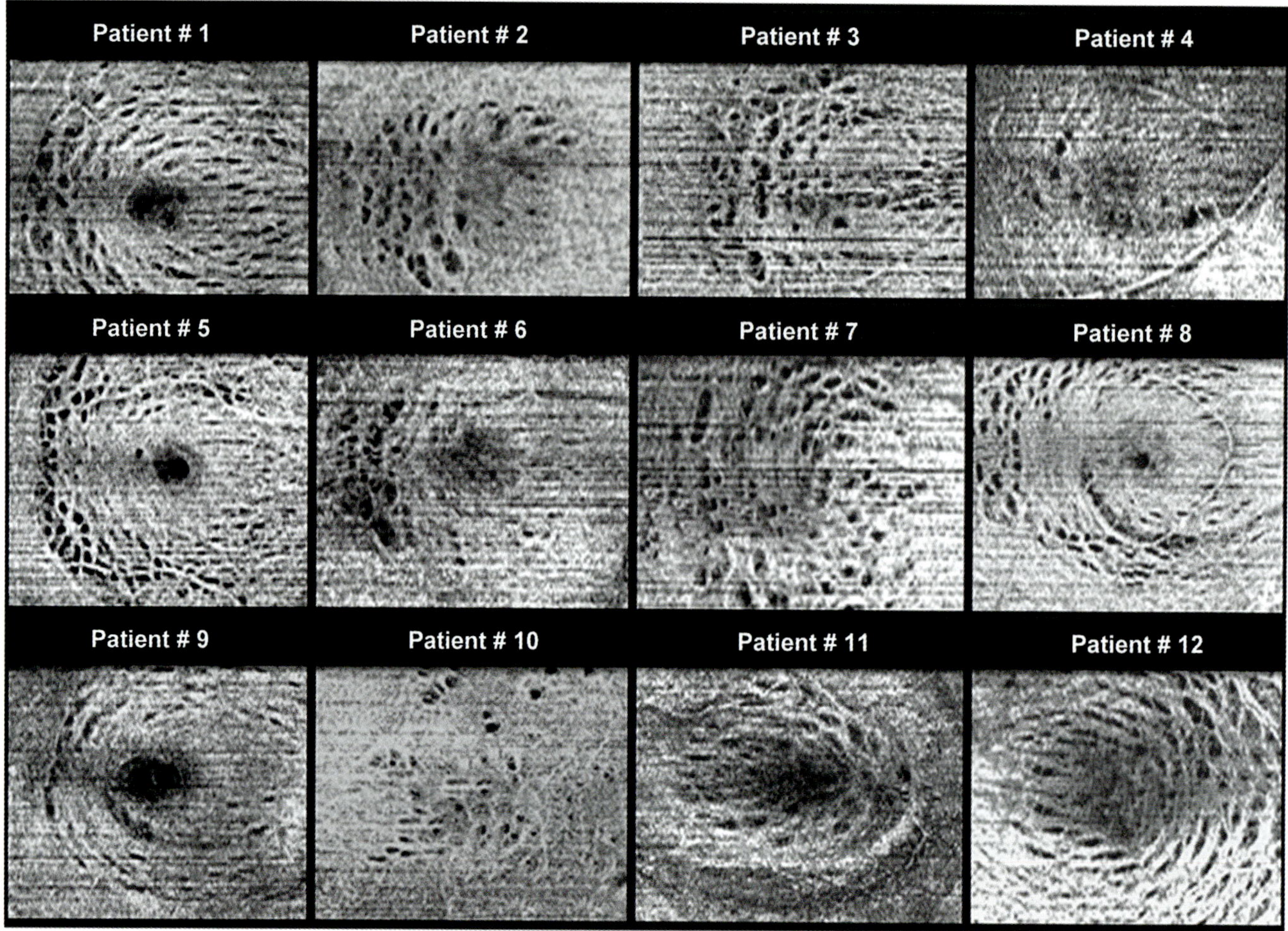

Figure 2: Postoperative *en face* optical coherence tomography (OCT) scans of 12 patients who underwent surgery with internal limiting membrane (ILM) peeling for idiopathic macular hole. A typical OCT pattern that the authors called concentric macular dark spots (CMDS) is clearly visible along the course of optic nerve fiber layer in the area of the ILM removal, corresponding to the dissociated optic nerve fiber layer (DONFL) previously described by Tadayoni et al[11]

[*Courtesy:* Cirrus HD-OCT 4000 (Carl Zeiss Meditec, Dublic, CA); IMO (Instituto de Microcirugia Ocular), Barcelona, Spain]

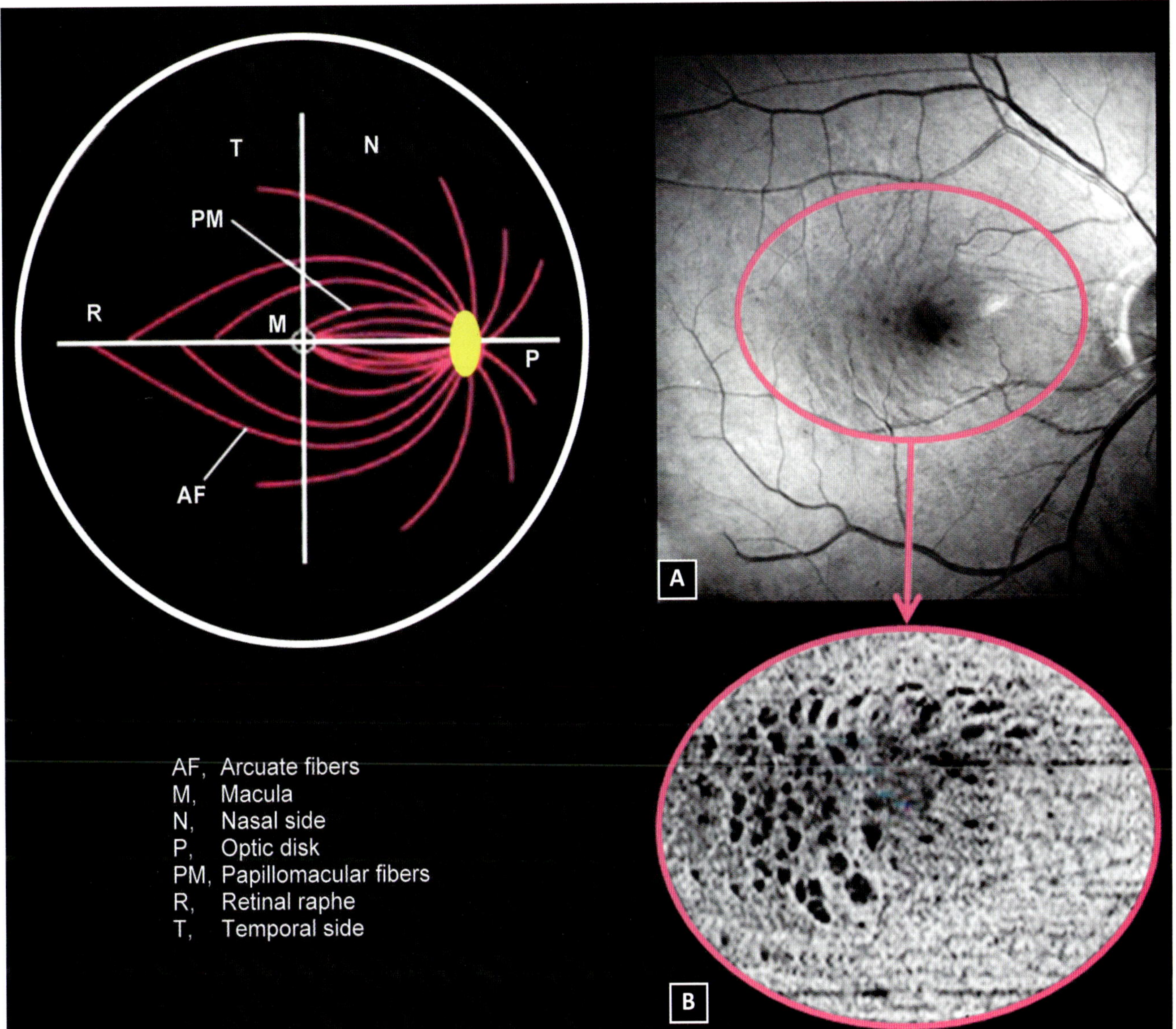

Figures 3A and B: Schematic diagram of the concentric macular dark spots appearance seen on Redfree image (Spectralis[TM] HRA+OCT. Heidelberg, Dossenheim, Germany) (A) and on the *en face* optical coherence tomography (RTVue-100®. Optovue Inc, Fremont, CA) (B) in the right eye. Note that the inner retinal defects seems to be related to the course of the arcuate fibers in the temporal side of the optic disk as shown in the upper left image
(*Courtesy:* San Giuseppe Hospital, University Eye Clinic, Milan, Italy)

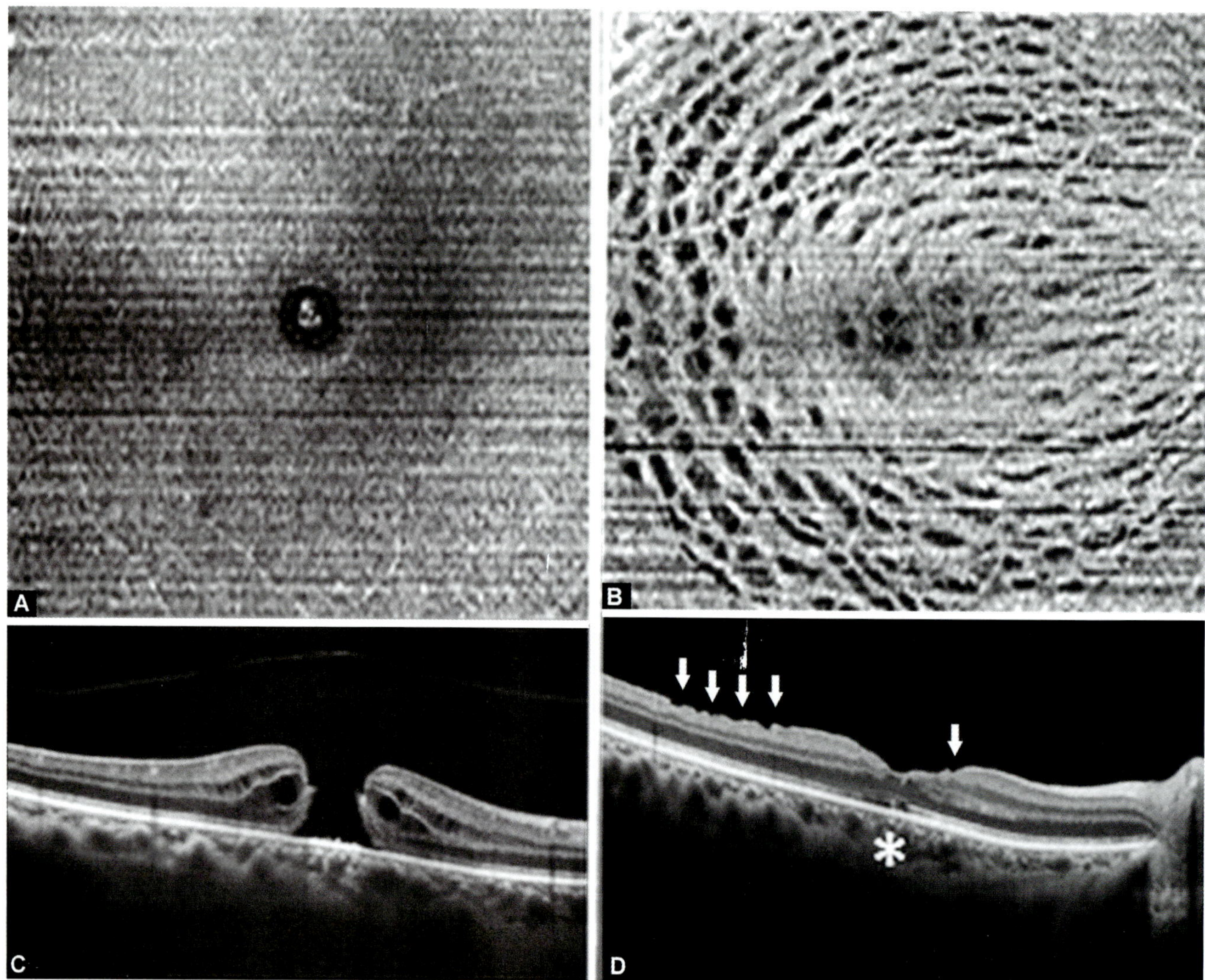

Figures 4A to D: Preoperative *en face* optical coherence tomography (OCT) (A) and horizontal B scan (B) of an idiopathic macular hole (MH). (C) *En face* C scan is also acquired 3 months after surgery showing a characteristic OCT pattern with the concentric macular dark spot appearance, which was not present preoperatively. Moreover, a complete MH closure (D) with an interrupted inner segment/outer segment line and an intact external limiting membrane was reported (asterisk). Some focal dehiscences corresponding to each dark spot, were visible within the thickness of the retinal nerve fiber layer (RNFL) on B scan OCT images (white arrows)

[*Reprinted with permission of the Authors from IOVS © ARVO;* Alkabes M, Salinas C, Vitale L, Burés-Jelstrup A, Nucci P, Mateo C. *En face* optical coherence tomography of inner retinal defects after internal limiting membrane peeling for idiopathic macular hole. Invest Ophthalmol Vis Sci. 2011 Oct 21;52(11):8349-55]

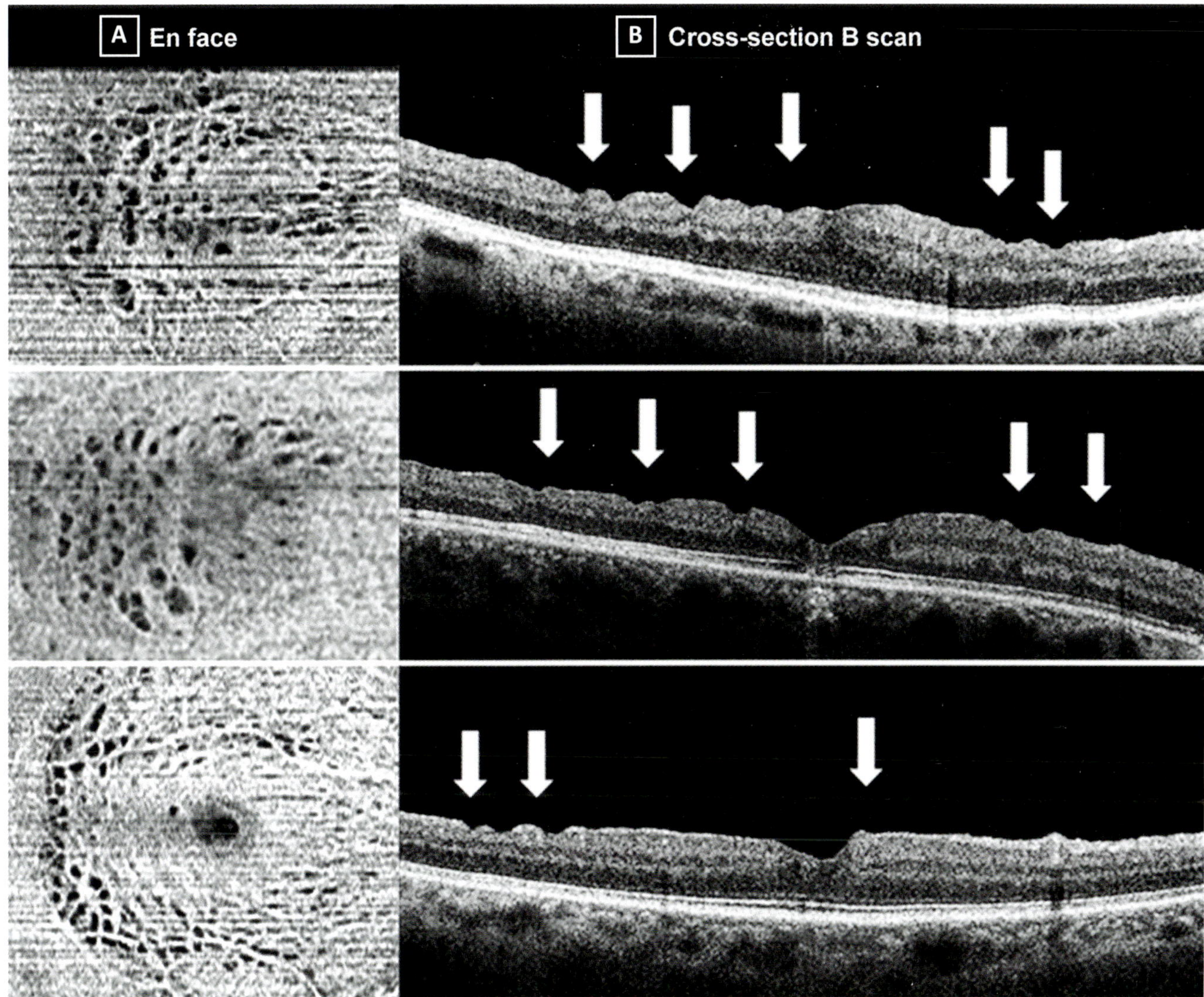

Figures 5A and B: Postoperative *en face* C scans (A) and corresponding B scans (B) of three patients who underwent pars plana vitrectomy (PPV) and internal limiting membrane peeling for idiopathic macular holes. Fine shallow dimples (white arrows) within the thickness of the retinal nerve fiber layer and corresponding to each concentric macular dark spots are evident on B scans

[*Courtesy:* Cirrus HD-OCT 4000 (Carl Zeiss Meditec, Dublic, CA); IMO (Instituto de Microcirugia Ocular), Barcelona, Spain]

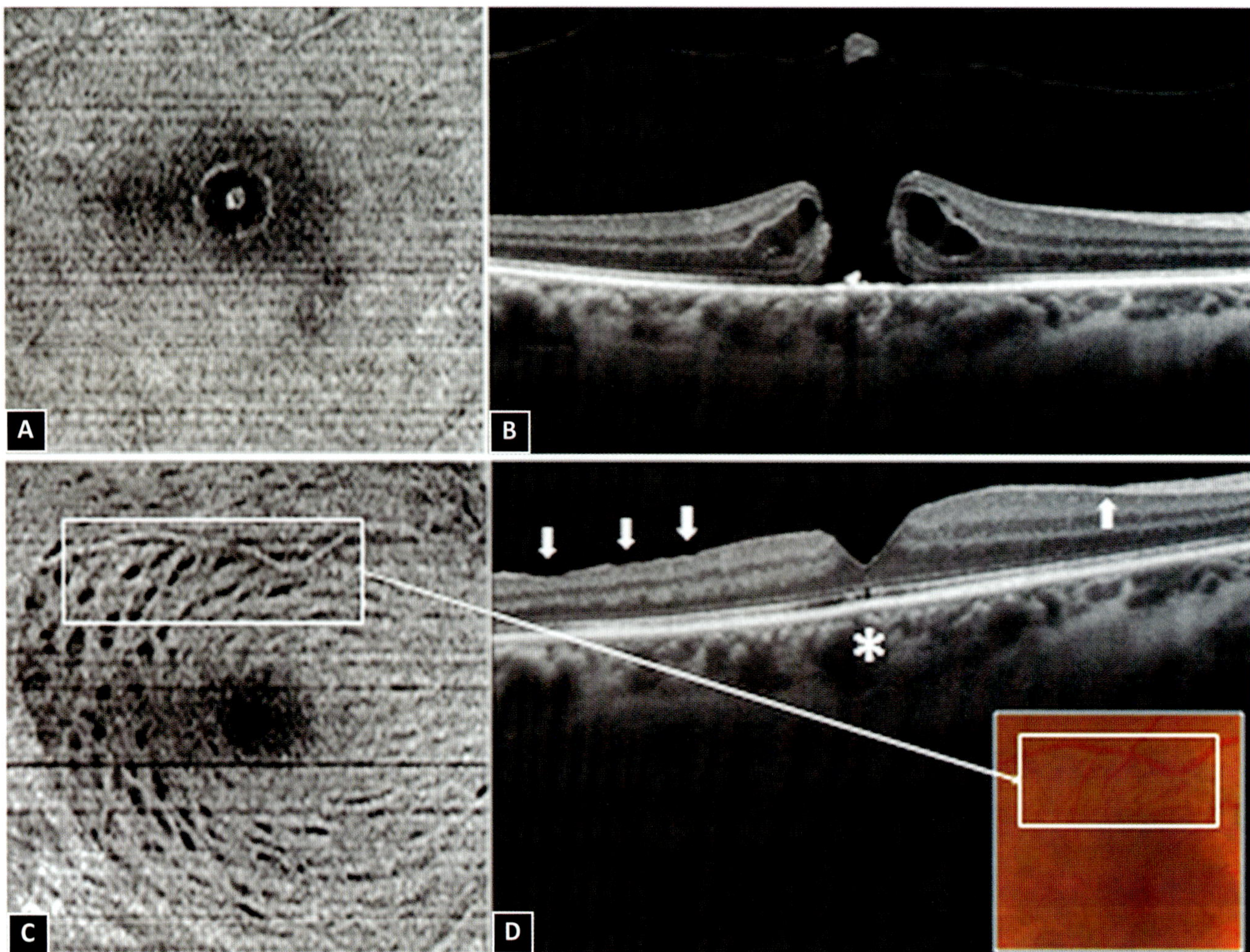

Figures 6A to D: Preoperative *en face* optical coherence tomography (OCT) scan (A) with no evidence of concentric macular dark spots (CMDS); (B) Corresponding horizontal B scan confirms the presence of a full-thickness macular hole with a retinal operculum on the posterior hyaloid. (C) After surgery, CMDS appearance was observed on the *en face* images, and it seemed to be in accordance to each stria on the corresponding color fundus photographs (D, *lower right, white square*). Furthermore, postoperative OCT B scan shows the typical dehiscences at the level of the optic nerve fibers layer less deep than its total thickness (white arrows) and some degree of interruption in the inner segment/outer segment line that often occurs during the healing process of macular hole surgery
[*Reprinted with permission of the Authors from IOVS © ARVO;* Alkabes M, Salinas C, Vitale L, Burés-Jelstrup A, Nucci P, Mateo C. *En face* optical coherence tomography of inner retinal defects after internal limiting membrane peeling for idiopathic macular hole. Invest Ophthalmol Vis Sci. 2011 Oct 21;52(11):8349-55]

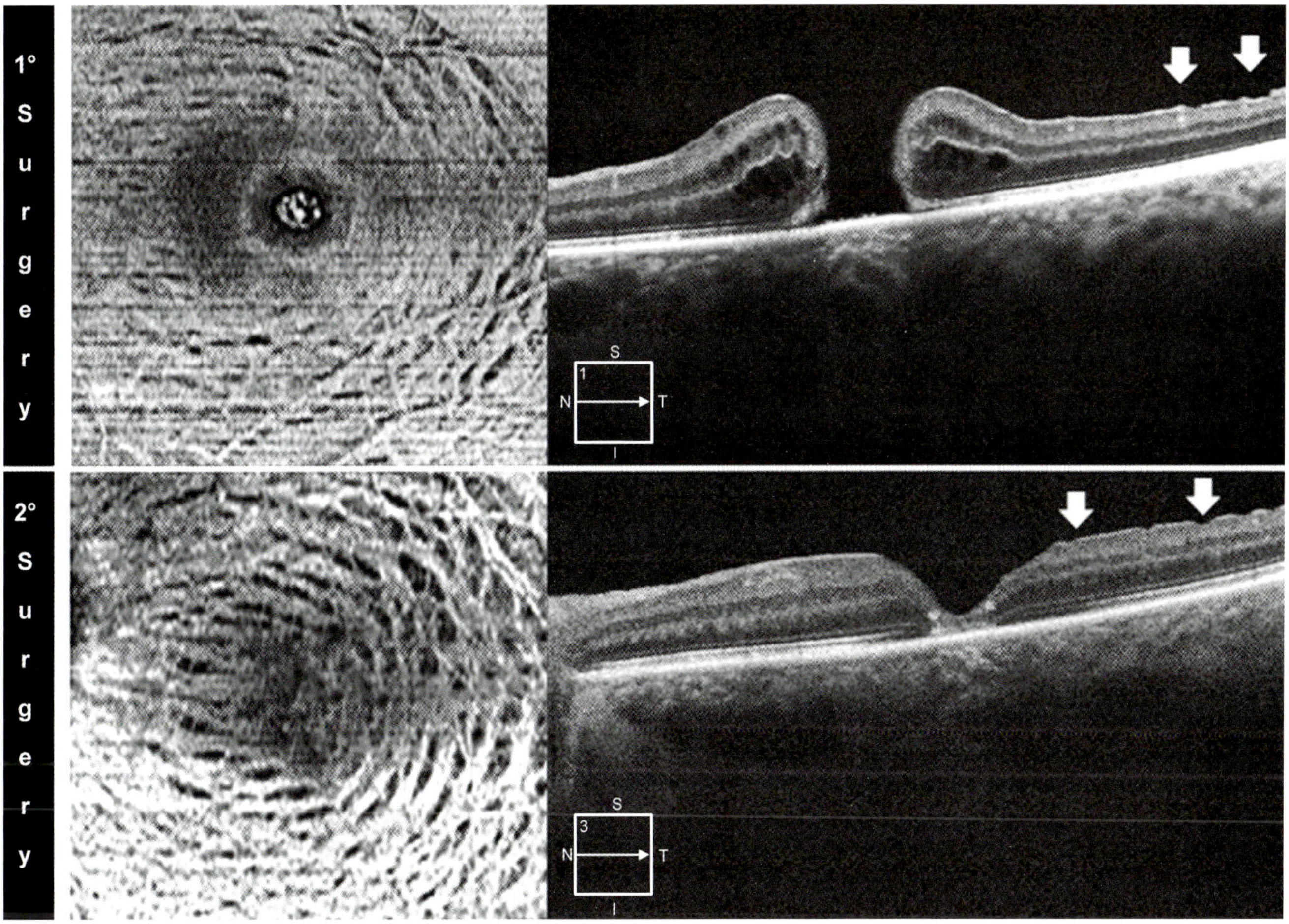

Figure 7: Optical coherence tomography (OCT) scans of a 65-year-old female patient with a persistent full-thickness macular hole who has been previously operated with pars plana vitrectomy PPV, internal limiting membrane (ILM) peeling and gas tamponade. Note that fine concentric macular dark spots are visible after the first surgery (4 months before), even if the macular hole (MH) is still open with elevated edge and some degree of intraretinal edema. A second surgery was necessary to achieve a complete MH closure. The typical OCT pattern was more clearly visible after an enlargement of the ILM removal up to the vascular arcades, since it has been observed to be still in part adherent to the retinal surface by intraoperative restaining
[*Courtesy:* Cirrus HD-OCT 4000 (Carl Zeiss Meditec, Dublic, CA); IMO (Instituto de Microcirugia Ocular), Barcelona, Spain]

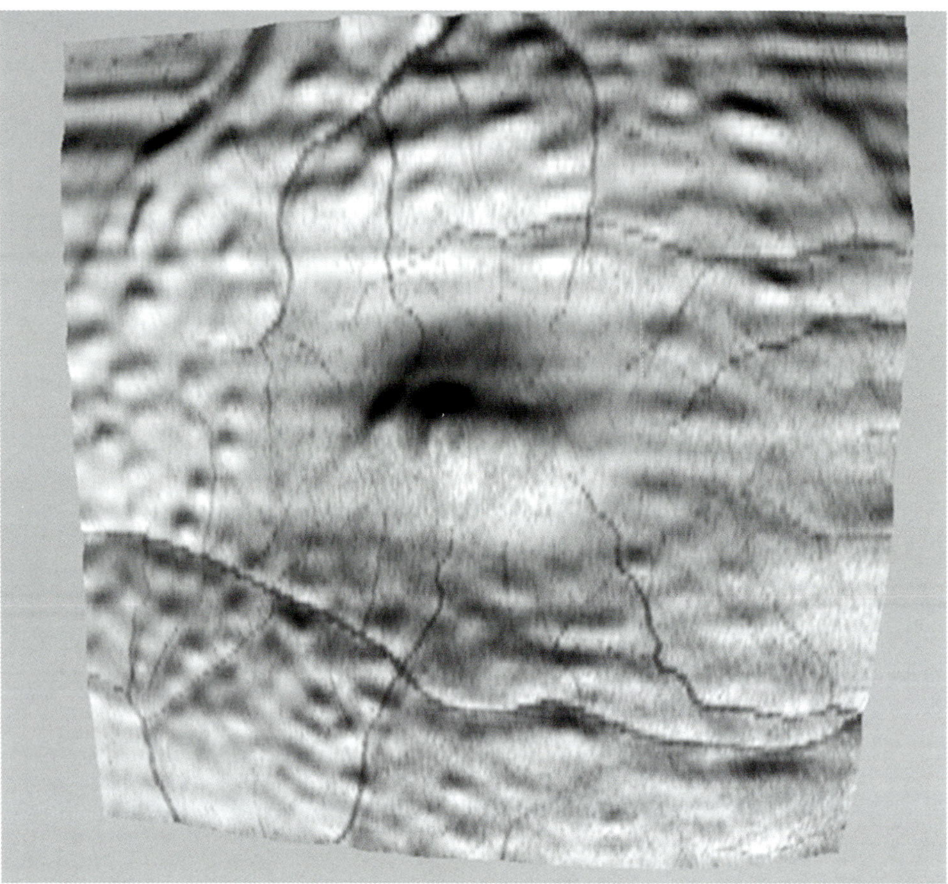

Figure 8: View of the inner retinal surface by the 3D visualization of the macular cube showing the characteristic concentric macular dark spots appearance (after setting adjustment)
[*Courtesy:* Cirrus HD-OCT 4000 (Carl Zeiss Meditec, Dublic, CA); IMO (Instituto de Microcirugia Ocular), Barcelona, Spain]

within the posterior pole along the course of optic nerve fibers using blue-filter photographs. However, in that series, this feature was observed only in 43% of patients after ILM removal but, even considering all the other studies, this rate was never greater than 62% using fundus photographs.[12]

If the authors compare all previous studies as reported in literature concerning the appearance of inner retinal changes after ILM extraction, their results could finally suggest that:

- *En face* OCT is a helpful and noninvasive technique to assess a complete ILM removal within the posterior pole if the CMDS appearance is reported (100% of our patients with idiopathic MH showed this appearance), even if they can be observed on color fundus photographs too **(Figures 6A to D)**.
- These inner retinal defects, not present preoperatively, are always detected by the *en face* technique 3 months after surgery, even if they can be priorly observed in pseudophakic and aphakic eyes too.
- This feature is not found in the surrounding unpeeled retina.

- Once CMDS are observed on *en face* OCT images, they remain stable over time **(Figures 9 and 10)**.
- *En face* OCT C scans should be considered more accurate than fundus photographs in detecting retinal surface changes in ILM-peeled eyes (100% vs 43% to 62.2% respectively).[11,12]

In addition, the ILM peeling seems to be effectively a successful procedure that increases the anatomical MH closure rate, especially in stage 3 or 4 idiopathic MH (100% MH closure rate in the authors' series).

But if these CMDS are not observed on the *en face* OCTs, does it always mean that the ILM has not been peeled off during MH surgery? Since this typical OCT pattern was observed in 100% of the authors' cases of idiopathic MHs, it may be inferred that should it not be present, the ILM could still be adherent to the retinal surface. However, this is what occurs in emmetropic eyes with full-thickness MH.

In high myopic eyes, MHs are often associated with a posterior staphyloma, with or without a retinoschisis **(Figures 11 to 15)**, which predisposes to an incorrect segmentation

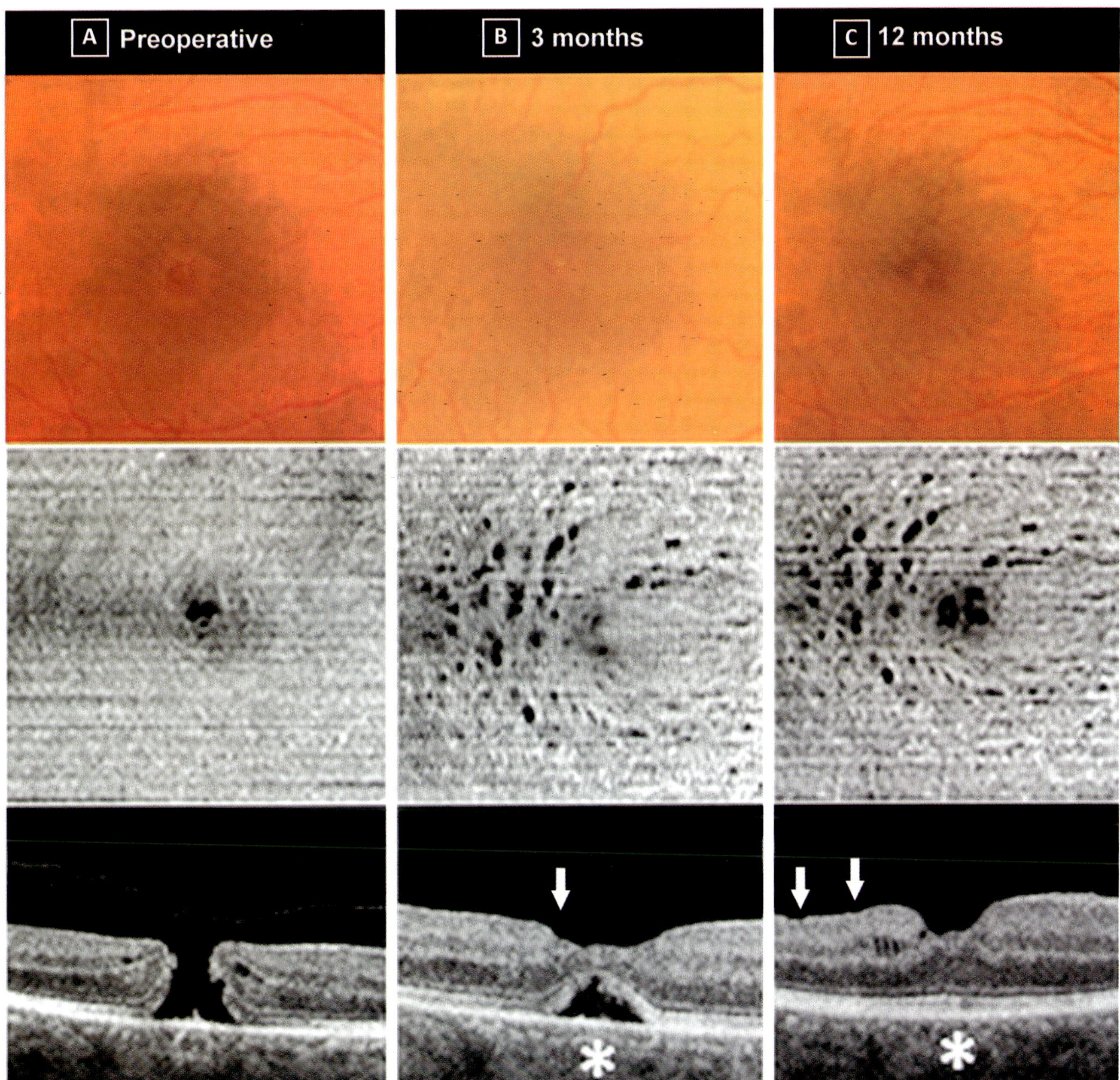

Figures 9A to C: Color fundus photographs (*top*), *en face* C scans (*middle*) and horizontal B scans (*bottom*) of a patient who underwent pars plana vitrectomy (PPV) with internal limiting membrane (ILM) removal for a full-thickness macular hole (FTMH) in the right eye. No concentric macular dark spots (CMDS) were evident before surgery on *en face* images (A, *middle left*). At 3 months they were visible along the course of the optic nerve fibers layer, except at the level of the fovea where some degree of subretinal fluid was still present (B, *middle*). Twelve months after surgery, when subfoveal fluid has disappeared and foveal detachment has completely resolved, these inner retinal defects became even more well defined (C, *middle right, bottom, left to right*). Optical coherence tomography B scans show a FTMH, its closure 3 months after surgery with a persistent foveal detachment and its finally complete closure with return to the normal foveal architecture 12 months after surgery (asterisks) with intact external limiting membrane and inner segment/outer segment line. Fine shallow dimples in the retinal nerve fiber layer were observed after ILM peeling (white arrows) [*Reprinted with permission of the Authors from IOVS © ARVO; Alkabes M, Salinas C, Vitale L, Burés-Jelstrup A, Nucci P, Mateo C. En face* optical coherence tomography of inner retinal defects after internal limiting membrane peeling for idiopathic macular hole. Invest Ophthalmol Vis Sci. 2011 Oct 21;52(11):8349-55]

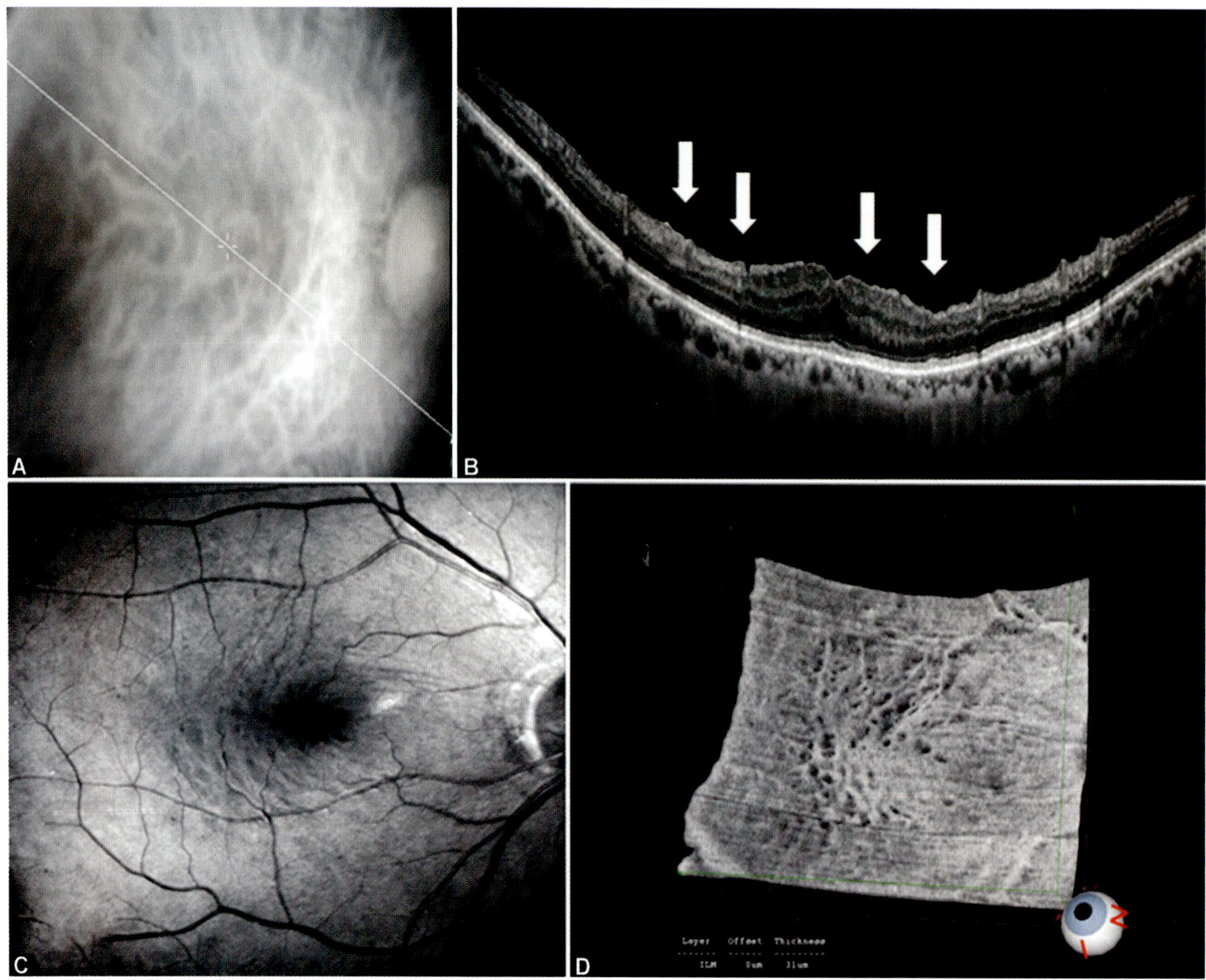

Figures 10A to D: Case of a 74-year-old female patient (A) who underwent pars plana vitrectomy with internal limiting membrane (ILM) removal for idiopathic full-thickness macular hole in 2001. Eleven years after surgery, mild concentric macular dark spots around the foveal region are observed on the redfree fundus photograph (Spectralis™ HRA+OCT. Heidelberg, Dossenheim, Germany) (C) corresponding to the typical OCT pattern as shown on 3D *en face* optical coherence tomography scan of the RTVue-100® (Optovue Inc, Fremont, CA) (D); Moreover, the characteristic dimples within the thickness of the retinal nerve fiber layer are evident on (B) the related cross-sectional B scan (white arrows) (*Courtesy:* San Giuseppe Hospital, University Eye Clinic, Milan, Italy)

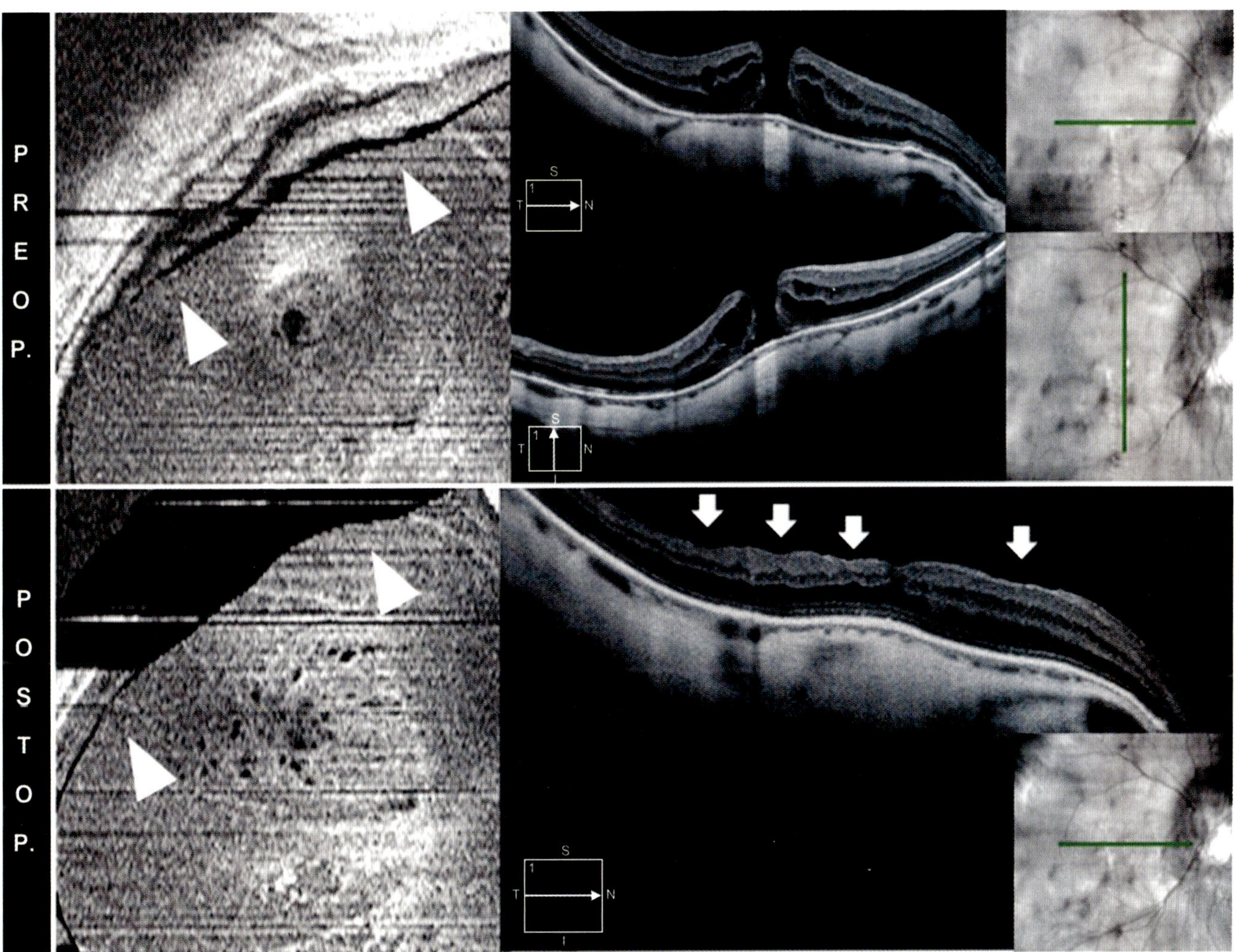

Figure 11: Preoperative optical coherence tomography scan of a 66-year-old myopic patient (Spherical Equivalent, SE -15.00 D) with a macular hole (MH) in her right eye, as shown on cross-sectional B scans. Three months after surgery a complete MH closure was reported by OCT B scan and fine shallow dimples appeared at the level of the retinal nerve fiber layer. Few visible concentric macular dark spots corresponding to each of these inner retinal defects are observed on the postoperative *en face* OCT, suggesting a complete internal limiting membrane removal. Note that an extensive "round off" artifact (arrowheads) appears on the upper left corner on the *en face* OCT image, due to the breakdown in the segmentation algorithm produced by any SD-OCT device provided with this acquisition protocol
[*Courtesy:* Cirrus HD-OCT 4000 (Carl Zeiss Meditec, Dublin, CA); IMO (Instituto de Microcirugia Ocular), Barcelona, Spain]

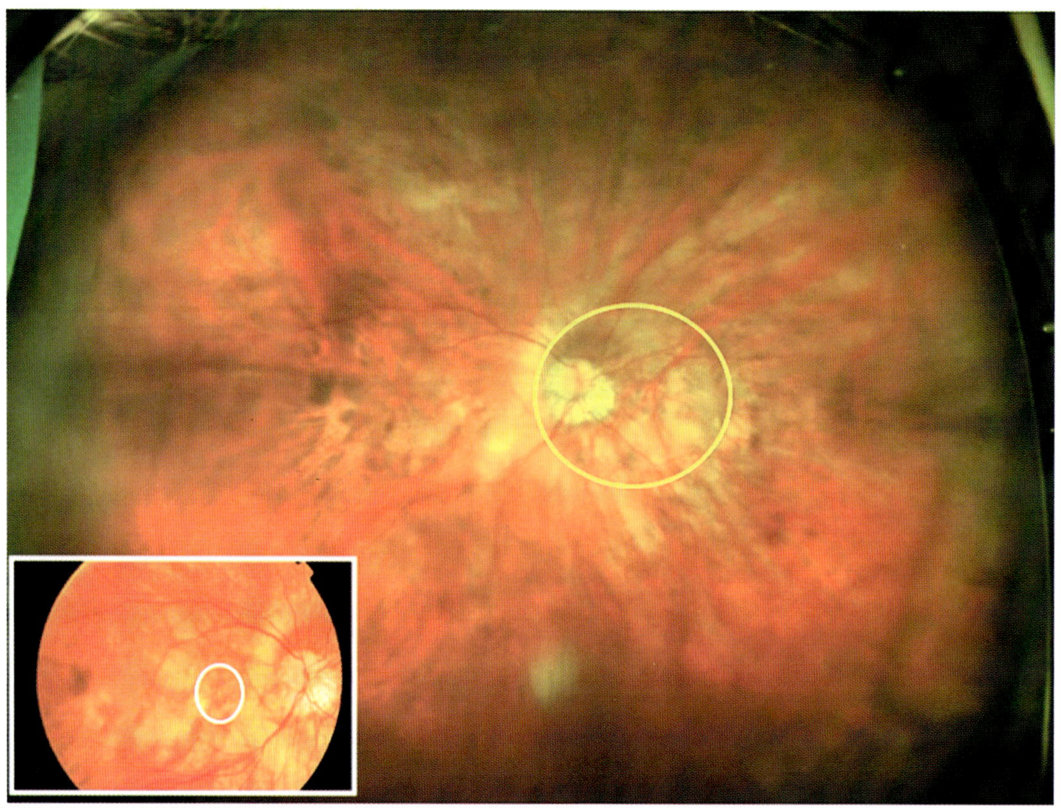

Figure 12: Color fundus photograph of the patient shown in Figure 10. The image was obtained with an ultra-wide-field scanning laser ophthalmoscope (SLO) with two laser wavelengths (Optomap 200MA; Optos PLC, Dunfermline, Fife, Scotland). Note the posterior staphyloma (yellow circle) nasal to the optic disk (Type IV according to the Curtin's Classification).[15] On the *bottom left*, a color photograph of the posterior pole was obtained using a mydriatic fundus camera (TRC-50DX type IA; Topcon, Tokyo, Japan). A full thickness MH within a wide area of retinal pigment epithelium changes can be observed (white circle) and the choroidal vessels are clearly visible through the thin retina
[*Courtesy:* IMO (Instituto de Microcirugia Ocular), Barcelona, Spain]

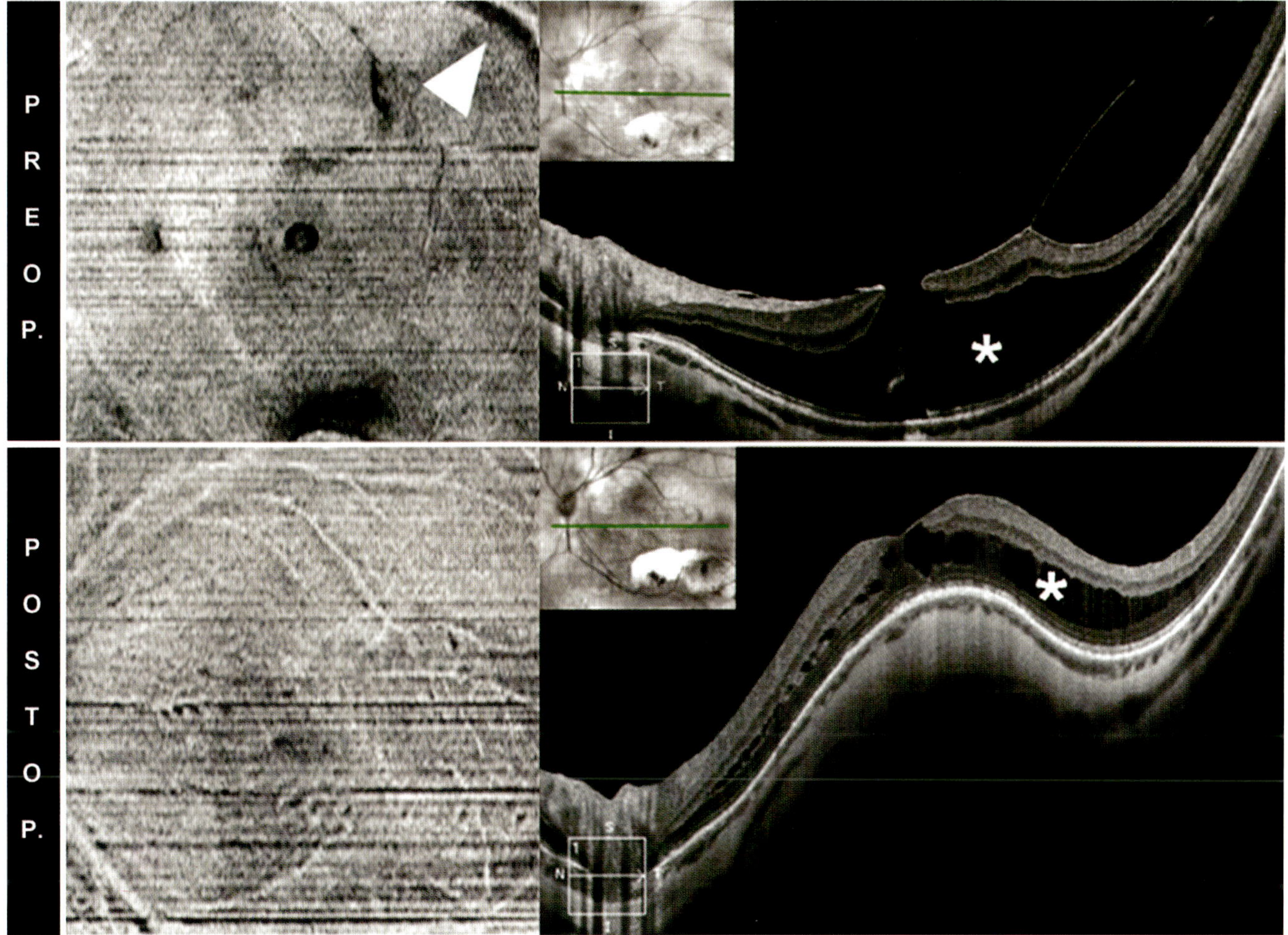

Figure 13: Preoperative optical coherence tomography scans (OCTs) of a 48-year-old myopic patient (Spherical equivalent, SE-19.75 D) with a macular hole (MH) and a concomitant retinoschisis in his left eye (asterisk), as shown on B scans. The posterior hyaloid is still adherent and can be observed temporally to the foveal region, causing some degree of vitreoretinal traction. Surgery consisted in pars plana vitrectomy, internal limiting membrane (ILM) peeling, gas tamponade and macular buckling. Three months after surgery, a complete MH closure and a thinner but persistent retinoschisis (asterisk) are reported on OCT B scans. Few visible concentric macular dark spots are observed on the postoperative *en face* OCT, suggesting a complete ILM removal, even if no dimples are detected at the level of the retinal nerve fiber layer on the corresponding cross-sectional B scan. Note the "round off" artifact (arrowhead) on the upper right corner on the *en face* OCT image, due to an error in the segmentation algorithm of the SD-OCT device
[*Courtesy:* Cirrus HD-OCT 4000 (Carl Zeiss Meditec, Dublic, CA); IMO (Instituto de Microcirugia Ocular), Barcelona, Spain]

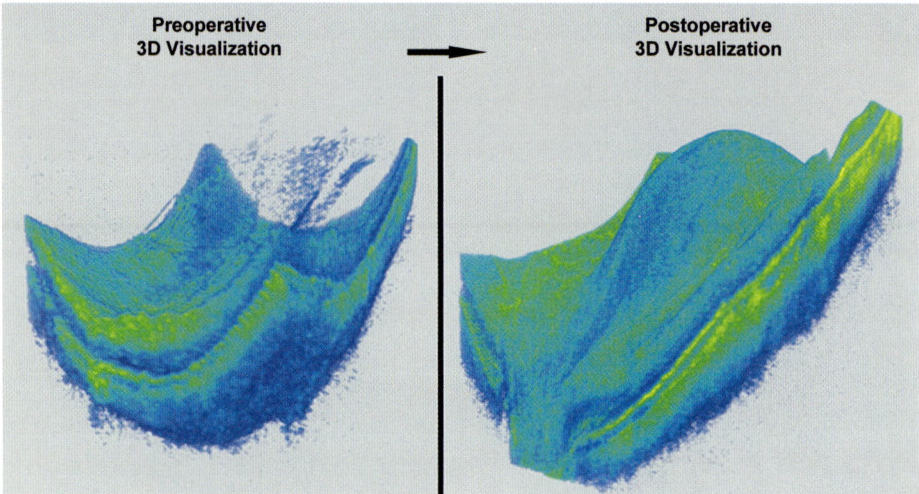

Figure 14: Three-dimensional visualization of the macular cube of the patient shown in Figure 12. A residual posterior hyaloid can be observed on the temporal side of the posterior pole corresponding to the hyper-reflective band as seen on preoperative B scan in Figure 12. Note the 3D elevation of the macular region due the presence of a posterior scleral buckle
[*Courtesy:* Cirrus HD-OCT 4000 (Carl Zeiss Meditec, Dublic, CA); IMO (Instituto de Microcirugia Ocular), Barcelona, Spain]

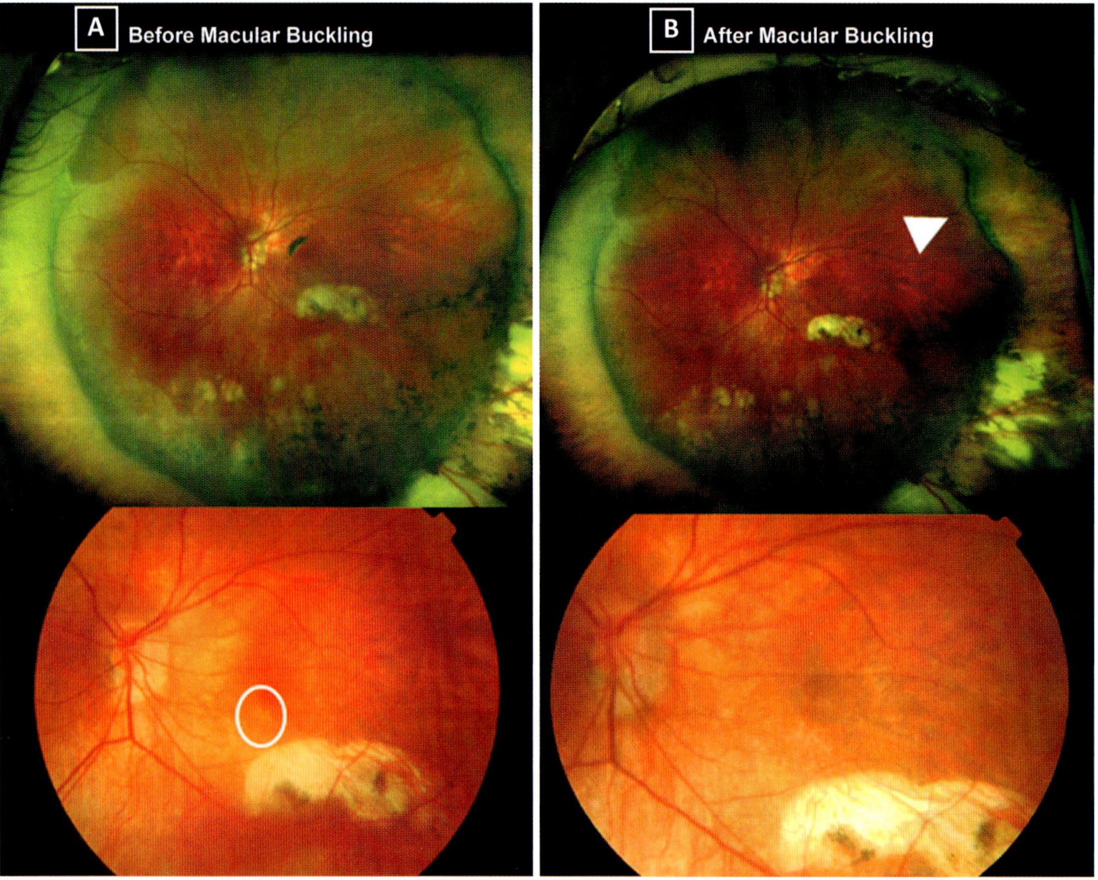

Figures 15A and B: Wide-field and posterior pole color fundus photographs of the patient described in Figures 12 and 13. (A, Left column) Fundus aspect with evidence of the encircling band for a prior rhegmatogenous retinal detachment. A full thickness macular hole is visible in the lower left image (white circle) with a zone of chorioretinal atrophy along to the inferior temporal vascular arcade; (B, Right column) Postoperative fundus appearance with the macular buckling visible in the superior temporal quadrant (arrowhead) and a complete macular hole closure. Note that the posterior scleral buckle was not so evident in the color fundus photograph of the macular region (bottom right)
[*Courtesy:* IMO (Instituto de Microcirugia Ocular), Barcelona, Spain]

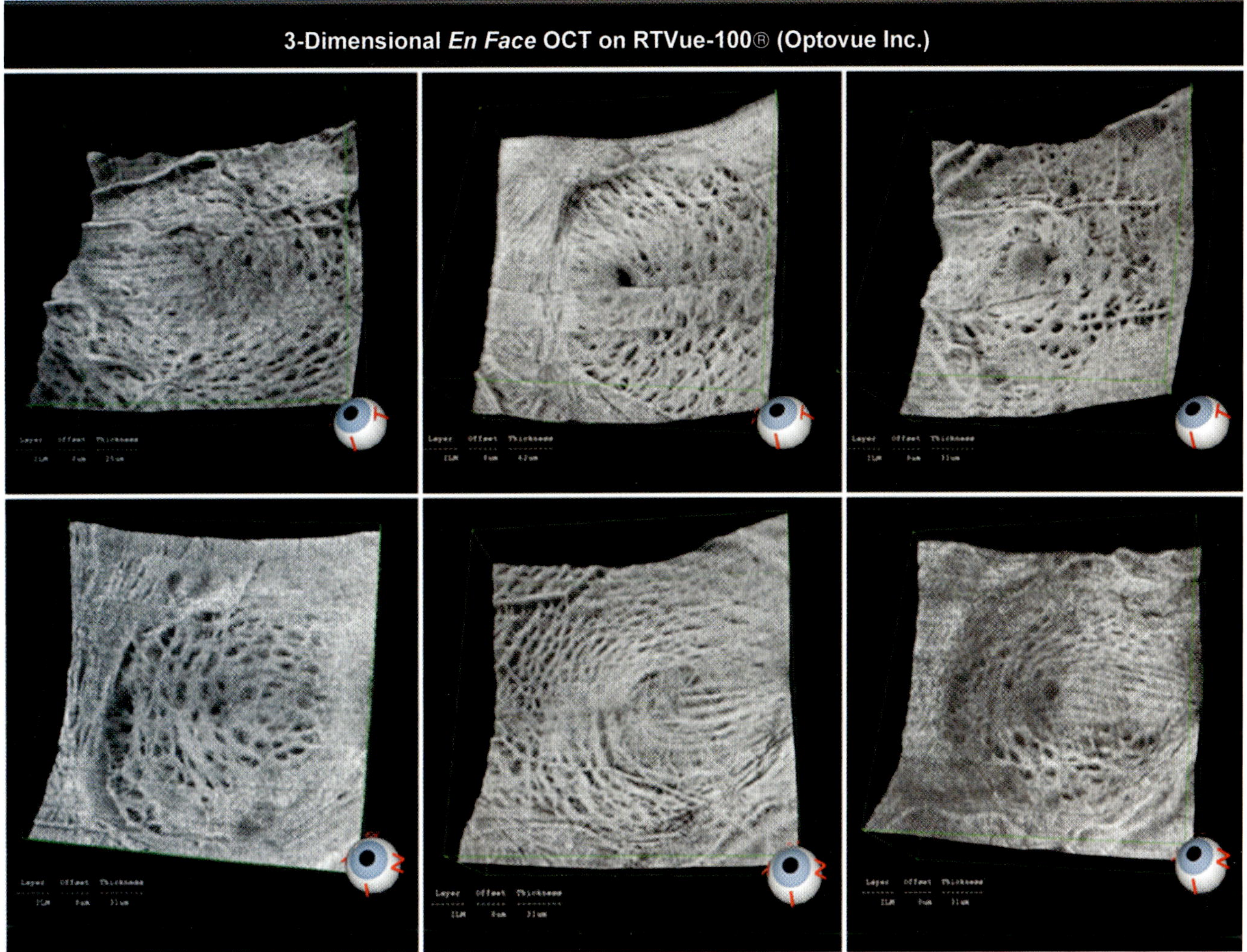

Figure 16: Postoperative 3D *en face* optical coherence tomography scans of nine patients who underwent surgery for idiopathic macular hole. The typical concentric macular dark spot appearance is clearly visible along the course of optic nerve fiber in the area of the internal limiting membrane (ILM) peeling, suggesting a complete ILM removal within the posterior pole
(*Courtesy:* San Giuseppe Hospital, University Eye Clinic, Milan, Italy)

software algorithm. This leads to incapacity of the SD-OCT to exactly identify the retinal boundaries, such as the RPE or the ILM, which is an essential condition to create the *en face* OCT C scans. The consequence is the appearance of some "round-off" or black spaces located often in the corner of the *en face* image **(Figures 11 and 13)** which are the transverse representation of the "mirror artifacts" usually seen on cross-sectional B scans in these patients.[13]

For these reasons and for the presence of a thinner RNFL in moderate and highly myopic individuals,[14] the ILM status preoperatively and postoperatively can be very difficult to assess and this may suggest that the CMDS' appearance, as described for idiopathic MHs, could not be so easy to evaluate in myopic population. Thus, operators should be aware that if CMDS are not observed postoperatively even after a long period, it does not mean that the ILM has not been peeled off during MH surgery in these patients.

Despite many circumstances in which the ILM is intraoperatively considered peeled off with the posterior hyaloid or with a concomitant epiretinal membrane, some of its fragments could be still detectable by restaining the retinal surface and do not allow the correct healing process. Thus, providing informations about the inner retinal surface and the ILM status, transverse *en face* OCT C scans may help in planning the best tailored approach to treat MHs, especially in cases of reopening or persistent MH in which the ILM may be still adherent even after previous surgery **(Figure 7)**.

Finally, this technique seems more useful and easier to perform in emmetropic rather than myopic eyes by any SD-OCT instrument which has an *en face* acquisition protocol **(Figures 10 and 16)**.

References

1. Sebag J. The vitreous. In: Hart WM (Ed). Adler's Physiology of the Eye, 9th edition. Baltimore: Mosby-Year Book; 1992. pp. 268-347.
2. Wollensak G, Spoerl E. Biomechanical characteristics of retina. Retina. 2004;24(6):967-70.
3. Wollensak G, Spoerl E, Grosse G, et al. Biomechanical significance of the human internal limiting lamina. Retina. 2006;26(8):965-8.
4. Ducournau D, Ducournau Y. A closer look to the ILM. Retinal Physician. 2008;5(Suppl. 6):4-15.
5. Gass JD. Idiopathic senile macular hole. Its early stages and pathogenesis. Arch Ophthalmol. 1988;106(5):629-39.
6. Kelly NE, Wendel RT. Vitreous surgery for idiopathic macular holes. Results of a pilot study. Arch Ophthalmol. 1991;109(5):654-9.
7. Schumann RG, Schaumberger MM, Rohleder M, et al. Ultrastructure of the vitreomacular interface in full-thickness idiopathic macular holes: a consecutive analysis of 100 cases. Am J Ophthalmol. 2006;141(6):1112-9.
8. Alkabes M, Salinas C, Vitale L, et al. *En face* optical coherence tomography of inner retinal defects after internal limiting membrane peeling for idiopathic macular hole. Invest Ophthalmol Vis Sci. 2011;52(11):8349-55.
9. Wolf S, Schnurbusch U, Wiedemann P, et al. Peeling of the basal membrane in the human retina: ultrastructural effects. Ophthalmology. 2004;111(2):238-43.
10. Mitamura Y, Suzuki T, Kinoshita T, et al. Optical coherence tomographic findings of dissociated optic nerve fiber layer appearance. Am J Ophthalmol. 2004;137(6):1155-6.
11. Tadayoni R, Paques M, Massin P, et al. Dissociated optic nerve fiber layer appearance of the fundus after idiopathic epiretinal membrane removal. Ophthalmology. 2001;108(12):2279-83.
12. Mitamura Y, Ohtsuka K. Relationship of dissociated optic nerve fiber layer appearance to internal limiting membrane peeling. Ophthalmology. 2005;112(10):1766-70.
13. Song Y, Lee BR, Shin YW, et al. Overcoming segmentation errors in measurements of macular thickness made by spectral-domain optical coherence tomography. Retina. 2012;32(3):569-80.
14. Rauscher FM, Sekhon N, Feuer WJ, et al. Myopia affects retinal nerve fiber layer measurements as determined by optical coherence tomography. J Glaucoma. 2009;18(7):501-5.
15. Curtin BJ. The posterior staphyloma of pathologic myopia. Trans Am Ophthalmol Soc. 1977;75:67-86.

chapter 37

Idiopathic Macular Holes

Nalin J Mehta

Introduction

Idiopathic macular holes are formed by a combination of tangential and anteroposterior tractional forces **(Figures 1A and B)**. Highly myopic eyes are also prone to macular hole formation. Vision can vary from 20/20 to less than 20/400, depending on the size and duration of the hole.

Surgical intervention is most often reserved for full-thickness holes **(Figures 1A and B)**, although surgical indications for partial-thickness (lamellar) holes are growing. *En face* imaging of these holes can be useful in anatomic differentiation, preoperative planning and postoperative prognostic determination of these holes **(Figures 2 to 7)**.[1,2]

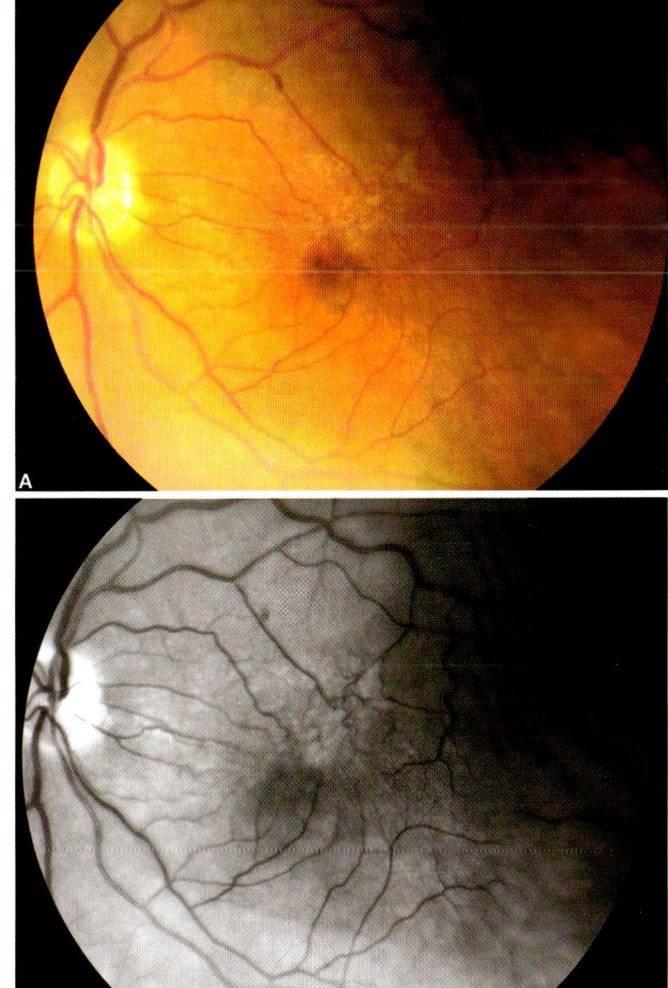

Figures 1A and B: A color and red-free fundus photo of a full-thickness macular hole with associated tangential traction from epiretinal membranous changes

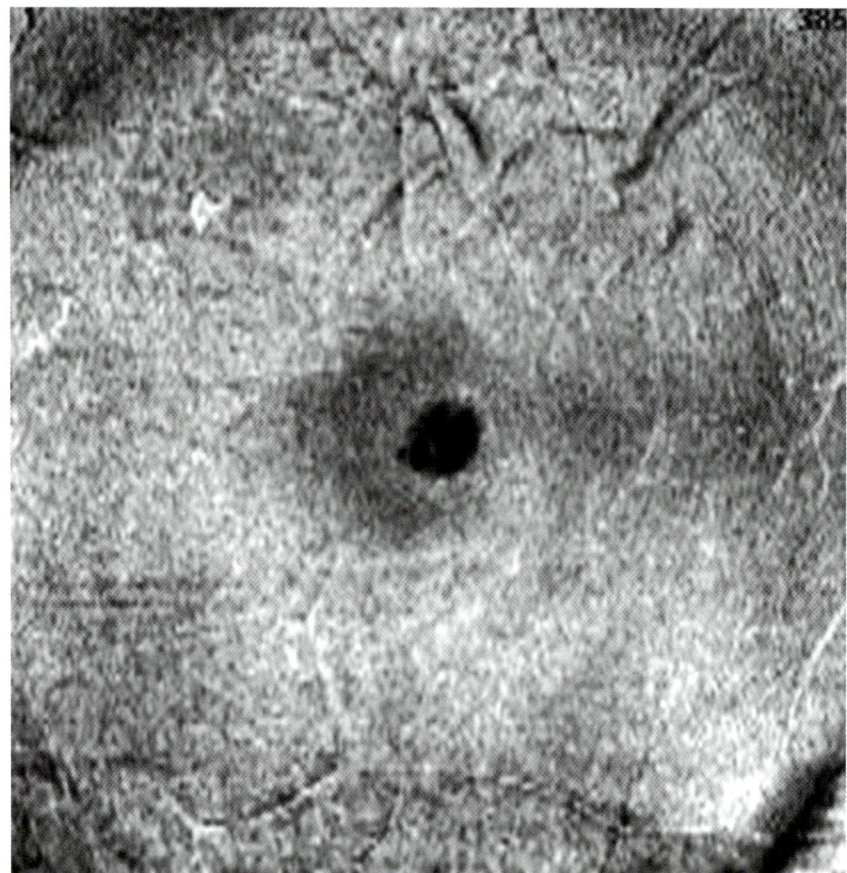

Figure 2: An *en face* view at the level of the internal limiting membrane. The puckering effect of the epiretinal membrane is seen superiorly. This view proves helpful in planning surgical intervention, which includes pars plana vitrectomy with removal of the epiretinal and sometimes internal limiting membrane

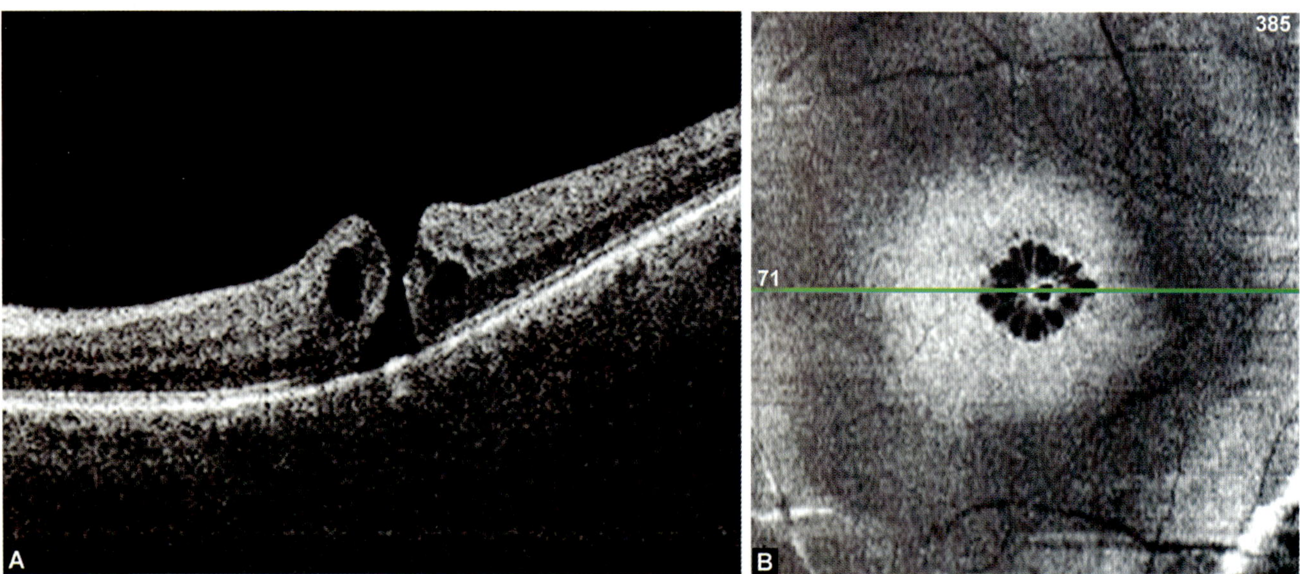

Figures 3A and B: B scan and *en face* views of the full-thickness macular hole. Note the cystoid edema at the edges associated with the edges of the hole; the *en face* view demonstrates a symmetric petalloid edematous pattern surrounding the hole

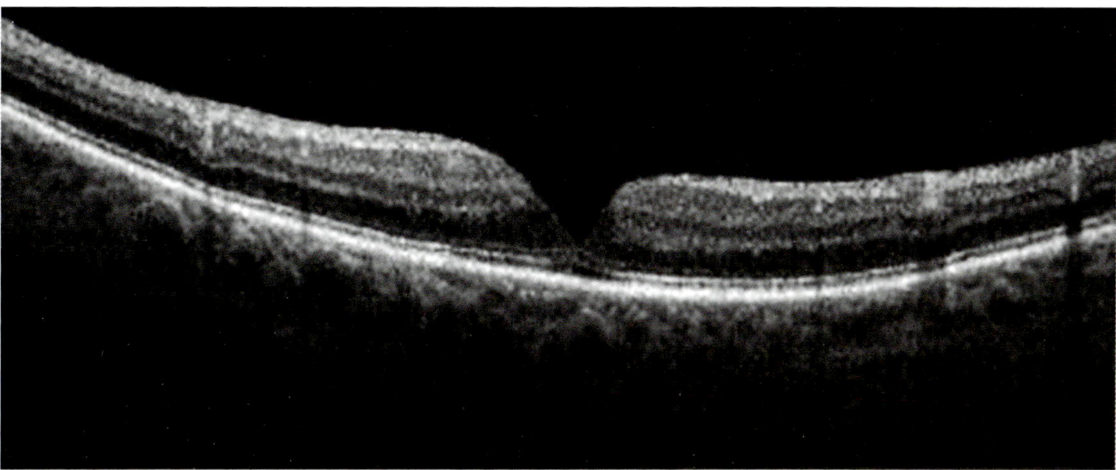

Figure 4: B scan of the macular hole after postoperative stabilization. Note a persistent defect in the inner segment/ outer segment line in the foveola, with outer segment signal loss

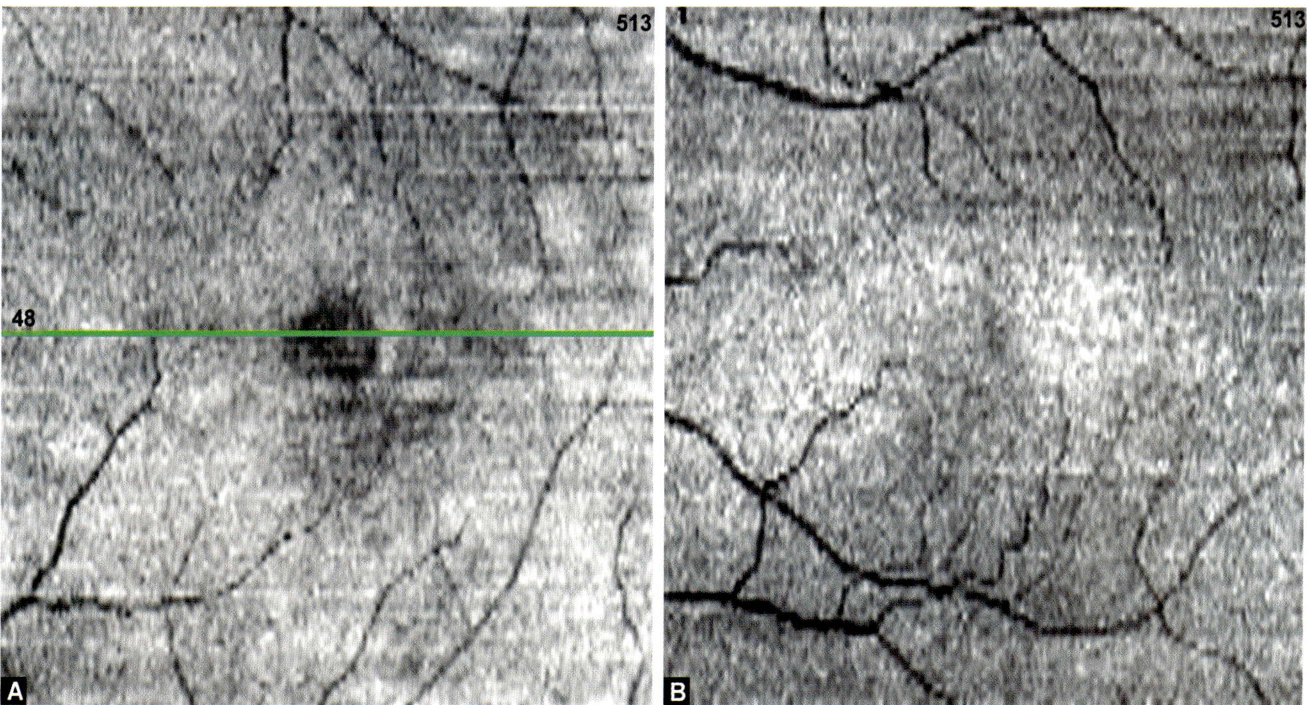

Figures 5A and B: Figure 5A shows the postoperative *en face* view of the macular hole in Figure 4 at the level of the outer segment, demonstrating a hyporeflective circular area of photoreceptor loss. This is in contrast to Figure 5B, which is located at the same level in a normal macula and may serve as a predictor of postsurgical visual outcome. *En face* postoperative imaging of the inner retina has furthermore been used to assess the completeness of internal limiting membrane removal[3]

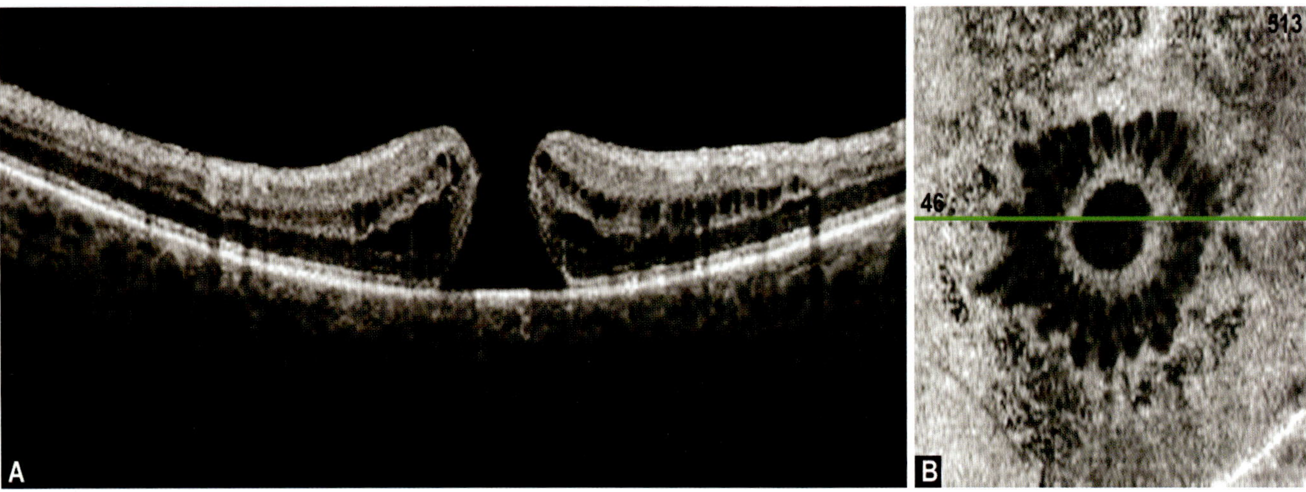

Figures 6A and B: Another full-thickness macular hole with the characteristic, relatively-symmetric, petalloid pattern surrounding the hole on the *en face* image. This pattern appears characteristic of full-thickness holes

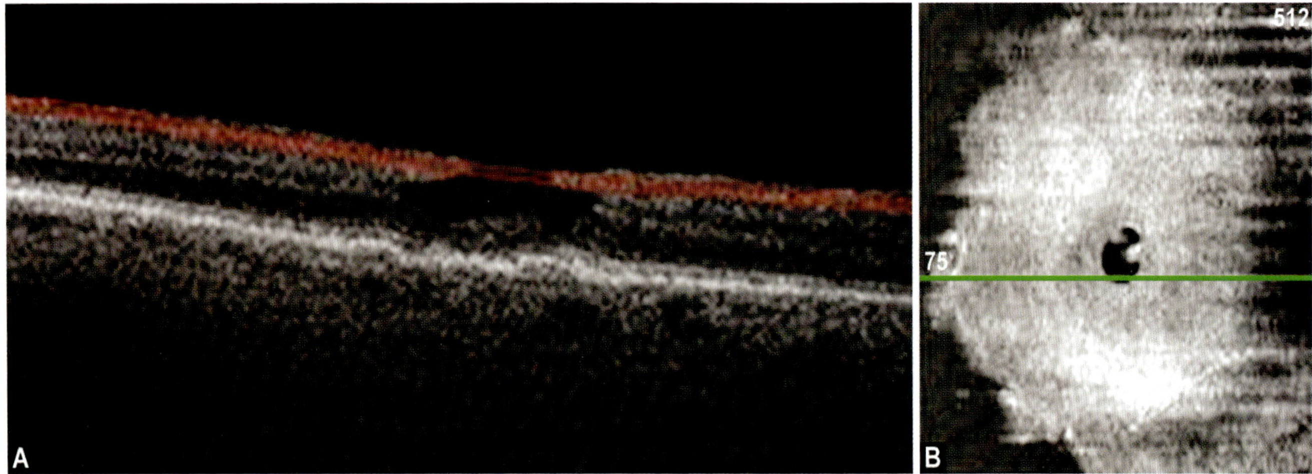

Figures 7A and B: Both lamellar holes (A and B, taken at the level of the nerve fiber layer) and pseudoholes do not usually show this type of symmetric petalloid pattern

References

1. Forte R, Pascotto F, Napolitano F, et al. *En face* optical coherence tomography of macular holes in high myopia. Eye (Lond). 2007;21(3):436-7.
2. Faghihi H, Hajizadeh F, Riazi-Esfahani M. Optical coherence tomographic findings in highly myopic eyes. J Ophthalmic Vis Res. 2010;5(2):110-21.
3. Alkabes M, Salinas C, Vitale L, et al. *En face* optical coherence tomography of inner retinal defects after internal limiting membrane peeling for idiopathic macular hole. Invest Ophthalmol Vis Sci. 2011;52(11): 8349-55.

chapter 38

Macular Pseudohole

Gezhi Xu, Min Wang

Introduction

The macular pseudohole is a round or oval defect of the epimacular membrane over the fovea. The pseudohole is formed by spontaneous contraction of an epiretinal membrane around the fovea. It is difficult to differentiate the pseudohole from real macular hole under the ophthalmoscope. But the *en face* optical coherence tomography (OCT) is able to detect the structural changes of the pseudohole.

Case Study 1

A 46-year-old female was diagnosed with macular pseudohole in her left eye. There is a pseudohole in the macula on fundus photo **(Figure 1)**. At the inner limiting membrane (ILM) level of *en face* OCT, there is a dark oval lesion that corresponds to the location of the pseudohole **(Figure 2)**. Epiretinal membrane (ERM) can be visualized on the temporal side of the pseudohole. At the inner plexiform layer (IPL) level, the shape of the pseudohole becomes round that matches the base of the pseudohole on OCT **(Figure 3)**. The pseudohole is not recognized on retinal pigment epithelium (RPE) and RPE reference level and this is the major difference from the real macular hole on *en face* OCT.

Case Study 2

A 38-year-old woman had the diagnosis of macular

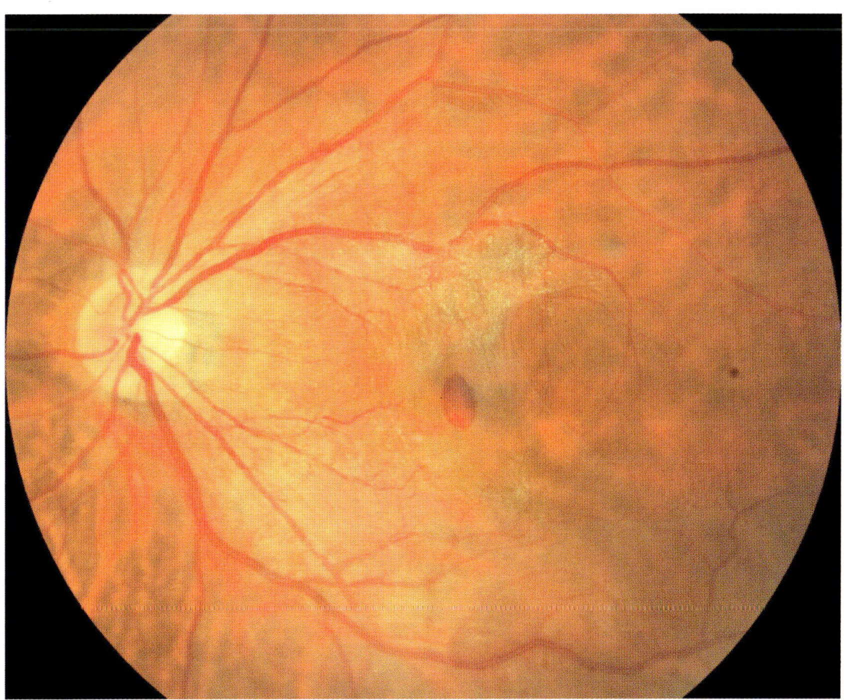

Figure 1: A 46-year-old female diagnosed with macular pseudohole in her left eye

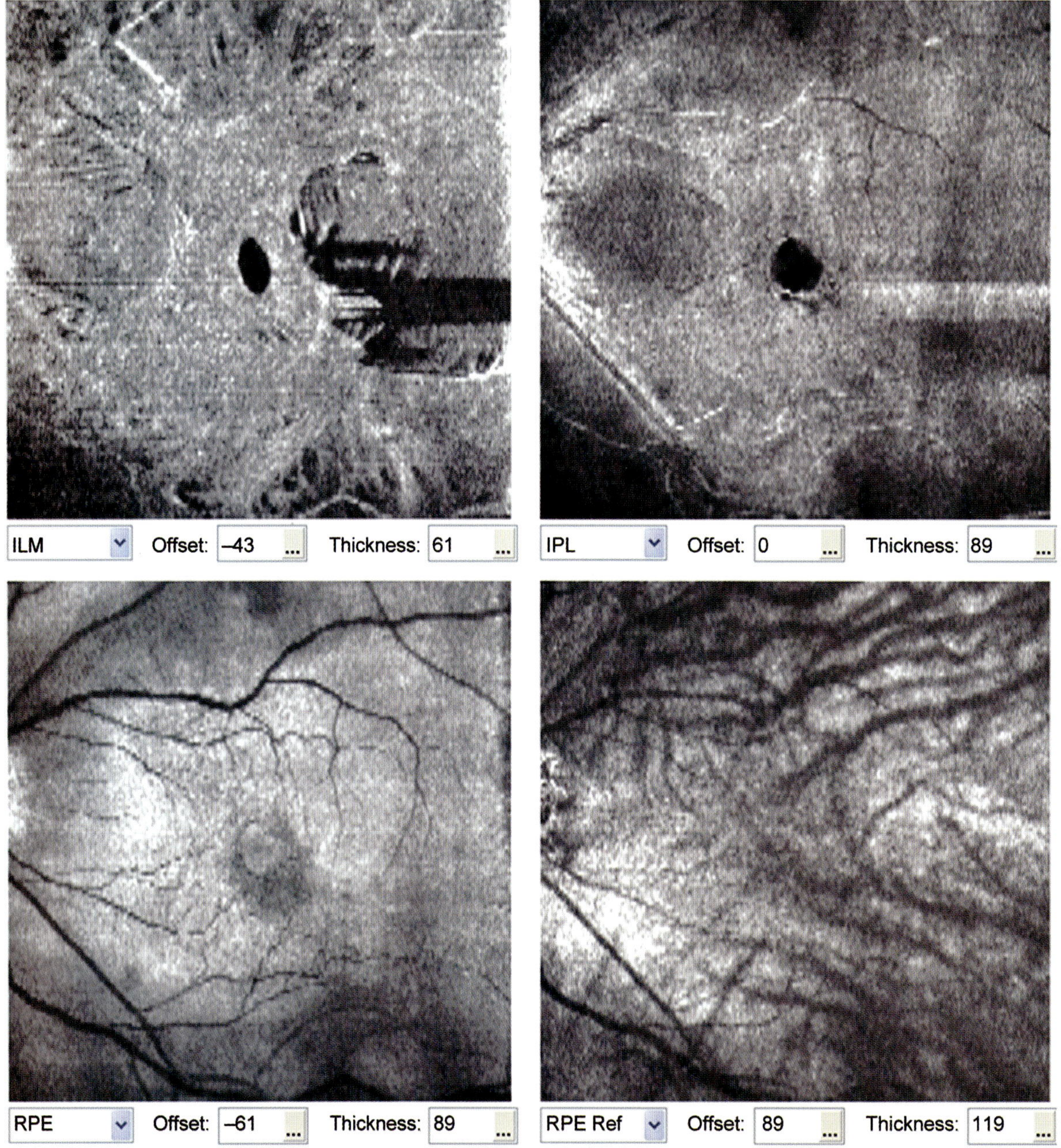

Figure 2: *En face* OCT showing a dark oval lesion at the ILM level

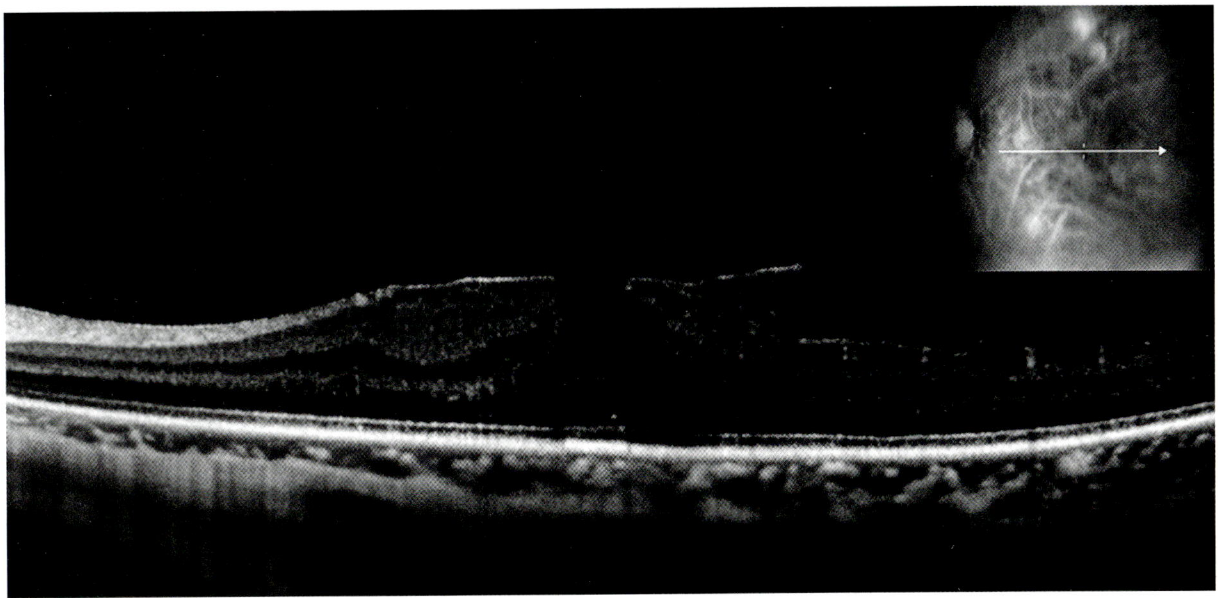

Figure 3: OCT line scan showing pseudohole and ERM

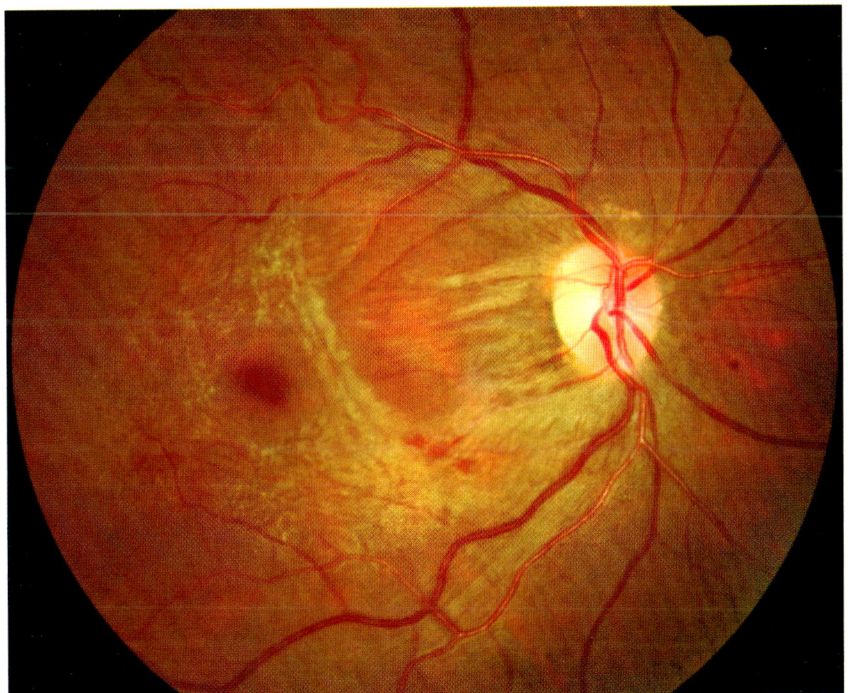

Figure 4: A 38-year-old woman diagnosed with macular pseudohole in her right eye. Macular pseudohole with epiretinal membrane can be observed

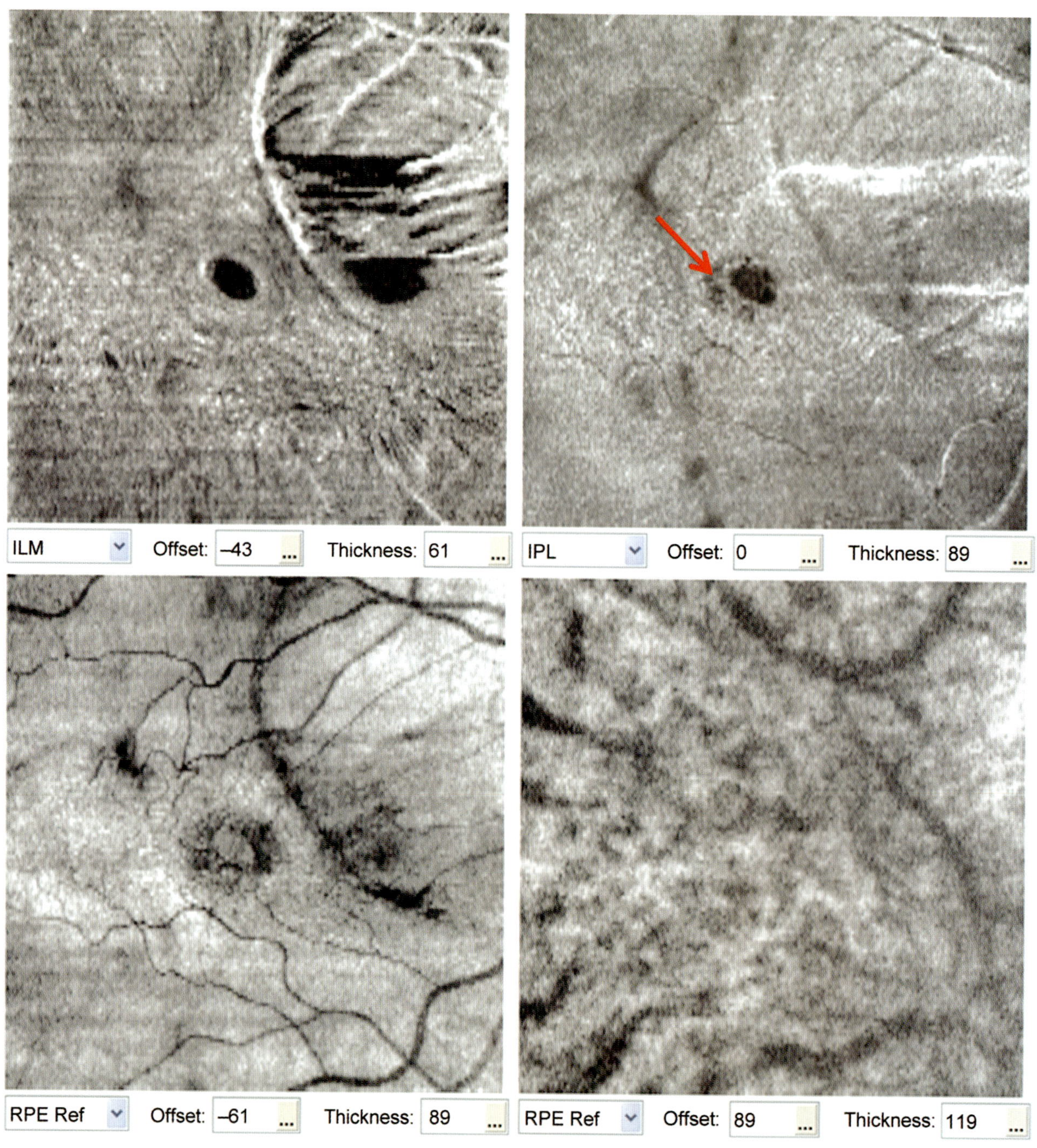

Figure 5: Pseudohole and ERM showing at ILM level and cystoid edema around pseudohole (red arrow) showing at IPL level

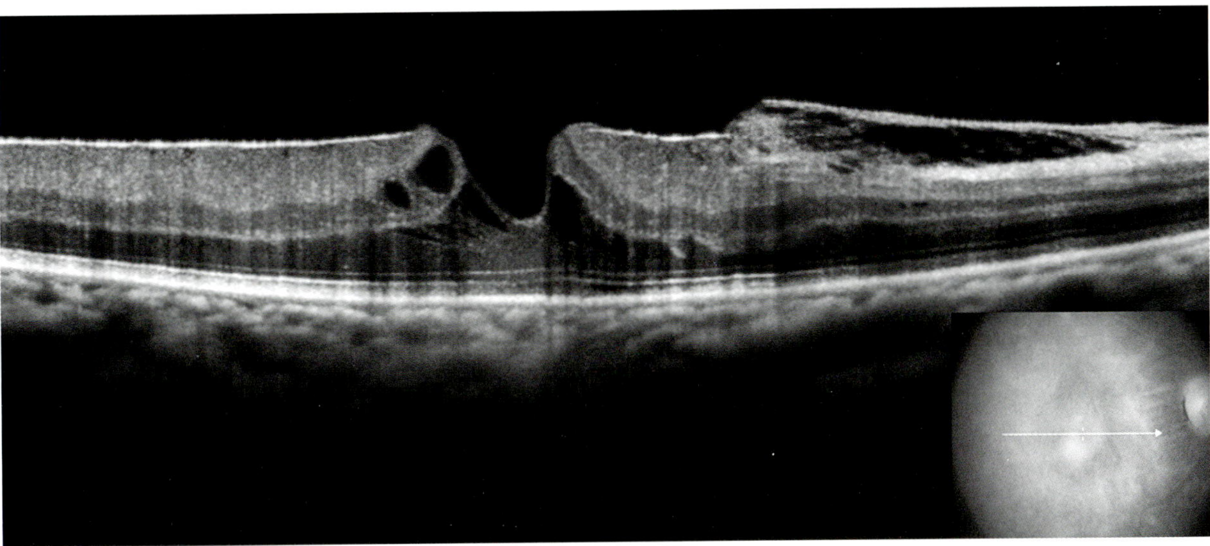

Figure 6: OCT line scan revealing pseudohole, cystoid edema and ERM

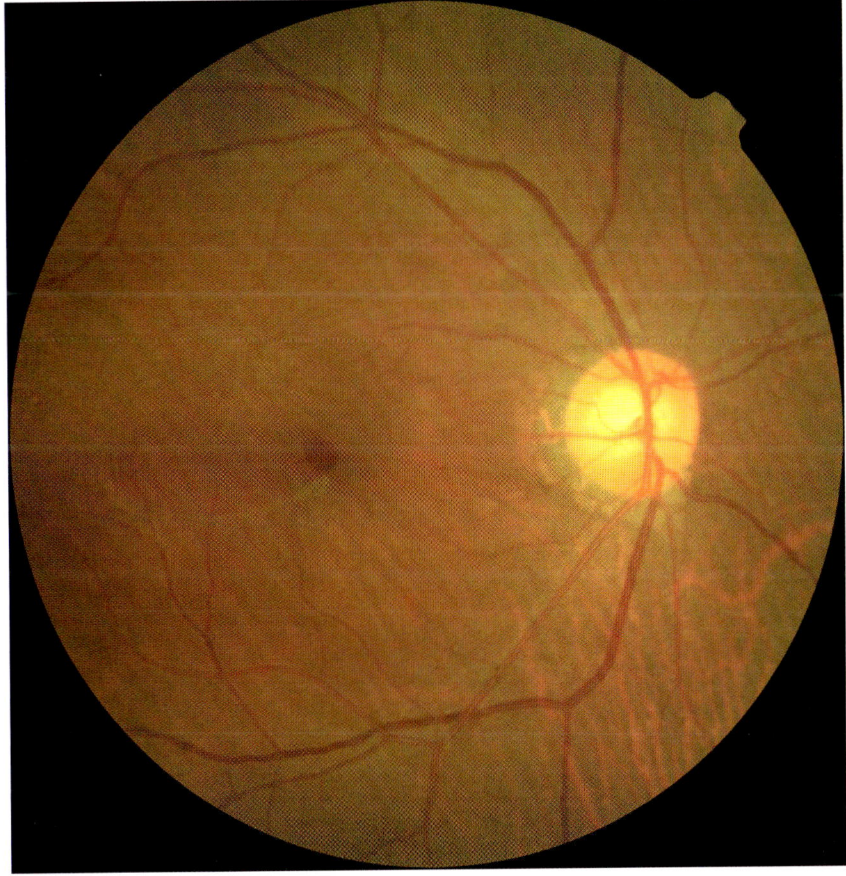

Figure 7: A 62-year old woman diagnosed with macular pseudohole in her left eye

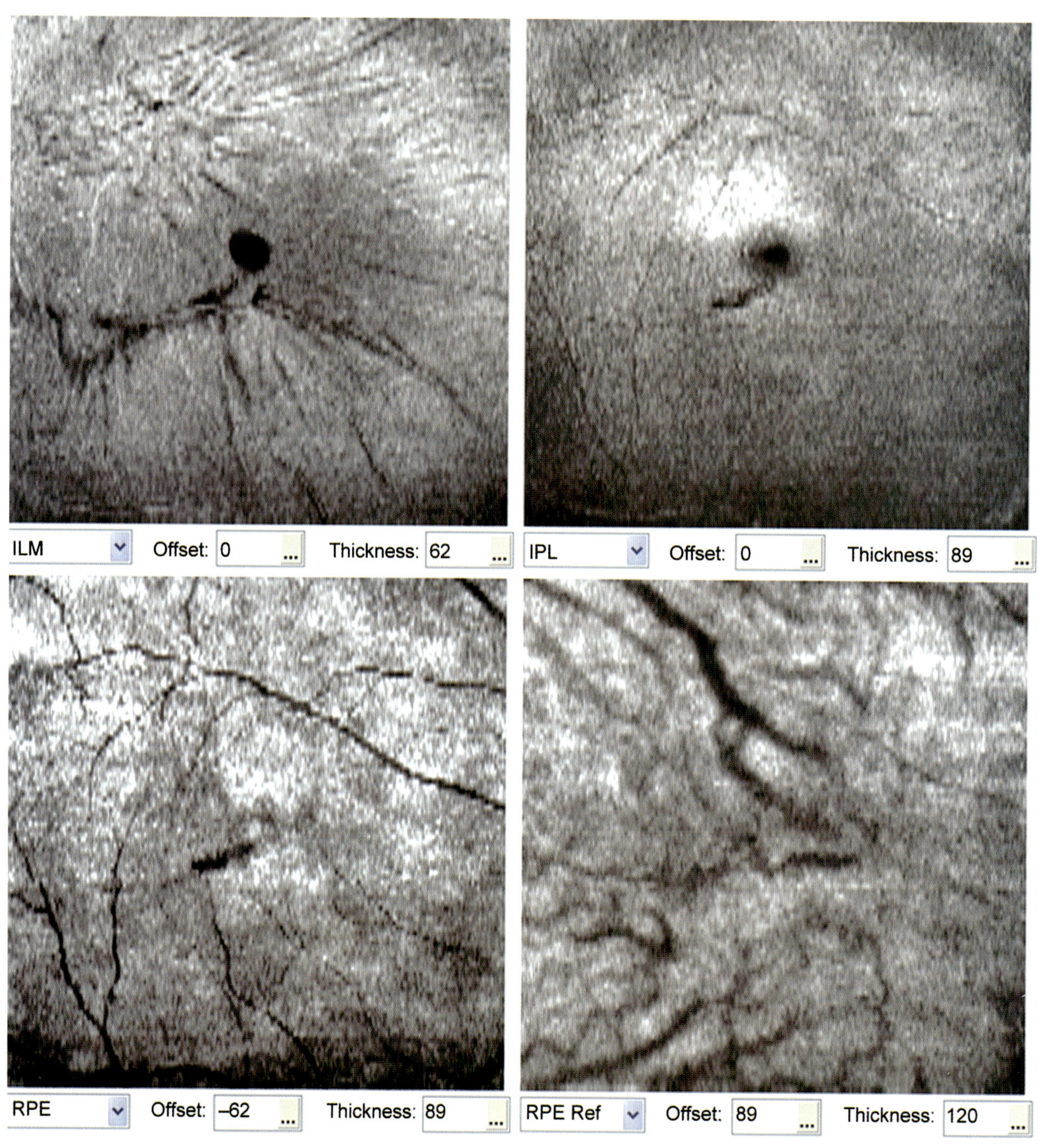

Figure 8: Pseudohole showing at ILM level

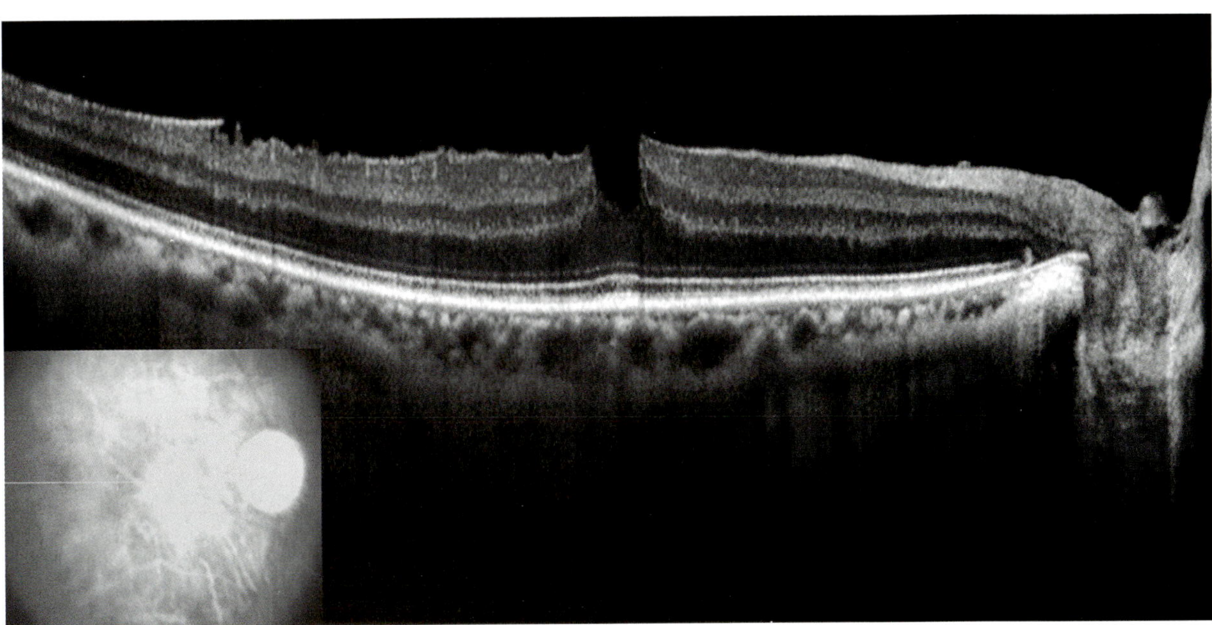

Figure 9: OCT line scan showing the pseudohole

pseudohole in her right eye. On the fundus photo, macular pseudohole with ERM can be observed (**Figure 4**). The pseudohole is demonstrated clearly at ILM level of *en face* OCT (**Figure 5**). The distribution of ERM around the pseudohole is displayed dramatically. At the IPL level, cystoid edema around the pseudohole (**Figure 5**, red arrow), which corresponds to the changes on OCT line scan (**Figure 6**) is recognized.

Case Study 3

A 62-year-old woman was diagnosed with macular pseudohole in her left eye (**Figure 7**). On *en face* OCT, ERM around the pseudohole is clearly observed at ILM level. The base of the pseudohole can be recognized at the level of IPL and not displayed at RPE and RPE reference levels (**Figure 8**). On OCT scan, the bottom of the pseudohole reaches the inner nuclear layer (INL) and the outer retinal layer remains normal (**Figure 9**).

chapter 39

Lamellar Holes

Bruno Lumbroso, Marco Rispoli, Chunhui Jiang

Introduction

In case of lamellar hole, retina loses its normal profile at level of the inner layers; the foveal depression is increased but the outer retinal layers seem intact.

Slits develop laterally, enlarging the hole, penetrating under the inner layers, sometimes simulating the retinoschisis wheel appearance. These asymmetric horizontal slits frequently dissociate the outer plexiform layer. The slit shape is determined by its position between parallel retinal layers that are dissociated from each other (**Figure 1**).

Minimal cavities and cystoid edema can be seen in the nuclear layers. The outer layers, photoreceptor nuclei, the external limiting membrane, the inner-outer photoreceptor segment junction and the pigment epithelium are frequently normal, thus explaining a good residual vision (**Figures 1 and 2**).

On *"en face"* scans typical lamellar holes may appear star and wheel shaped. These lesions follow the radial structure of Henle fibers and Müller cells (**Figure 2**). *En face* optical coherence tomography (OCT) shows lesions corresponding to schisis cavities in the inner and outer nuclear layer, and in the inner plexiform layer (**Figures 3 to 6**).

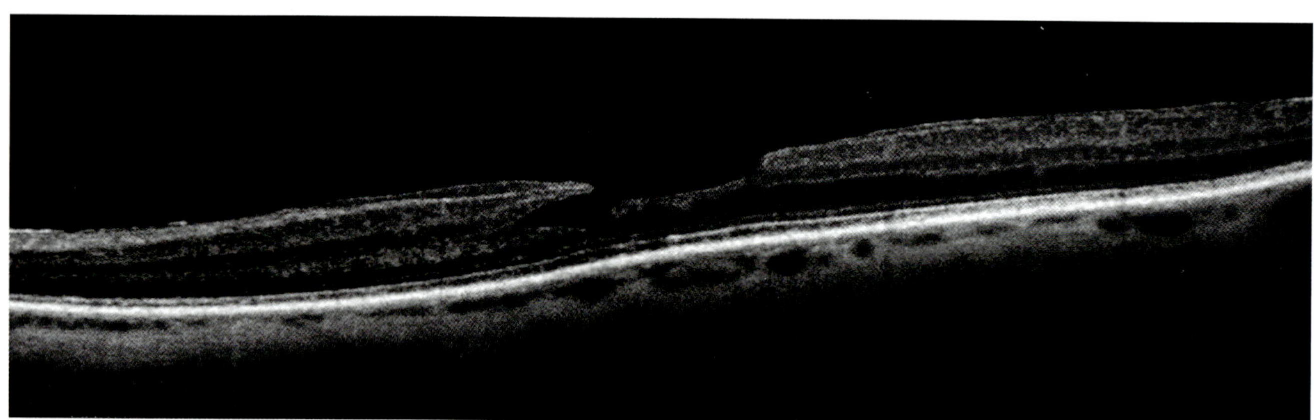

Figure 1: Lamellar hole B scan. The retina has lost its normal profile. Fissures enlarge, laterally, the lamellar hole, penetrating under the inner layers. An asymmetric horizontal slit can be observed dissociating the outer plexiform layer. Minimal cavities, associated to cystoid edema, can be seen in the nuclear layers. The slit shape is determined by its position between parallel retinal layers that separate from each other. The outer retinal layers are preserved, explaining a good residual vision (Optovue RTVue)

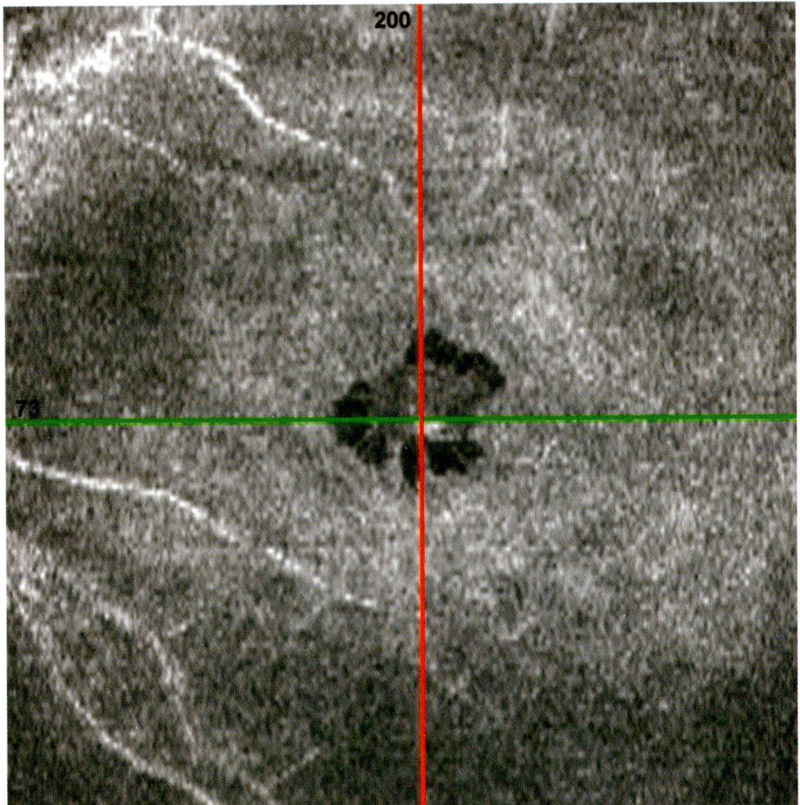

Figure 2: Lamellar hole *en face* scan. In this case *en face* scan fissures enlarge laterally the lamellar hole, penetrating under the inner layers, simulating the retinoschisis wheel shaped appearance. On *"en face"* scans lamellar holes can appear star and wheel shaped, following the radial structure of Henle fibers and Müller cells (Optovue RTVue)

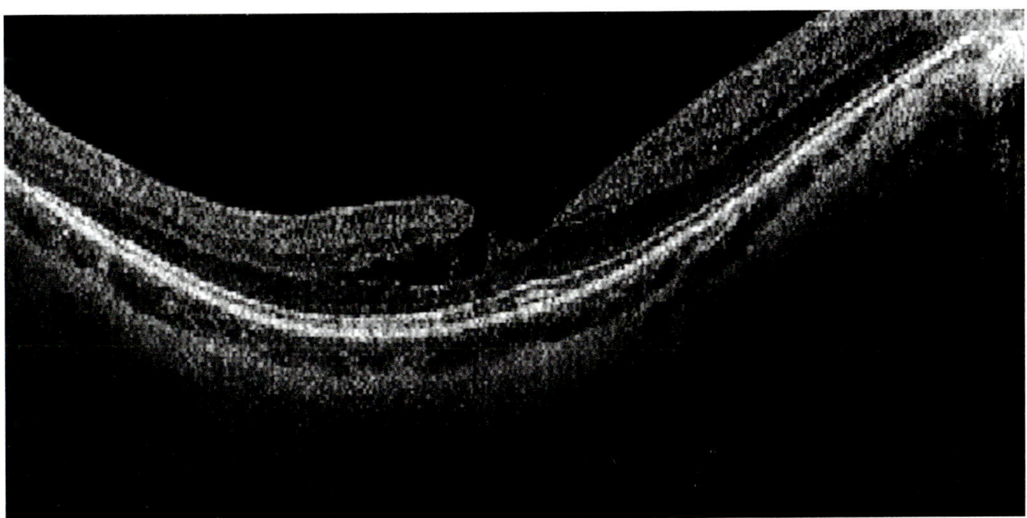

Figure 3: Lamellar hole B scan. The B scan shows a lamellar hole with cyst or cleft like structure at the outer plexiform layer (Optovue RTVue)

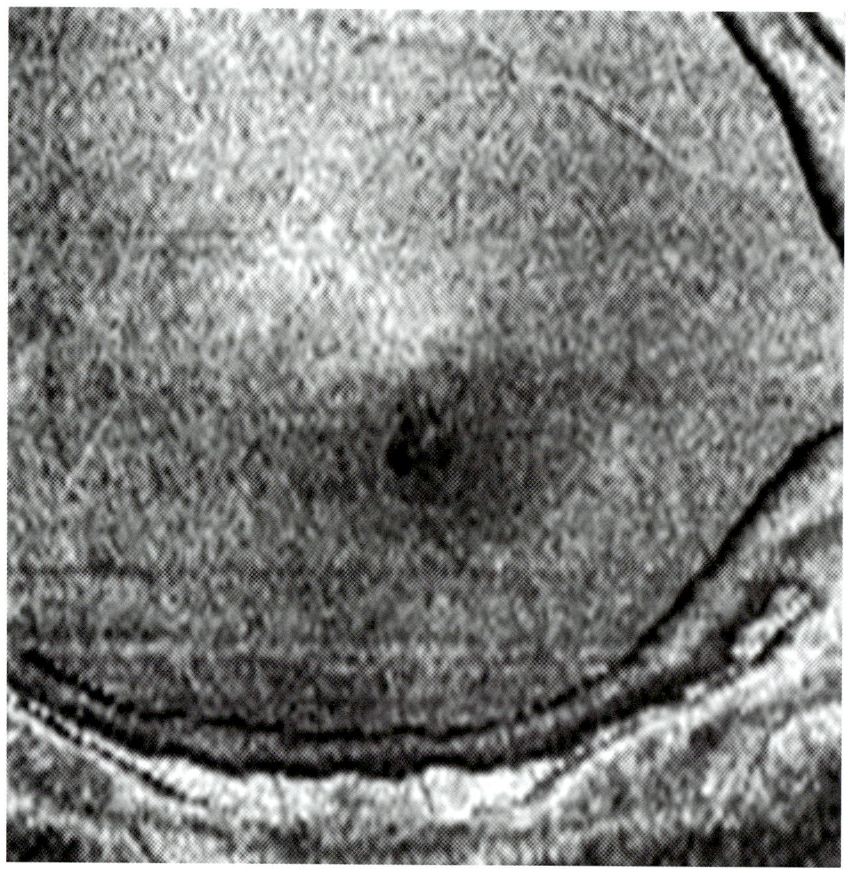

Figure 4: Lamellar hole *en face* scan. From the same patient as Figure 3 a small defect is at the center of a rather even retinal surface, except the black line at the inferior which is the result of posterior staphyloma (Optovue RTVue)

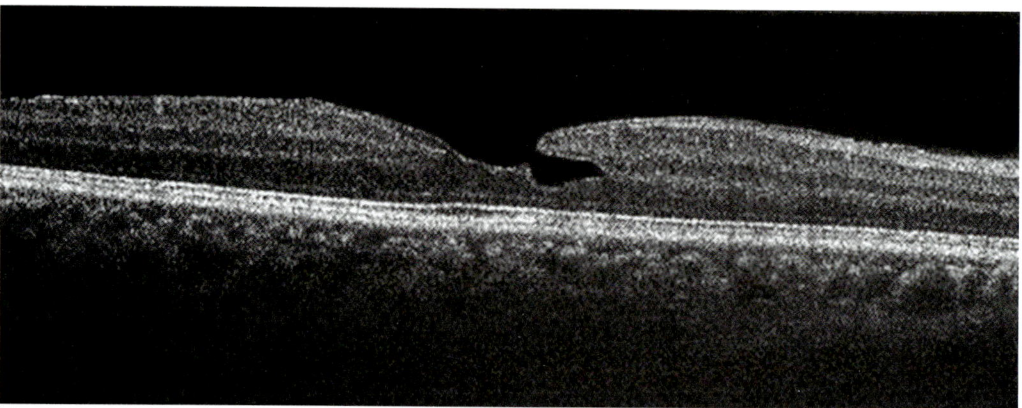

Figure 5: Lamellar hole B scan. The B scan shows a lamellar hole with cleft-like structure at the nasal side (right to the fovea) (Optovue RTVue)

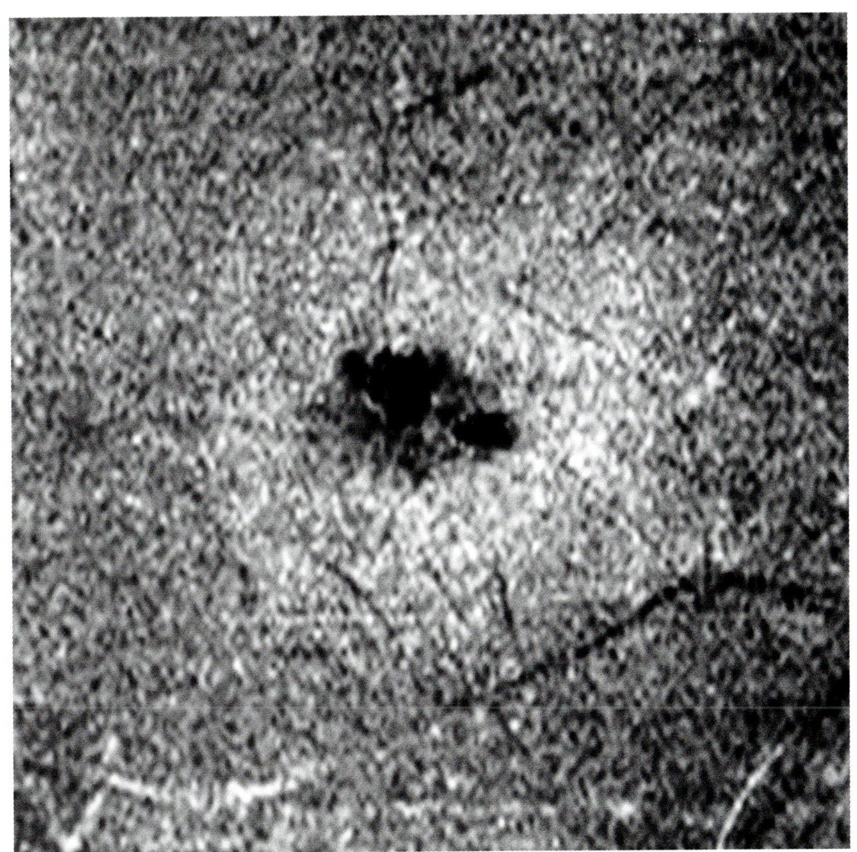

Figure 6: Lamellar hole *en face* scan. From the same patient as Figure 5, due to the irregular contour of the lamellar hole, the dark defect at the center is divided into two by a rather large tissue column (Optovue RTVue)

Section 10

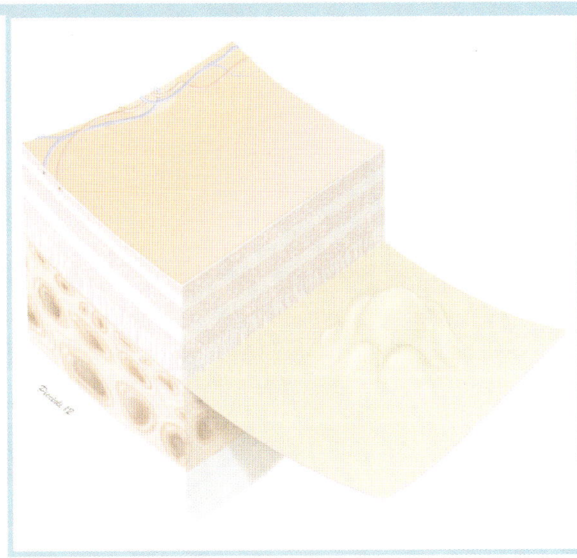

Choroid

Evaluation of Intrachoroidal Cavitation (Peripapillary Detachment) in Pathologic Myopia with *En Face* Optical Coherence Tomography

Gilda Cennamo, Giuseppe de Crecchio

Introduction

The peripapillary detachment of the retinal pigment epithelium (RPE) and retina, also known as peripapillary intrachoroidal cavitation, is an arcuate, subretinal, orange-yellowish lesion, more commonly located under the optic disk **(Figures 1A, 2A and 3A)**.

Freund et al[1] first described it with optical coherence tomography (OCT) as a localized retinal pigment epithelium (RPE) detachment around the optic disk and called it peripapillary detachment in pathologic myopia (PDPM) **(Figures 1E, 2D and 3E)**. Toranzo et al[2] have renamed this abnormality "peripapillary intrachoroidal cavitation".

The incidence in high myopic eyes is about 5%. The finding is often casual, not being associated with any decrease in terms of visual acuity. Nevertheless, visual field defects are detectable in 70% of the eyes, may be related with the passage of nerve fibers through the involved area. Most of the cases are not diagnosed because located inside a large peripapillary atrophic area.

In accordance with the extent around the optic disk or myopic conus, this peripapillary dome-shaped lesion has been classified as:

- Grade 1 (less than a semicircle)
- Grade 2 (more than a semicircle but less than three-fourth of circle)
- Grade 3 (more than three fourths).

At fluorescein angiography (FA), this area shows early hypofluorescence and late staining without dye pooling **(Figures 1B, 2B and 3B)**, whereas at indocyanine green angiography (ICGA), it is hypofluorescent throughout the entire sequence **(Figures 1C, 2C and 3C)**.

En face OCT scans have allowed to visualize the lateral extent of the peripapillary sub-RPE nonreflective area and to measure its thickness. The origin of this sub-RPE hyporeflectivity could be ascribed to the deep excavation of the myopic conus and the consequent impossibility for the retina-RPE to follow this steep fall. They would detach from the choroid and would return to a more normal level, thus creating a space between the retina-RPE and the choroid. *En face* OCT scans show the retinal hole, the posterior detachment and the vascular tractions, that are further manifestations of the ocular stretching taking place in highly myopic eyes **(Box 1)**. *En face* OCT also detects the gravitational enlargement of the intrachoroidal widening.[3-7] Thus, many authors suggest that the passage of vitreous underneath the pigment epithelium could represent a further etiologic factor **(Figures 1D, 2D and 3D)**.[5-7]

Box 1: Intrachoroidal cavitation on *en face* optical coherence tomography

- Nonreflective peripapillary sub-RPE area very similar to indocyanine green angiography image
- Determine the size and grading of the lesion
- Detect anomalous communication from the edge of cavitation and vitreous space
- Show vascular tractions

Conclusion

In conclusion *en face* OCT has allowed to evaluate the thickness and the lateral extent of the peripapillary detachment. Therefore, its use could be important in

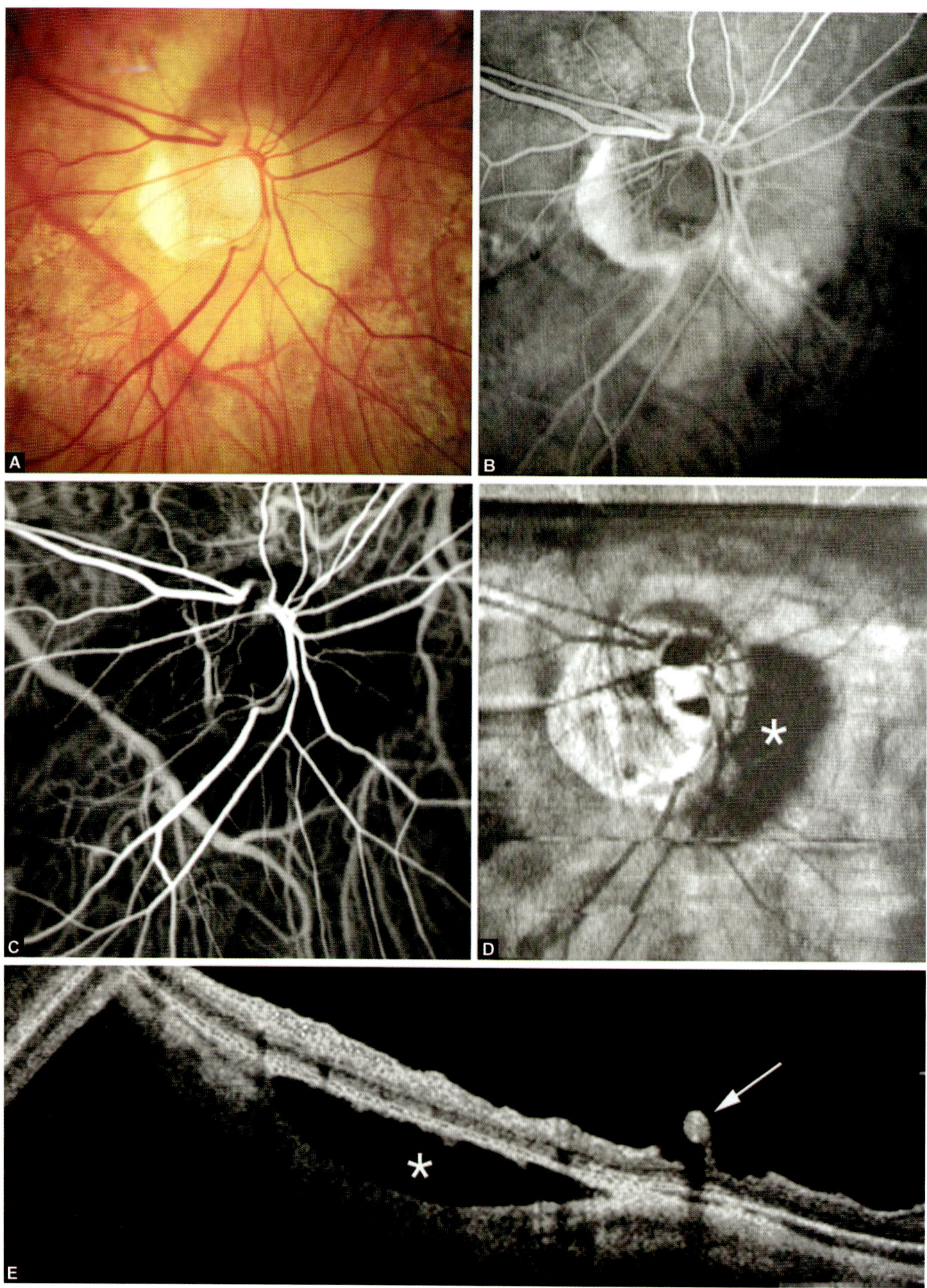

Figures 1A to E: (A) Fundus image of the right eye shows a deep excavation of the myopic conus, with tilting of the optic disk and yellow-orange peripapillary area; (B and C) Fluorescein angiography and indocyanine green angiography show a peripapillary hypofluorescent area; (D and E) *En face* optical coherence tomography and longitudinal B scan show a grade 1 sub-RPE nonreflective area (asterisk) and the vascular tractions (arrow)

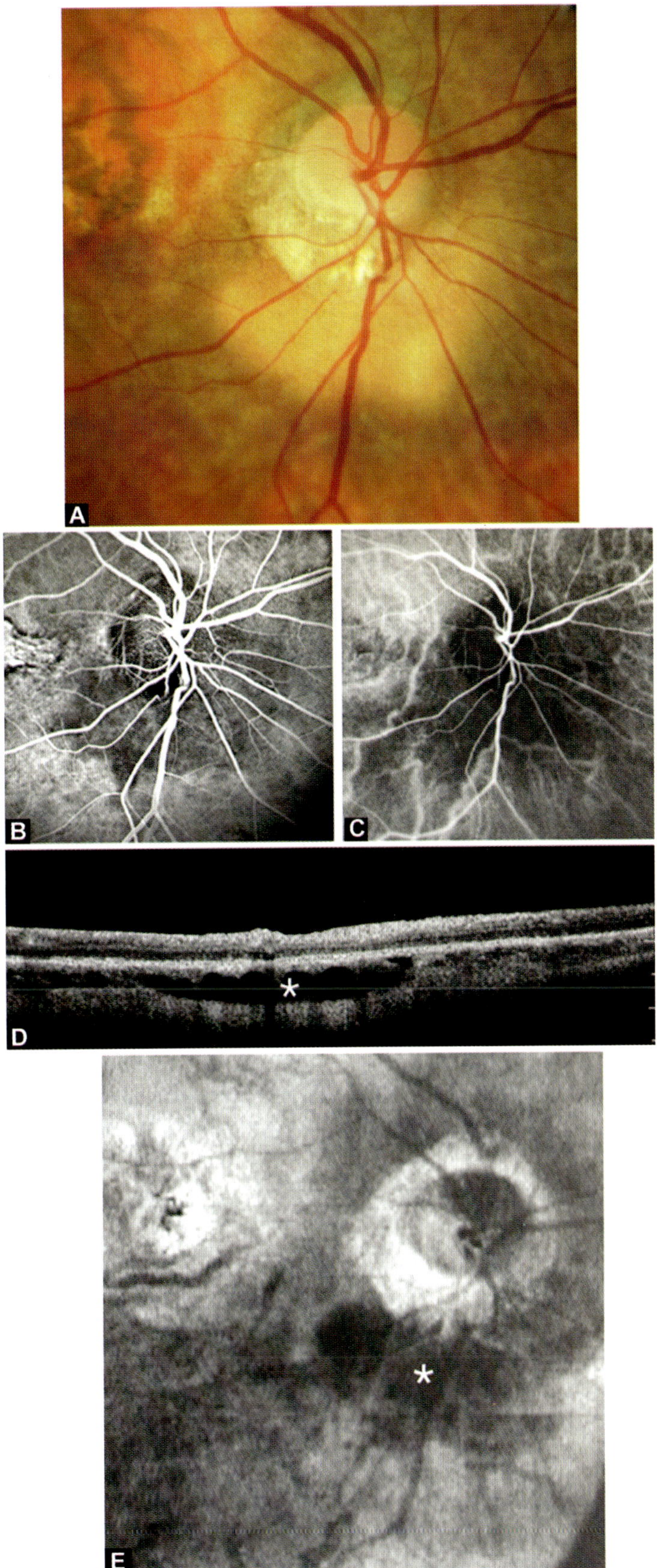

Figures 2A to E: (A to C) Fundus image, fluorescein angiography and indocyanine green angiography show the peripapillary lobulated area; (D and E) *En face* optical coherence tomography and longitudinal B scans show a grade 3 sub-RPE normoreflective area (asterisk)

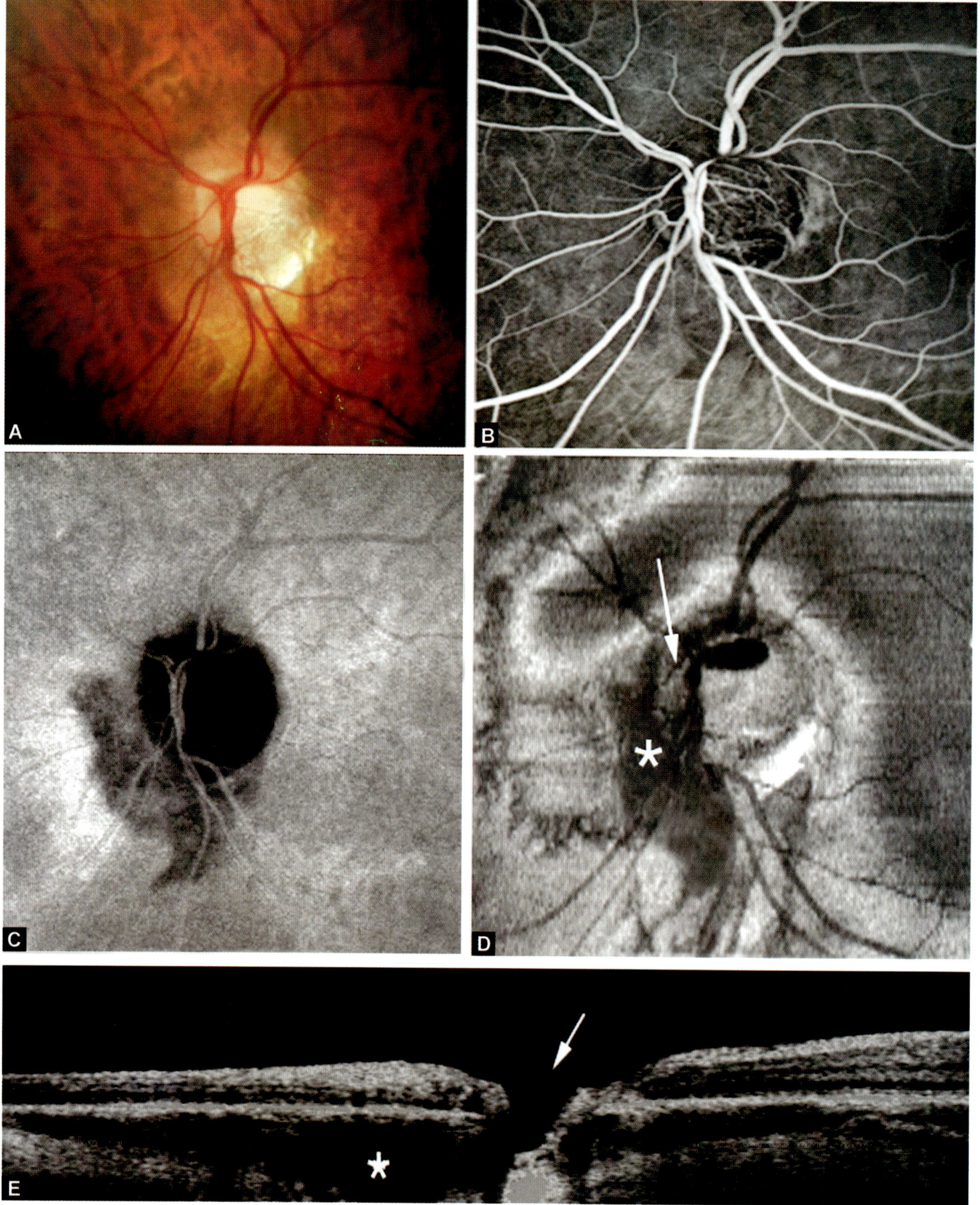

Figures 3A to E: (A) Fundus image shows the peripapillary lobulated area; (B and C) Fluorescein angiography and indocyanine green angiography show a peripapillary hypofluorescent area; (D and E) *En face* optical coherence tomography and longitudinal B scans show a sub-RPE normoreflective area (asterisk) and a full-thickness defect in the retina-RPE layers is detectable at both cross-sectional and coronal scans (arrow)

determining the size and grading of these lesions at the first visit, and to detect minimal changes of width and thickness during follow-up as an alternative to FA.

References

1. Freund KB, Ciardella AP, Yannuzzi LA, et al. Peripapillary detachment in pathologic myopia. Arch Ophthalmol. 2003;121(2):197-204.
2. Toranzo J, Cohen SY, Erginay A, et al. Peripapillary intrachoroidal cavitation in myopia. Am J Ophthalmology. 2005;140(4):731-2.
3. Van Velthoven ME, Verbraak FD, Yannuzzi LA, et al. Imaging the retina by *en face* optical coherence tomography. Retina. 2006;26(2):129-36.
4. Forte R, Pascotto F, Soreca E, et al. Posterior retinal detachment without macular hole in high myopia: visualization with *en face* optical coherence tomography. Eye (Lond). 2007;21(1):111-3.
5. Forte R, Pascotto F, Cennamo G, et al. Evaluation of peripapillary detachment in pathologic myopia with *en face* optical coherence tomography. Eye (Lond). 2008; 22(1):158-61.
6. Forte R, Cennamo G, Pascotto F, et al. *En face* optical coherence tomography of the posterior pole in high myopia. Am J Ophthalmol. 2008;145(2):281-8.
7. Shimada N, Ohno-Matsui K, Yoshida T, et al. Characteristics of peripapillary detachment in pathologic myopia. Arch Ophthalmol. 2006;124(1):46-52.

chapter 41

En Face Optical Coherence Tomography of Choroidal Nevi and Melanomas

Gilda Cennamo

Introduction

Choroidal nevi are the most common intraocular tumors.[1] Population studies reveal that these tumors are more prevalent in Caucasians (6.5%) than in Asians (1.4%).[1] Nevi are typically pigmented (**Figures 1A, 3A and 6A**). They have smooth margins and overlying drusen, and measure less than 5 mm in basal diameter and 3 mm in thickness. Usually, they do not cause visual symptoms and, more importantly, they are generally benign. Factors predictive of nevus transformation into melanoma are thickness greater than 3 mm, the presence of subretinal fluid, orange pigment, juxtapapillary location and symptoms of blurred vision or photopsia (**Figures 6A to E**). The presence of any one of these factors confers a relative risk of 1.9, three factors a relative risk of 7.4 and the presence of all five confers a relative risk of 27.1.[1,2]

Uveal melanoma is the most common primary intraocular malignancy and 90% develop in the choroid. Most choroidal melanomas can be differentiated from nevi because melanomas are much larger. They often present as a pigment and subretinal fluid (**Figures 4, 5 and 7**). Subretinal fluid associated with melanoma shifts with positioning and may cause intermittent blurred vision or flashes (**Figure 5D**).[1,2]

Fourier-domain optical coherence tomography (FD-OCT) provides information about the effects of choroidal nevus and melanoma on the retinal architecture, which include retinal edema, subretinal fluid, retinal atrophy, photoreceptor loss, outer retinal thinning, and retinal pigment epithelial detachment.[3-7]

At FD-OCT examination, choroidal nevi appear as a highly reflective band within the choriocapillaris layer with posterior shadowing (**Figures 1D, 2D, 3C and 6E**), whereas choroidal melanomas show a highly reflective band in the anterior choroid with lack of visibility of both the choroidal vessels and the inner sclera (**Figures 4D, 5D and 7D**).[3]

Thus far, there are no reports about the use of *en face* OCT to investigate choroidal nevi or melanoma.

In their department, the authors are studying choroidal nevi and melanoma with *en face* OCT. In fact, *en face* scan OCT is able to localize very small nevi and to detect structural and morphologic details. *En face* OCT imaging of choroidal nevi shows a well demarcated, flat, sub-RPE hyporeflectivity area. This area is predominantly circular, and the wall aspect is frequently uniform due to hyperpigmentation of the lesion (**Figures 1C, 2B, 3B and 6D**). Differently, *en face* OCT of choroidal melanomas show a sub-RPE highly reflective area. The shape of this area is predominantly circular but the wall aspect is slightly irregular perhaps due to vascular tissue inside the tumor (**Figures 4D, 5F and 7C**).

In conclusion, *en face* OCT of choroidal nevi and melanomas could be used to visualize and determine the tumor area, and represents an alternative to echographic examination to detect minimal morphologic changes during follow-up.

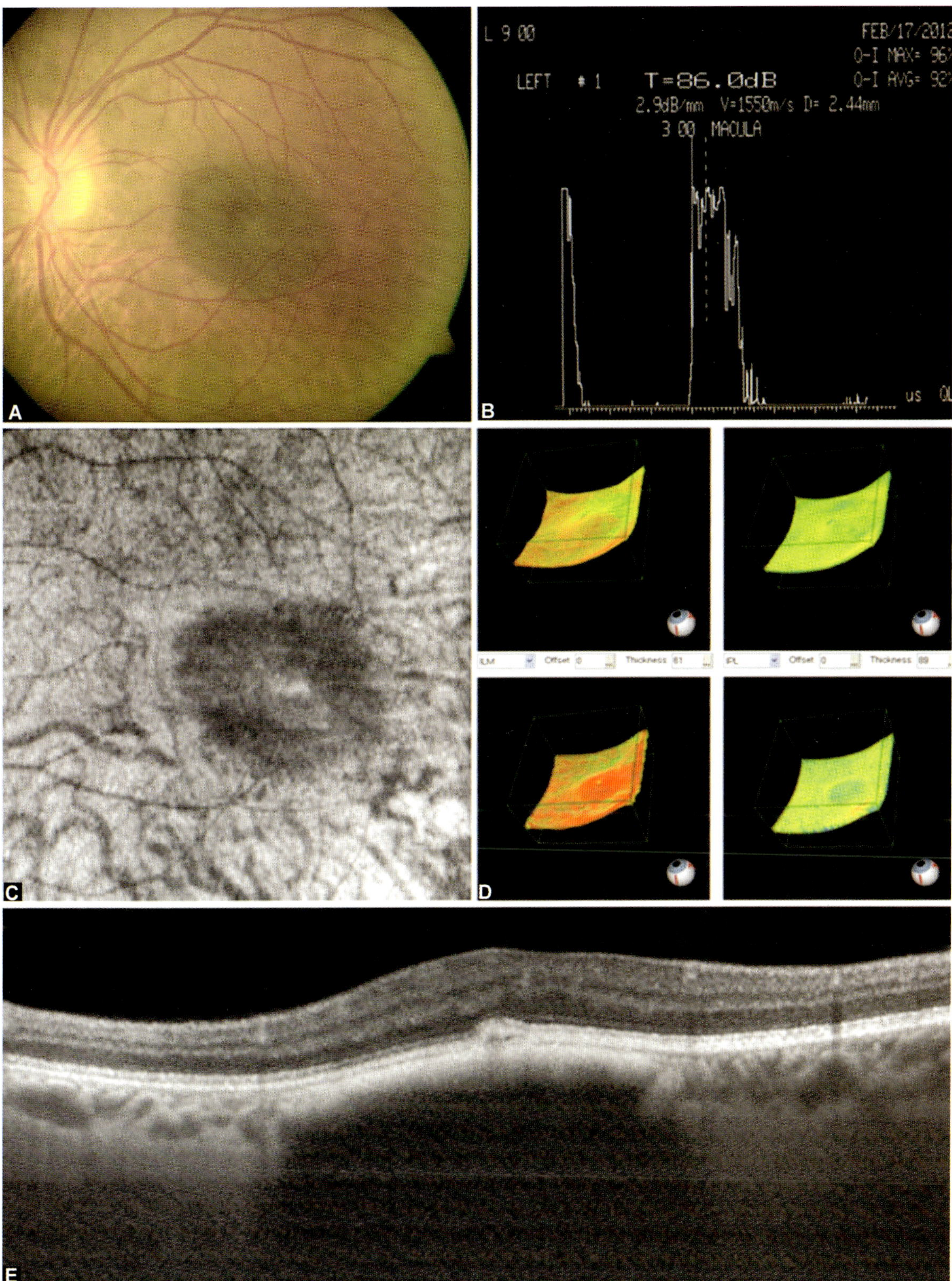

Figures 1A to E: Choroidal nevus (A) Color fundus image showing a flat and well-demarcated melanocytic nevus; (B) A standardized echographic scan showing high reflectivity of the lesion; (C) *En face* optical coherence tomography image showing a well demarcated hyporeflectivity area; (D) Three-dimensional Fourier-domain optical coherence tomography shows a flat choroidal lesion; (E) Fourier-domain optical coherence tomography. The lesion is distinguished from the surrounding normal choroid as highly reflective band with posterior shadowing. A thin hyporeflective line separates the retinal pigment epithelium and the anterior tumor surface

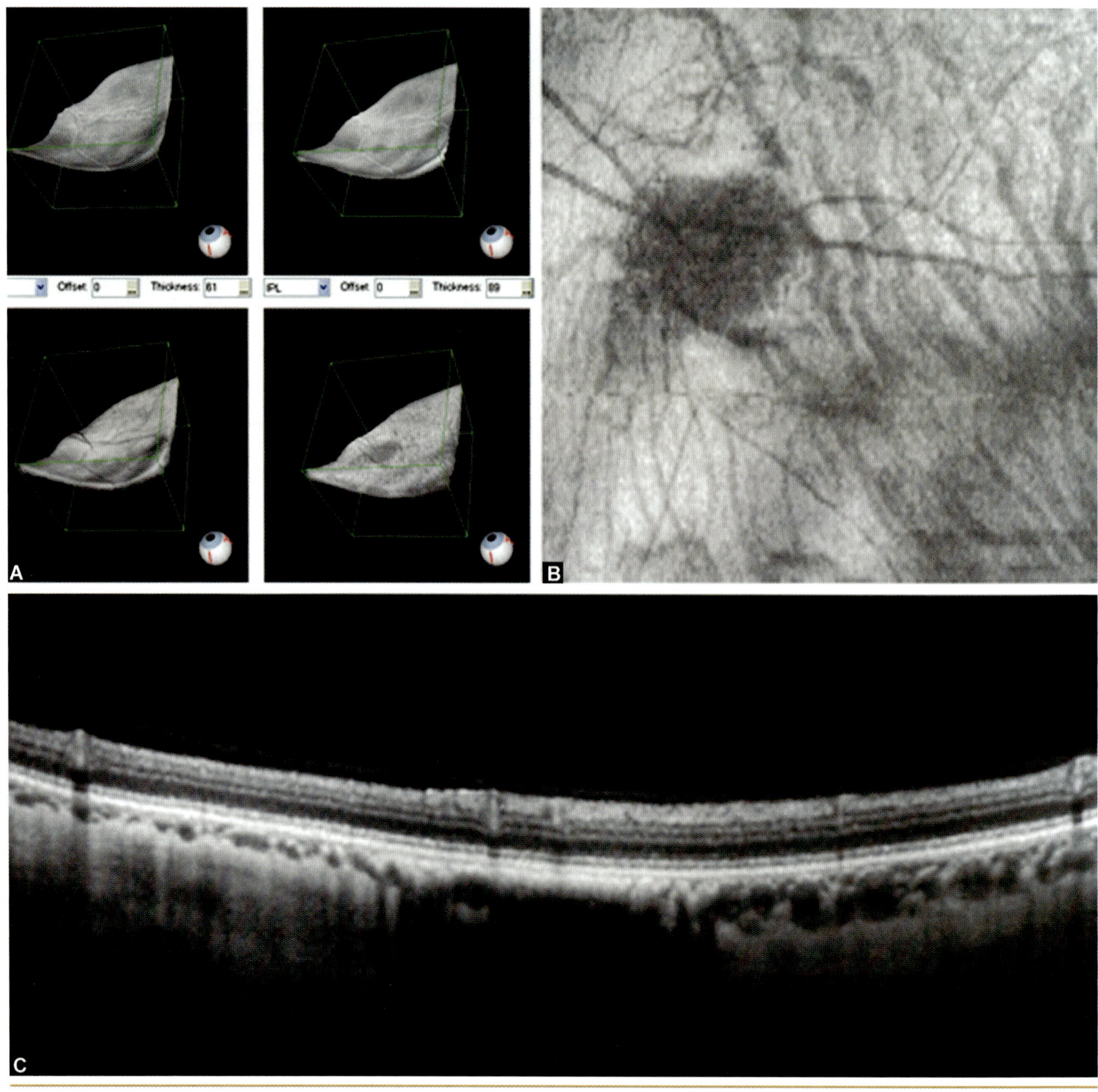

Figures 2A to C: Choroidal nevus. (A) Three-dimensional Fourier-domain optical coherence tomography of the lesion; (B) *En face* optical coherence tomography shows a flat hyporeflectivity area; (C) Fourier-domain optical coherence tomography image: note the loss of choriocapillaris over the lesion

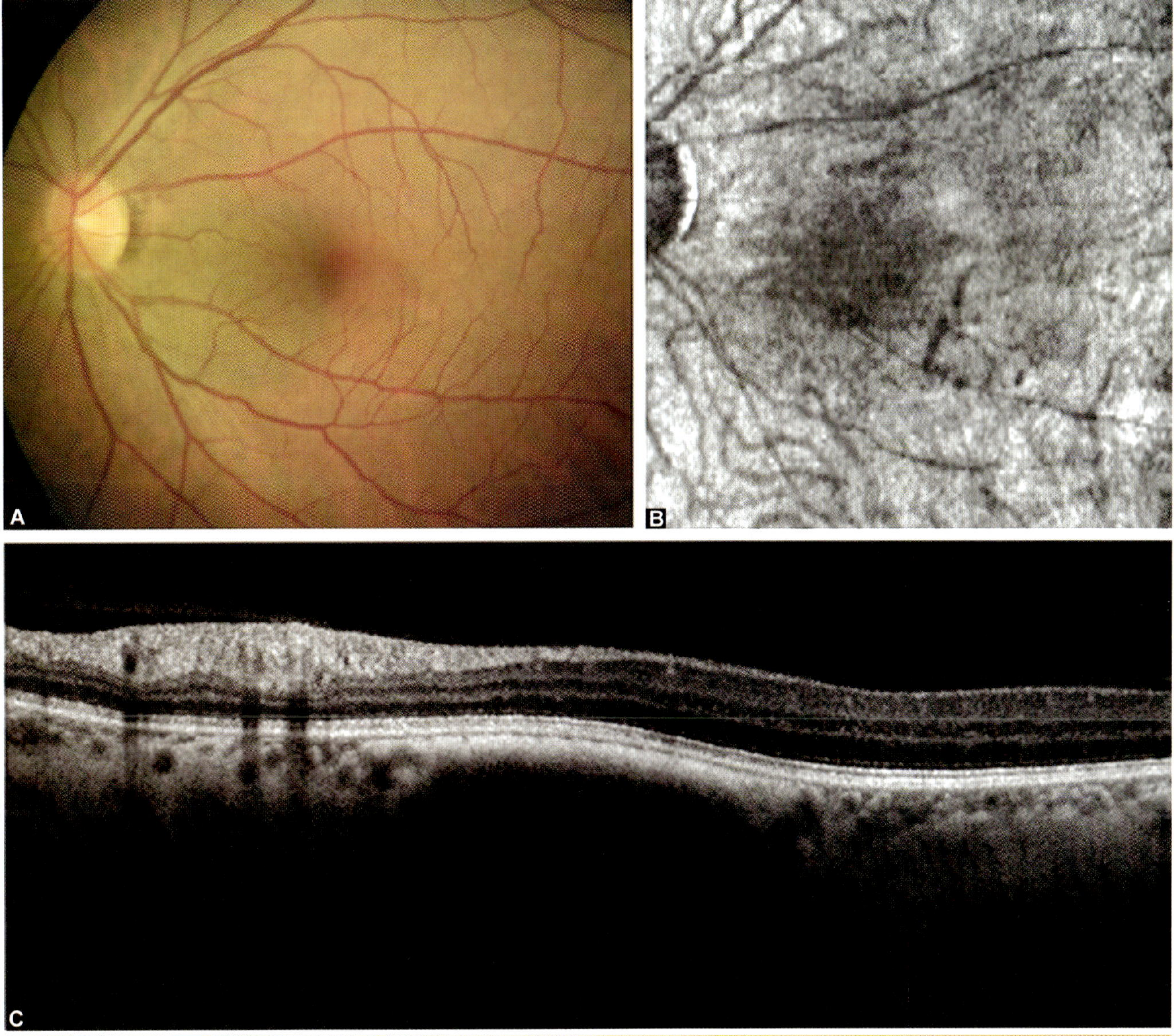

Figures 3A to C: Choroidal nevus. (A) Color fundus photograph showing a pigmented choroidal nevus; (B) *En face* optical coherence tomography showing a hyporeflective lesion; (C) The lesion appears as a sharply highly reflective band at the Bruch's/retinal pigment epithelium/choriocapillaris layer and posterior shadowing

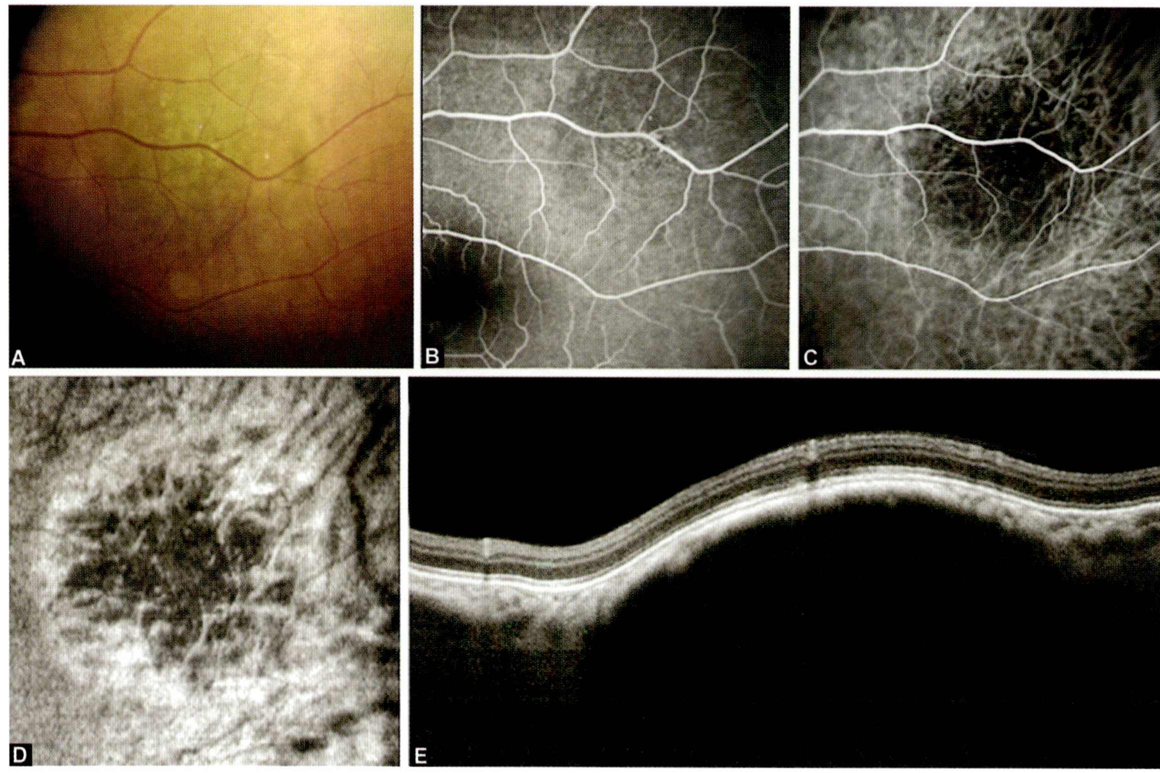

Figures 4A to E: Choroidal melanoma. (A) Color fundus photograph showing a mildly elevated and pigmented choroidal lesion; (B and C) At fluorescein angiography and indocyanine green angiography, this area shows light hyperfluorescence; (D) *En face* optical coherence tomography showing a hypo-/hyper-reflective area due to vascular tissue; (E) Fourier-domain optical coherence tomography shows elevation of the retina-choroid complex and thinning of choriocapillaris

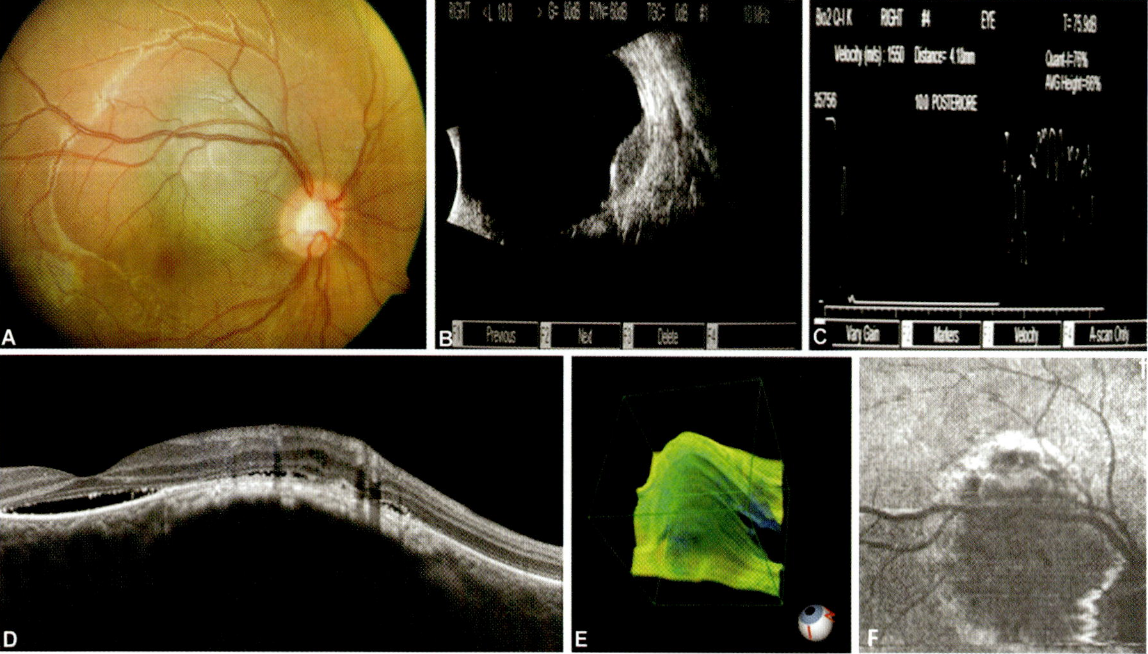

Figures 5A to F: Choroidal melanoma. (A) Color fundus photograph showing a choroidal melanocytic tumor; (B) B scan ultrasound shows a slightly irregular dome shaped mass; (C) An A scan standardized echography shows a medium-low reflectivity of the lesion; (D) Fourier-domain optical coherence tomography clearly demonstrates subretinal fluid in foveal region; overlying the dome-shaped elevation of the choroid is a thickened irregular RPE and thickening of the outer retinal layers; (E) Three-dimensional Fourier-domain optical coherence tomography shows an elevation of retina/choroid complex; (F) *En face* optical coherence tomography shows a hyporeflective area with irregular and hyper-reflective edge

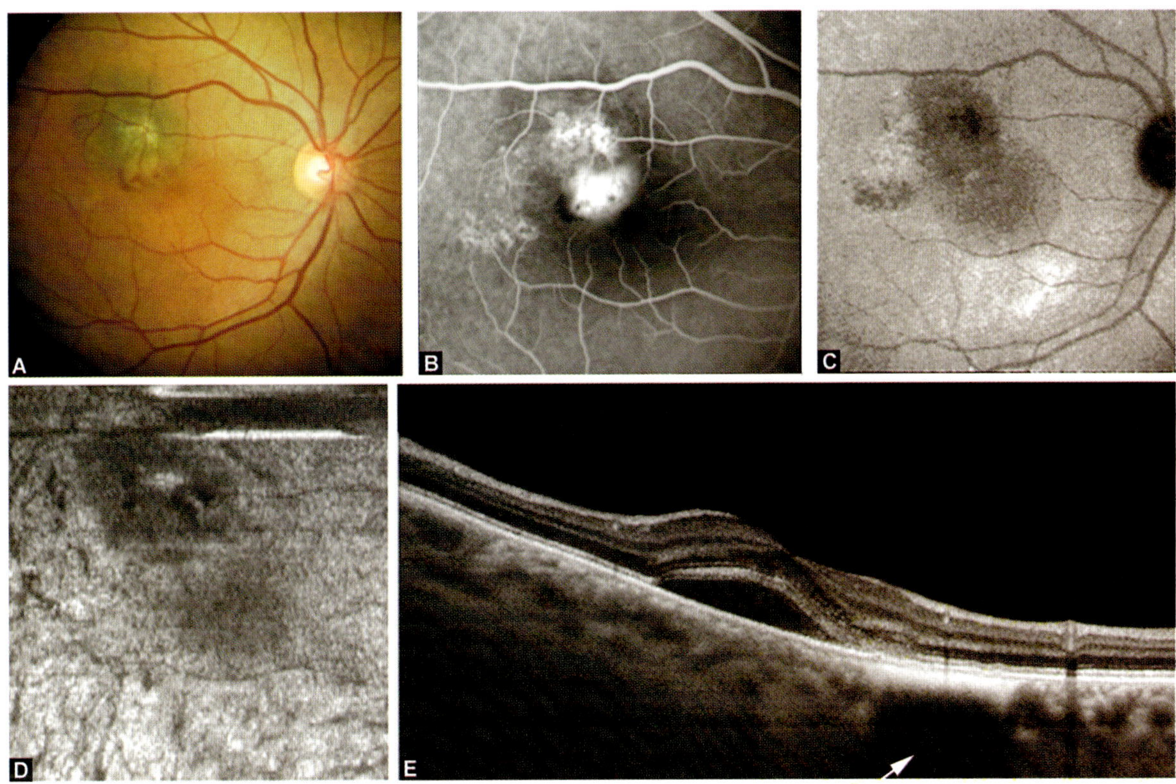

Figures 6A to E: Choroidal nevus with choroidal neovascularization. (A) Fundus photograph shows choroidal nevus with exudative retinal detachment; (B and C) Fluorescein angiography and indocyanine green angiography show choroidal nevus with choroidal neovascularization; (D) *En face* optical coherence tomography shows a hyporeflective area; (E) Fourier-domain optical coherence tomography shows a highly reflective band with posterior shadowing (arrow) and foveal detachment

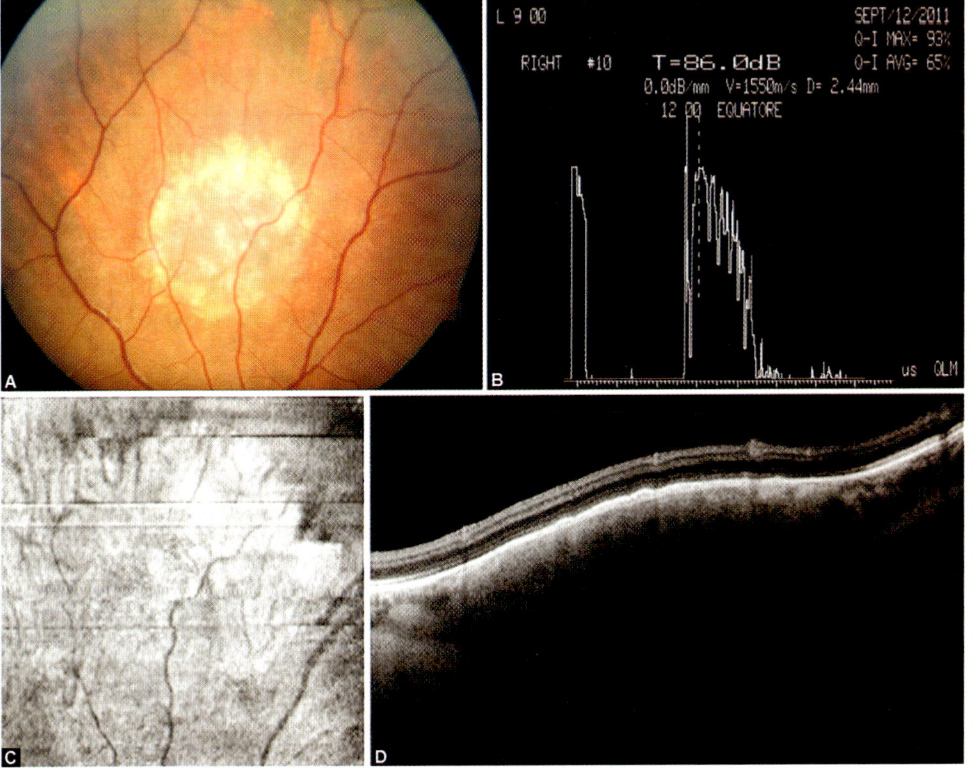

Figures 7A to D: Choroidal melanoma. (A) Pigmented, elevated choroidal mass with associated orange pigment; (B) A scan standardized echography shows low internal reflectivity of the lesion; (C) *En face* optical coherence tomography shows a hyper-reflective area. (D) Fourier-domain optical coherence tomography shows a middle elevation of choroid/retina complex. Note the medium reflective choroidal band and some vessels under retinal pigment epithelium layer in the tumor area

References

1. Say EA, Shah SU, Ferenczy S, et al. Optical coherence tomography of retinal and choroidal tumors. J Ophthalmol. 2011;2011:385058. Epub 2011 Jul 18.
2. Torres VL, Brugnoni N, Kaiser PK, et al. Optical coherence tomography enhanced depth imaging of choroidal tumors. Am J Ophthalmol. 2011;151(4):586-93.e2. Epub 2011 Jan 22.
3. Shields CL, Materin MA, Shields JA. Review of optical coherence tomography for intraocular tumors. Curr Opin Ophthalmol. 2005;16(3):141-54.
4. Muscat S, Parks S, Kemp E, et al. Secondary retinal changes associated with choroidal naevi and melanomas documented by optical coherence tomography. Br J Ophthalmol. 2004;88(1):120-4.
5. Shah SU, Kaliki S, Shields CL, et al. Enhanced depth imaging optical coherence tomography of choroidal nevus in 104 cases. Ophthalmology. 2012;119(5):1066-72. Epub 2012 Jan 31.
6. Sayanagi K, Pelayes DE, Kaiser PK, et al. 3D Spectral domain optical coherence tomography findings in choroidal tumors. Eur J Ophthalmol. 2011;21(3):271-5.
7. Singh AD, Belfort RN, Sayanagi K, et al. Fourier domain optical coherence tomographic and auto-fluorescence findings in indeterminate choroidal melanocytic lesions. Br J Ophthalmol. 2010;94(4):474-8.

Section 11

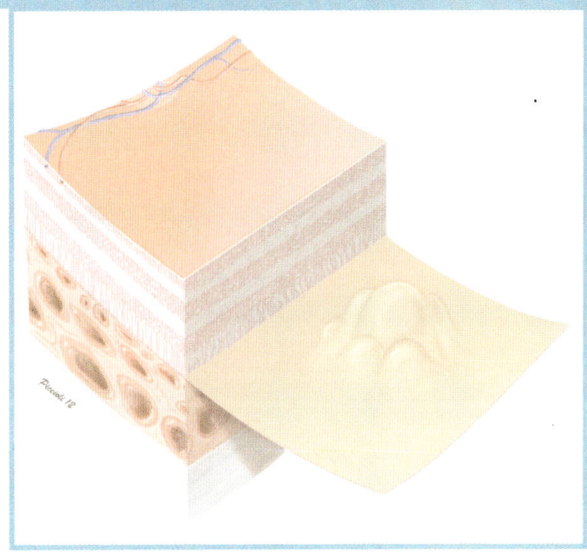

Glaucoma and
Optic Nerve

Inner Nuclear Layer Cystic Degeneration, in the Macular Area of Glaucomatous Patients, on *En Face* and B Scan Optical Coherence Tomography

Adil El Maftouhi, Michel Puech, Maddalena Quaranta-El Maftouhi

Introduction

The measurement of the perifoveal ganglion cell layer (GCL) has recently emerged as a new diagnostic parameter in detecting early structural damage in glaucoma. Indeed, glaucomatous damage occurs in retinal ganglion cells (RGCs) and their axons, leading to the characteristic changes in the structure of the optic disk.[1] The structural loss of RGCs often precedes, at a preperimetric stage, functional glaucomatous visual field defects.

The ganglion cell complex is defined as the three innermost retina layers: the retinal nerve fiber layer (RNFL), the GCL and the inner plexiform layer.[2] Glaucoma preferentially affects these inner layers rather than the whole retinal layers in the macular area because they contain axons, cell bodies and dendrites of ganglion cells (**Figure 1**).

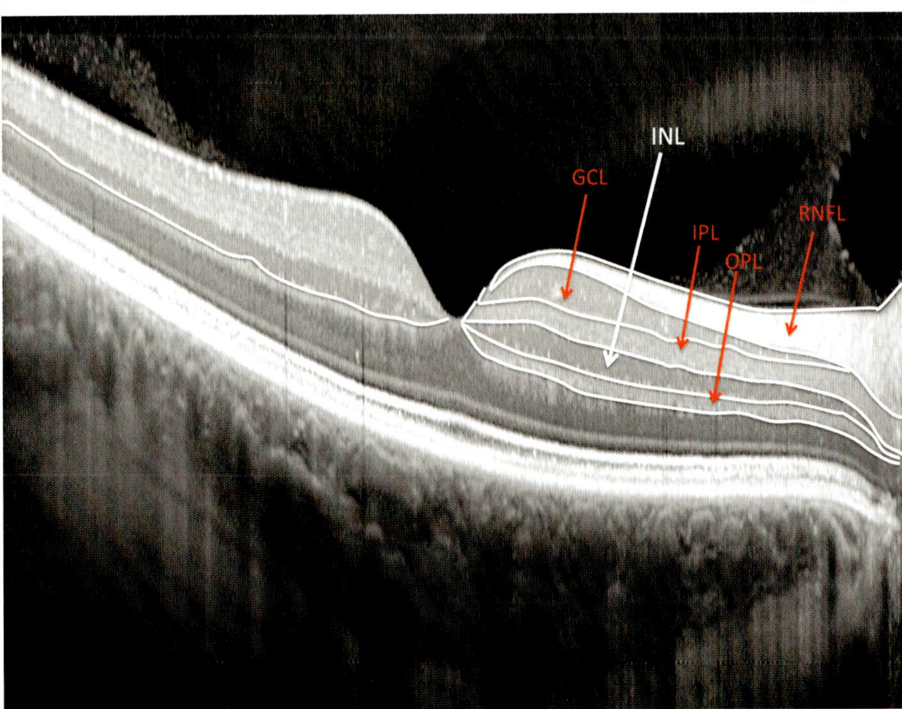

Figure 1: Optical coherence tomography B scan of a normal retina depicting good quality segmentation. Inner nuclear layer (INL) is mildly reflective. (CGL: Ganglion cell layer; IPL: Inner plexiform layer; OPL: Outer plexiform layer; RNFL: Retinol nerve fiber layer)

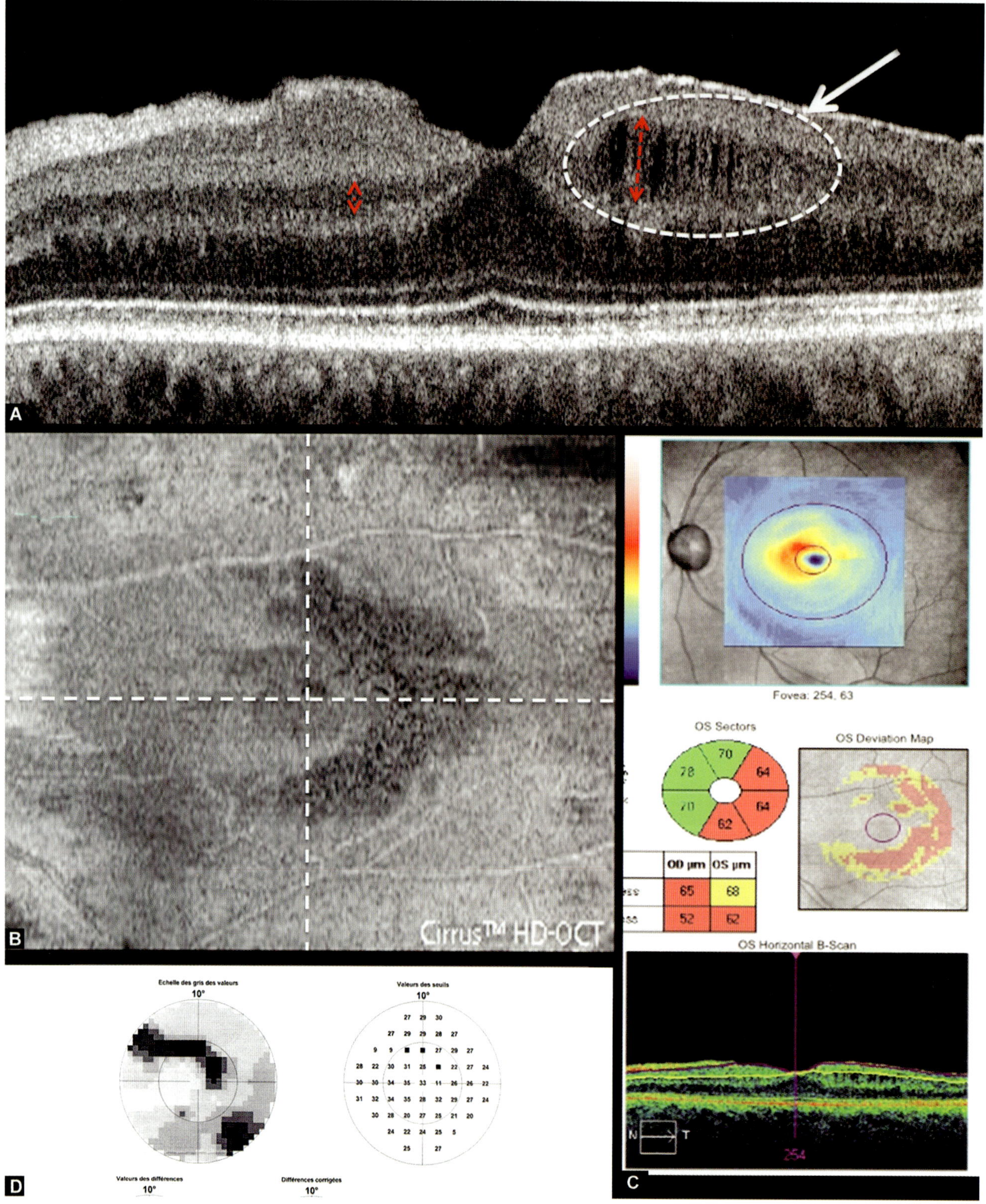

Figures 2A to D: (A) Optical coherence tomography B scan (CIRRUS, Carl Zeiss Meditec) of the retina of a glaucomatous eye shows spindle-shaped cysts in the macular inner nuclear layer (INL). The temporal part of the INL, where the cystic changes are (dotted circle) shown, appears thickened when compared with the nasal part; (B) C scan image shows the topography of the inner retinal cystic degeneration that appears as a temporal shady zone; (C) Ganglion cells analysis demonstrates the thinning of ganglion cell complex layers predominantly in the temporal area as compared with the normal age-matched database; (D) Central visual defect corresponding to the cystic area

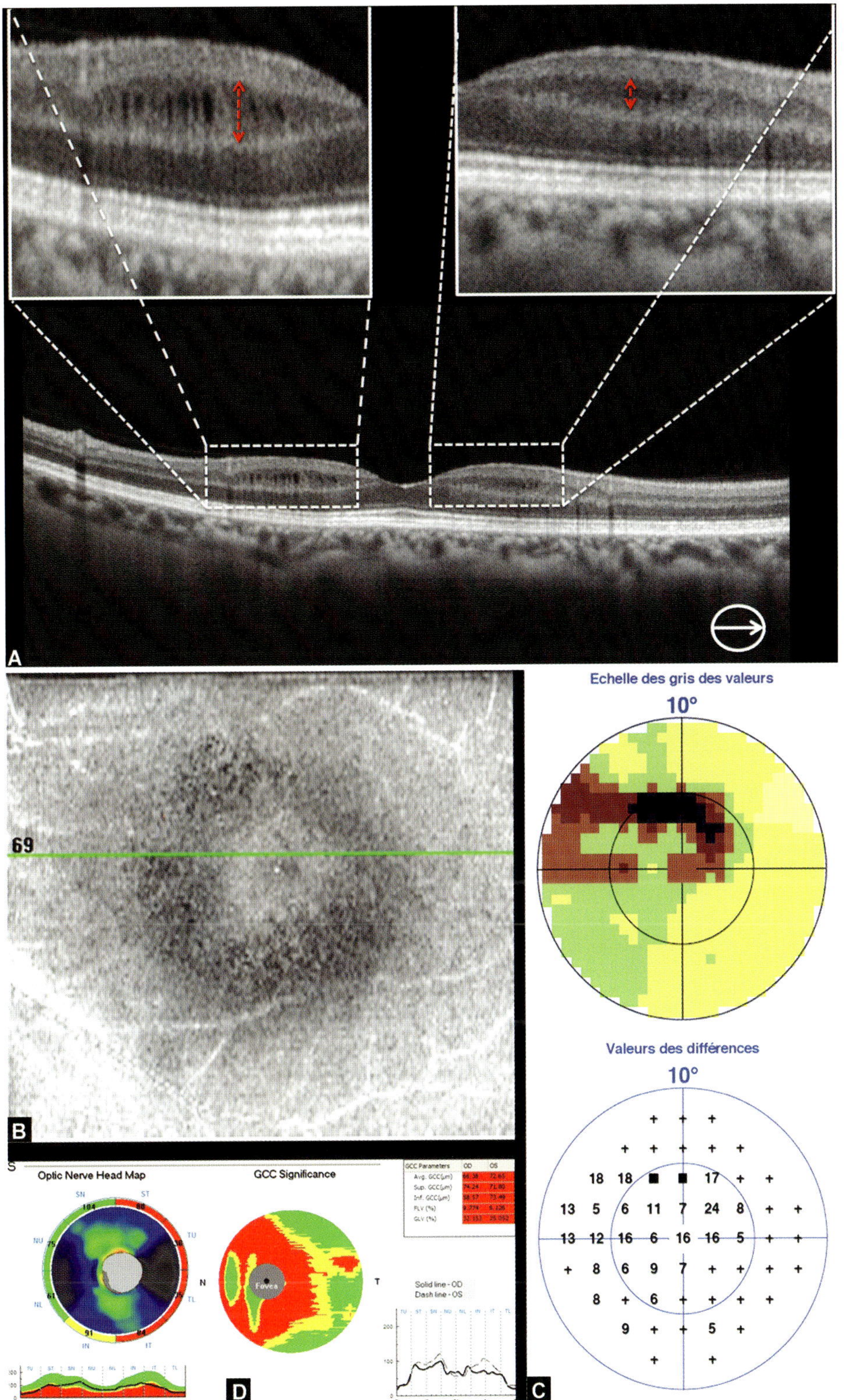

Figures 3A to D: (A) Optical coherence tomography B scan (RTVUE, Optovue, Inc, Fremont CA) of a glaucomatous patient with cystic degeneration of the inner nuclear layer (INL). Thickness of the INL seems to be proportional to the size of cysts and appears more pronounced temporal to the fovea; (B) C scan topography of the INL presents a shady appearance of the INL, more evident in the inferior part of the macula; (C) This feature corresponds to a defect in the superior part of the central visual field; (D) Ganglion cells complex (GCC) analysis shows a decrease in thickness of the GCC complex. This is associated with retinal nerve fiber layer thinning that is more pronounced in the temporal and especially in the inferotemporal region

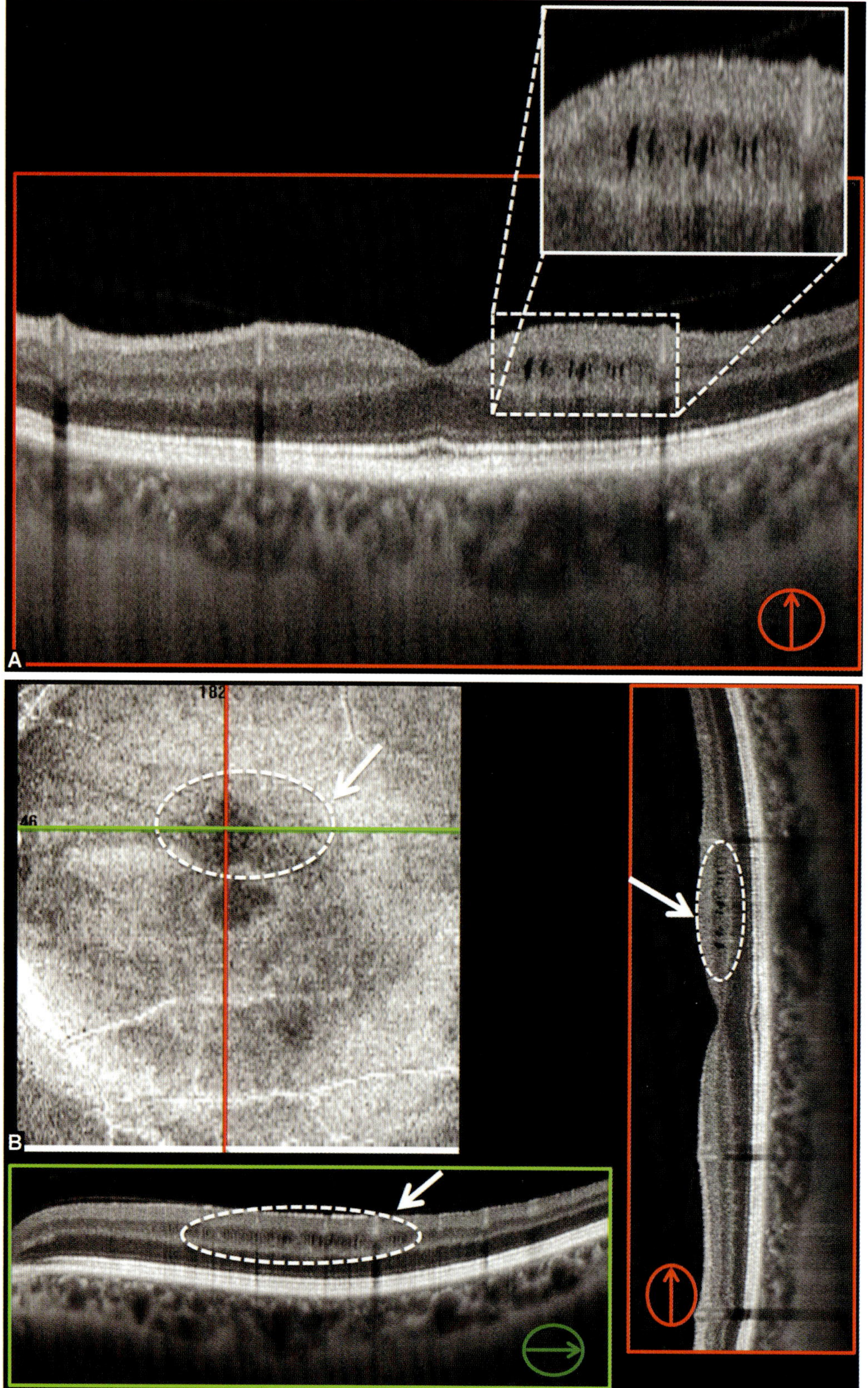

Figures 4A and B: (A) Optical coherence tomography B scan (RTVUE, Optovue, Inc) showing cystic appearance of the inner nuclear layer (INL) in the superior part of the fovea in a glaucoma patient. Note the spindle shape of the cysts; (B) C scan of the INL precisely displays the topography and distribution of cystic changes

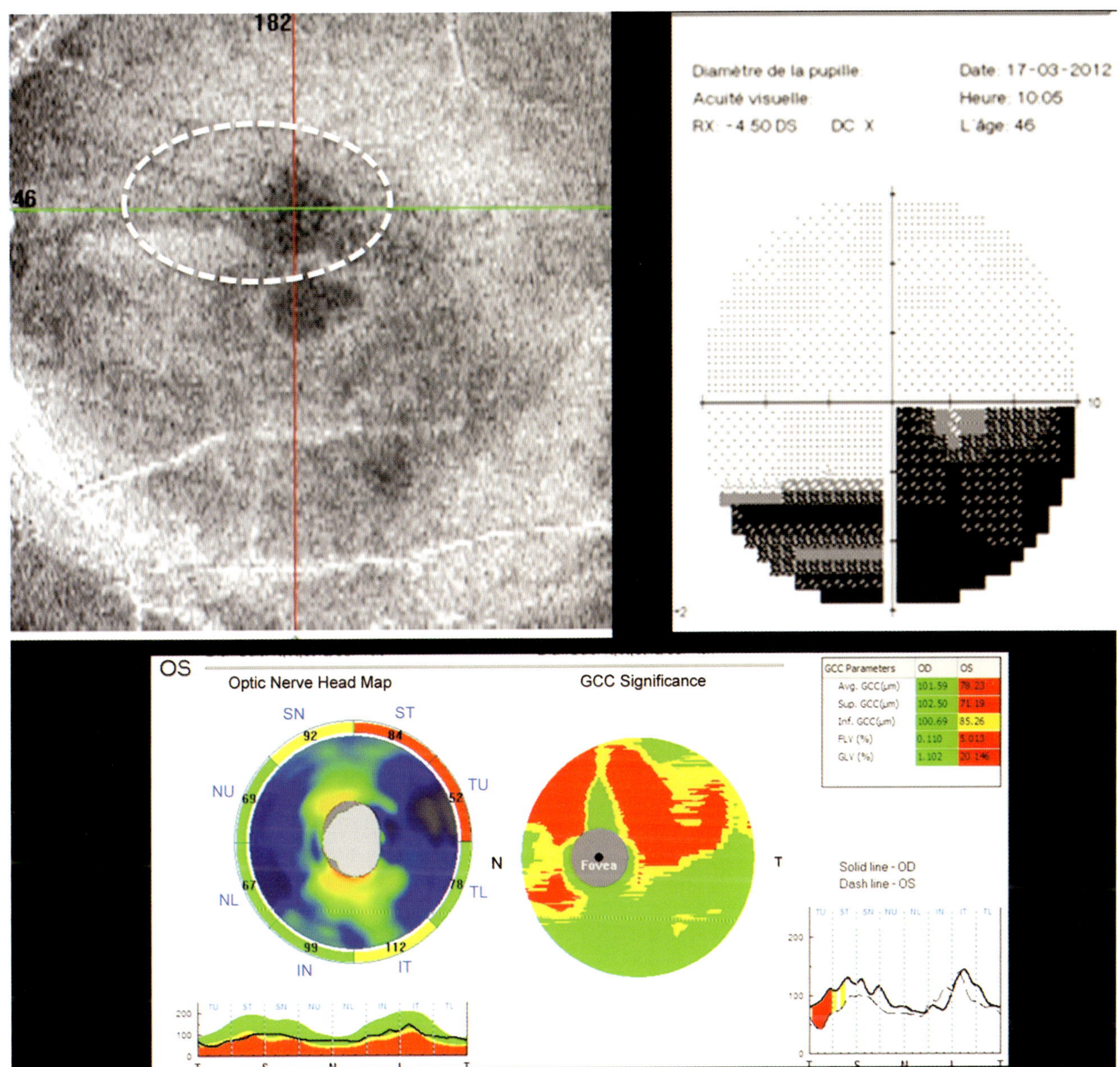

Figure 4C: Ganglion cells complex (GCC) analysis shows thinning of the GCC, superior to the macula. This zone exactly corresponds to the location of the cystic changes of the INL and to the visual field defect

High-resolution spectral domain optical coherence tomography (SD-OCT) enhances visualization and improves segmentation of the retinal layers, providing a higher degree of accuracy in the identification of subtle changes. In glaucomatous patients, the authors recently described a microcystic appearance of the macular inner nuclear layer (INL) on SD-OCT (**Figure 2A**). This change was observed during retrospective analysis of the SD-OCT scans that are routinely performed in their clinic to assess the GCL complex and RNFL in glaucomatous patients.

On *en face* OCT scans, focused on the INL, the authors observed several punctuate microcystic defects in the perifoveal area, depicting a shady zone. Central visual field defects were always present and correlated with the location of the cysts.[3] Analyzing the B scans of this region, we found microcystic changes in the macular INL. Inner nuclear layer was visibly thickened. The microcysts were spindle-shaped, with the major axis perpendicular to retinal surface. Their size was proportional to INL thickness. The GCL and RNFL were always thinned. This OCT finding seems to be related to intraretinal degeneration at the level of INL, in relation with GCL thinning (**Figures 2 to 4**).

In human and experimental glaucoma models, histological evidence supports neuronal loss in the other layers of the retina outside the retinal GCL, including the loss of horizontal cells, amacrine cells and the associated thinning of the INL.[4,5] Hollander et al. demonstrated, after optic nerve axotomy, that pathological changes were restricted to the innermost layers of the retina, especially INL thinning.[6,7] However, Sriram et al. demonstrated no significant INL thinning despite severe RGC loss.[8] Their data could be due to a lack of accuracy in the segmentation of retinal layers. In fact, the segmentation software algorithm could not precisely recognize modified or degenerated retinal layers. The inaccuracy of SD-OCT technology, used by various companies, in measuring GCL loss shows how difficult it is to provide precise retinal segmentation.

Using multiphoton confocal microscopy, Yuan Lei described neural loss in the INL and outer nuclear layer (ONL).[9] In their patients, the authors could not find any structural changes in the ONL using OCT scanning. If GCL and RNFL changes are well known, this case report is the first describing B scan and *en face* OCT, INL modifications in glaucomatous patients using SD-OCT.

The INL includes not only the nuclei of bipolar cells, but also horizontal cells, amacrine cells, interplexiform cells and supportive Müller cells. On OCT B scans, the INL appeared to be thickened due to the presence of the cystic abnormalities (**Figure 3A**). This sort of "degenerative swelling" could precede the atrophic changes and INL thinning.

The loss of GCL could initiate a cascade of transneuronal degeneration, and intraretinal cystic alterations in the INL could be the result of trans-synaptic retinal degenerative processes as the GCL extends. The described OCT finding would be in favor of this hypothesis and would be initiated by ganglion cells loss.[10]

This is the first *in vivo* report of degenerative cystic processes in the INL in glaucomatous patients. This new OCT finding in glaucoma could be related to the severity of optic neuropathy and must be differentiated from any other form of cystic appearance or edema.

The superficial analysis of automatic software images of GCL and RNFL are insufficient to disclose the cystic

changes of the INL and points out, once more, the importance of thoroughly examining each single B scan and *en face* OCT for a better understanding of each pathologic process. An accurate and comprehensive study of the clinical characteristics of the patients presenting with cystic degeneration of the INL, as well as experiments using animal models of trans-synaptic degeneration are required to better understand this new SD-OCT finding.

References

1. Zeimer R, Asrani S, Zou S, et al. Quantitative detection of glaucomatous damage at the posterior pole by retinal thickness mapping. A pilot study. Ophthalmology. 1998;105(2):224-31.
2. Kim NR, Lee ES, Seong GJ, et al. Structure-function relationship and diagnostic value of macular ganglion cell complex measurement using Fourier-domain OCT in glaucoma. Invest Ophthalmol Vis Sci. 2010;51(9):4646-51.
3. Holländer H, Bisti S, Maffei L, et al. Electroretinographic responses and retrograde changes of retinal morphology after intracranial optic nerve section. A quantitative analysis in the cat. Exp Brain Res. 1984;55(3):483-93.
4. Guo L, Normando EM, Nizari S, et al. Tracking longitudinal retinal changes in experimental ocular hypertension using the cSLO and spectral domain-OCT. Invest Ophthalmol Vis Sci. 2010;51(12):6504-13.
5. Sriram P, Graham SL, Wang C, et al. Trans-synaptic retinal degeneration in optic neuropathies: optical coherence tomography study. Invest Ophthalmol Vis Sci. 2012;53(3): 1271-5.
6. Lei Y, Garrahan N, Hermann B, et al. Quantification of retinal transneuronal degeneration in human glaucoma: a novel multiphoton-DAPI approach. Invest Ophthalmol Vis Sci. 2008;49(5):1940-5.
7. Cho JW, Sung KR, Lee S, et al. Relationship between visual field sensitivity and macular ganglion cell complex thickness as measured by spectral-domain optical coherence tomography. Invest Ophthalmol Vis Sci. 2010; 51(12):6401-7.
8. Holcombe DJ, Lengefeld N, Gole GA, et al. Selective inner retinal dysfunction precedes ganglion cell loss in a mouse glaucoma model. Br J Ophthalmol. 2008;92(5):683-8.
9. Gunn DJ, Gole GA, Barnett NL. Specific amacrine cell changes in an induced mouse model of glaucoma. Clin Experiment Ophthalmol. 2011;39(6):555-63.
10. Lebrun-Julien Frederic, Di Polo A. Le rôle des cellules de Müller dans la mort des cellules ganglionnaire par des mécanismes cellulaires non-autonomes. Thèse de pathologie et biologie cellulaires. 2010.

PART III

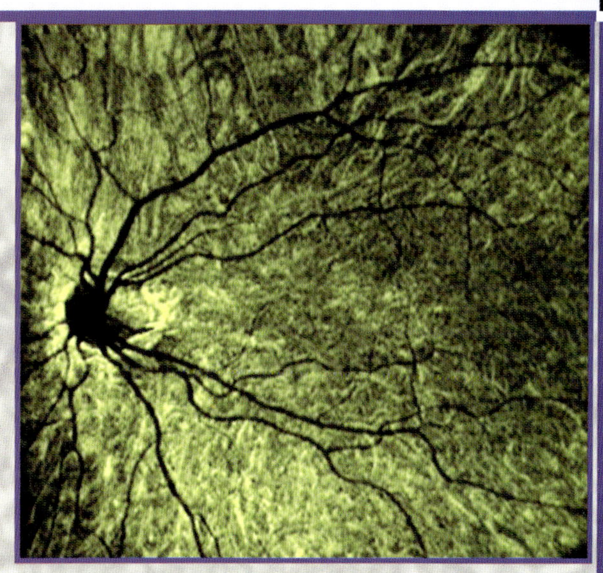

CLINICAL *EN FACE* OCT
FUTURE DEVELOPMENTS

Section 12

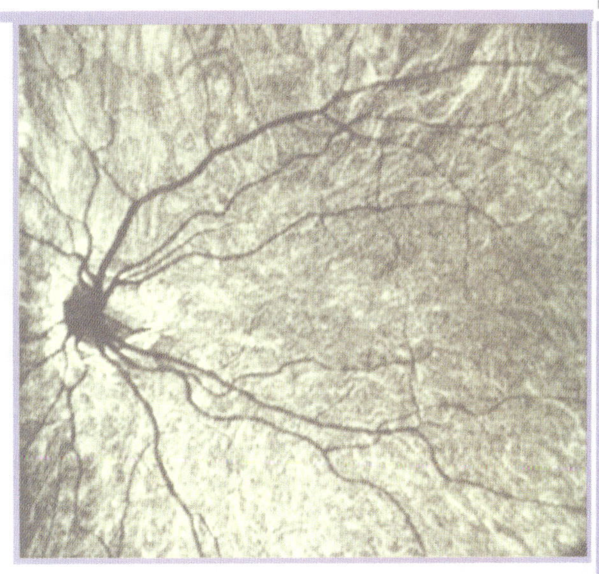

Future Developments in *En Face* Optical Coherence Tomography

En Face Angiography of the Retinal, Choroidal and Optic Nerve Head Circulation with Ultrahigh-Speed Optical Coherence Tomography

Yali Jia, David Huang, James G Fujimoto, Joachim Hornegger, Martin F Kraus

Introduction

Examination of ocular circulation is important for the assessment of eye diseases. Diabetic retinopathy,[1] age-related macular degeneration,[2] and glaucoma[3] are leading causes of blindness that are all associated with impaired circulation. For understanding and diagnosing these typical eye diseases, label-free, three-dimensional (3D) imaging of the retinal, choroidal, and optic nerve head (ONH) circulation would be very helpful.

At present, the most widely used technique for examining ocular circulation abnormalities is fundus fluorescein angiography (FA) in which intravenously injected dye is detected. This is an invasive procedure, and the dye injection has potential side effects, such as nausea and anaphylaxis. Additionally, FA cannot distinguish choroidal vessels from retinal vessels or detect the lamina cribrosa perfusion deep inside the ONH. Other existing noninvasive imaging techniques, such as scanning laser Doppler flowmetry and scanning laser speckle flowmetry are also limited to 2D imaging of the superficial perfusion.[3]

We have developed a new 3D angiography method using ultrahigh-speed optical coherence tomography (OCT). The algorithm is called split-spectrum amplitude-decorrelation angiography (SSADA). By splitting the full OCT spectrum into several narrower bands, SSADA reduces OCT axial resolution and consequently reduces its susceptibility to axial motion noise. These changes result in improved detection of the flow signal, which in the ocular fundus is predominantly in the transverse dimension. With a ~3 second scan using our 100 kHz swept-source OCT prototype, SSADA provides a high-quality 3 × 3 × 3 mm 3D angiogram. By selecting the maximum value along the axial (Z) direction or by slicing the angiographic volume at each layer, 3D OCT angiography can produce different types of *en face* X-Y projection angiograms for retinal, choroidal, and ONH circulation. In the following sections, the system and theory of OCT angiography and its performance will be demonstrated.

Optical Coherence Tomography Angiography

System Setup

Our OCT angiography studies use an ultrahigh-speed swept-source OCT system recently developed by a group at the Massachusetts Institute of Technology[4] for 3D *in vivo* imaging of the human eye. To enhance the choroidal penetration and increase imaging depth, we use a light source with a central wavelength of 1050 nm. The laser tuning range is 100 nm, providing an axial resolution of 5.3 µm (full-width-half-maximum amplitude profile) and a total depth range of 2.9 mm in the tissue. The laser tuning cycle has a repetition rate of 100 kHz. The emitted radiation from the laser is split into the sample and reference arms. In the sample arm, a focused spot of 18 µm diameter (full-width-half-maximum amplitude profile) is achieved on the retinal plane. The light returning from the reference and sample arms interferes and is detected by a balanced receiver.

Scan Pattern

The scanning protocol has been optimized to implement the SSADA. For example, in the fast transverse scan (X) direction, the B scan contains 200 A lines covering 3 mm. With this configuration, the B scan frame rate of the system is 500 frames per second. In the slow transverse scan (Y) direction, 200 sampling positions covering 3 mm are used to capture a 3D data set, with 8 repeated B scans at every position. The 8 repeated B-frames (M-B-frames) are used for the SSADA calculation to obtain both the structure and blood flow images. Therefore, 1600 B scans are acquired to form a 3D data cube within an acquisition time of 3.2 seconds.

Split-Spectrum Amplitude Decorrelation

Speckle decorrelation has long been used in ultrasound[5,6] and in the laser speckle technique[7] to detect optical scattering from moving particles such as red blood cells. This phenomenon is also clearly exhibited by the real-time OCT reflectance images. The scattering pattern of blood flow varies rapidly over time. This is because the flow stream drives randomly distributed blood cells through the imaging volume (voxel). This results in decorrelation of the received backscattered signals that are a function of scatterer displacement over time. The contrast between the decorrelation of blood flow and static tissue can be used to extract flow signals for angiography.

Amplitude decorrelation measurement is sensitive to transverse flow and immune to phase noise in comparison to Doppler and other phase-based approaches in Fourier domain OCT. However, the high axial resolution of swept-source OCT makes it very sensitive to the pulsatile bulk motion noise in the axial direction. In the fundus, ocular pulsation mainly occurs along the axial direction and is driven by the retrobulbar orbital tissue in relation to the heart beat. The high sensitivity in that direction results in unacceptable signal-to-noise ratio (SNR). To overcome this limitation, we created the novel SSADA algorithm based on the decorrelation of OCT signal amplitude due to flow.

The full OCT spectrum is split into several narrower spectral bands, resulting in the OCT resolution cell in each band being isotropic and less susceptible to axial motion noise (**Figure 1**). The basic procedures of SSADA are shown in **Figure 2**. The high resolution OCT amplitude frames (M-B frames) transformed by the full spectrum are not used for amplitude decorrelation computation. The key step of SSADA (**Figure 2**, purple shadow) is splitting the raw full spectrum into a new spectrum with narrow bands. New bandwidth is intentionally created to lower the OCT axial resolution. This minimizes the noise along the axial direction and optimizes flow detection along the transverse direction. After narrower spectrums are Fourier-transformed, low resolution OCT amplitude frames are used to calculate decorrelation. Inter-B scan decorrelation can be determined at each of the narrower spectral bands separately and then averaged. Recombining the decorrelation images from the spectral bands yields angiograms that use the full information in the entire OCT spectral range. The recent work shows that such images produced significant improvement of SNR for both flow detection and connectivity of microvascular networks when compared to other amplitude decorrelation techniques.[8] Further, creation of isotropic resolution cells having equal sensitivity to axial and transverse flow can be useful for quantifying flow. In the other words, OCT angiography extracts flow information that can be further processed for quantification because the flow value generated by the isotropic resolution cell is a function of the flow velocity regardless of direction. This concept has been under investigation in our group.

En Face Angiogram

The 3D SSADA data set comprises a stack of 200 averaged decorrelation cross-sectional images, along with the associated

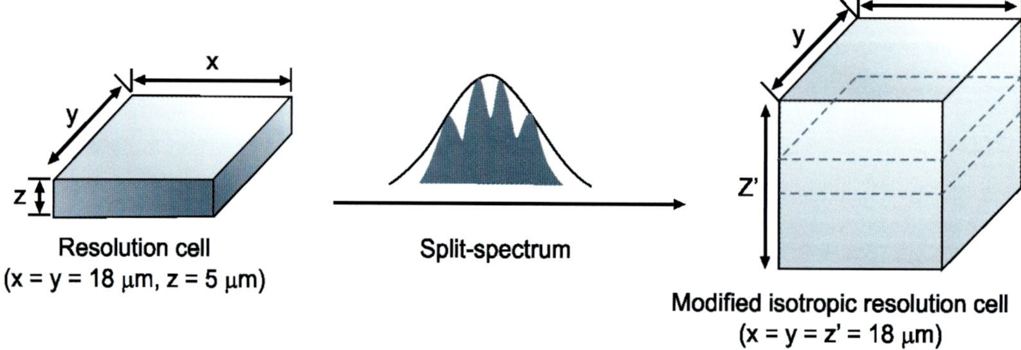

Figure 1:.Diagram of the modification of the OCT imaging resolution cell using the split-spectrum method. The resolution cell (x = y > z) in the current configuration can be modified into a new resolution cell (x = y = z)

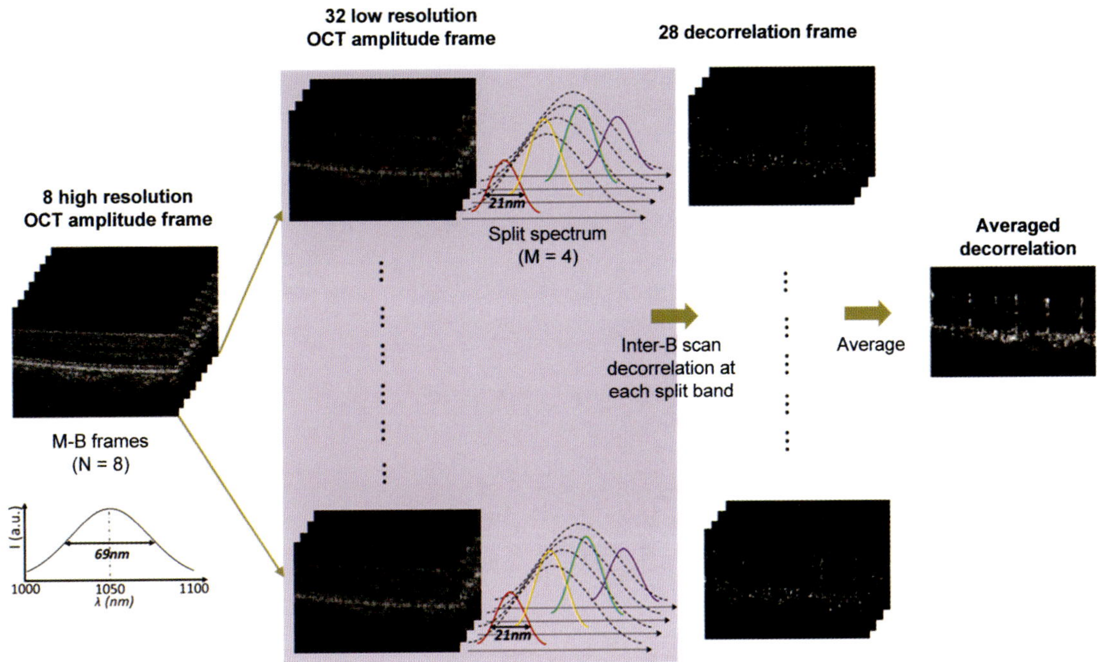

Figure 2: Flow chart detailing the basic steps of the SSADA method. Eight high-resolution OCT amplitude frames are transformed into 32 low-resolution frames by splitting the raw full spectrum into 4 new spectrum bands. After inter-B scan decorrelation of each split band, the 28 decorrelation frames are averaged

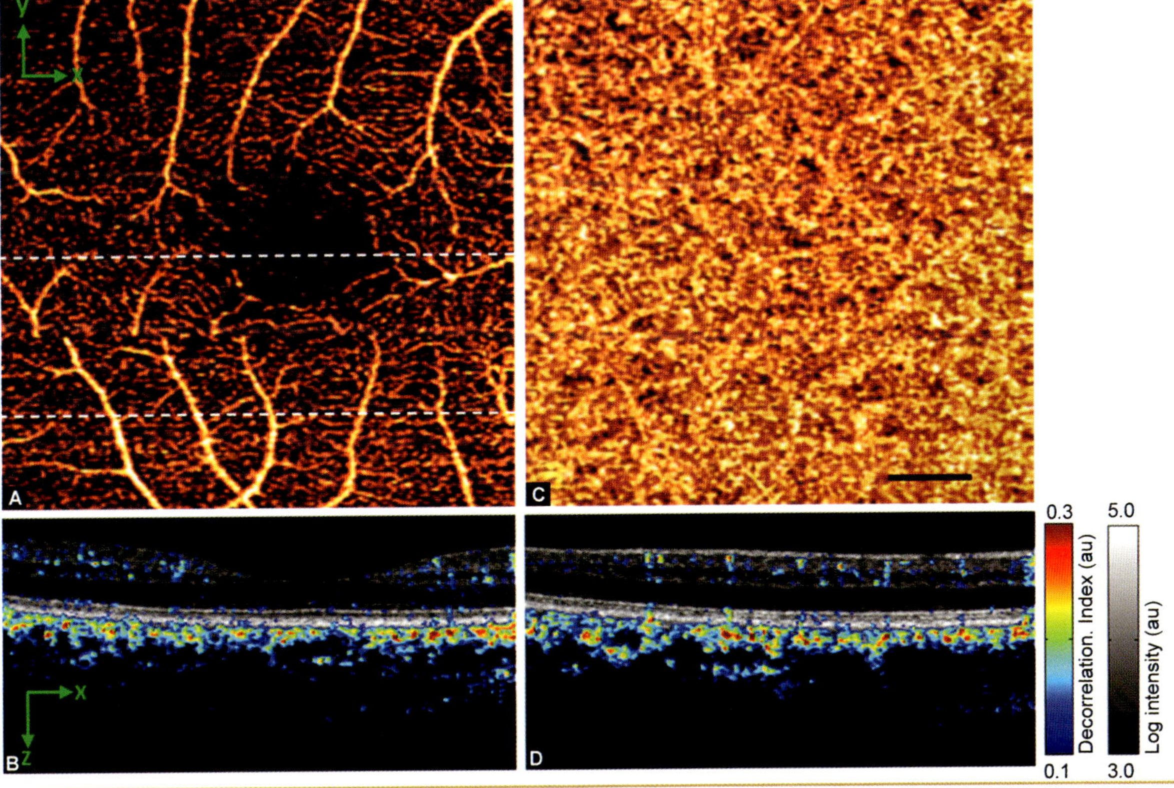

Figures 3: *In vivo* 3D volumetric OCT of the macula processed with the SSADA algorithm. The dimensions are [3.0 (x) × 3.0 (y) × 2.9 (z) mm], except for panels (B) and (D) where the images are cropped from 2.9 mm to 1.5 mm axially. (A) *En face* maximum decorrelation projection angiogram of the retinal circulation; (B) Horizontal OCT cross-section through the foveal center (upper dashed line in A) with merged flow and structure information; (C) *En face* maximum decorrelation projection angiogram of the choroidal circulation. Black bar, 500 μm; (D) Merged horizontal cross-section of the inferior macula (lower dashed line in A)

averaged reflectance images, that together span 3 mm in the slow transverse scan (Y) direction. The 3D data is separated into retinal and choroidal regions with the dividing boundary set at the retinal pigment epithelium (RPE). The depth (Z direction) of the highly reflective RPE is identified through the analysis of the reflectance and reflectance gradient profiles.[9] The region above the RPE is the retinal layer and the region below is the choroidal layer. The *en face* X-Y projection angiograms are produced by selecting the maximum decorrelation value along the axial (Z) direction in each layer. In ONH scans, the RPE depth just outside the disk boundary is used to set an interpolated RPE plane inside the disk. Additionally, the transverse scans, also referred to as coronal scans, C scans, or *en face* scans, are produced in the X-Y plane at a fixed "Z" coordinate.

Macular Region Retinal and Choroidal Circulation

The macular region of the fundus is responsible for central vision. Capillary dropout in the macular region due to diabetic retinopathy is a major cause of vision loss. Focal loss of the choriocapillary is a possible causative factor in the pathogenesis of both dry and wet age-related macular degeneration,[10] the leading cause of blindness in industrialized nations.[11] Thus macular angiography is important. The SSADA is used to demonstrate macular angiography of both the retinal and choroidal circulations in a normal eye (**Figures 3A to D**). The flow pixels form a continuous microcirculatory network in the retina. The vascular network is absent in the foveal avascular zone (**Figure 3A**) of approximately 600 µm diameter, in agreement with known anatomy. There are some disconnected apparent flow pixels within the foveal avascular zone (**Figure 3A**) due to noise. Inspection shows these false flow pixels to be decorrelation noise in the high reflectance layers of the RPE and photoreceptors (**Figure 3B**). The choriocapillaris layer forms a confluent overlapping plexus,[12] so it is to be expected that the projection image of the choroidal circulation shows confluent flow (**Figure 3C**).

By overlaying flow signals (color scale) on the structure signals (gray scale), the cross-sections (**Figures 3B and D**) show retinal vessels from the nerve fiber layer (NFL) to the outer plexiform layer, in agreement with known anatomy.[13] Based on the decorrelation seen in the color scale, the flow in the inner choroid has higher velocity. The volume is also greater than the retinal circulation, again consistent with known physiology that the choroidal circulation has much higher flow than the retinal circulation.[12] There are signal voids in the outer choroid that may be due to fringe washout from high flow velocity and the shadowing effect of overlying tissue. The cross-sections also show a few spots of decorrelation in the RPE layer. These must be artifacts

because the RPE is avascular. This is likely due to the projection of flow decorrelation in a proximal layer (i.e. inner retinal layers) onto distal layers with a strong reflected signal (i.e. RPE).

Another way to separately demonstrate retinal and choroidal circulation is by *en face* angiograms (C scan) at each Z coordinate. Inevitably, there are saccadic motion artifacts in the 3D dataset. This can be reduced by the use of 3D registration algorithms[14] for the better viewing of C scans. In C scans sliced along the X-Y plane parallel to the RPE layer, the RPE coordinate is set to zero (**Figure 4**). In this figure, there is no attempt to display the blood vessel network within anatomical layers. Therefore, we select the C scans at different Z coordinates showing diverse depth-encoded blood perfusion maps and provide our estimates based on the specific appearances of vessel networks.[15] The −290 µm slice includes the radial peripapillary vessels that are located in the inner part of the retina (NFL and ganglion cell layer). The −220 µm slice shows denser capillary network in the inner plexiform layer. The −150 µm slice shows the deeper capillaries around the outer plexiform layer. The +30 µm slice is just below the choriocapillary layer. The small, dense vessels in this layer form a confluent overlapping plexus. The +90 µm slice contains the medium sized arteries and venules in the Sattler's layer. Lastly, the +150 µm, +210 µm, and +270 µm slices correspond to the larger outer arteries and veins in the Haller's layer.[15]

Optic Nerve Head Circulation

From one 3D volumetric data set, both reflectance intensity images and decorrelation (angiography) images can be obtained. For the ONH scan, the *en face* maximum projection of reflectance intensity shows the major retinal blood vessels and the second order branches, but finer branches and the microcirculation of the retina, choroid, and optic disk are not visible (**Figure 5A**). In the vertical cross-sectional intensity image, the connective tissue struts (bright) and pores (dark) of the lamina cribrosa are visualized deep within the optic disk (**Figure 5B**). Around the disk, the retina, choroid, and sclera can also be delineated.

The ONH angiogram obtained by the SSADA shows both many orders of vascular branching as well as the microcirculatory network. The *en face* maximum decorrelation projection angiogram (**Figure 5C**) shows the major retinal branch vessels as well as many fine branches that could not be visualized well on the *en face* intensity image. Interestingly, the angiogram also shows a cilioretinal artery that emerges at the nasal disk margin. This artery is not part of the central retinal circulation, but arises from the posterior ciliary artery and can be recognized by its fish-hook shape just inside the disk margin.[16]

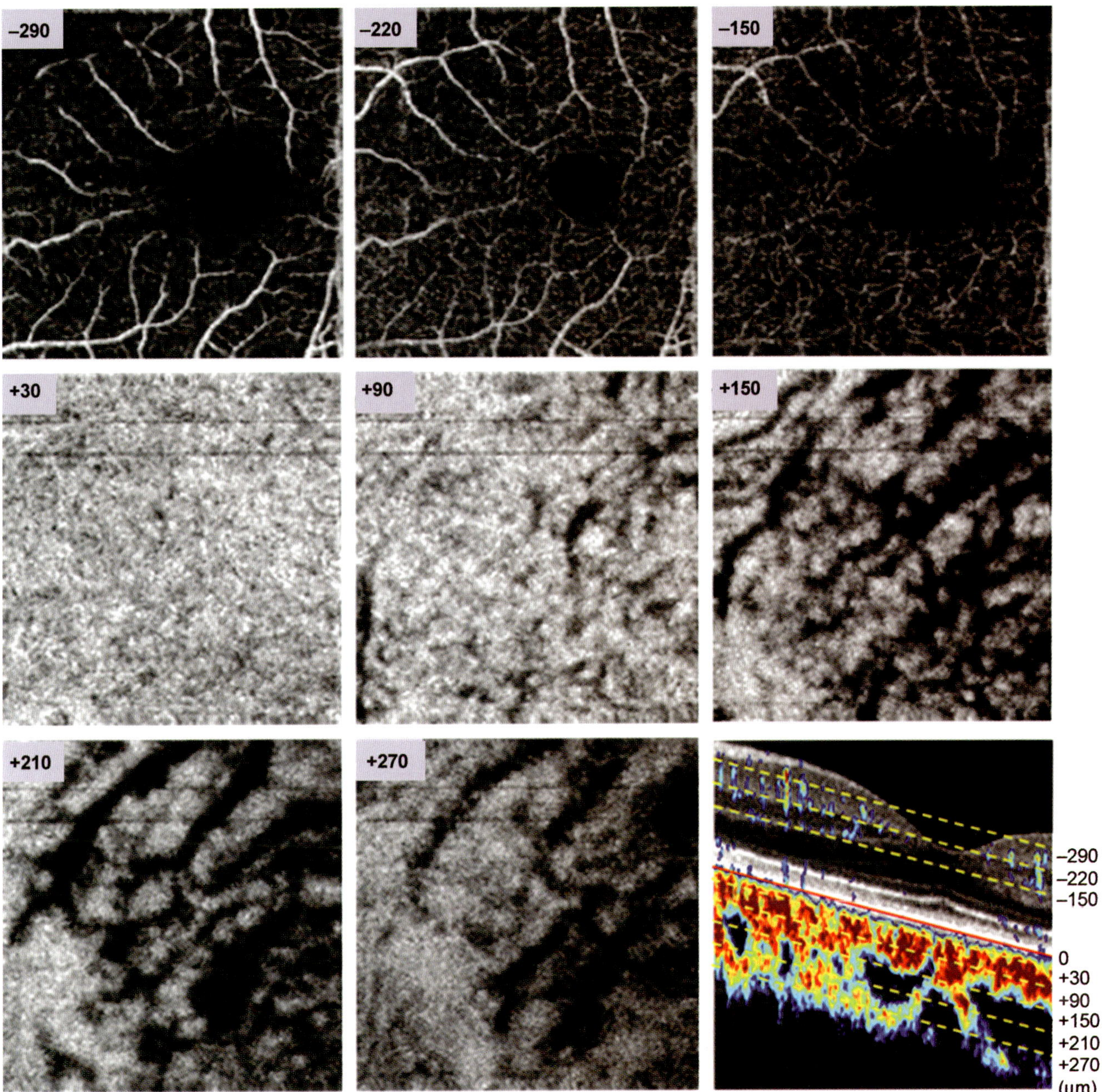

Figure 4: *En face* retinal and choroidal angiograms at different Z coordinates that have been tilted to be approximately perpendicular to the RPE X-Y plane. The Z coordinate of the RPE is set to be zero and other *en face* slices are defined by their distances (µm) away from the RPE location along Z

To separately view the retinal vessels and superficial disk vessels, we remove pixels below the level of the peripapillary RPE. The resulting *en face* angiogram **(Figure 5D)** shows the superficial vascular network that nourishes the disk edges at the disk boundary. By comparison, the choroidal circulation forms an almost continuous sheet of blood flow under the retina **(Figure 5B)**. The *en face* images **(Figures 5A to C)** show RPE atrophy in a temporal crescent just outside the disk margin. Inside the crescent there is also a small region of choriocapillaris atrophy **(Figure 5B)**. The structure-flow merged image shows that the major retinal branch vessels are at the level of the peripapillary NFL **(Figure 5E)**. It also shows the blood flow within the full thickness of the choroid. The combined image also reveals that the deeper disk circulation resides primarily in the pores of the lamina cribrosa and not in the connective tissue struts.

By use of the same 3D registration and slicing procedures as applied on macular scans, *en face* ONH angiography can be performed at different depths **(Figure 6)**. Because there are no superficial large vessels that block light penetration

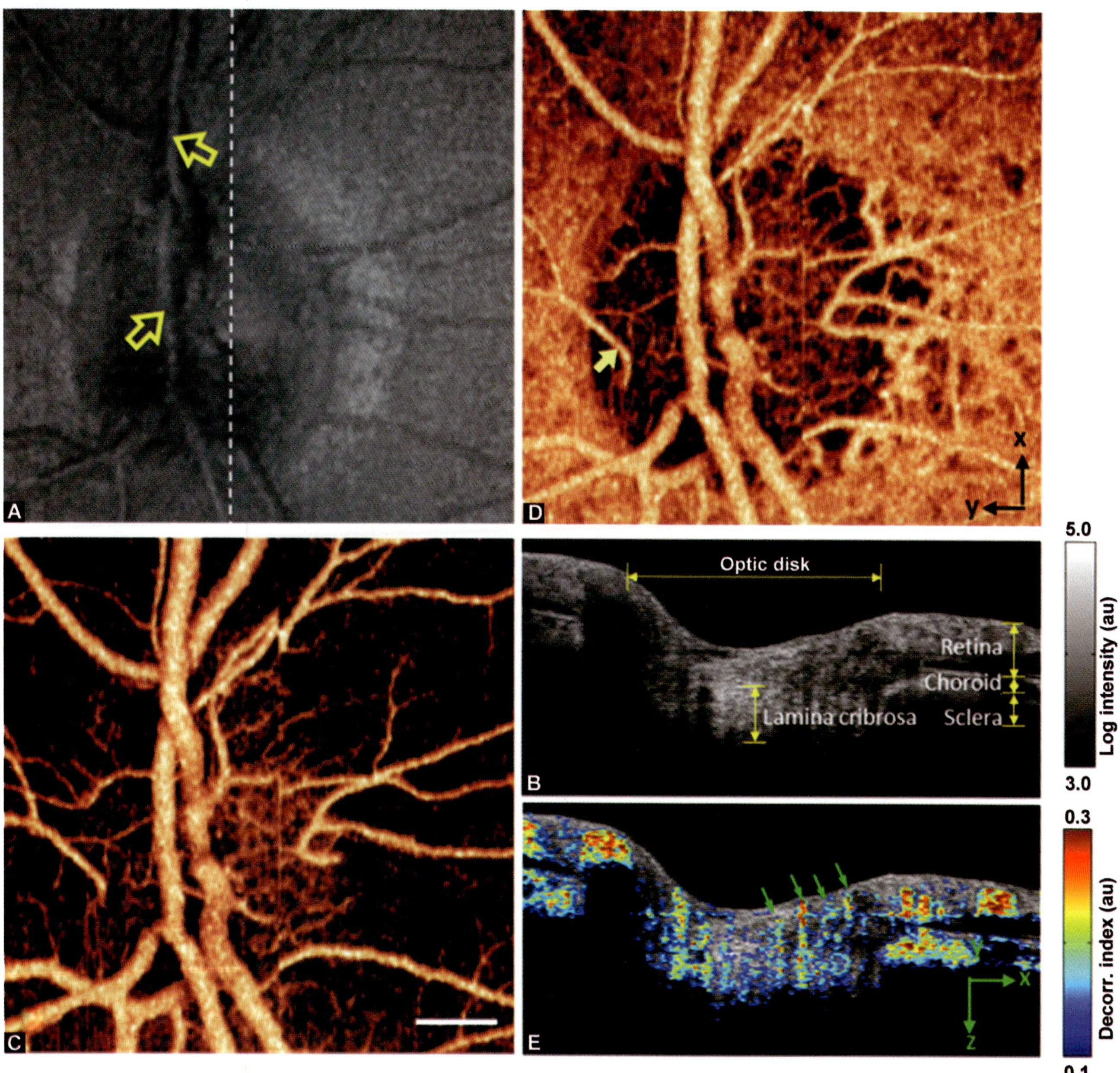

Figures 5A to E: *In vivo* 3D volumetric OCT of the ONH in the right eye of a myopic individual. The dimensions are [3.0 (x) × 3.0 (y) × 2.9 (z) mm], except for panels (D) and (E) where the images are cropped from 2.9 mm to 1.5 mm axially. (A) *En face* maximum reflectance intensity projection shows branches of the central retinal vessels; (B) OCT cross-section at the plane marked by white dashed line in (A); (C) *En face* maximum decorrelation projection angiogram computed with the SSADA algorithm. The arrow shows a cilioretinal artery that emerges at the nasal disk margin; (D) *En face* maximum decorrelation projection angiogram after removing the choroid. White bar, 500 µm; (E) The merged cross-section (same plane as D) shows in a 3D volumetric fashion the perfusion of the disk, retina, and choroid

of the temporal sector, the ONH perfusion is clearly displayed by OCT angiography. The –240 µm slice crossing the NFL layer shows the major retinal vessels **(Figure 6)**. The –120 µm slice shows the absence of retinal vessels in the outer nuclear layer, contrasted with the dense vascular network within the disk. In the following 5 slices, from +30 µm to +390 µm, the choroidal networks look similar to those of the macular region. Below 300 µm, peripapillary scleral vessels are not discernible except for a small patch below a patch of temporal RPE atrophy. Due to the tilt of the disk, the nasal portion of the lamina cribrosa was overshadowed by the RPE and choroid, whereas the lamina cribrosa in the superior and inferior poles are overshadowed by major retinal vessels. But in the temporal quadrant, vessels

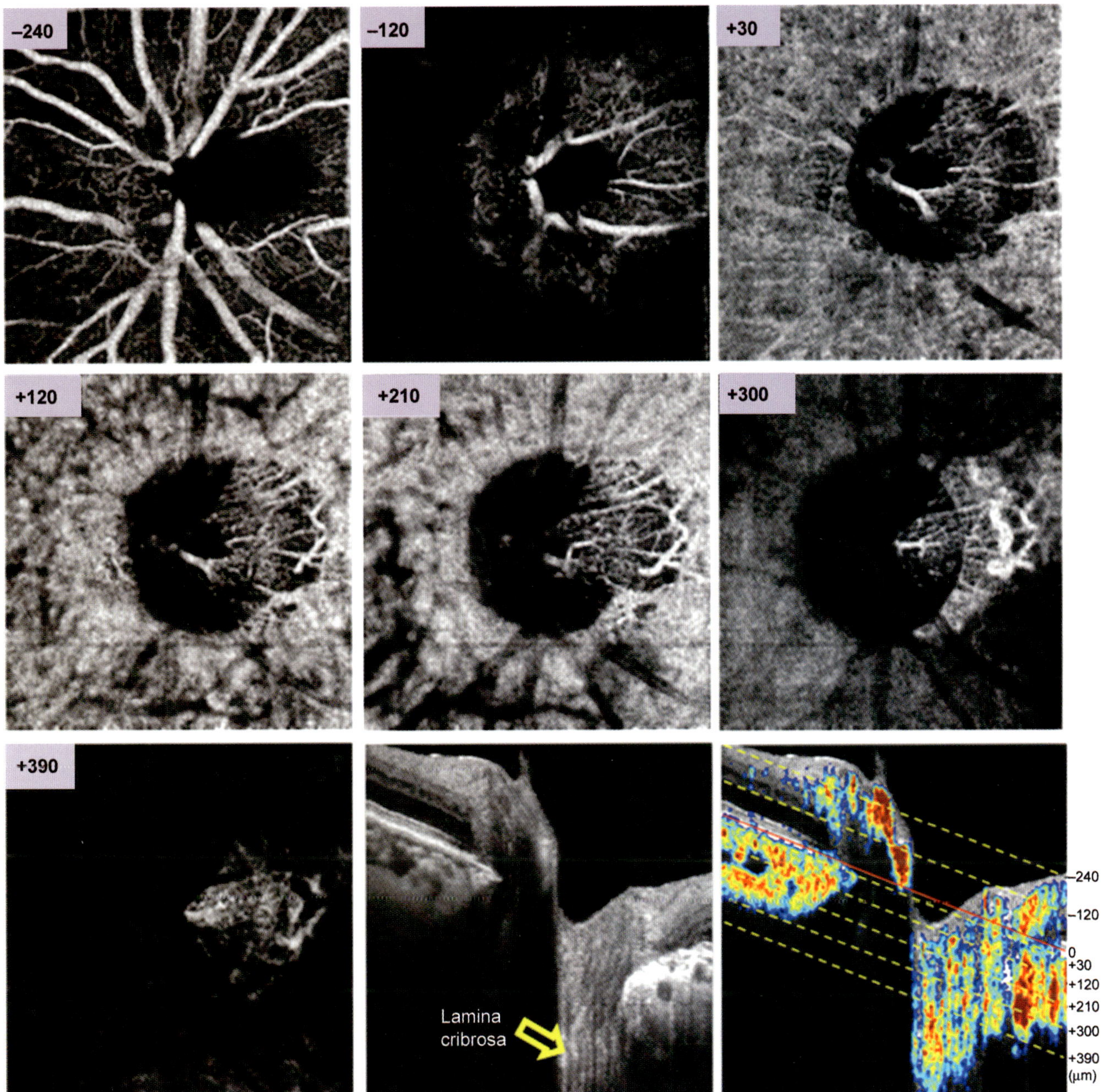

Figure 6: *En face* ONH angiograms at different Z coordinates that have been tilted to be approximately perpendicular to the RPE X-Y plane. The Z coordinate of RPE is set to be zero and other *en face* slices are defined by their distances (µm) away from the RPE location along Z

in the lamina cribrosa could be visualized down to the plane of the sclera. To our knowledge, this is the first time that the disk microcirculation has been visualized noninvasively in such a comprehensive manner.

Summary

We developed a novel optical angiography technique that can be used noninvasively to visualize the vasculature and blood flow at the posterior part of the eye. This technique is based on the decorrelation of OCT signal amplitude due to blood flow. By splitting the full OCT spectral interferograms into several spectral bands, the OCT resolution cell in each band is less susceptible to axial motion noise. Recombining the decorrelation images from the spectral bands yields angiograms that use the full information in the entire OCT spectral range. This is a step towards developing a new evaluation system for eye diseases.

Compared to fluorescein/Indocyanine green (ICG) angiography, OCT angiography performed by SSADA has the following advantages: First, it is a 3D imaging method that easily separates disk, retinal, and choroidal circulations and also flexibly produces sections and projections along any plane. Second, it is quantitative, using the flow index values that are proportional to the blood flow rate. We are now working on the specific algorithm to quantify the blood flow in the retinal, choroidal, and ONH vasculature and investigating its relationship to eye abnormalities. Third, it does not require dye injection, and therefore has no potential side effects such as nausea and anaphylactic reaction. Certainly, there are some limitations to OCT angiography. First, our current prototype provides a small imaging field (3 mm); however, that field will increase with higher speed OCT. Second, it cannot visualize leakage and stain, but fluid space and thickening are readily detectable. Overall, OCT angiography is faster, more sensitive, and has deeper depth penetration than other angiography modalities. Soon it may enable comprehensive investigation of blood flow in the whole eyeball.

References

1. Patel V, Rassam S, Newsom R, et al. Retinal blood flow in diabetic retinopathy. BMJ. 1992;305:678-83.
2. Friedman E. A hemodynamic model of the pathogenesis of age-related macular degeneration. Am J Ophthalmol. 1997;124:677-82.
3. Flammer J, Orgül S, Costa VP. The impact of ocular blood flow in glaucoma. Prog Retin Eye Res. 2002;21:359-93.
4. Potsaid B, Baumann B, Huang D, et al. Ultrahigh speed 1050 nm swept source/Fourier domain OCT retinal and anterior segment imaging at 100,000 to 400,000 axial scans per second. Opt Express. 2010;18:20029-48.
5. Hein IA, WD O'Brien Jr. Current time-domain methods for assessing tissue motion by analysis from reflected ultrasound echoes—a review. IEEE Trans Ultrasonics, Ferroelectrics and Frequency Control. 1993;40(2):84-102.
6. Hoeks AP, Arts TG, Brands PJ, et al. Comparison of the performance of the RF cross correlation and Doppler autocorrelation technique to estimate the mean velocity of simulated ultrasound signals. Ultrasound Med Biol. 1993;19:727-40.
7. Dainty JC. Laser speckle and related phenomena. Springer-Verlag: New York. 1984.
8. Jia Y, Tan O, Tokayer J, et al. Split-spectrum amplitude-decorrelation angiography with optical coherence tomography. Opt. Express. 2012;20:4710-25.
9. An L, Wang RK. *In vivo* volumetric imaging of vascular perfusion within human retina and choroids with optical micro-angiography. Opt. Express. 2008;16:11438-52.
10. Zhao J, Frambach DA, Lee PP, et al. Delayed macular choriocapillary circulation in age-related macular degeneration. International Ophthalmology. 1995;19(1):1-12.
11. Bressler NM. Age-Related Macular Degeneration is the Leading Cause of Blindness. JAMA. 2004;291(15):1900-01.
12. Roh S, Weiter JJ. Retinal and Choroidal Circulation in Ophthalmology. In: Yanoff M, Duker JS (Eds). Mo: Mosby Elsevier, St. Louis. 2008.
13. Funk RH. Blood supply of the retina. Ophthalmic Res. 1997;29:320-5.
14. Kraus M, Mayer M, Bock R, et al. Motion Artifact Correction in OCT Volume Scans Using Image Registration, in Association for Research in Vision and Ophthalmology. ARVO, Fort Lauderdale. 2010.
15. Henkind P, Hansen RI, Szalay J. Ocular circulation in Physiology of the Human Eye and Visual System. In: Records RE (Ed). Harper & Row: New York; 1979. pp. 99-155.
16. Hayreh SS. Posterior ciliary artery circulation in health and disease: the Weisenfeld lecture. Invest Ophthalmol Vis Sci. 2004;45:749-57.

chapter 44

Development and Advances in *En Face* OCT Using Spectral and Swept Source/Fourier Domain Technologies

James G Fujimoto, Jay S Duker

Introduction

En face OCT imaging is a powerful imaging modality which provides many advantages for visualizing, diagnosing and monitoring the progression of retinal and choroidal pathology. However, *en face* imaging is one of the most technically demanding OCT imaging methods because it requires extremely high imaging speeds in order to generate high quality *en face* images. For this reason, improvements in *en face* OCT imaging are strongly dependent on advances in fundamental OCT detection and imaging technology. This chapter presents an overview of the development of *en face* imaging, how OCT works and the different methods for image detection that enabled advances in *en face* imaging performance.

The most commonly used imaging modality in ophthalmology, retinal fundus imaging via a camera, is inherently an *en face* modality. The scanning laser ophthalmoscope (SLO) developed by Webb et al in 1980 was one of the earliest applications of advanced technology for *en face* retinal imaging.[1,2] Scanning laser ophthalmoscope images are generated by illuminating the retina with a laser beam which is rapidly scanned in a two dimensional "raster" pattern. Images of the retina are generated by detecting the backscattered and backreflected light as the laser is scanned over different positions on the retinal fundus. SLO images are generated electronically, by displaying the detected light signal as a gray scale on a monitor, similar to the way early generation televisions operated. In fact, early publications described the SLO as a "flying spot TV ophthalmoscope".[1] Scanning laser ophthalmoscope can generate excellent quality, high contrast images of the retinal fundus even in the presence of ocular opacities, because the electronic image detection can reject unwanted scattered light. The scanning laser can also be used to excite fluorescence from intrinsic retinal fluorophores or from extrinsic dyes such as fluorescein or indocyanine green. However, the depth resolution for SLO imaging is limited because it detects all of the backscattered or backreflected light from the retina, without time resolving light echoes from different delays or axial range.

The concept of detecting echo time delays for *en face* imaging dates back even earlier than the SLO, to work by Duguay et al in 1971.[3,4] Working at AT&T Bell Laboratories in the field of optics and lasers, Duguay developed high speed photography with picosecond (10^{-12} second) time resolution using a short pulse laser activated shutter (**Figure 1A**). The shutter consisted of a cell containing CS2 placed between crossed polarizers (**Figure 1B**). When the CS2 is excited by a short infrared laser pulse, it rotates the polarization of light, opening the shutter. The shutter speeds that Duguay achieved were so high that it was possible to photograph light pulses in flight (**Figure 1B**). This landmark publication also demonstrated another key concept, "gated picture ranging", detecting images at different axial range or depth by time resolving the backscattered or backreflected light. **Figures 1C to E** show gated picture ranging of an AT&T logo behind a scattering screen. Illuminating the AT&T logo with a short laser pulse and photographing the image with a precisely timed high speed shutter, it was possible to reject the unwanted scattered light from the screen (which arrives earlier) and detect only light which comes from the AT&T logo behind the screen. This study demonstrated that it is possible to generate images from structures which are hidden by unwanted scattered light by time resolving echoes of light.

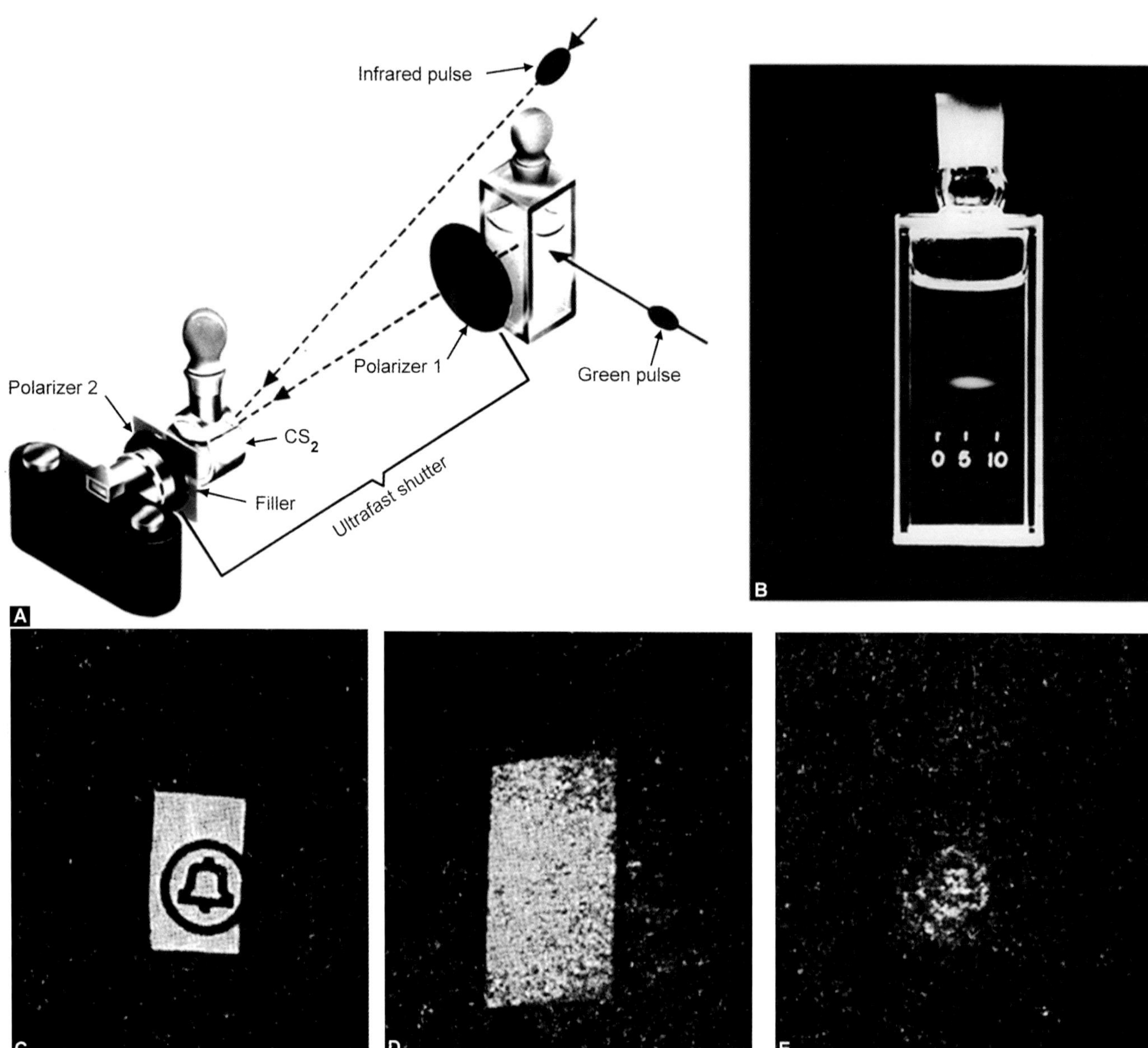

Figures 1A to E: Photographing light in flight and gated picture ranging. (A) An ultrafast optical shutter using a short laser pulse to induce transient polarization rotation between crossed polarizers achieves 10 picosecond resolution; (B) Photograph of an ultrashort laser pulse propagating through a cell of scattering liquid. The pulse duration is 10 picoseconds and appears localized in space. Gated picture ranging showing (C) an AT&T logo; (D) the logo behind a scattering screen photographed using an ordinary camera and (E) the logo photographed using ultrashort pulse illumination with an ultrafast shutter timed to transmit only light from the AT&T logo (arriving later than the unwanted scattered light from the screen). These early results suggested that time resolved detection could be used to see inside biological tissues by rejecting unwanted scattered light (*Source*: Adapted from Duguay MA and Mattick AT. Ultrahigh speed photography of picosecond light pulses and echoes. Applied Optics. 1971;10:2162-70.)

HOW SPECTRAL/FOURIER DOMAIN OCT DETECTION WORKS

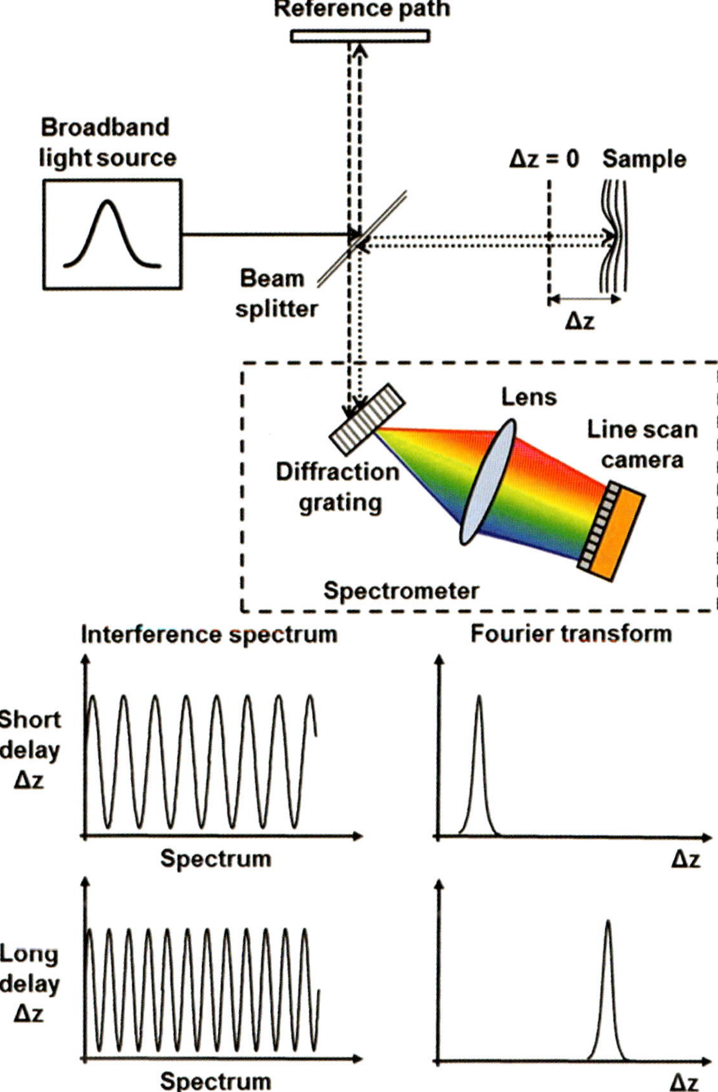

Figure 2: Shows a schematic of how spectral/Fourier domain OCT detection works. Spectral/Fourier domain detection uses a broadband light source, an interferometer and a spectrometer with a high speed, line scan camera. In spectral/ Fourier domain detection, different echo time delays of light are encoded as different oscillation frequencies in the interference spectrum. The echo time delays can be measured by Fourier transforming the interference spectrum, which essentially measures the oscillation frequencies. Spectral/ Fourier domain can be understood by noting that an interferometer acts like a periodic frequency filter, where the periodicity of the frequency filter depends on the delay difference Δz between the sample and reference paths. The output from a broadband light source is split into two paths. One light path is directed onto the tissue to be imaged and light is backreflected or backscattered from structures at different depths. The second light path is reflected from a fixed (not scanned) reference mirror at a reference delay position. The signal path and the reference path have a relative time delay given by the path length difference (Δz) or the depth of the structure in the tissue. When light from the tissue and the reference path interferes, the interference signal will have oscillations in its spectrum because different frequency/wavelength components will constructively or destructively interfere. The modulation or oscillation in the spectrum can be measured using a spectrometer and the frequency of this oscillation will be related to the echo time delay Δz. Larger echo delays will produce higher frequency oscillations in the interference spectrum. The echo magnitude and time delay can then be extracted by Fourier transforming the interference signal to produce an axial scan or A scan. The Fourier transform is a mathematical operation which measures the frequency content of a signal. Multiple axial scans are acquired by repeatedly reading the spectrometer with the line scan camera and Fourier transforming the interference spectra.

Optical coherence tomography (OCT) performs cross-sectional and three dimensional imaging by measuring the echo time delay and magnitude of backscattered or backreflected light.[5] Detecting the time delay of optical echoes is at the core of OCT imaging technology, and this time resolved detection, which can distinguish light from different distances or axial range, is key to achieving cross-sectional and three dimensional imaging. OCT imaging was developed and first reported by Huang et al in 1991.[5] It employs low coherence interferometry to detect the magnitude and time delay of light.[6] Unlike the high speed shutter that Duguay demonstrated, which generated a full field photographic like image, OCT uses a scanning laser beam and detects the magnitude and echo time delay of backscattered or backreflected light along the direction of the scanning beam, analogous to an axial scan or A scan in ultrasound. Optical coherence tomography cross-sectional images or B scans are generated by scanning the OCT optical beam in the transverse direction and acquiring successive axial scans. In order to generate *en face* images, the beam must be scanned in two transverse directions, in a manner analogous to the SLO. Typically, the OCT beam is scanned in a "raster" pattern which acquires sequential cross-sectional images or B scans to form a three dimensional 3D data set. The 3D-OCT data sets are volumetric and analogous to CT or MR images.

One of the inherent challenges in OCT has been image acquisition speed. The first generation OCT technology developed in 1991 used time domain detection and could acquire several hundred axial scans per second, enough to generate multiple individual cross-sectional images. However, these speeds were insufficient for three dimensional imaging and *en face* OCT. This problem was solved by a novel detection method developed by Podoleanu et al in 1997.[7,8] This method achieved *en face* imaging by detecting the backreflected or backscattered light from a specific distance or axial range while scanning the OCT beam in a raster pattern on the retina. This technique did not require detecting all of the light echoes from different time delays and therefore could achieve high sensitivity and high speed. This advance enabled the generation of *en face* OCT retinal images for the first time. However, the limitation of detecting light from a specific distance or axial range is that the *en face* OCT images are generated in a specific image plane at this fixed range. Because of the eye and retina are curved, fixed range *en face* images intercept the eye in a circular contour, similar to latitude contours on the globe. In order to display *en face* images conforming to the retinal curvature, multiple *en face* planes at different distances or ranges must be acquired in order to generate a 3D data set. Curved *en face* OCT images which match the retinal contour can then be extracted from this 3D volumetric data.

High Speed Spectral/Fourier Domain OCT

Spectral/Fourier domain detection was a critical advance for *en face* OCT because of the need to acquire 3D volumetric data. Spectral/Fourier domain OCT achieves a sensitivity increase of ~20 dB, enabling imaging ~50 to 100 times faster than previous generation OCT systems which used time domain detection. High speed spectral/Fourier domain OCT has many advantages, including improved image quality, preservation of true retinal topography, improved retinal coverage and accurate registration of OCT cross-sectional images to fundus features. For a given acquisition time, high-speed imaging can increase the number of axial scans or transverse pixels per image to yield high definition images, as well as increase the number of cross-sectional images acquired to improve retinal coverage. Spectral/Fourier domain OCT was a key advance for *en face* OCT because each pixel in the *en face* OCT image requires an axial scan and therefore increasing the number of pixels in an *en face* image requires a dramatic increase in imaging speed.

The concepts of spectral/Fourier domain detection were proposed by Fercher et al. in 1995.[9] However, at that time retinal imaging could not be performed due to limitations in electronic camera technology. The first demonstration of retinal imaging was reported by Wojtkowski et al in 2002.[10] In 2003, three different independent research groups demonstrated that Fourier domain detection has a powerful sensitivity advantage over previous generation time domain detection, since Fourier domain detection essentially measures all of the echoes of light simultaneously.[11-13] The sensitivity is improved by approximately the ratio of the axial resolution to the imaging depth range. This yields a sensitivity increase of 50 to 100 times and corresponding increases in imaging speeds. Spectral/Fourier domain OCT studies in 2004 demonstrated video rate retinal imaging using at 29,000 axial scans per second with 6 μm axial resolution, as well as ultrahigh resolution imaging with ~2 μm axial resolution at 19,000 axial scans per second.[14,15] These and other advances stimulated rapid growth in OCT research and commercial development.

Spectral/Fourier domain OCT imaging enables the acquisition of 3D-OCT data sets in a time comparable to that of previous time domain OCT protocols that acquired multiple individual cross-sectional images. **Figures 3A to F** show 3D-OCT raster scan imaging of the optic disk from Wojtkowski et al in 2005.[16] The 3D-OCT volumetric data set contains comprehensive structural information. An *en face* OCT fundus image, identical to a standard retinal fundus view, can be generated by summing the signal in the axial direction.[16-18] This has the advantage that individual cross-

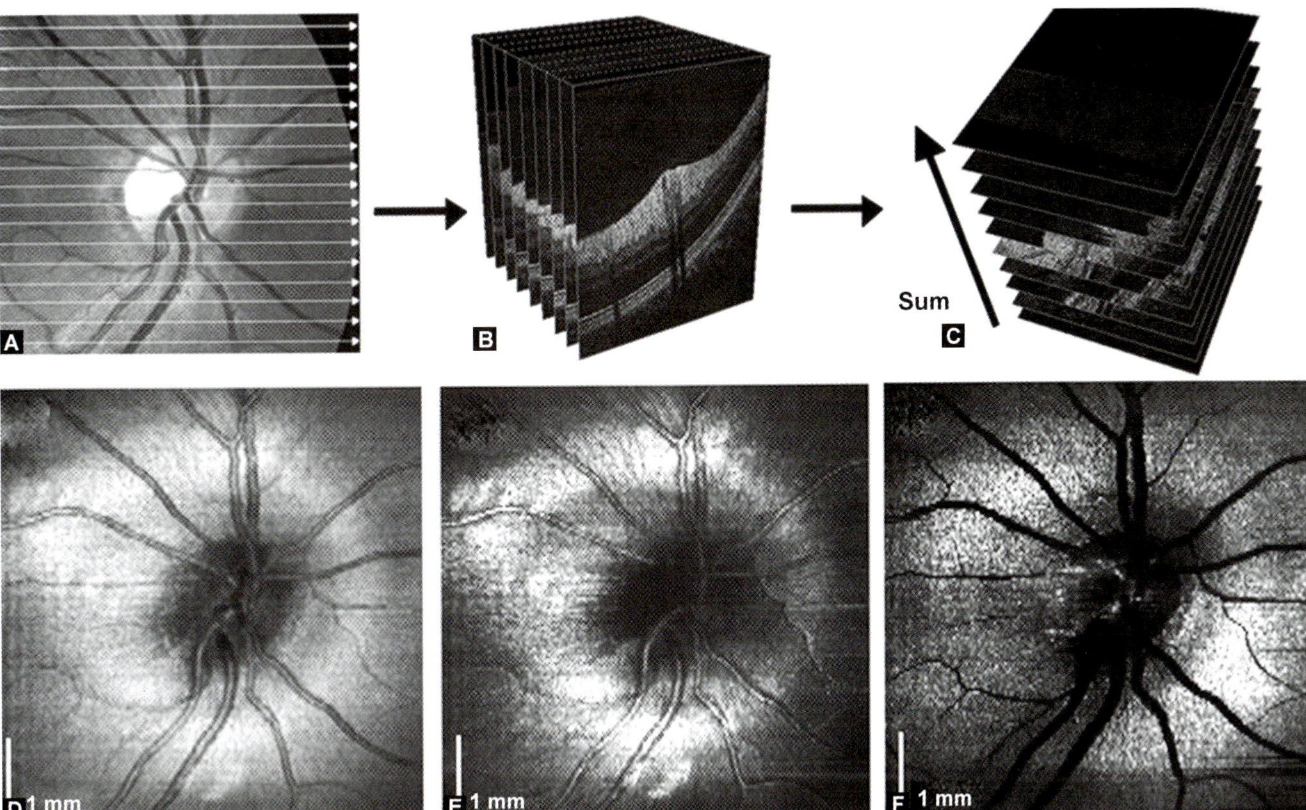

Figures 3A to F: *En face* OCT imaging using 3D volumetric data. (A) Fundus image showing positions of OCT raster scan; (B) 3D volumetric data consisting of sequential cross-sectional imaging (B scans); (C) Summing signal in the axial direction generates *en face* OCT images from the 3D data; (D) Summing entire axial range generates an OCT fundus image equivalent to fundus photograph. Different *en face* OCT images can be generated by summing depth levels around; (E) the nerve fiber layer and; (F) retinal pigment epithelium; (F) *En face* OCT images enable cross-sectional images to be precisely and reproducibly registered with respect to fundus features (*Source*: Adapted from Wojtkowski M, Srinivasan V, Fujimoto JG, et al. Three-dimensional retinal imaging with high-speed ultrahigh-resolution optical coherence tomography. Ophthalmology. 2005;112:1734-46.)

sectional OCT images (B scans) can be precisely and reproducibly registered to *en face* features of the retina. In addition to summing the backreflected or backscattered light from all depths, it is possible to select signals from specific depth levels or axial ranges to create projection OCT fundus images with enhanced contrast. **Figures 3E and F** show examples of *en face* OCT images created by summing signals from a depth levels corresponding to the nerve fiber layer and the retinal pigment epithelium (RPE).

En face OCT using 3D volumetric OCT data sets allows multiple *en face* images corresponding to different depth levels or axial ranges to be generated from a single data set. **Figures 4A and B** show how *en face* images are generated with example images from a normal subject.[19] In order to generate *en face* images which conform to the retinal curvature, an anatomical feature such as the RPE, choroid or vitreoretinal interface is identified by image processing segmentation. The backscattered or backreflected light from

specific axial ranges or depth levels relative this reference anatomic surface is summed (projected) and displayed. **Figures 4A and B** show different *en face* OCT images from depth levels at the choroid, RPE, photoreceptor outer segments, outer nuclear layer and photoreceptor inner segments, and inner retinal levels. Shadowing produced by retinal vasculature is evident on the *en face* images of the deeper retinal levels. *En face* images from the normal retina are relatively homogenous.

En face OCT imaging can be used to rapidly visualize the extent of retinal pathology as well as to identify specific cross-sectional images for further examination. At the same time, disruptions in normal retinal morphology from pathology cause retinal features to appear in different depth levels or axial ranges. Therefore, special care and experience is required for image interpretation. **Figures 5A and B** show examples of *en face* OCT imaging of an 83-year-old female subject with dry age-related macular degeneration (AMD).[19]

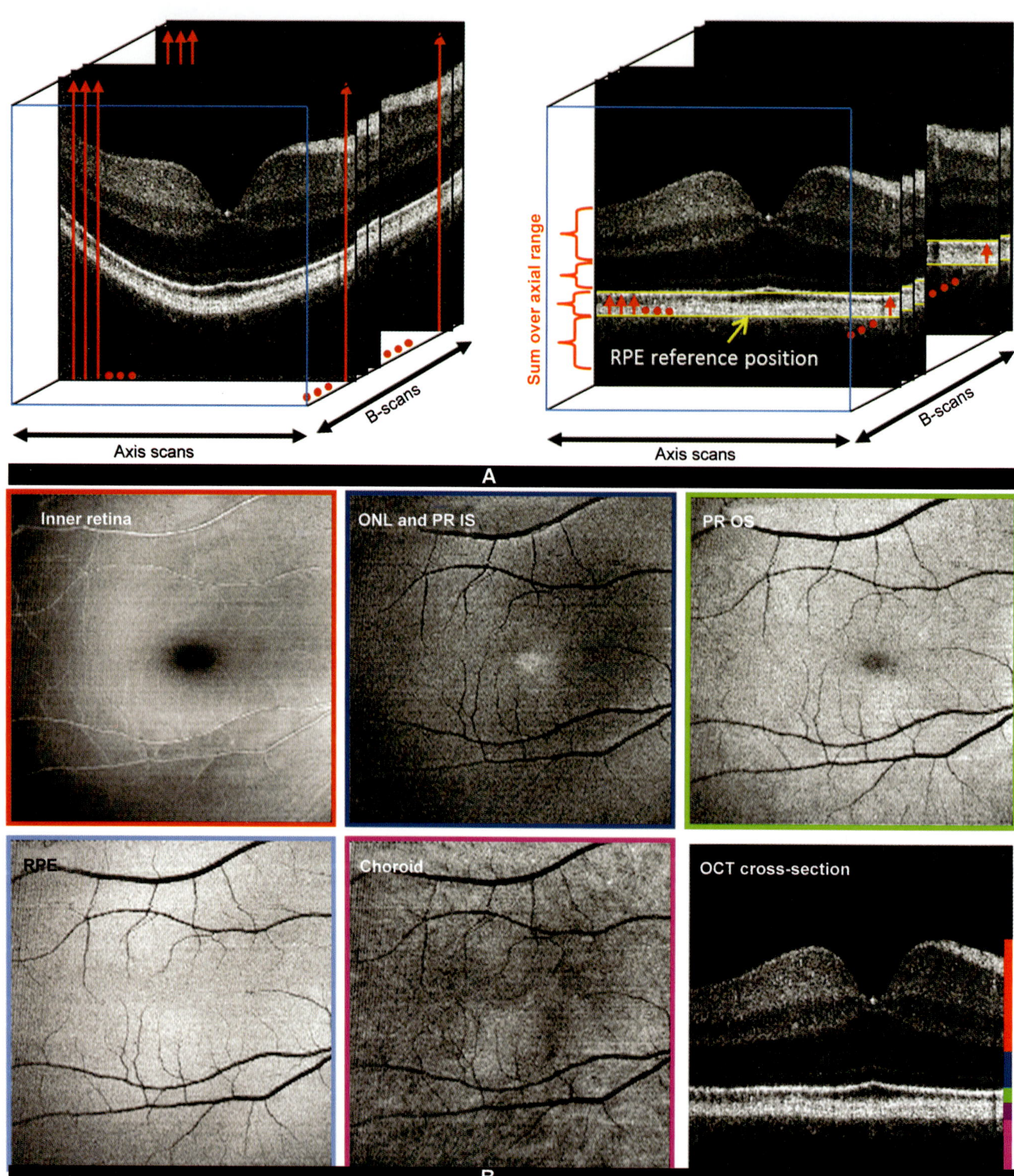

Figures 4A and B: Generation of *en face* OCT images in the normal retina. (A) 3D volumetric data consisting of sequential cross-sectional images; (B) Retinal contour from the RPE and choroid is identified and used as a reference surface. Different axial ranges corresponding to different depth levels in the retina are summed to create *en face* OCT images. Examples show depth levels corresponding to the inner retina, outer nuclear layer (ONL) and photoreceptor inner segments (PR IS), photoreceptor outer segments (PR OS), retinal pigment epithelium (RPE) and choroid. Representative cross-sectional image shows depth levels over which axial summation is performed. Color coded ranges match to *en face* images. Imaging was performed at 840 nm and image size is 6 mm x 6 mm

The images were acquired with a spectral/Fourier domain OCT system at 840 nm wavelength. The red free fundus photograph and late phase fluorescein angiogram show drusen with RPE atrophy and pigment clumping. Displaying *en face* OCT images from different levels improves contrast and differentiation of pathology. Hyper-scattering features visible in the ONL level may indicate inner retinal changes and atrophy of the ONL as well as pigment migration. Hyper-scattering areas in the photoreceptor outer segment level image show drusen that has extended into the photoreceptors. Dark areas in the photoreceptor outer segment level image correspond to drusen free regions in the ONL level and may indicate disruptions of the photoreceptors. Changes at the RPE level image indicate areas of drusen and RPE disruption. Hyper-scattering regions in the choroidal level suggest RPE atrophy. The *en face* choroidal level image is especially interesting because it allows regions of geographic atrophy to be identified and mapped. The *en face* images enable visualization of important features across the fundus and guide which cross-sectional images should be selected for detailed viewing. It is important to note that the *en face* OCT images display features which are at specific depths from RPE, choroid or ILM, rather than in specific anatomical retinal layers. The position of the RPE or choroid can be easily identified in normal eyes. However, it is much more difficult to reliably automatically identify and segment specific retinal layers if they are disrupted by pathology. Therefore, *en face* images do not necessarily conform to individual retinal layers, but instead show disruptions of retinal features at specific levels. Interpretation of *en face* images, especially on an individual basis, is challenging because pathology causes the displacement of retinal layers from their normal depth positions. Interpretation is improved if multiple *en face* images at different depth levels can be viewed sequentially. In addition, both *en face* OCT images as well as corresponding cross-sectional OCT images are helpful for definitive interpretation of pathology. This suggests the orthoplane viewing, analogous to methods used in CT or MR data sets would be helpful in OCT imaging.

It is important to note that the data in this example was acquired with a prototype spectral/Fourier domain OCT instrument at 840 nm with an ultrahigh 3.5 μm axial resolution, but at imaging speeds of 29,000 axial scans per second which is comparable to standard OCT instruments. The data consisted of 180 cross-sectional images (B scans) with 500 axial scans each, covering a 6 mm × 6 mm region of the retina and was acquired in ~4 seconds. This acquisition time is longer than typically used in clinical OCT imaging. Optical coherence tomography (OCT) instruments without eye tracking using acquisition times of ~2 seconds or less in order to avoid excessive eye motion. Although acquisition times in this example are long, this points out the role of imaging speed and *en face* image quality. The 3D-OCT data sets consist of 180 × 500 axial scans which yield *en face* OCT images with 90,000 pixels. In contrast, most commercial OCT instruments acquire a volume consisting of 200 × 200 axial scans within ~2 seconds. This yields *en face* OCT images with 40,000 pixels, which have lower quality than the images shown in this example.

Fortunately, there have been recent advances in line scan camera technology which enable higher speed image acquisition using spectral/Fourier domain OCT. Imaging speeds scale according to the number of pixels in the camera. Larger numbers of pixels are required in order to support finer axial image resolution or longer imaging range. Therefore, there is an inherent trade-off between axial image resolution or axial range, versus imaging speed. Faster imaging speeds can be obtained by sacrificing image resolution or range. In addition, increasing the imaging speed reduces detection sensitivity because the camera exposure times must be shorter and less light is detected. Record imaging speeds of over 300,000 axial scans per second (~10x faster than standard commercial OCT instruments) with ~9 μm axial resolution, < 1 mm imaging ranges and ~90 dB sensitivity were achieved by Potsaid et al in 2008.[20] These speeds are useful in research prototype instruments and can enable visualization of small retinal features as well as large area retinal coverage. However, in order to maintain sufficient resolution, image range and sensitivity for general clinical use, it is likely that future generations of spectral/Fourier domain OCT instruments will operate at slower speeds in the range of 100,000 axial scans per second, which are still factors of 2–3× faster than current instruments. This increased speed will yield corresponding improvements in *en face* OCT image quality.

Ultrahigh Speed Swept Source/Fourier Domain OCT (Figure 6)

The most promising approach for achieving even faster imaging speeds is another OCT detection technique known as swept source/Fourier domain detection. Swept source/Fourier domain detection uses an interferometer with a narrow bandwidth light source which is frequency swept in time, rather than a broadband light source, spectrometer and line scan camera.[21,22] Swept source /Fourier domain OCT has several important advantages for ophthalmic imaging. Since it uses high speed detectors instead of a spectrometer and line scan camera, the inherent detection efficiency can be higher because there are no spectrometer or camera losses. In addition, it is possible to perform imaging at longer wavelengths of 1050 nm, which are difficult to detect using

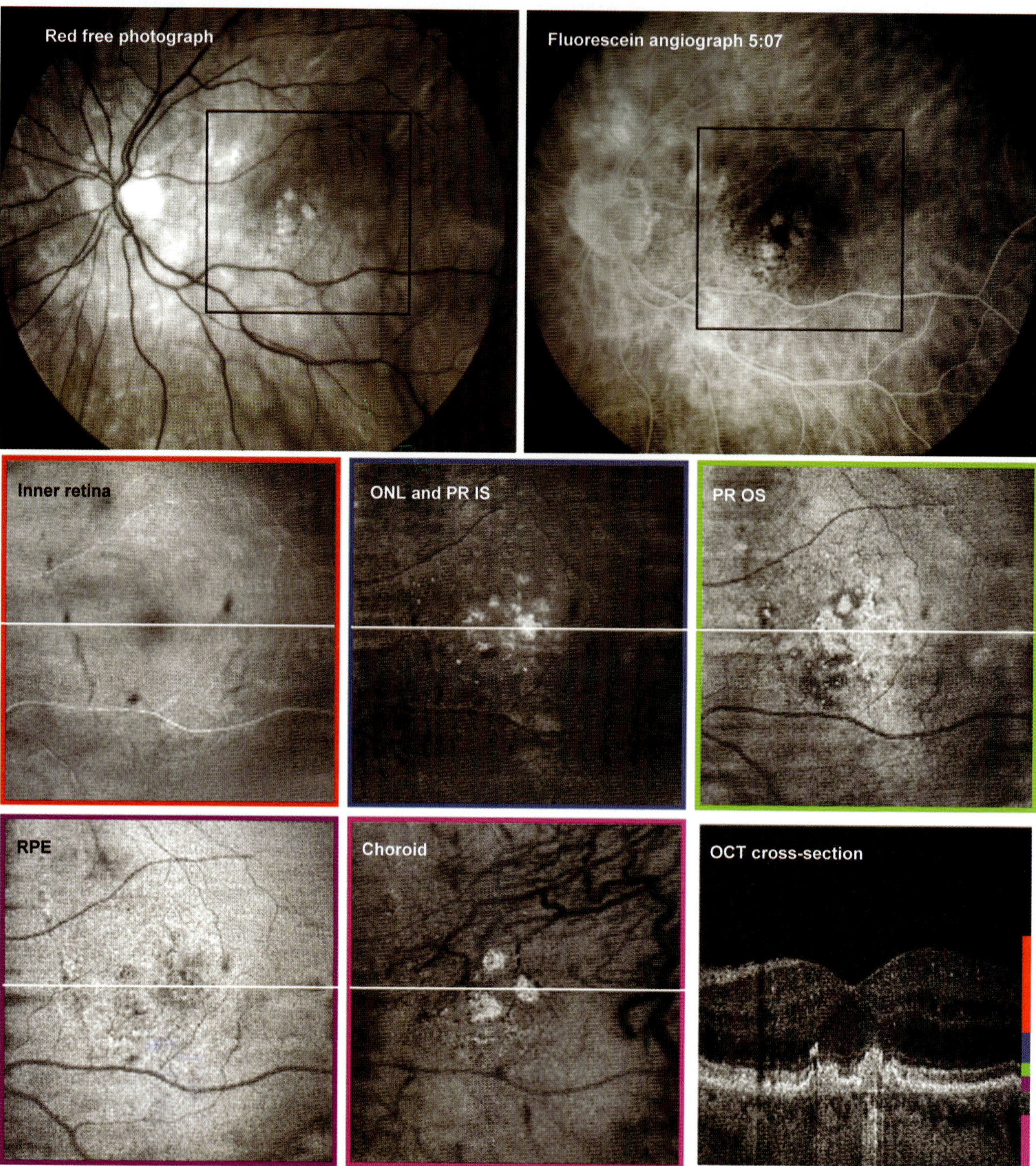

Figures 5A and B: *En face* OCT images in dry AMD. (A) Red-free photograph; (B) Fluorescein angiograph. *En face* OCT images from depth levels corresponding to the inner retina, outer nuclear layer (ONL) and photoreceptor inner segments (PR IS), photoreceptor outer segments (PR OS), retinal pigment epithelium (RPE) and choroid. Cross-sectional image at position indicated on the *en face* images. *En face* images provide increased contrast and show disruption of normal structure caused by drusen and RPE atrophy. Choroid level images show regions of RPE atrophy from increased light penetration into the choroid. Imaging was performed at 840 nm and image size is 6 mm x 6 mm (*Source*: Adapted from Gorczynska I, Srinivasan VJ, Vuong LN, et al. Projection OCT fundus imaging for visualizing outer retinal pathology in non-exudative age-related macular degeneration. Br J Ophthalmol. 2009;93(5): 603-9.)

HOW SWEPT SOURCE/FOURIER DOMAIN OCT DETECTION WORKS

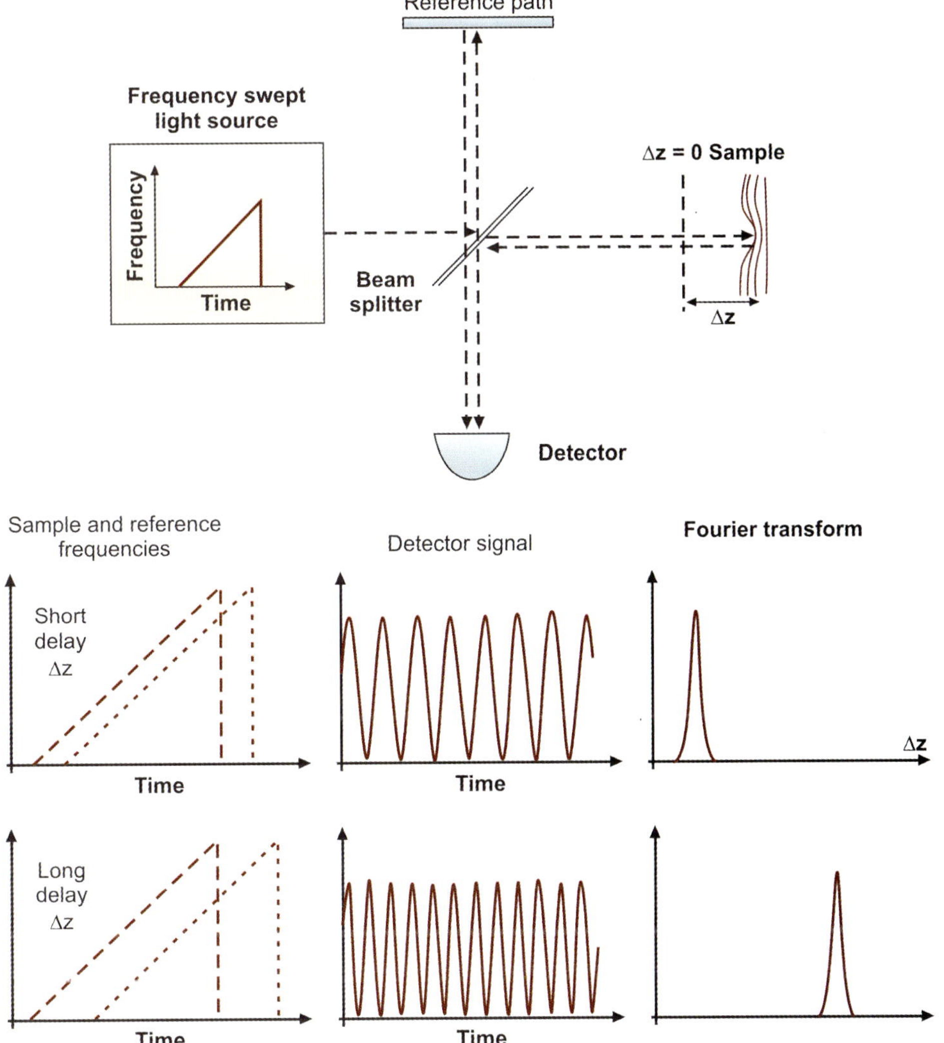

Figure 6: Shows a schematic of how swept source/Fourier domain detection works. Swept source/Fourier domain detection uses a narrow bandwidth, frequency swept light source as an input into an interferometer. The output of the interferometer is detected with a high speed photodetector without the need for a spectrometer and line scan camera. In swept source/ Fourier domain detection, different echo time delays of light are encoded as different oscillation frequencies in time when the laser light source is frequency swept. The echo time delays can be measured by Fourier transforming the detector signal to extract the oscillation frequencies. Swept source/Fourier domain detection can also be understood by noting that the frequency sweep in the light source essentially labels different times with different frequencies of light. The output from the swept light source is split into two paths. One light path is directed onto tissue and light is backreflected or backscattered from structures at different depths. The second light path is reflected from a fixed (not scanned) reference mirror at a given delay. The signal path from the tissue and the reference path have a relative time delay Δz related to the depth of the structure in the tissue. The interference of the two light paths will produce an oscillation or beat frequency because there is a frequency difference between the two light waves at the detector. The oscillation frequency will be related to the echo time delay Δz. Larger echo delays will produce higher frequency oscillations. Similar to spectral/ Fourier domain detection, the echo delays or axial scans can be measured by Fourier transforming the detector signal acquired over one frequency sweep of the light source. Each frequency sweep of the light source generates one axial scan and the axial scan imaging rate is determined by the sweep repetition rate of the light source.

line scan cameras. Imaging with longer wavelengths near 1050 nm has the advantage that scattering loss from cataracts and ocular opacities are reduced and image penetration is improve compared to 800 nm wavelengths used in commercial OCT instruments.[23,24] In addition, safe ocular exposure limits for 1050 nm are slightly higher than for 850 nm, allowing higher incident light levels to be used for imaging. These combined advantages enable swept source/Fourier domain OCT to achieve ultrahigh imaging speeds as well as to image deep retinal structures, such as the choroid and optic nerve head.

Swept source/Fourier domain OCT has a long history of development leading up to its present iteration. Swept source detection techniques were used 20 years ago to perform measurements in fiber optics and photonics components. Swept source/Fourier domain OCT was demonstrated by our group as early as 1997 by Chinn et al[22] and Golubovic et al,[21] but performance was limited by the available laser technology. Advances in swept source OCT imaging speed have been closely related to advances in laser technology because axial scan rates are determined by the laser sweep repetition rate. Studies by Yun et al. in 2003 demonstrated OCT imaging with 19,000 axial scans per second and 13–14 μm axial resolution in free space.[25] Imaging speeds of 115,000 axial scans per second were achieved in 2005 using swept laser technology with a diffraction grating and rotating polygon mirror tuner.[26] The development of a new swept laser technology known as Fourier domain modelocking or FDML (not related to Fourier domain OCT) by Huber et al in 2006 overcame many of the fundamental limitations to laser sweep speed and enabled dramatic increases in swept source OCT imaging speeds.[27]

Figures 7A and B and **8A to E** show examples of record imaging speed results from Srinivasan et al in 2008.[28] Images were acquired with a laboratory prototype instrument using an FDML laser at 249,000 axial scans per second and 1050 nm wavelength with an axial resolution of 8 μm in tissue. **Figures 7A and B** show a 3D volumetric image of the optic nerve head with 512 × 450 axial scans (more than 4x greater than standard 200 × 200 volumetric data sets in current ophthalmic instruments) which was acquired in only ~1 second. The 3D rendering and cross-sectional image shows deep image penetration into the optic nerve head and lamina cribrosa. Sequential *en face* OCT images generated from the 3D volumetric data show the lamina cribrosa at different depths. Pore size decreases with depth relative to the RPE and larger pores are observed in the superior and inferior portions of the lamina. **Figures 8A to E** show a 3D volumetric image of the retina with 512 × 850 axial scans which was acquired in ~2 seconds. In this example,

different retinal layers or boundaries were detected and segmented to better display *en face* OCT images corresponding to retinal layers. *En face* OCT images from the retinal nerve fiber layer show the orientation of the nerve fibers. Images from the ganglion cell layer and inner nuclear/inner plexiform layer show retinal vasculature and capillary networks. Visualization of small features such as capillaries requires higher pixel density images and larger numbers of axial scans. These results highlight the importance of increases in image acquisition speeds which enable higher pixel density *en face* imaging.

Commercially available swept lasers at 1050 nm using polygon mirror tunable filter technology were employed for swept source OCT retinal imaging at 28,000 axial scans per second and 10 μm axial resolution.[30] Swept lasers using microelectromechanical systems (MEMS) tunable filter technology could achieve higher imaging speeds of 100,000 to 200,000 axial scans per second with 7 μm axial resolution.[31] The most recent advances in swept laser technology have been using vertical cavity surface emitting laser (VCSEL) technology. Imaging speeds of 580,000 axial scans per second have been recently demonstrated at 1050 nm wavelength with 9 μm axial resolution. These imaging speeds enable a 1024 × 1024 axial scan volumetric data set to be acquired in only ~1.8 seconds.[32] **Figures 9A to E** show an example of wide field swept source/ Fourier domain retinal imaging. The 3D rendering is shown without motion correction and has relatively little motion artifact due to the rapid acquisition time. The long wavelengths enable deep image penetration and *en face* OCT images from the choriocapillaris and choroid show vasculature behind the RPE. The extremely high imaging speeds are essential in order to acquire the large numbers of axial scans needed to generate high pixel density *en face* OCT images.

Optical coherence tomography (OCT) imaging using FDML swept laser technology has continued to advance and imaging speeds of ~680,000 and ~1,300,000 axial scans per second at 1050 nm with 12 μm and 19 μm axial resolutions, respectively were demonstrated in 2011.[33] These ultrahigh imaging speeds enable wide field retinal coverage, however there are trade-offs in image resolution and range. In addition, for any system, there is an ultimate trade off in sensitivity versus imaging speed. It is likely that practical imaging speeds for clinical ophthalmic imaging will be in the range of 200,000 to 500,000 axial scan per second because of sensitivity requirements. Imaging speeds for these future clinical instruments will be slower than laboratory prototype instruments, but should still be factors of 10 times faster than current commercial instruments.

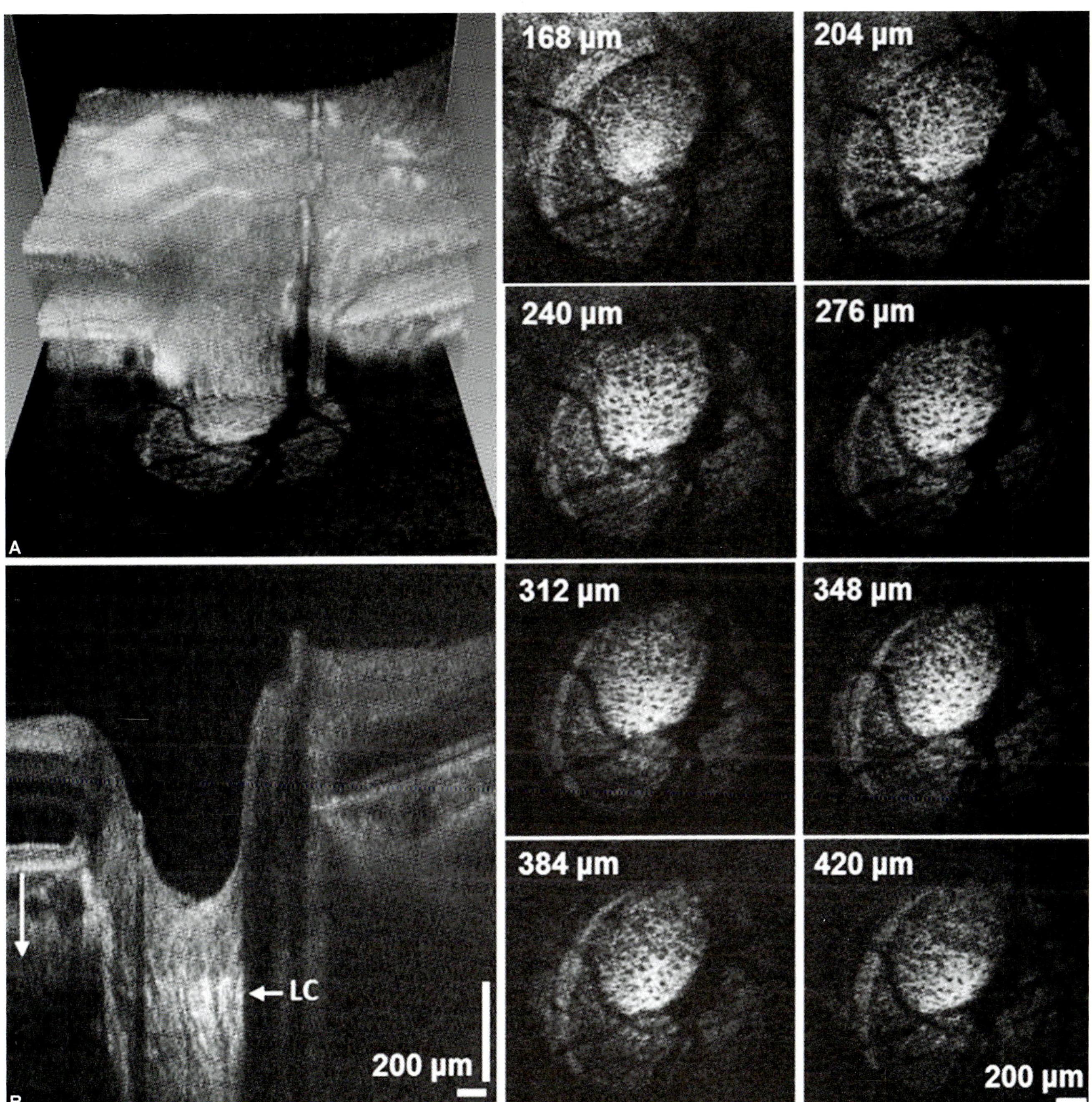

Figures 7A and B: Ultrahigh speed swept source/Fourier domain OCT imaging of the optic nerve head. Imaging was performed using an FDML laser at 249,000 axial scans per second and 1050 nm wavelength. (A) 3D rendering of volumetric data of the normal optic nerve heard; (B) Representative cross-sectional image showing deep image penetration depth in the lamina cribrosa (LC). Series of eight, *en face* OCT images in the optic nerve head at different depth levels relative to the RPE (arrow in B). Images consist of 512 x 450 axial scans and were acquired in ~1 second (*Source*: Adapted from Srinivasan VJ, Adler DC, Chen YL, et al. Ultrahigh-Speed Optical Coherence Tomography for Three-Dimensional and *En face* Imaging of the Retina and Optic Nerve Head. Investigative Ophthalmology & Visual Science. 2008;49:5103-10.)

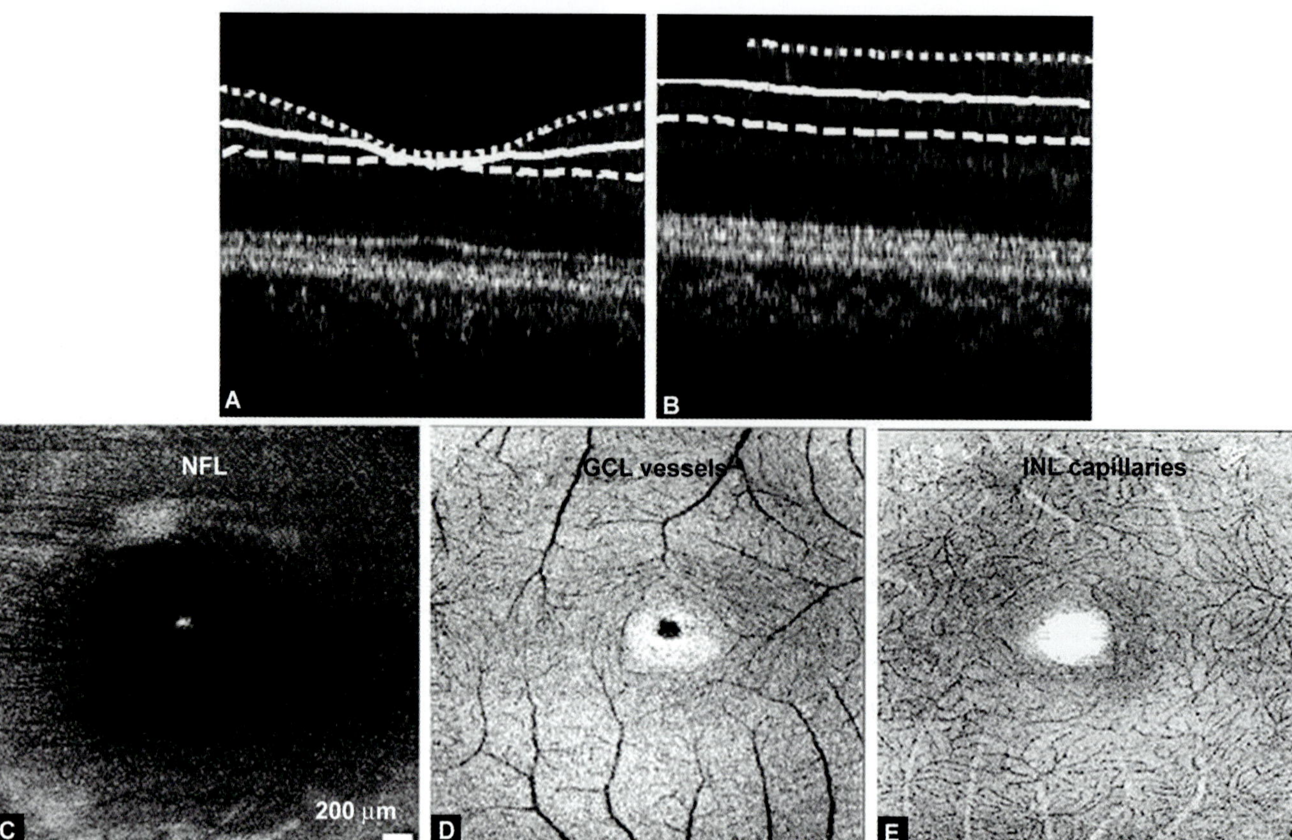

Figures 8A to E: Ultrahigh speed swept source/Fourier domain OCT retinal imaging. Imaging was performed using an FDML laser at 249,000 axial scans per second and 1050 nm wavelength. (A and B) Different retinal layers or boundaries are delineated and used as reference surfaces for axial summation. *En face* OCT images from (C) retinal nerve fiber layer, (D) ganglion cell layer and (E) inner nuclear/plexiform layer. Images are displayed with an inverted gray scale. Imaging was performed over a 3 mm x 3 mm area with 512 x 850 axial scans acquired in ~2 seconds (*Source*: Adapted from Srinivasan VJ, Adler DC, Chen YL, et al. Ultrahigh-Speed Optical Coherence Tomography for Three-Dimensional and *En face* Imaging of the Retina and Optic Nerve Head. Investigative Ophthalmology & Visual Science. 2008;49:5103-10.)

Increasing Image Acquisition Time Using Motion Tracking and Compensation

Sensitivity constraints limit the ultimate acquisition speeds for OCT instrumentation, even using the most advanced spectral or swept source/Fourier domain technologies. However, another approach for acquiring larger numbers of axial scans is to increase the imaging time by reducing or compensating for the effects of eye motion. Eye tracking techniques enable eye motion to be measured in real time and the OCT beam to be scanned to compensate for eye motion.[34,35] Eye motion can be measured using a separate tracking beam which scans landmark features on the retina or by using a fundus image generated by an SLO or video camera and these methods have different accuracies and response times. Eye tracking has been implemented in several

commercial OCT instruments and enables increased image acquisition times of several seconds. Eye tracking is also extensively used in combination with image averaging, where multiple OCT scans are performed on a tracked location of the fundus in order to improve sensitivity and image quality by reducing speckle noise.

Software based registration techniques are another approach for compensating motion artifacts in OCT data. Software methods have the advantage that they typically do not require special hardware that is used for eye tracking. Early time domain OCT systems used cross-correlation methods on sequential axial scans in order to compensate for axial eye motion within a cross-sectional image or B scan.[6] Since OCT images are typically expanded in the axial direction for display purposes, they are very sensitive to distortion from micron scale axial eye motion. Axial scan motion correction produced smooth retinal images, but

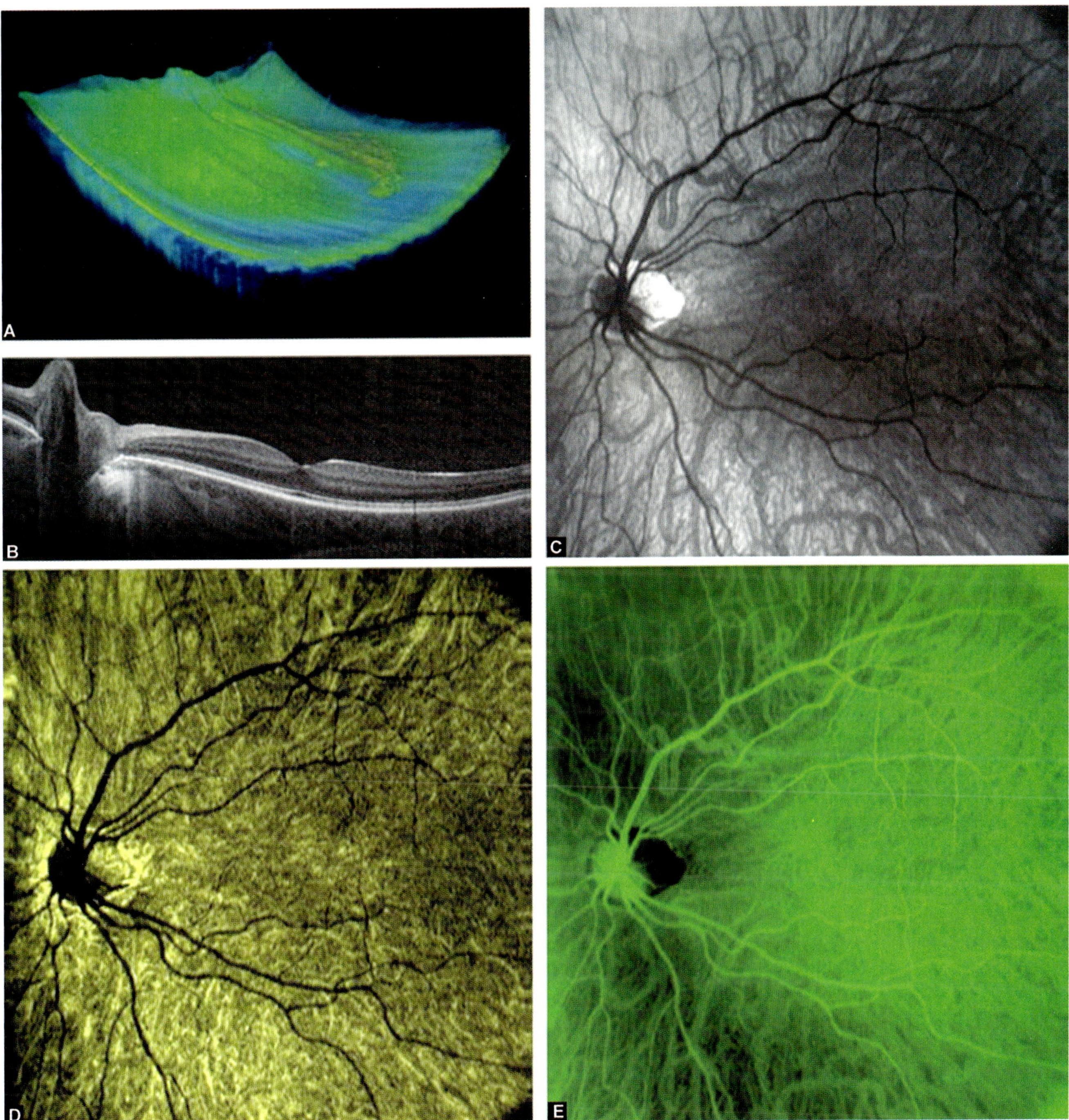

Figures 9A to E: Wide field, ultrahigh speed swept source/Fourier domain OCT retinal imaging. Imaging was performed using VCSEL light source at 580,000 axial scans per second and 1050 nm wavelengths. (A) 3D rendering of volumetric wide-field data set; (B) Cross-sectional image showing deep image penetration and ability to visualize choroid; (C) *En face* OCT image from summing entire axial range showing 12 mm x 12 mm field; (D) *En face* OCT image summing 30 µm below the RPE; (E) *En face* OCT image summing the entire choroid. Color has been added for emphasis (*Courtesy* of I Grulkowski.)

resulted in loss of retinal contour and topography. With the development of spectral/Fourier domain OCT which could acquire cross-sectional images or B scans within a few thousandths of a second, motion within a single B scan became negligible. However, acquisition of volumetric data sets by raster scanning still requires an acquisition time of seconds and therefore axial as well as transverse motion which occurs from B scan to B scan can produce significant motion artifacts.

Recently a software based method for compensating transverse as well as axial motion was developed by Kraus et al.[36] **Figure 10** shows a schematic of how this software motion correction method works. Two 3D volumetric data sets are acquired using complementary scan patterns, with a horizontal raster and a vertical raster. The effects of motion are different in each data set and motion is estimated and compensated for the horizontal and vertical raster scan data sets. The motion estimates are calculated under the assumption

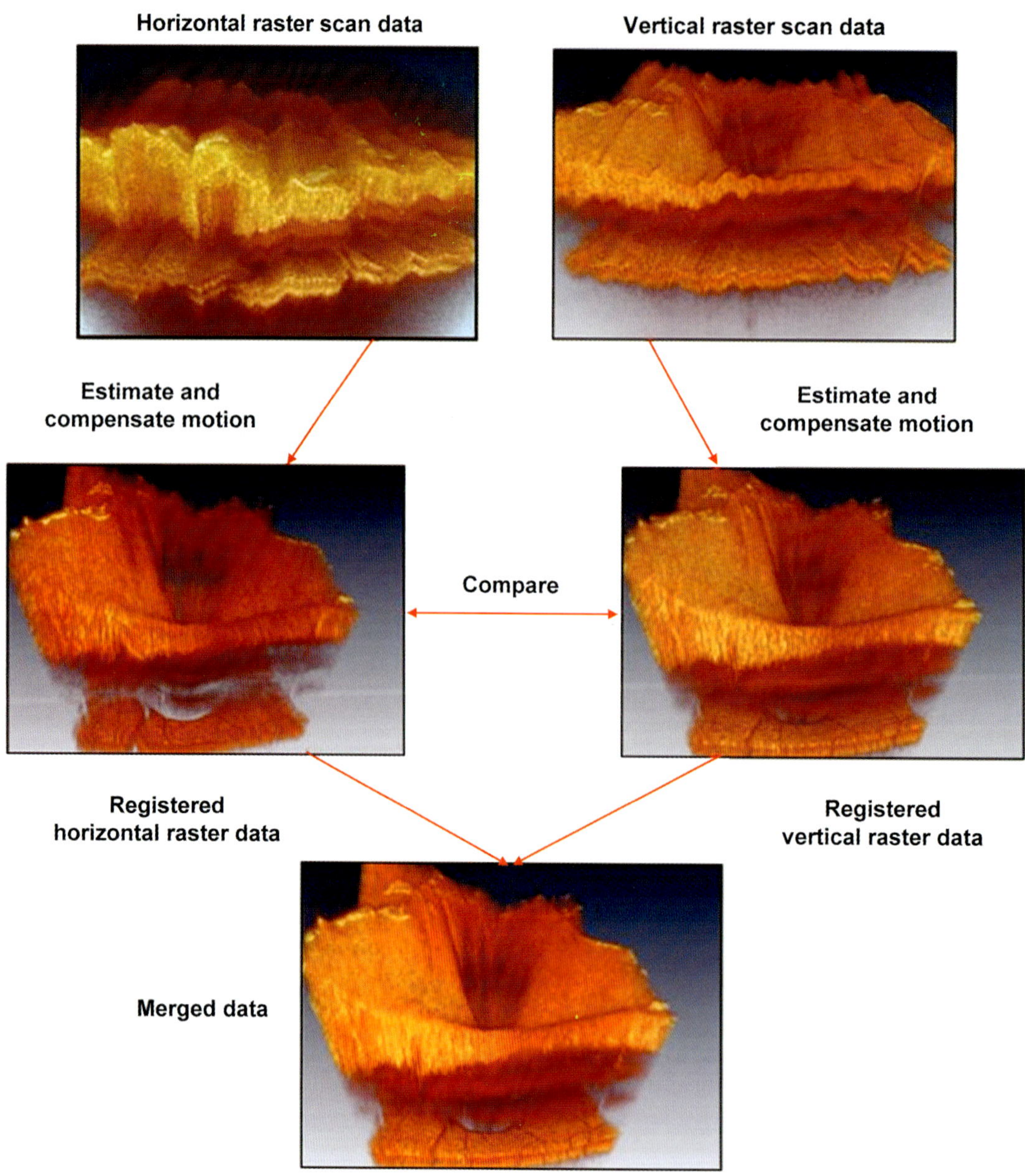

Figure 10: Software based motion correction. The method uses two input volumes acquired with orthogonal raster scans. Motion is estimated by iteratively compensating the motion in the two volumes and comparing them under the assumption that the motion corrected volumes should be similar as similar as possible. Motion corrected volumetric data sets are merged to create a motion corrected data set with improved signal and image quality (*Courtesy* of J Hornegger and M Kraus.)

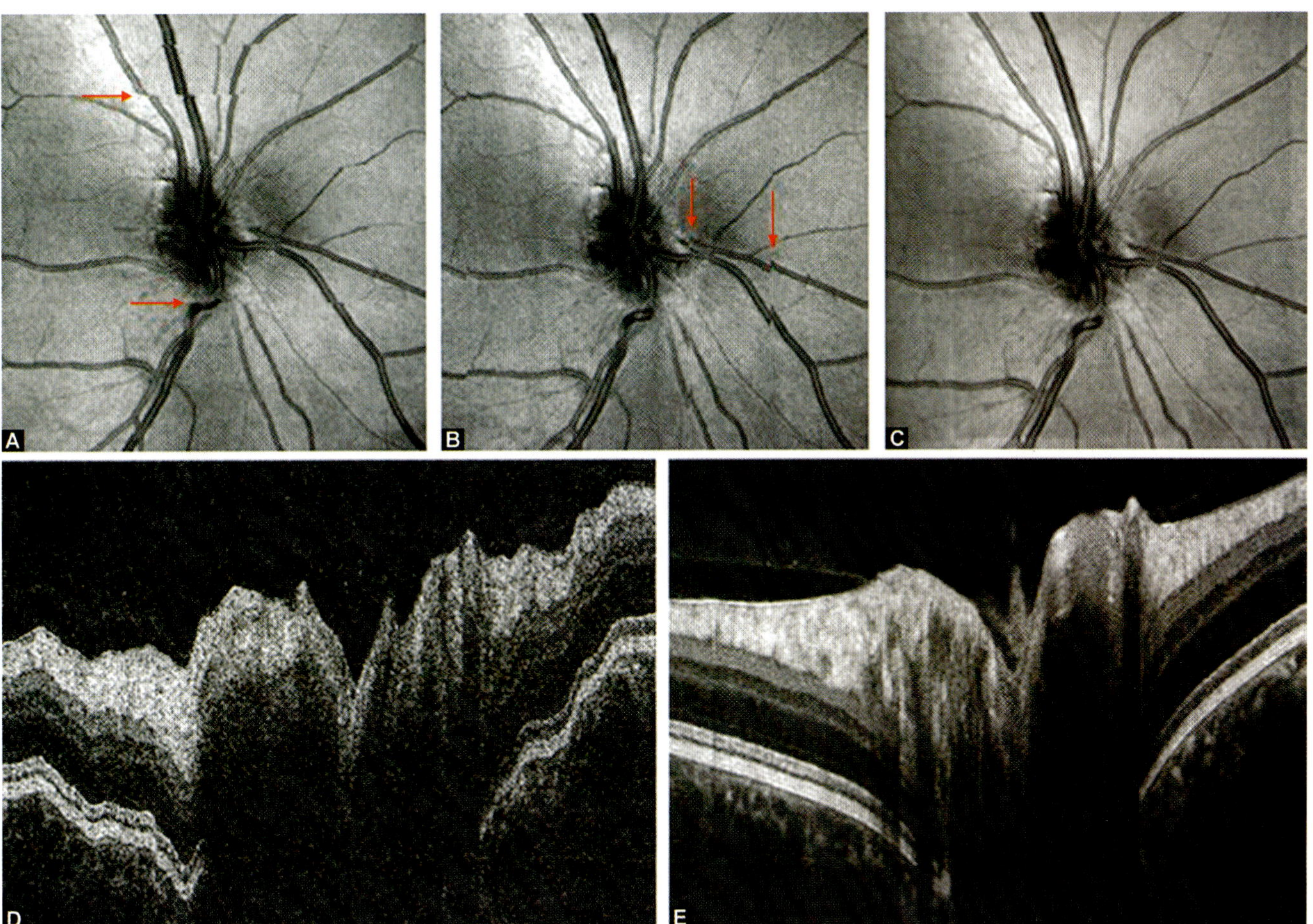

Figures 11A to E: Motion correction on a volumetric optic nerve head data set. (A and B) _En face_ OCT image of volumetric data from horizontally and vertically oriented raster scans; (C) _En face_ OCT of motion corrected merged volumetric data showing compensation of motion distortion; (D) Representative cross-sectional image from the input data set with the cross section taken perpendicular to the B scan direction to show motion; (E) Representative cross-sectional image from the motion corrected volume (_Courtesy_ of J Hornegger and M Kraus.)

that the motion corrected data sets should be as similar as possible, but with the constraint that the eye motion is limited as a function of time. The two motion corrected volumetric data sets can then be combined or merged into a single volumetric data set which has improved signal and reduced noise.

Figures 11A to E show an example of motion correction. (A and B) show _en face_ OCT images of horizontal and vertical raster scan volumes. Transverse eye motion is visible as discontinuities in the _en face_ images. The _en face_ OCT of the registered merged volume; (C) shows a corrected _en face_ OCT image without motion distortion; (D) shows a representative vertical cross-sectional image from the horizontal raster scan image of **Figure 11A**. The image is in the direction perpendicular to the B scans and significant motion distortion is present; (E) shows a cross-sectional image from the same location in the registered and motion corrected

data set. The image demonstrates that the effects of axial eye motion have been corrected. In addition, the sensitivity and image quality is improved because two volumetric data sets have been combined and merged to create the motion corrected volumetric data set.

Software motion correct is relatively new and still requires validation on subjects with retinal pathologies. However, this example suggests that software motion correction methods can play an important role in future OCT imaging. Motion correction is important for _en face_ OCT because it can enable longer acquisition times required to generate large numbers of axial scans for high definition _en face_ images. Combined with ultrahigh speed imaging speed OCT instrumentation, these methods promise to enable the acquisition of _en face_ OCT images with multi-megapixel resolution corresponding to volumetric data sets with multi-gigavoxel size. In addition, motion correction promises to

EN FACE OCT IMAGING IN ART CONSERVATION

En face OCT imaging can be applied in a wide range of applications outside of ophthalmology. **Figures 12A to E** show *en face* OCT in the field of art conservation.[29] Imaging was performed using a swept source OCT system at 42,000 axial scans per second operating at 1300 nm wavelength with an axial resolution of 9 µm in air (corresponding to ~6 µm in paint or varnish). The long 1300 nm wavelengths in the infrared enable image penetration through paints or pigments which are opaque at visible wavelengths. Imaging was performed using a microscope with a 30 mm working distance and a 30 µm spot using 10 mW of incident power. 3D volumetric OCT datasets consisted of 1024 × 1024 axial scans over a 6 mm × 6 mm region of the painting. The figure shows a color photograph of the painting, an infrared photograph of the underdrawing, drawn in charcoal before the application of pigments. The *en face* OCT images are the summed signals from various depths showing surface and internal features. *En face* OCT imaging in art conservation is an interesting analog to ophthalmic retinal imaging, because imaging must be performed non-destructively. *En face* OCT enables visualization of internal features in the painting which are hidden by surface reflection and scattering and validates Duguay's original proposal of "gated picture ranging".[4]

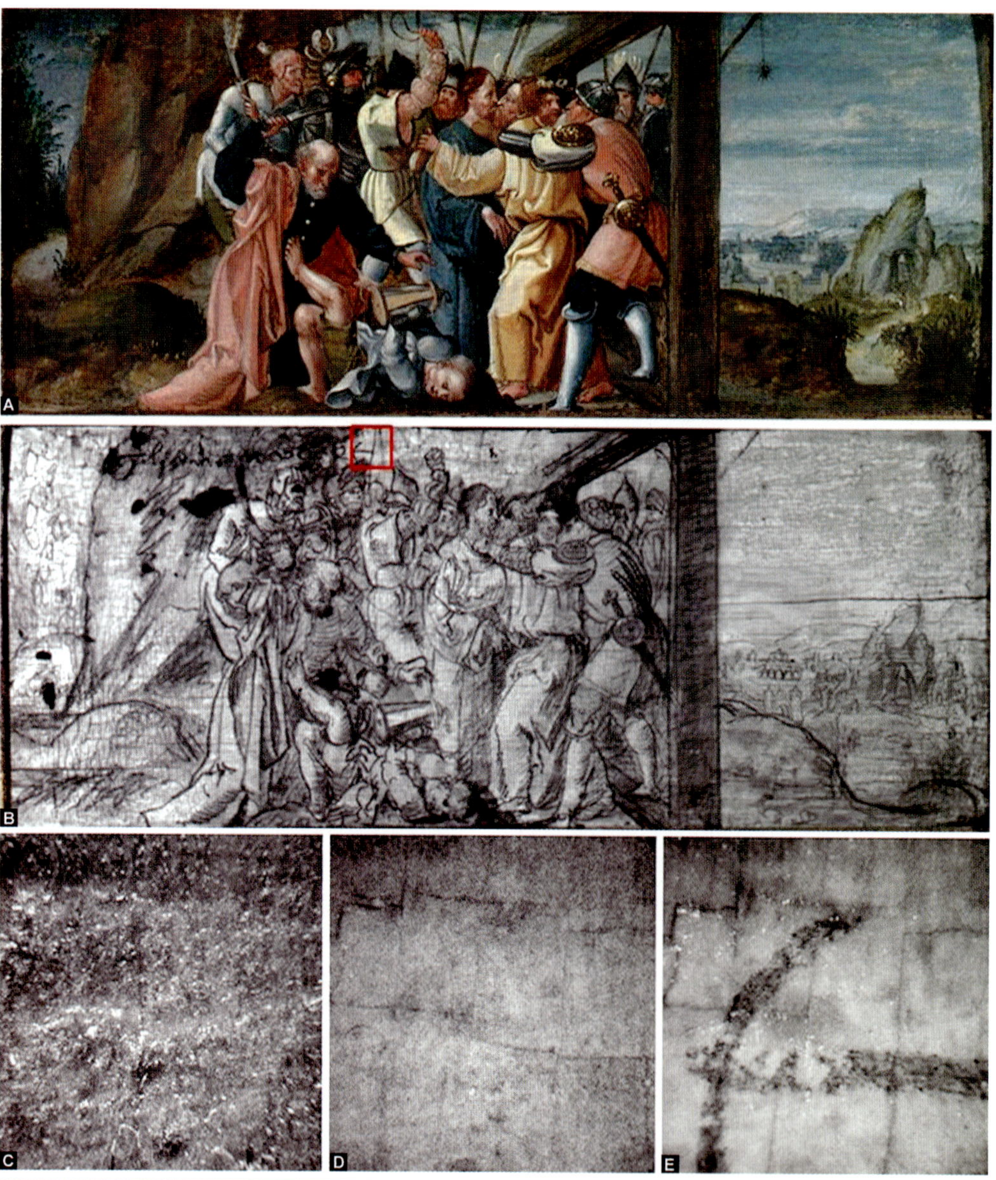

Figures 12A to E: *En face* OCT of painting "Arrest of Christ," circa 1520. (A) Color photograph. (33.8 cm x 13.5 cm); (B) Infrared photograph of the underdrawing, with red box showing region of OCT. *En face* OCT images of (C) varnish layer; (D) paint layer and (E) underdrawing layer. *En face* OCT images provide enhanced contrast of subsurface features. Imaging was performed at 1300 nm wavelength over a 6 mm x 6 mm area with 1024 x 1024 axial scans (*Source:* Adapted from Adler DC, Stenger J, Gorczynska I, et al. Comparison of three-dimensional optical coherence tomography and high resolution photography for art conservation studies. Optics Express 2007;15:15972-86.)

improve the reproducibility of quantitative measurements such as nerve fiber layer or retinal layer thickness. Improved reproducibility, combined with the ability to compare features in volumetric data sets over time, from different patient visits, promises to improve the sensitivity for measuring disease progression and response to therapy. These advances are particularly interesting for pharmaceutical development, because improved sensitivity can reduce clinical trial times.

Summary

En face OCT is a powerful and intuitive method for visualizing retinal pathology. However, from a technological viewpoint it is one of the most demanding imaging modalities because each *en face* OCT image pixel requires one axial scan in a 3D volumetric data set. Furthermore, in order to increase retinal coverage, retinal area increases as the square of the linear dimension scanned, placing severe demands on imaging speeds and data size. The development of new spectral and swept source/Fourier domain detection technologies promises to increase imaging speeds by 10 times compared with current clinical instrumentation. However, the development process for clinical instrumentation is complex and demanding because of engineering and regulatory requirements. Therefore, the translation of new technology from laboratory prototype to widespread clinical practice can move slowly. However, software methods for motion correction are also a promising area of development and software advances can often progress more rapidly than hardware advances. Methods for motion correction can significantly extend image acquisition times and represent another complementary approach for obtaining large volumetric data sets needed for high definition, high pixel density *en face* OCT imaging. These complementary approaches promise to enable continued advances for *en face* OCT imaging, improving image quality as well as the ability to more sensitively diagnose disease and assess progression and response to therapy.

References

1. Webb RH, Hughes GW, Pomerantzeff O. Flying Spot TV Ophthalmoscope. Applied Optics. 1980;19:2991-7.
2. Webb RH, Hughes GW, Delori FC. Confocal Scanning Laser Ophthalmoscope. Applied Optics. 1987;26:1499.
3. Duguay MA. Light photographed in flight. American Scientist. 1971;59:551-6.
4. Duguay MA, Mattick AT. Ultrahigh speed photography of picosecond light pulses and echoes. Applied Optics. 1971;10:2162-70.
5. Huang D, Swanson EA, Lin CP, et al. Optical coherence tomography. Science. 1991;254:1178-81.
6. Swanson EA, Izatt JA, Hee MR, et al. In vivo retinal imaging by optical coherence tomography. Optics Letters. 1993;18:1864-6.
7. Podoleanu AG, Dobre GM, Webb DJ, et al. Simultaneous en-face imaging of two layers in the human retina by low-coherence reflectometry. Opt Lett. 1997;22:1039-41.
8. Podoleanu AG, Seeger M, GM Dobre, et al. Transversal and longitudinal images from the retina of the living eye using low coherence reflectometry. Journal of Biomedical Optics. 1998;3:12-20.
9. Fercher AF, Hitzenberger CK, Kamp G, et al. Measurement of intraocular distances by backscattering spectral interferometry. Optics Communications. 1995;117:43-8.
10. Wojtkowski M, Leitgeb R, Kowalczyk A, et al. In vivo human retinal imaging by Fourier domain optical coherence tomography. Journal of Biomedical Optics. 2002;7:457-63.
11. de Boer JF, Cense B, Park BH, et al. Improved signal-to-noise ratio in spectral-domain compared with time-domain optical coherence tomography. Optics Letters. 2003;28:2067-9.
12. Choma M, Sarunic M, Yang C, et al. Sensitivity advantage of swept source and Fourier domain optical coherence tomography. Optics Express. 2003;11:2183-9.
13. Leitgeb R, Hitzenberger CK, Fercher AF. Performance of Fourier domain vs. time domain optical coherence tomography. Optics Express. 2003;11:889-94.
14. Nassif N, Cense B, Park BH, et al. In vivo human retinal imaging by ultrahigh-speed spectral domain optical coherence tomography. Opt Lett. 2004;29:480-2.
15. Wojtkowski M, Srinivasan VJ, Ko TH, et al. Ultrahigh-resolution, high-speed, Fourier domain optical coherence tomography and methods for dispersion compensation. Optics Express. 2004;12:2404-22.
16. Wojtkowski M, Srinivasan V, Fujimoto JG, et al. Three-dimensional retinal imaging with high-speed ultrahigh-resolution optical coherence tomography. Ophthalmology. 2005;112:1734-46.
17. Wojtkowski M, Bajraszewski T, Gorczynska I, et al. Ophthalmic imaging by spectral optical coherence tomography. Am J Ophthalmol. 2004;138:412-9.
18. Jiao S, Knighton R, Huang X, et al. Simultaneous acquisition of sectional and fundus ophthalmic images with spectral-domain optical coherence tomography. Optics Express. 2005;13.
19. Gorczynska I, Srinivasan VJ, Vuong LN, et al. Projection OCT fundus imaging for visualising outer retinal pathology in non-exudative age-related macular degeneration. British Journal of Ophthalmology. 2009;93:603-9.
20. Potsaid B, Gorczynska I, Srinivasan VJ, et al. Ultrahigh speed Spectral/Fourier domain OCT ophthalmic imaging at 70,000 to 312,500 axial scans per second. Optics Express. 2008;16:15149-69.
21. Golubovic B, Bouma BE, Tearney GJ, et al. Optical frequency-domain reflectometry using rapid wavelength tuning of a Cr4+:forsterite laser. Optics Letters. 1997;22:1704-06.

22. Chinn SR, Swanson EA, Fujimoto JG. Optical coherence tomography using a frequency-tunable optical source. Optics Letters. 1997;22:340-2.

23. Unterhuber A, Povazay B, Hermann B, et al. In vivo retinal optical coherence tomography at 1040 nm-enhanced penetration into the choroid. Optics Express. 2005;13: 3252-8.

24. Povazay B, Hermann B, Unterhuber A, et al. Three-dimensional optical coherence tomography at 1050 nm versus 800 nm in retinal pathologies: enhanced performance and choroidal penetration in cataract patients. Journal of Biomedical Optics. 2007;12.

25. Yun SH, Tearney GJ, Bouma BE, et al. High-speed spectral-domain optical coherence tomography at 1.3 mu m wavelength. Optics Express. 2003;11:3598-3604.

26. Oh WY, Yun SH, Tearney GJ, et al. 115 kHz tuning repetition rate ultrahigh-speed wavelength-swept semiconductor laser. Optics Letters. 2005;30:3159-61.

27. Huber R, Wojtkowski M, Fujimoto JG. Fourier Domain Mode Locking (FDML): A new laser operating regime and applications for optical coherence tomography. Optics Express. 2006;14:3225-37.

28. Srinivasan VJ, Adler DC, Chen YL, et al. Ultrahigh-Speed Optical Coherence Tomography for Three-Dimensional and *En face* Imaging of the Retina and Optic Nerve Head. Investigative Ophthalmology & Visual Science. 49:2008; 5103-10.

29. Adler DC, Stenger J, Gorczynska I, et al. Comparison of three-dimensional optical coherence tomography and high resolution photography for art conservation studies. Optics Express. 2007;15:15972-86.

30. Yasuno Y, Hong YJ, Makita S, et al. In vivo high-contrast imaging of deep posterior eye by 1-mu m swept source optical coherence tomography and scattering optical coherence angiography. Optics Express. 2007;15: 6121-39.

31. Potsaid B, Baumann B, Huang D, et al. Ultrahigh speed 1050 nm swept source/Fourier domain OCT retinal and anterior segment imaging at 100,000 to 400,000 axial scans per second. Optics Express. 2010;18:20029-48.

32. Grulkowski I, Liu J, Potsaid B, et al. Retinal, anterior segment and full eye imaging using ultrahigh speed swept source OCT with vertical-cavity surface emitting lasers. Biomedical Optics Express. 2012;3:2733-51.

33. Klein T, Wieser W, Eigenwillig CM, et al. Megahertz OCT for ultrawide-field retinal imaging with a 1050 nm Fourier domain mode-locked laser. Optics Express. 2011;19:3044-62.

34. Ferguson RD, Hammer DX, Paunescu LA, et al. Tracking optical coherence tomography. Optics Letters. 2004;29: 2139-41.

35. Hammer DX, Ferguson RD, Magill JC, et al. Active retinal tracker for clinical optical coherence tomography systems. Journal of Biomedical Optics. 2005;10:24038-41.

36. Kraus MF, Potsaid B, Mayer MA, et al. Motion correction in optical coherence tomography volumes on a per A scan basis using orthogonal scan patterns. Biomedical Optics Express. 2012;3:1182-99.

chapter 45

Adaptive Optics Fundus Imaging: Application to Age-related Macular Degeneration

Kyioko Gocho, Michel Paques

Introduction

Fundus imaging using adaptive optics (AO) has been developed in the last two decades by several teams in the world. Adaptive optics is basically an optoelectronic technique based on the dynamic adaptation of a deformable mirror to match the optical aberrations of the ocular milieu; this increases the lateral (albeit not the axial) resolution of images. Technically, AO may be combined to any fundus imaging system; either flood imaging, scanning laser ophthalmoscopy or optical coherence tomography (OCT). Current AO systems for fundus images allow a 1–5 μm lateral resolution. The actual resolution depends on a number of factors, among them the number of actuators of the deformable mirror.

Adaptive optics technology is reaching technological maturity, hence it can be expected that commercially available systems will soon enter clinical routine. The primary contribution of AO to clinical retinal imaging has been the observation of the cone photoreceptor mosaic (Liang et al).[1] Indeed, current concepts of the optical properties of the retina suggest that the outer segments of photoreceptors have a particularly high reflectance index as compared to other retinal structures; and, since in the posterior pole cones are larger than rods, the former are more easily detected. However, AO imaging has not yet entered routine clinical practice. This is partly due to the fact that interpretation of AO images in retinal diseases is not as straightforward as OCT; it is indeed sometime challenging because a number of factors may interfere with the obtained image. Among these factors are the level of pigmentation of the fundus, the transparency of the retina, the presence of other sources of light dispersion in diseased retina, the spatial and temporal variability of photoreceptor reflectance, and the variable orientation of photoreceptor outer segments. Current softwares for photoreceptor counting are therefore affected by significant intersession variability.

Despite the above mentioned difficulties, most studies of AO imaging focused on photoreceptor imaging. This may have overshadowed other possible applications of AO imaging. Most AO imaging systems uses infrared light, which is highly absorbed by melanin (Keilhauer and Delori).[2] It can be assumed that pigment redistribution reflect to some extent the degree of alteration of the retinal pigment epithelium (RPE), as shown by histological studies. To our knowledge there has been no AO imaging study of melanin dispersion. While performing AO images on patients with geographic atrophy, the dry form of age-related macular degeneration, the authors noted that even if photoreceptors were sometime hardly detectable because of media opacities, a strikingly precise mapping of melanin redistribution could be obtained in most cases. Indeed, it is known that the RPE is involved early in the process of age-related maculopathy, even before the occurrence of atrophy *per se*. The authors present here some examples of AO imaging of geographic atrophy which highlights these findings.

This study was sponsored by the INSERM, received academic funding from the Agence Nationale de la Recherche and was approved by an Ethics Committee. All patients gave informed consent to participate. The AO camera that we used (rtx1 camera, Imagine Eye, France) probes wavefront aberrations with a 750 nm superluminescent diode and corrects them with a 52 actuator AO system operating in a closed loop. The fundus is illuminated with a temporally low coherent light emitting diode flashed flood source operating at 840 nm. The lateral resolution of the system is approximately 3 μm, whereas its depth of field is approximately 40 μm. For image acquisition, the patient is positioned on a standard ophthalmic chin rest, with or without pupil dilation. A live video display of the pupil allows alignment of the pupil with the incident light. A live display of fundus image allows brightness, contrast and focus to be adjusted. A focus range of 800 μm enables to adjust the focus plane. Once the region of interest has been chosen and the focus adjusted, a stack of fundus images are acquired at a rate of 9.5 frames per second over 2 seconds in a 4° × 4° area by a charged coupled device camera (Roper Scientific, Tucson, AZ). It is estimated that in emmetropic eyes each image covers a 1.2 × 1.2 mm area. Each acquisition consists of a stack of 19 images, out of which 10 are digitally averaged to increase the signal to noise ratio. The minimal interval between the acquisitions of two images is approximately 1 minute.

An example of photoreceptor imaging in a normal subject is shown in **Figure 1**. By AO imaging, drusen were not directly visible. However, since they displaced the photo-receptor layer, they locally modified the reflectance of outer segments and hence became visible through a local Stile-Crawford effect **(Figure 2)**.

Patients with geographic atrophy (GA), with severities ranging from mild to extensive atrophy have been examined.

In all cases, AO imaging revealed in fine details the dispersion of melanin within GA lesions **(Figures 3 to 5)**. At higher magnification, such dispersion appeared as melanin clumps of variable size. Thanks to the higher contrast of melanin dispersion, borders of GA lesions could be delineated with greater precision than by scanning laser ophthalmoscope (SLO) imaging.

Our preliminary experience suggests that AO imaging in GA eyes is of particular interest in two situations:

- In presence of very small GA lesions; indeed, these areas could be followed-up at a small spatial scale, which is of obvious clinical interest.
- In presence of foveal sparing, in which there is a very small central island of retinal tissue supporting central vision **(Figures 5A and B)**.

At such level of resolution, histology is of significant help to interpret the images. A number of phenotypic changes occur in RPE cells during GA (Penfold, Curcio).[3,4] We found that many features reported by them, such as the presence of ectopic RPE cells and the accumulation of pigment at borders, beared many similarities with *in vivo* images. Also, such studies showed that melanosomes can be present

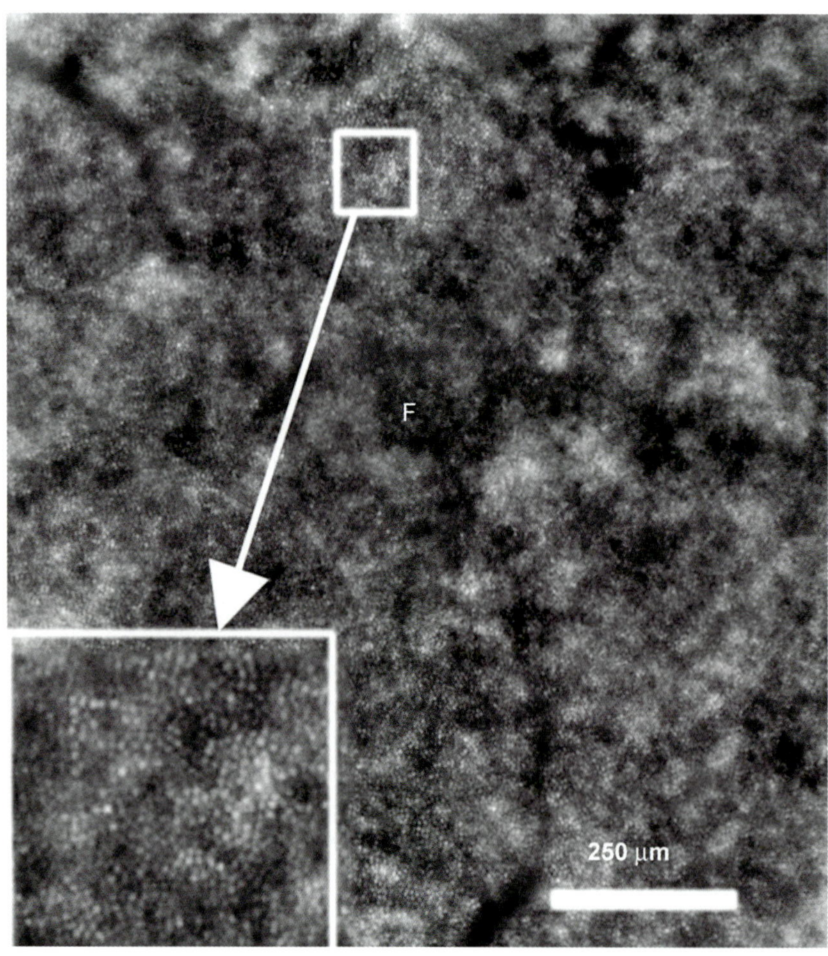

Figure 1: Typical image of the cone mosaic in a healthy retina of 66-year-old woman (F: fovea)

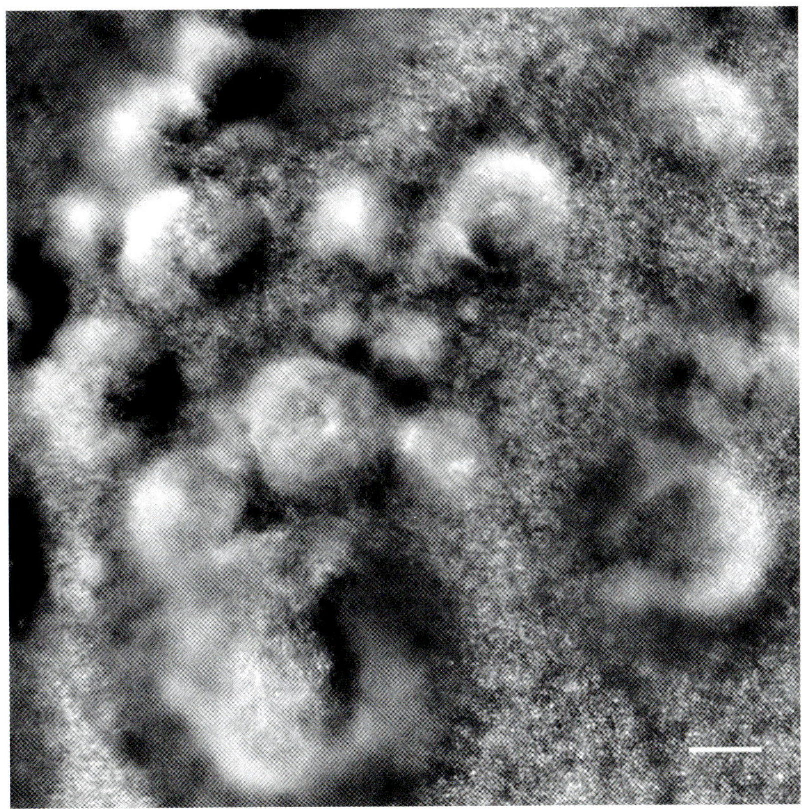

Figure 2: Typical aspect of drusens by adaptive optics imaging (Bar, 100 μm)

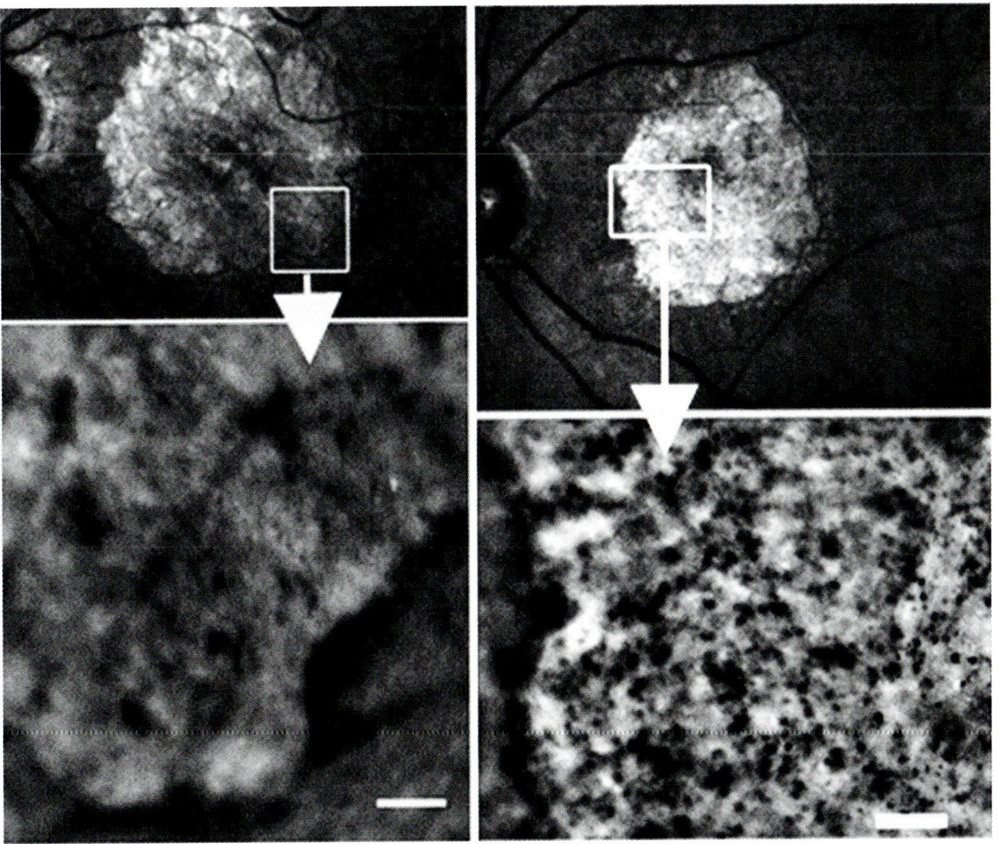

Figure 3: Comparison of scanning laser ophthalmoscopy infrared imaging (top) and adaptive optics imaging (bottom) in two cases of geographic atrophy (bars, 200 μm)

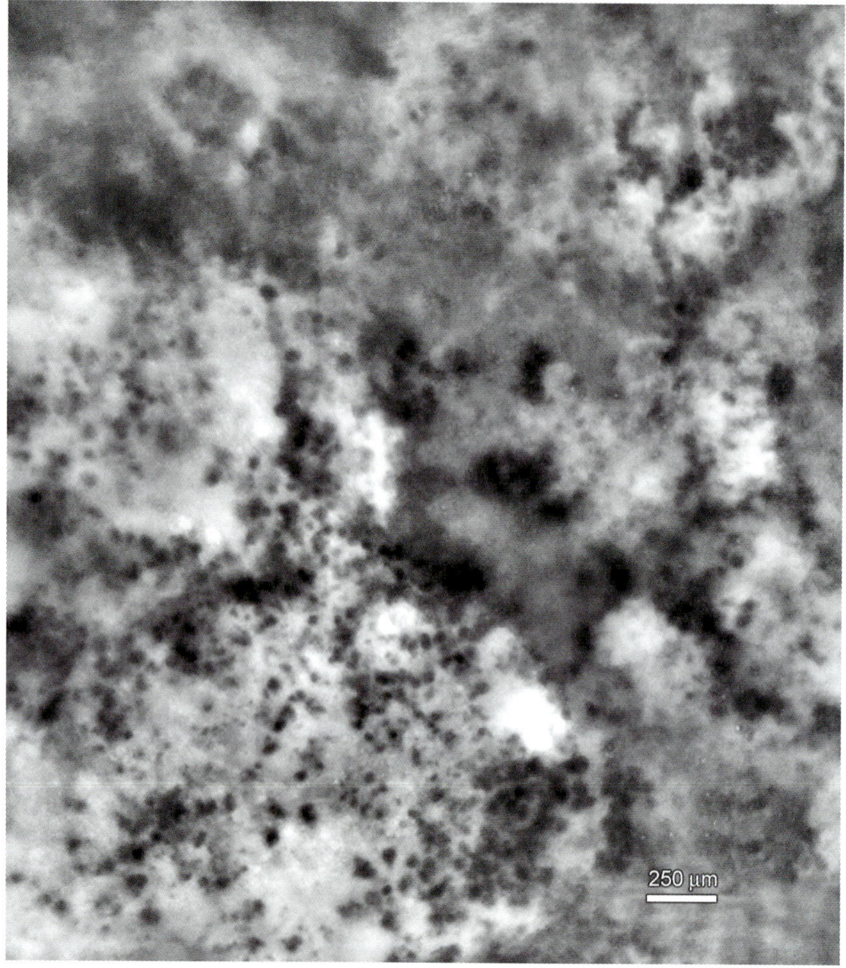

Figure 4: Adaptive optics image of a case of geographic atrophy showing extensive melanin dispersion within the atrophic area

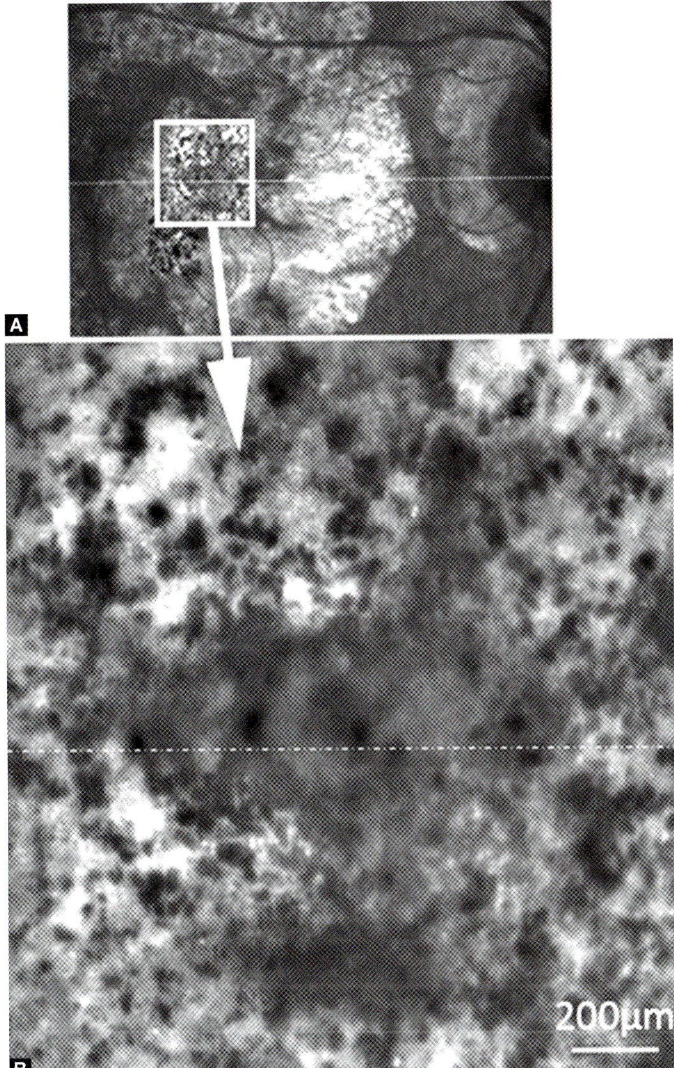

Figures 5A and B: Adaptive optics imaging of a case of geographic atrophy with foveal sparing. (A) Scanning laser ophthalmoscopy infrared reflectance image; (B) Adaptive optics imaging. The fovea is in the center of the image

intracellularly or extracellularly. The latter situation is described histologically as "pigment debris", which may account for the disseminated dust-like aspect of many GA lesions by *in vivo* imaging.

The authors experience shows that AO NIR imaging can therefore document microscopic features of GA at a small temporal and spatial scale, and is well suited for the documentation and follow-up of small GA lesions. Accurate characterization of the progression of atrophic lesions during GA is important for the estimation of its long-term prognosis and consequently for the evaluation of therapeutic results. More generally, our findings highlight the fact that AO imaging may bring information about the fundus of diseased eyes beyond photoreceptor detection. Further investigations are going on to identify other retinal structures that may benefit from AO imaging.

References

1. Liang J, Williams DR, Miller DT. Supernormal vision and high-resolution retinal imaging through adaptive optics. J Opt Soc. Am A Opt Image Sci Vis. 1997;14(11):2884-92.
2. Keilhauer CN, Delori FC. Near-infrared autofluorescence imaging of the fundus: visualization of ocular melanin. Invest Ophthalmol Vis Sci. 2006;47(8):3556-64.
3. Penfold PL, Killingsworth MC, Sarks SH. Senile macular degeneration. The involvement of giant cells in atrophy of the retinal pigment epithelium. Invest Ophthalmol Vis Sci. 1986;27(3):364-71.
4. Curcio CA, Medeiros NE, Millican CL. The Alabama Age-Related Macular Degeneration Grading System for donor eyes. Invest Ophthalmol Vis Sci. 1998;39(7):1085-96.

chapter 46

Near Adaptive Optics Quality Scanning Laser Ophthalmoscopy— Optical Coherence Tomography

Imaging Using Ultra-high Resolution Confocal Microscopy and Ultra-high Speed Spectral Domain Optical Coherence Tomography

Richard Rosen, Rishard Weitz, Mark Hathaway

Introduction

Retinal imaging has undergone tremendous advances since Helmholtz's ophthalmoscope provided the first glimpse of the fundus. It was clear from this first device that the *en face* or coronal orientation provided wealth of useful data for the clinician. Gullstrand's invention of slit lamp in 1911 added the capability of optical cross-sections, but the retina's transparency limited the doctor's grasp of the internal detail. With the introduction of infrared optical coherence tomography (OCT) in 1991, the ability to define layers within the transparent retina demonstrated the possibility of a histological-level examination and potentially cellular imaging in the clinic.[1-4]

Cellular-level imaging has an increasing number of clinical applications as treatment options expand. Measurement of photoreceptor loss or rescue could be very useful in the evaluation of new pharmaceuticals, gene therapies or stem cell implants. The ability to reliably detect microscopic progression of geographic atrophy could also significantly help shorten clinical trials, limiting prolonged studies of dead-end approaches, saving time, money and effort.

The optics of the eye has been a major limiting factor in achieving lateral resolution capable of detecting cellular boundaries. Cones range in size from 4.0 microns down to 0.5 microns in the foveal center, while rods are typically 2.5 microns in diameter. Williams, Liang, and Miller implemented adaptive optics, a technology first conceived for astronomy in 1953 to overcome atmospheric distortions, into an adaptive optics scanning laser ophthalmoscope (SLO) in 1997,[5,11] allowing the visualization of the cone mosaic

in the living eye. More recently in 2011, Dubra and Carroll have advanced the optical design to 2 micron lateral resolution enabling clear images of rods.

Despite the exceptional resolution of the adaptive optics SLO, its complexity, size and cost still pose significant barriers to its implementation as a workaday clinical tool. Investigating alternative solutions, Podoleanu, who first introduced *en face* optical coherence tomography with simultaneous SLO imaging in 1998,[6] and Hathaway conceived of a technique to achieve higher resolution with conventional SLO. They demonstrated the possibility of enhancing resolution by reducing the scanning angle. At scanned fields reduced to 6.5°or less, it was possible to see clearly defined cone bodies at a location eccentric to the fovea (**Figure 1**).

A clinical prototype, based on a modified commercial Opko-OTI SD-OCT/SLO, was developed by Hathaway and Weitz in 2009 which could exploit this enhanced resolution. Using an ultrafast spectrometer, with capabilities of capturing 100 frames/second at scanning field sizes ranging from 300 microns to 15,000 microns, the system was compact and simple enough for conventional clinical imaging. The added speed allowed acquisition of three-dimensional (3D) data sets capable of producing reformatted *en face* C scans which demonstrated exceptional detail to the level of cone mosaic resolution at the smallest field sizes. Utilizing the integrated OCT/SLO approach originally pioneered by Podoleanu, Jackson, Rogers, Dunne, and Weitz in the earlier OTI systems,[7-10] the current prototype allows consistent orientation at different levels of zoom and correlation between OCT cross-sectional features, SLO *en face* landmarks and flattened reformatted C scan OCT slices (**Figures 2 and 3**).

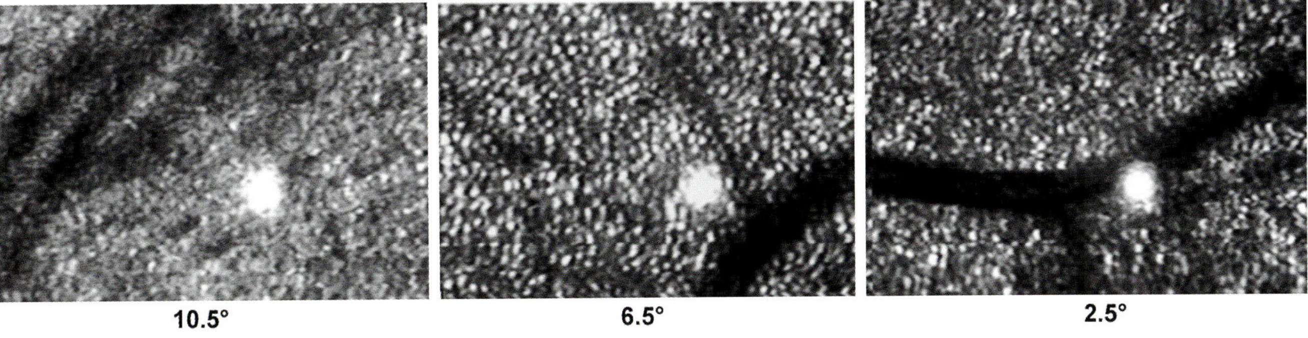

Figure 1: Progressively smaller fields captured with a full field scanning laser ophthalmoscope achieving magnification to the level of the cone mosaic by utilizing the full resolution of the standard scanning angle at reduced scanning angle (Podoleanu, Hathaway 2007)

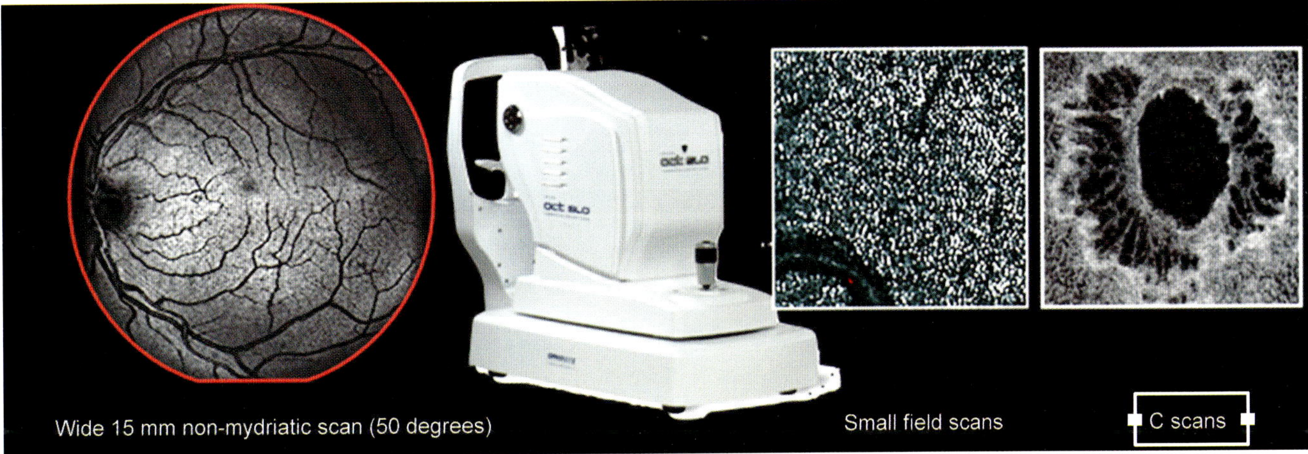

Figure 2: Ultra-high speed SD-OCT/SLO system with near-adaptive optics quality variable field scanning. Left image shows the widest view. Right images show small field and C scan examples

The resolving capability of this zooming technique compares favorably with the current generation of commercially available Adaptive Optics Imager (Imagine Eyes™), which has been optimized for cone counting (**Figure 4**).

One of the most clinically useful features of the system is the dense 3D data set which provides resolution sufficient to allow reconstruction of flattened C scan slices. These slices allow the examiner to interpret the depth information in relation to the surrounding fundus features. The higher speeds have the particular advantage of reducing movement artifacts which plagued the time-domain *en face* OCT images and the reconstruction process allows flattening which enables segmentation of layers. **Figure 5** demonstrates the sequence of representative segmented layers from 4 mm scans through a normal macula.

Reconstructed *En Face* C Scan Tomographic Dissection of the Retina

By reducing the scanning angle even further to 1 mm or 3.3° it is possible to see details of the deeper capillary beds of the retina (**Figures 5 and 6**).

The clinical value of this level of resolution is demonstrated in a case of a 36-year-old man who complained of a persistent positive scotoma noted following a particularly strenuous basketball workout. Conventional imaging with fluorescein angiography and spectral domain (SD)-OCT did not clearly corroborate his complaints, however, microperimetry testing showed some evidence of decreased sensitivity in the area of complain, small field OCT/SLO

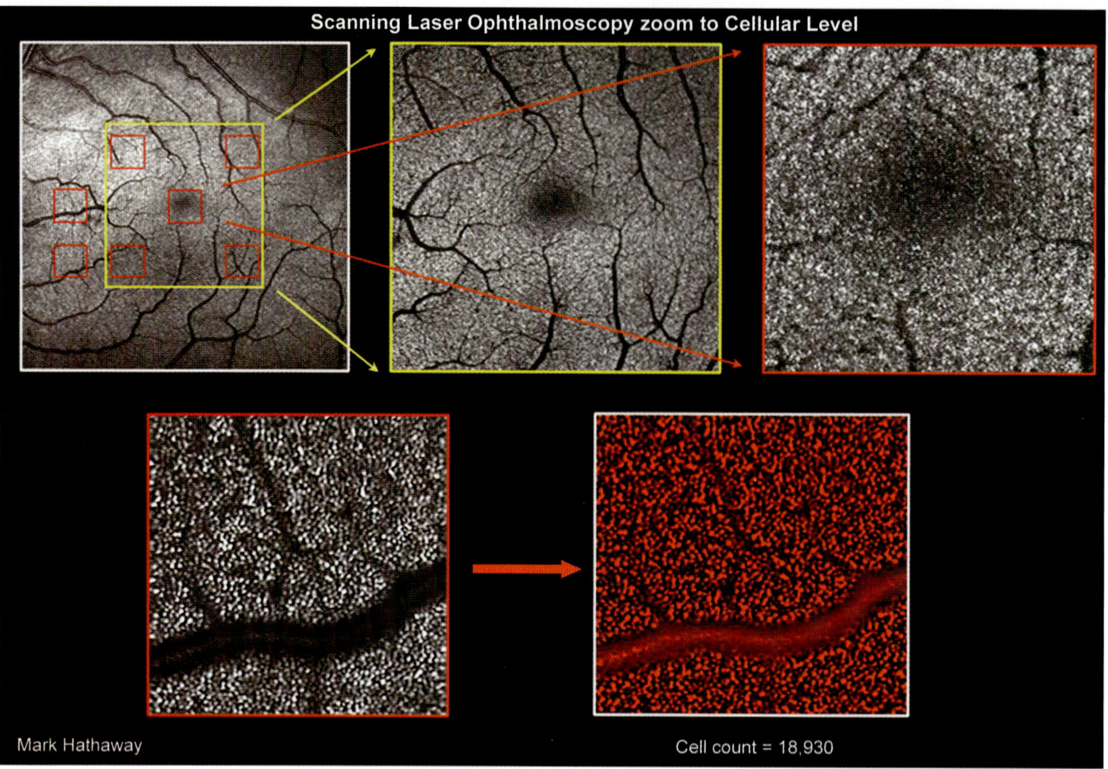

Figure 3: Variable magnification achieved by alteration of scanning laser ophthalmoscope scanning angle. When the scanning resolution of the 25° wide-field image (upper left) is reduced to 1° (lower row), the perimacular cone mosaic becomes evident and accessible to postprocessing counting algorithms

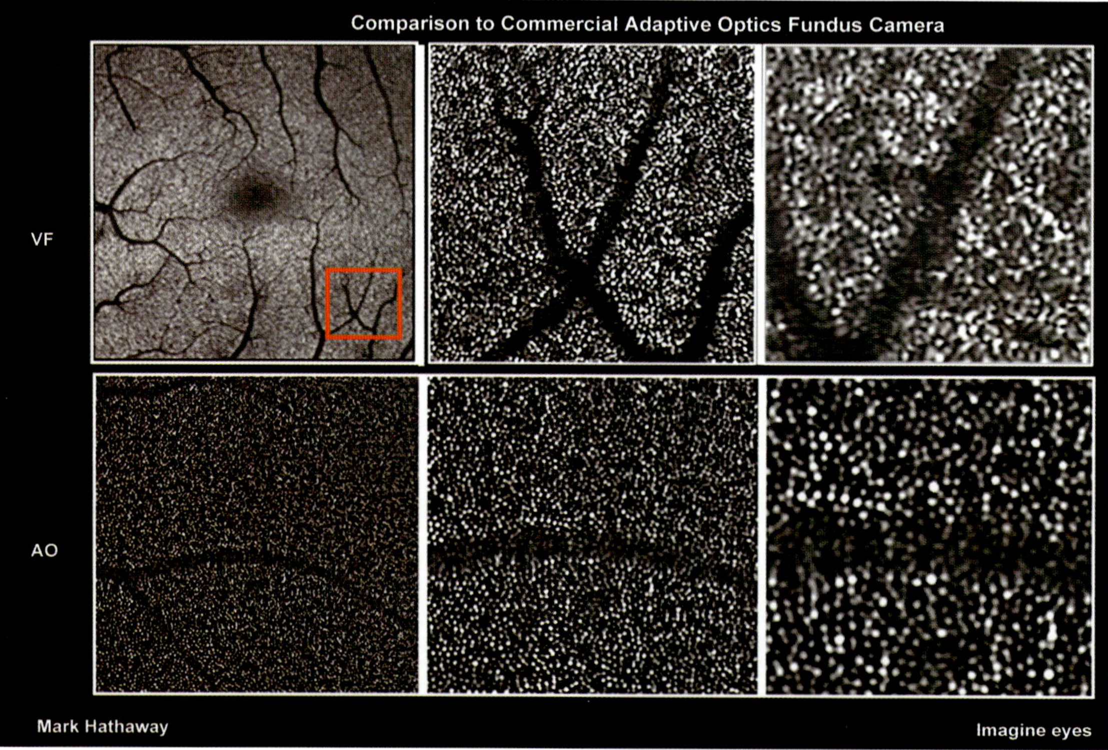

Figure 4: Comparison of variable field SLO/OCT imaging of cones to current generation adaptive optics fundus camera. The ability to resolve the cone mosaic in the eye of an optimal subject using the SD OCT/SLO prototype approaches the level of the Imagine Eyes™ Adaptive Optics Fundus Camera
(*Abbreviations:* VF: Variable field OCT/SLO; AO: Adaptive optics)

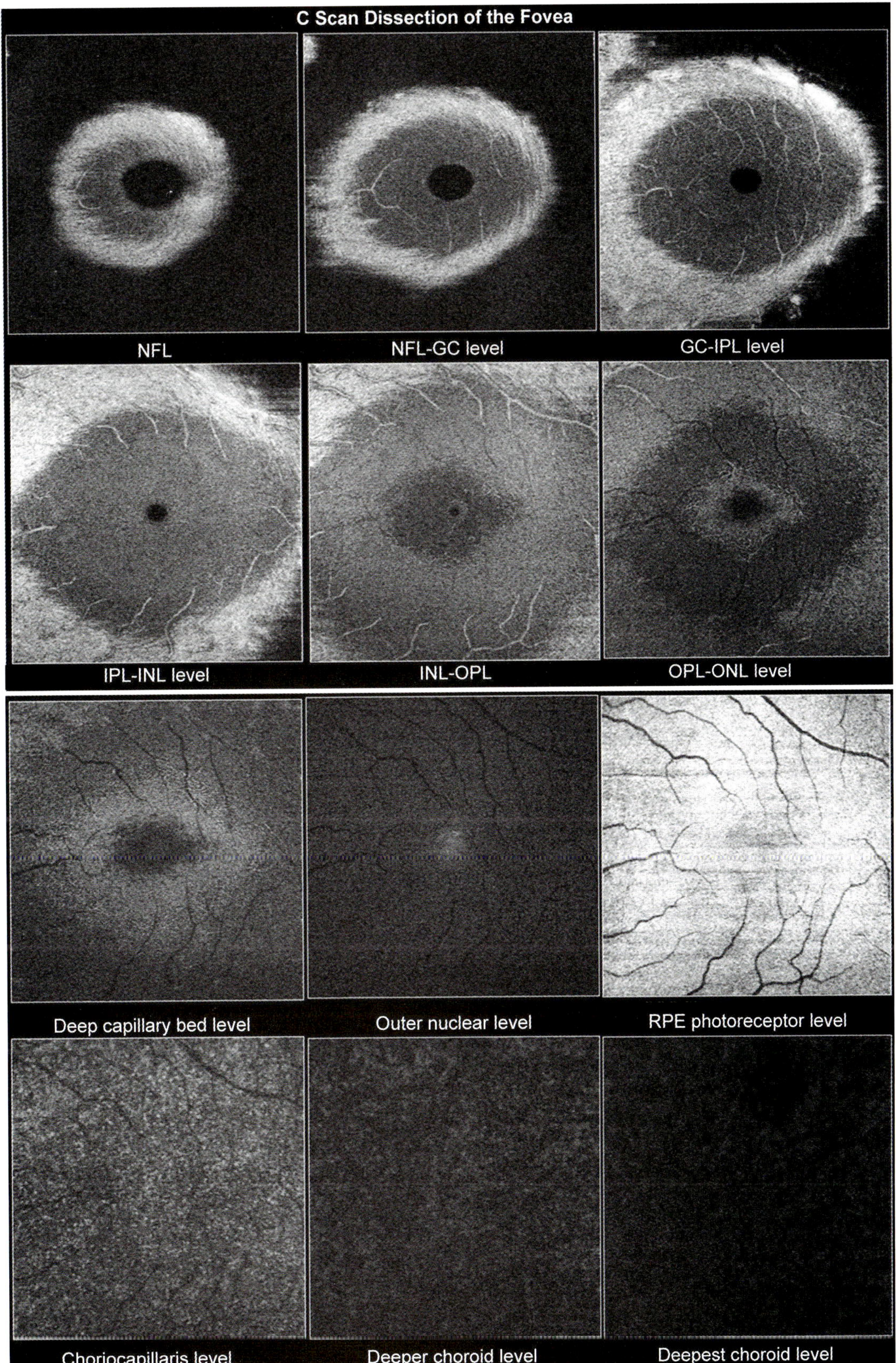

Figure 5: *En face* C scan slices through a normal macula. These are representative slices from a series of 400 taken through a normal macula. The scan size is 4.5 mm or 14°
(*Abbreviations:* NFL: Nerve fiber layer; GC: Ganglion cell; IPL: Inner plexiform layer; INL: Inner nuclear layer; OPL: Outer plexiform layer; ONL: Outer nuclear layer; RPE: retinal pigment epithelium)

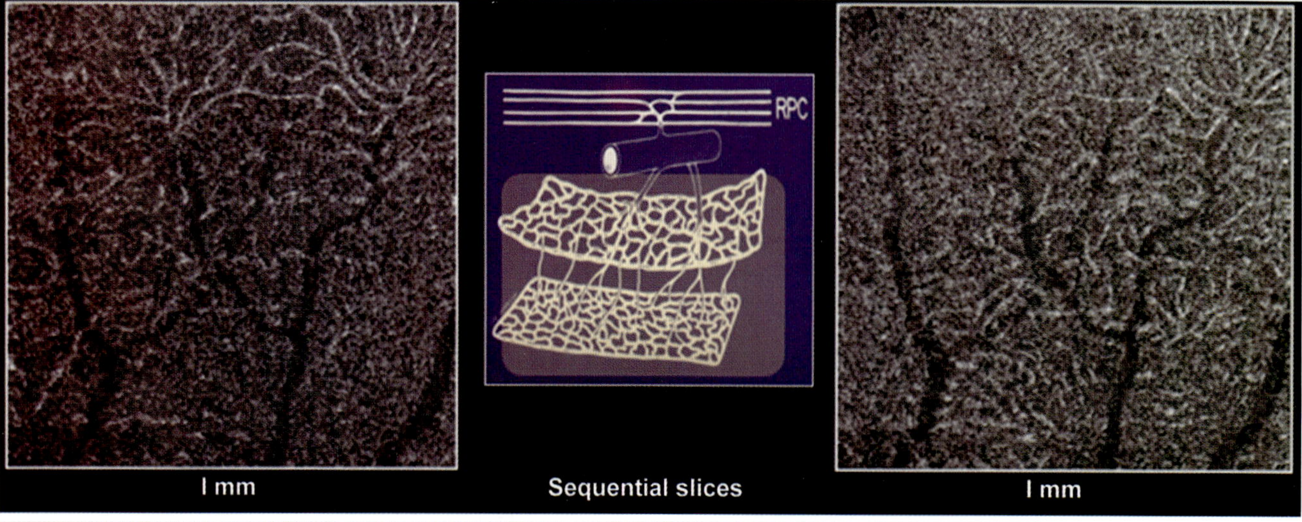

Figure 6: Deep capillary beds revealed in 1 mm C scans of the macula. At the smaller scanning angle of 3.3°, the details of the smallest capillaries of the fundus become evident

reconstructed C scans clearly demonstrated an area of infarct in the outer capillary bed which matched the patients description of a "galloping horse" (**Figures 7A to F**).

In a case with more extensive branch arteriole infarct the *en face* C scan view reveals the relationship between the edema and the capillary bed and more clearly documents the extent of vascular bed compromise than the fluorescein (**Figures 8A to D**).

The ability of *en face* C scans to correlate with fluorescein angiography is further demonstrated in the following next example of central serous retinopathy. In this disorder the nature on the contrast leakage is at the level of the outer blood retinal barrier, rather than the retinal vasculature. The perspective of the C scan matches the fluorescein image localizing the leakage to specific anatomic points of RPE disturbance (**Figures 9A to H**).

In a more chronic example of central serous retinopathy (**Figure 10**) the enhanced resolution of the small field SLO is able to document the loss of cones in the area of the previous lesion as compared to unaffected areas elsewhere in the same fundus.

The enhanced resolution also extends to vitreous-retina interface as demonstrated in the case of macular hole (**Figures 11A to C**). The *en face* C scan perspective provides new information regarding the potential forces at work in the development of the macular hole as demonstrated by taut lines within the middle retinal layers extending ut radially. It also exposes features at the edge of the hole (**Figures 11A to C**) which may help predict the successful return of vision following surgery.

The enhanced magnification and ability to explore the features of the hole in depth from the normal ophthalmoscopic perspective provides a better idea of the extent of damage at the edge of the hole and may be helpful in predicting prognosis for visual recovery following surgery (**Figures 12A to D**).

Summary

The marriage of high speed SD-OCT to a variable field SLO in a compact unit offers new options for higher resolution imaging, including the capability of generating *en face* C scan tomographic sequences of retinal internal anatomy. Small angle scanning provides near adaptive optics quality at a substantial saving in operation and maintenance costs. What it lacks in the ultra-resolution of the adaptive optics ophthalmoscope it makes up in speed and simplicity of operation as well as the presence of integrated OCT.

Limitations of the technique are similar to those of any higher resolution system. Patients must have the ability to cooperate, possess clear media and a stable tear film. Operator skills are currently somewhat more demanding than standard systems and the very large data sets generated require adequate computer and storage capabilities.

The ability to zoom in on small lesions offers an unprecedented clinical view of histology and the OCT C scan tomographies allow dissection of the retina from a clinically familiar perspective. Refinement of the cellular density analysis holds the promise of earlier recognition of disease which will hopefully allow new proactive therapeutic interventions.

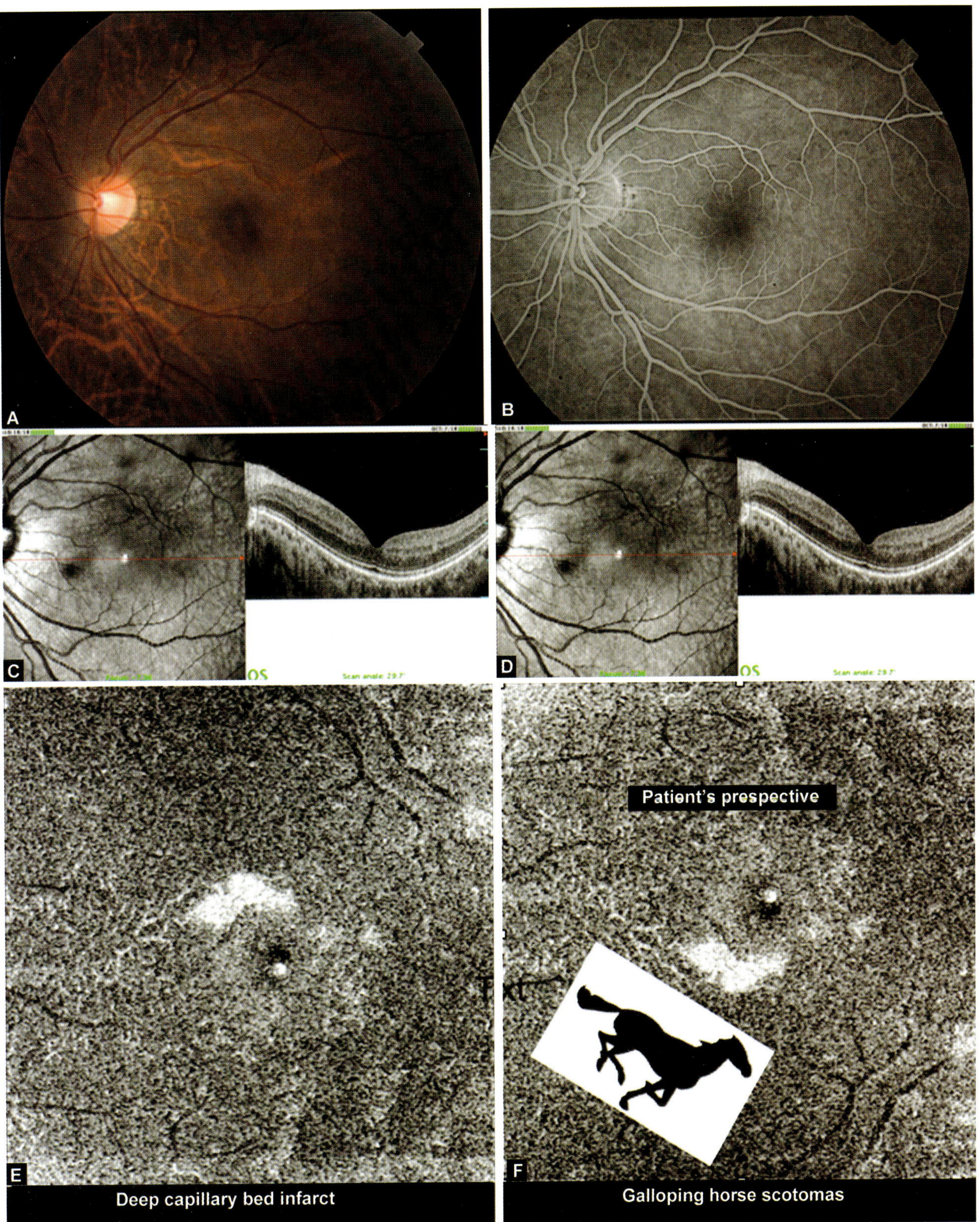

Figures 7A to F: Galloping horse scotoma due to infarct in the deep capillary bed. (A) Fundus image; (B) Fluorescein image; (C and D) Horizontal and vertical OCT/SLO slices; (E) Capillary bed infarct (bright perifoveal lesion); (F) Inverted detail compared to galloping horse image

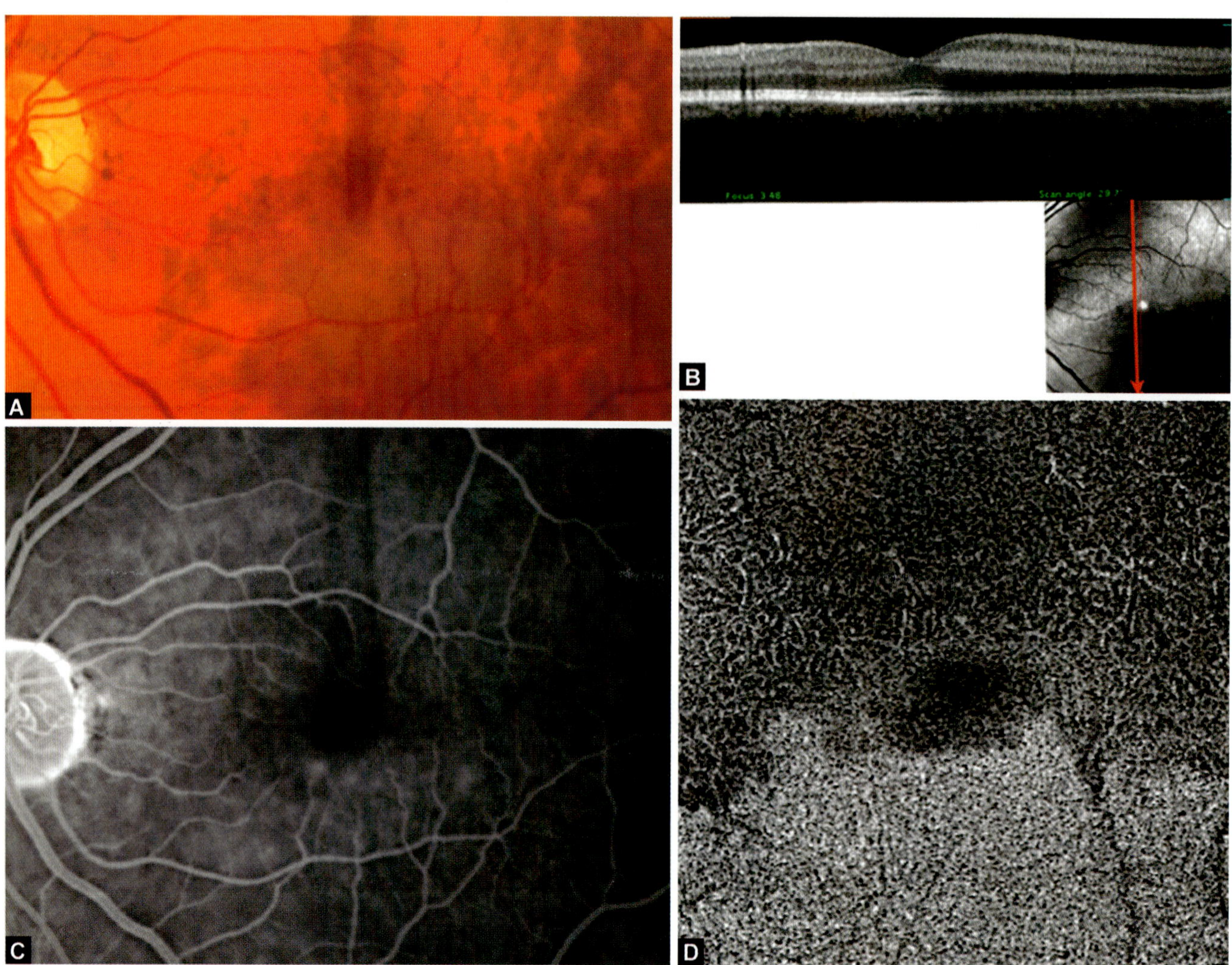

Figures 8A to D: Branch retinal artery occlusion. (A) Fundus photo showing small area of edema below the fovea; (B) Vertical B scan optical coherence tomography (OCT) revealing hyperfluorescence of middle retinal layers with no disturbance of the foveal profile; (C) Fluorescein angiogram at 5:27 showing some mild leakage in the area of edema; (D) C scan OCT revealing more extensive involvement of middle capillary bed

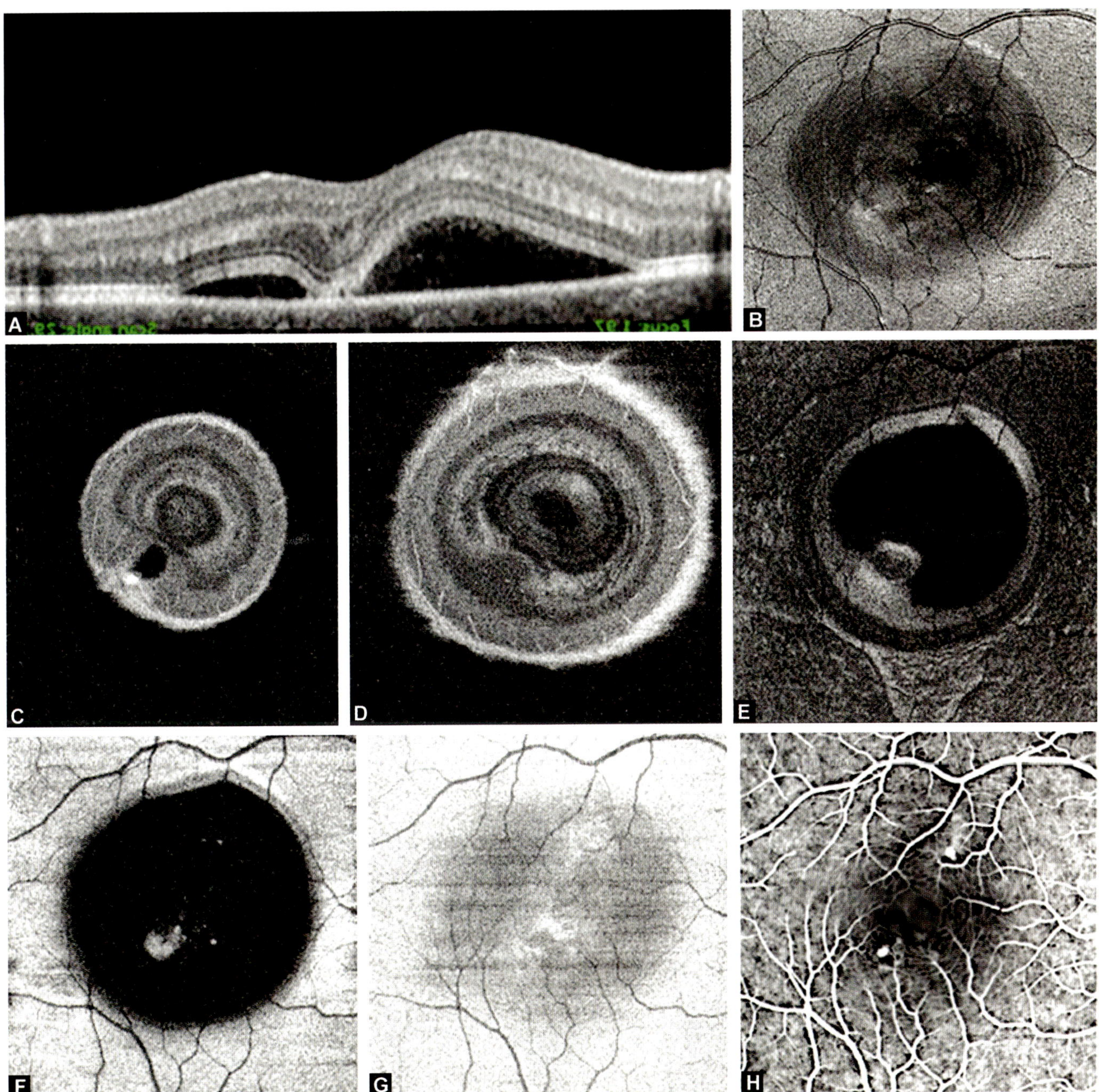

Figures 9A to H: Central serous retinopathy. A 34-year-old man with central distortion in his left eye. (A) B scan optical coherence tomography (OCT) showing irregular serous detachment of the macula; (B) Scanning laser ophthalmoscopy image showing abnormal foveal reflex; (C to G) C scan tomographic dissection of serous elevation; (H) Fluorescein angiogram frame showing leakage at corresponding areas of retinal pigment epithelium disturbance

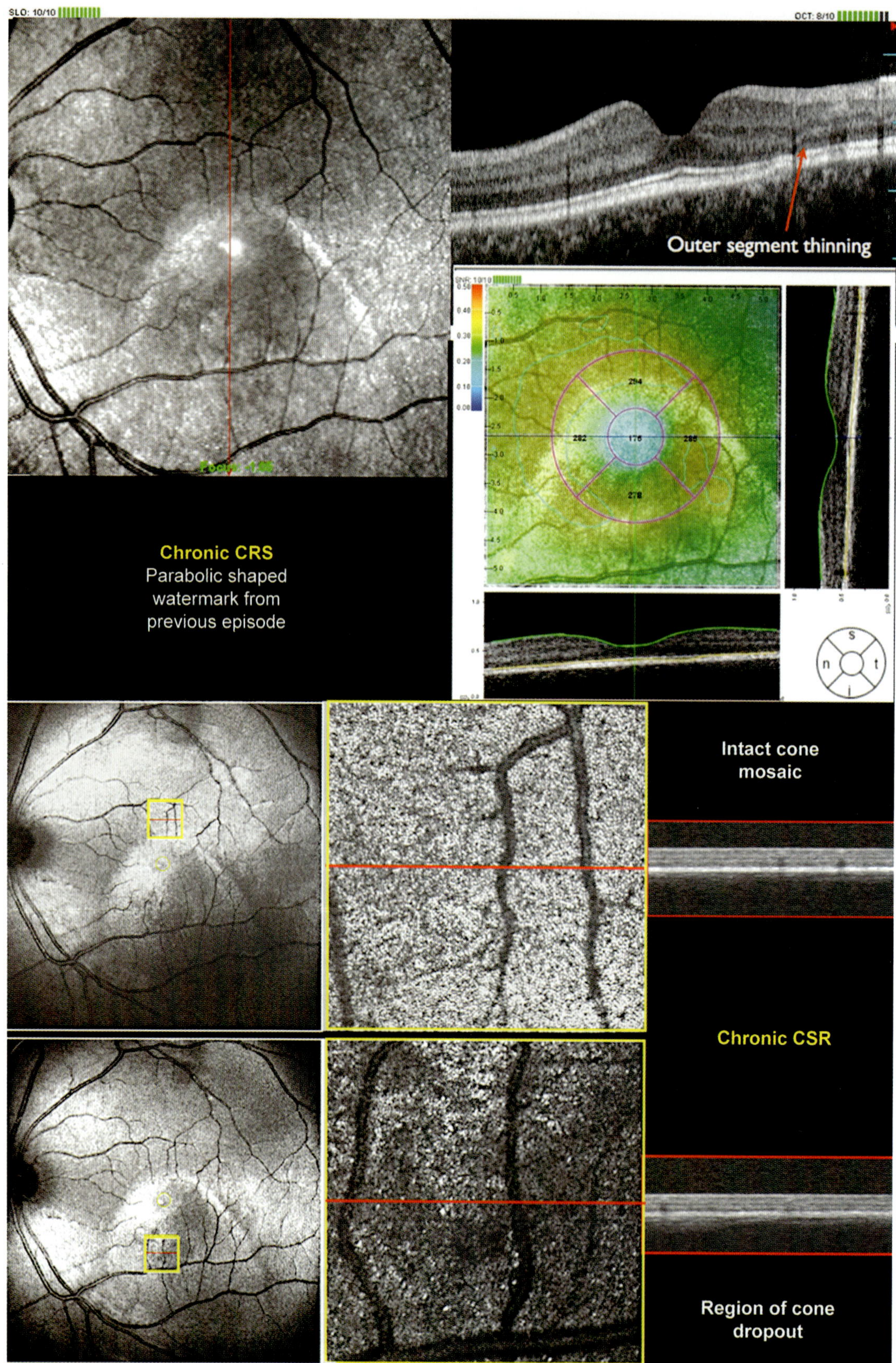

Figure 10: Chronic central serous retinopathy. Parabolic watermarked area of previous episode appears slightly thinner on spectral domain optical coherence tomography as confirmed by topography map. Small field scans in affected areas show dropout of cones as compared to normal cone mosaic in adjacent unaffected retina

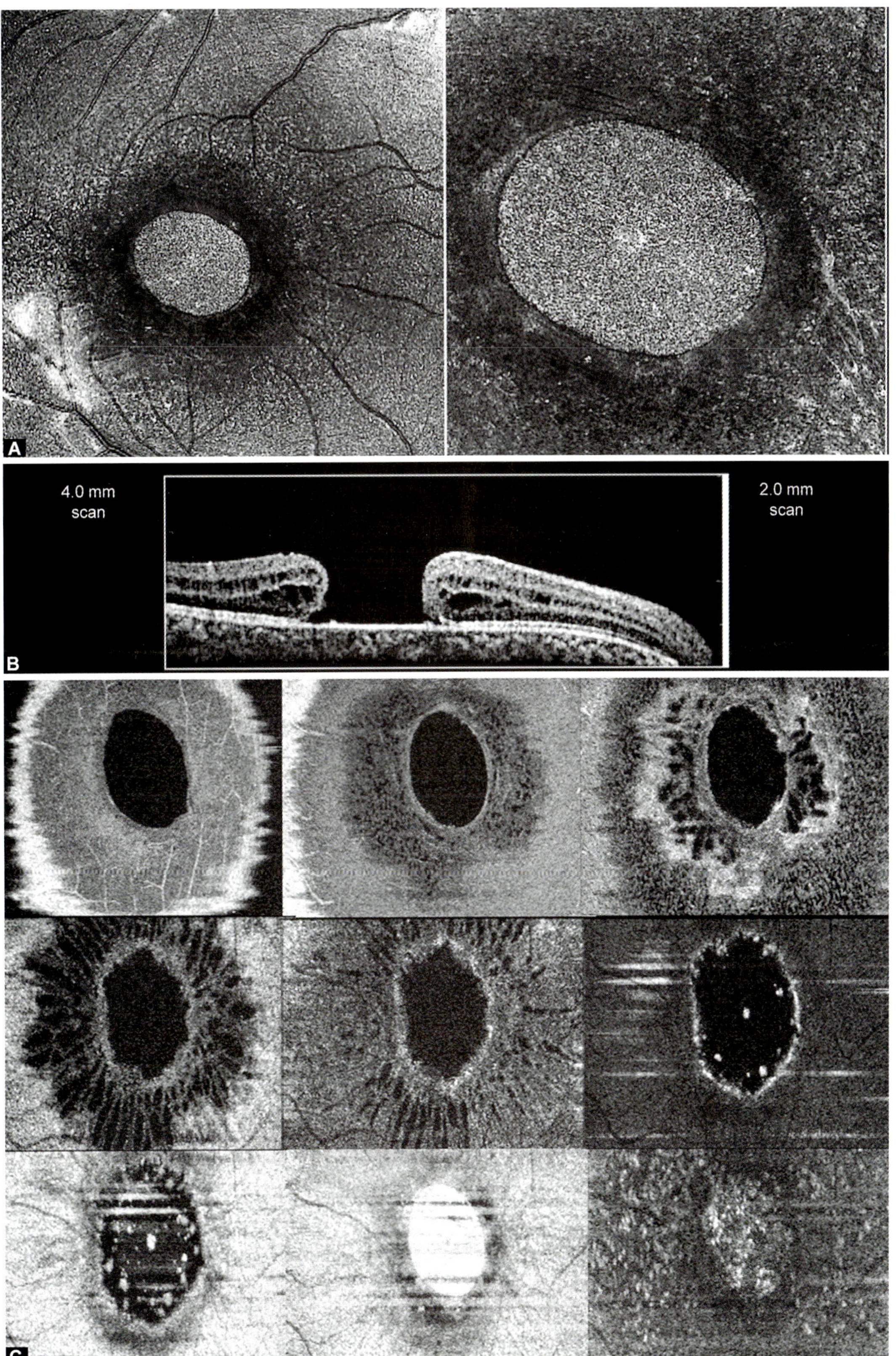

Figures 11A to C: Macular hole. (A) Variable field scanning laser ophthalmoscope (SLO) images reveal the texture of the retinal surface and the granularity of exposed retinal pigment epithelium (RPE) uncovered by the hole; (B) Spectral domain OCT/SLO cross-section of the hole showing cystic changes and basal drusen (Klein's tags); (C) *En face* C scan tomographic sequence from the retinal surface to the base and beyond to the RPE level and then below at the choriocapillaris level

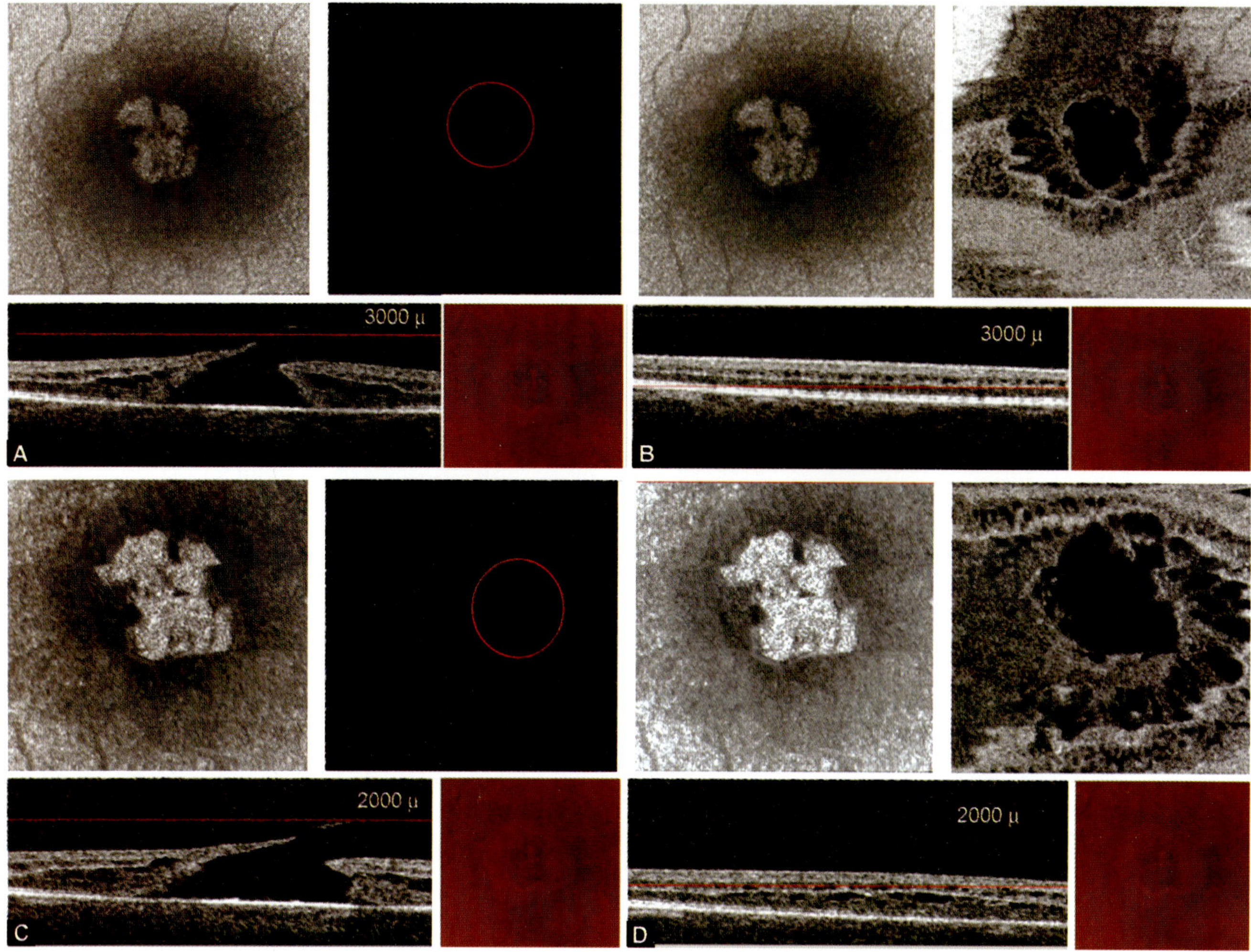

Figures 12A to D: Macular hole with irregular edge and persistent traction. (A) 3000 μ scan superficial to the retinal surface revealing persistent vitreoretinal traction; (B) 3000 μ scan deeper within the middle retinal layers showing network of radial fibers and a moth-eaten edge to the hole; (C and D) 2000 μ scans magnify the irregular features seen in A and B which define this hole

References

1. Huang D, Swanson EA, Lin CP, et al. Optical coherence tomography. Science. 1991;254(5035):1178-81.
2. Izatt JA, Hee MR, Swanson EA, et al. Micrometer-scale resolution imaging of the anterior eye *in vivo* with optical coherence tomography. Arch Ophthalmol. 1994; 112(12): 1584-9.
3. Wojtkowski M, Srinivasan V, Ko T, et al. Ultrahigh-resolution, high-speed, Fourier domain optical coherence tomography and methods for dispersion compensation. Opt Express. 2004;12(11):2404-22.
4. Cense B, Nassif N, Chen T, et al. Ultrahigh-resolution high-speed retinal imaging using spectral-domain optical coherence tomography. Opt Express. 2004;12(11):2435-47.
5. Liang J, Williams DR, Miller DT. Supernormal vision and high resolution retinal imaging through adaptive optics. J Opt Soc Am A Opt Image Sci Vis. 1997;14: 2884-92.
6. Podoleanu A, Rogers J, Jackson D, et al. Three-dimensional OCT images from retina and skin. Opt Express. 2000;7(9): 292-8.
7. Podoleanu AG, Dobre GM, Cucu RG, et al. Combined multiplanar optical coherence tomography and confocal scanning ophthalmoscopy. J Biomed Opt. 2004;9(1): 86-93.
8. Rosen RB, van velthoven ME, Garcia PM, et al. Ultrahigh-resolution combined coronal optical coherence tomography confocal scanning ophthalmoscope (OCT/SLO): A pilot study. Spektrum Augenheilkd. 2007;21(1):17-28.
9. van Velthoven ME, Verbraak FD, Yannuzzi LA, et al. Imaging the retina by *en face* optical coherence tomography. Retina. 2006;26(2):129-36.
10. Podoleanu AG, Rosen RB. Combinations of techniques in imaging the retina with high resolution. Prog Retin Eye Res. 2008;27(4):464-99.
11. Williams DR. Imaging single cells in the living retina. Vision Res. 2011;51(13):1379-96.

Index

Page numbers followed by *f* for figure and *t* for table, respectively.